FSC
www.fsc.org
MIX
Papier aus verantwortungsvollen Quellen
Paper from responsible sources
FSC® C105338

Imprint of Infinite Science GmbH,
Technikzentrum | MFC 1
Maria-Goeppert-Straße 1
23562 Lübeck, Germany

Cover Design and Illustration: Uli Schmidts, metonym
Editorial and Copy Editing: University of Lübeck

Publisher: Infinite Science GmbH, Lübeck, www.infinite-science.de
Printed in Germany, BoD, Norderstedt

ISBN: 978-3-945954-65-2

Bibliografische Information der Deutschen Nationalbibliothek:
Die Deutsche Nationalbibliothek verzeichnet diese Publikation in der Deutschen Nationalbibliografie; detaillierte bibliografische Daten sind im Internet über http://dnb.d-nb.de abrufbar.

Student Conference Proceedings 2021

10th Conference on Medical Engineering Science
6th Conference on Medical Informatics
4th Conference on Biomedical Engineering
3rd Conference on Auditory Technology
1st Conference on Biophysics
1st Conference on Robotics and Autonomous Systems

Lübeck, March 10-12, 2021

Editors in Chief

T. M. Buzug, H. Handels, C. Hübner, S. Klein, A. Mertins, P. Rostalski

Associate Editors

C. Debbeler, K. Gräfe, J.-H. Wrage, C. Droigk, K. Ehlers, Y.-H. Song, S. Venker

Editors

E. Barth, M. Berekovic, M. Beyerlein, H. Botterweck, R. Brinkmann, T. M. Buzug, C. Damiani, A. Drews, S. Ensminger, F. Ernst, T. Franke, B. Fujita, V. García Vázquez, K. Gräfe, J. Groppe, M. Grzegorzek, T. Gutsmann, H. Hamann, H. Handels, M. Heinrich, R. Huber, C. Hübner, H. Husstedt, G. Hüttmann, J. Ingenerf, T. Jürgens, M. Kallinger, S. Karpf, S. Klein, M. Leucker, N. Linz, A. Madany Mamlouk, S. Meier, A. Mertins, E. Mohammadi, R. Moll, S. Müller, A. Neumann, H. Paulsen, M. Rafecas, R. Rahmanzadeh, F. Reinholz, P. Rostalski, E. Rückert, G. Schildbach, A. Schrader, A. Schweikard, Y.-H. Song, F. Spitzenberger, M. Stille, J. Tchorz, M. Urban, W.-H. Wang, D. Warnack, R. Wendlandt, D. Willkomm, C. Zechel, M. Zille

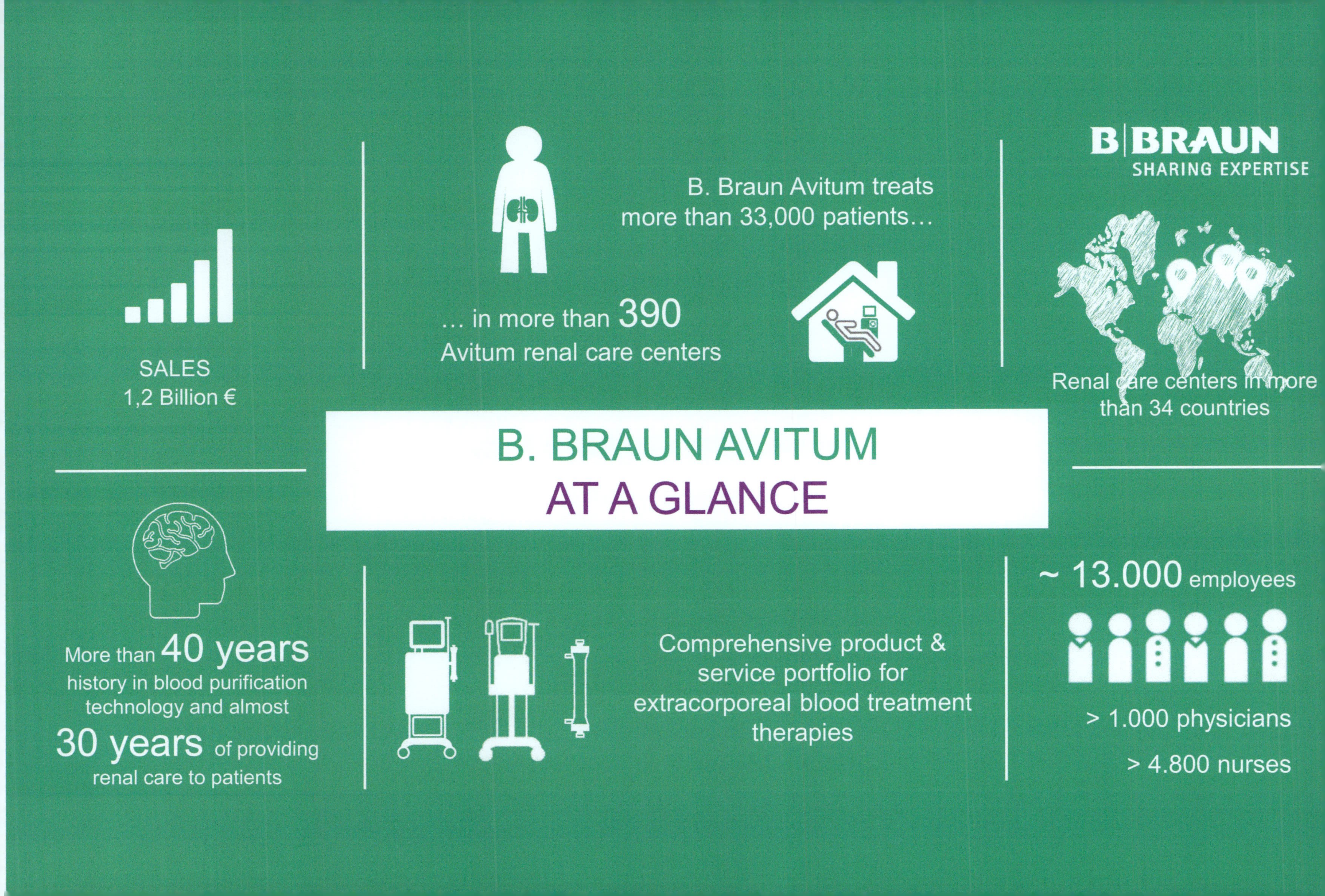
B. BRAUN AVITUM
AT A GLANCE
SALES
1,2 Billion €
B. Braun Avitum treats
more than 33,000 patients…
… in more than 390
Avitum renal care centers
B|BRAUN
SHARING EXPERTISE
Renal care centers in more
than 34 countries
More than 40 years
history in blood purification
technology and almost
30 years of providing
renal care to patients
Comprehensive product &
service portfolio for
extracorporeal blood treatment
therapies
~ 13.000 employees
> 1.000 physicians
> 4.800 nurses

IHK Lübeck

Mein UNTERNEHMEN ZUKUNFT

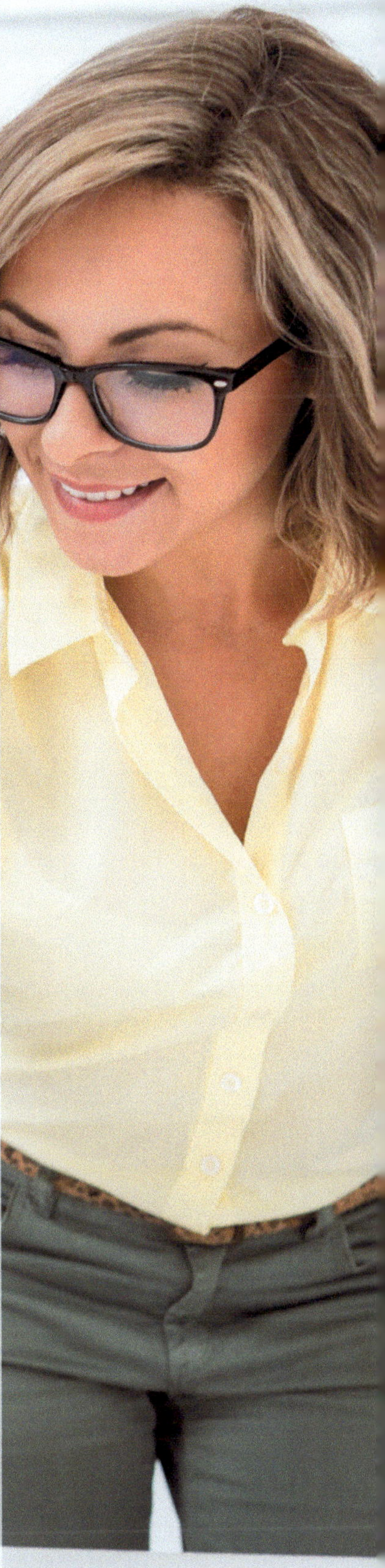

Angebote der IHK zu Lübeck für Studierende

Erst das Studium und dann... Über den besten Studienplatz, interessante Praktikumsplätze, Finanzierung und Förderung sowie die Möglichkeiten, sich selbstständig zu machen und von gestandenen Unternehmerinnen und Unternehmern zu lernen, unter www.Mein-Unternehmen-Zukunft.de

Best of ...

Karrieretag

Der Karrieretag ist eine gemeinsame Veranstaltung der Universität zu Lübeck, der Technische Hochschule Lübeck, der BioMedTec Management GmbH sowie der IHK zu Lübeck und richtet sich an Studentinnen und Studenten, Absolventinnen und Absolventen. Beim Karrieretag stellen Sie die Weichen für Ihre berufliche Zukunft und knüpfen Kontakte zu zukünftigen Arbeitgebern. Mehr unter: www.ihk-sh.de/karrieretag

Praktikumsbörse

Die IHK-Praktikumsbörse www.praktikum-sh.de bietet Schülern und Studierenden die kostenlose Möglichkeit, Praktikumsplätze bei Unternehmen in Schleswig-Holstein zu finden.

Beratung StudiLe

Das Studium mit integrierter Lehre (StudiLe) ist ein duales Studienmodell, welches eine betriebliche Ausbildung mit einem Bachelorstudium an der Fachhochschule Lübeck verbindet. In circa vier Jahren können somit zwei berufsqualifizierende Abschlüsse erworben werden. Nähere Informationen finden Sie unter www.studile.de.

Informationen für Studienabbrecher

Die IHK zu Lübeck engagiert sich im Netzwerk „Zweifel am Studium?" und steht Studienabbrecherinnen und Studienabbrechern für individuelle berufliche Beratungsgespräche zur Verfügung. Eine erste Orientierungsberatung zur Studiensituation und dem persönlichen Profil bietet die Handwerkskammer Lübeck im Studentenwerk auf dem Campus der Lübecker Hochschulen an: www.kurswechsel-machen.de
Zusätzliche Informationen finden Sie unter: www.ihk-sh.de/studienabbrecher

Existenzgründung und Unternehmensförderung

Ob Sie eine Firma gründen, die Wettbewerbsfähigkeit Ihres Unternehmens für die Zukunft sichern oder die Nachfolge regeln möchten – wir stehen von Anfang an an Ihrer Seite und begleiten Ihr Unternehmen von der Gründung bis zur Übergabe. Mehr zu finden unter: www.ihk-sh.de/starthilfe
Für Studierende bieten wir Informationsveranstaltungen und -gespräche zur Existenzgründung sowie individuell zugeschnittene Finanzierungs- und Förderberatungen an.

Mehr Informationen finden Sie unter www.Mein-Unternehmen-Zukunft.de

Student Conference Proceedings 2021

Conference Chairs

Thorsten M. Buzug	Institute of Medical Engineering, Universität zu Lübeck
Heinz Handels	Institute of Medical Informatics, Universität zu Lübeck
Christian Hübner	Institute of Physics, Universität zu Lübeck
Stephan Klein	Medical Sensors and Devices Laboratory, Lübeck University of Applied Sciences
Alfred Mertins	Institute for Signal Processing, Universität zu Lübeck
Philipp Rostalski	Institute for Electrical Engineering in Medicine, Universität zu Lübeck
Hartmut Gehring	Department of Anesthesiology, UKSH, Lübeck

Local Coordination

Christina Debbeler	Institute of Medical Engineering, Universität zu Lübeck
Ksenija Gräfe	Institute of Medical Engineering, Universität zu Lübeck
Jan-Hinrich Wrage	Institute of Medical Informatics, Universität zu Lübeck
Christine Droigk	Institute for Signal Processing, Universität zu Lübeck
Kristian Ehlers	Institute of Computer Engineering, Universität zu Lübeck
Young-Hwa Song	Institute of Physics, Universität zu Lübeck
Silke Venker	Medical Sensors and Devices Laboratory, Lübeck University of Applied Sciences

Scientific Program Committee

Barth, Prof. Dr. Erhardt	Institute for Neuro- and Bioinformatics, Universität zu Lübeck
Berekovic, Prof. Dr.-Ing. Mladen	Institute of Computer Engineering, Universität zu Lübeck
Beyerlein, Prof. Dr. Mathias	Department of Applied Natural Sciences, Lübeck University of Applied Sciences
Botterweck, Prof. Dr. Henrik	Department of Applied Natural Sciences, Lübeck University of Applied Sciences
Brinkmann, Dr. Ralf	Medizinisches Laserzentrum Lübeck GmbH and Institute of Biomedical Optics, Universität zu Lübeck
Buzug, Prof. Dr. Thorsten M.	Institute of Medical Engineering, Universität zu Lübeck
Damiani, Dr. Christian	Medical Sensors and Devices Laboratory, Lübeck University of Applied Sciences
Drews, Prof. Dr. André	Department of Mechanical Engineering and Business Administration, Lübeck University of Applied Sciences
Ensminger, Prof. Dr. Stephan	Department of Cardiac and Thoracic Vascular Surgery, University Hospital of Schleswig-Holstein, Lübeck
Ernst, Prof. Dr. Floris	Institute for Robotics and Cognitive Systems, Universität zu Lübeck
Franke, Prof. Dr. Thomas	Institute for Multimedia and Interactive Systems, Universität zu Lübeck
Fujita, Dr. Buntaro	Department of Cardiac and Thoracic Vascular Surgery, University Hospital of Schleswig-Holstein, Lübeck
García Vázquez, Dr. Verónica	Institute for Robotics and Cognitive Systems, Universität zu Lübeck
Gehring, Prof. Dr. Hartmut	Department of Anesthesiology, University Medical Center Schleswig-Holstein, Lübeck
Gräfe, Dr.-Ing. Ksenija	Institute of Medical Engineering, Universität zu Lübeck
Groppe, Dr. Jinghua	Institute of Information Systems, Universität zu Lübeck
Grzegorzek, Prof. Dr. Marcin	Institute of Medical Informatics, Universität zu Lübeck
Gutsmann, Prof. Dr. Thomas	Research Center Borstel, Leibniz Lungcenter
Hamann, Prof. Dr.-Ing. Heiko	Institute of Computer Engineering, Universität zu Lübeck

Scientific Program Committee - Cont'd

Handels, Prof. Dr. Heinz	Institute of Medical Informatics, Universität zu Lübeck
Heinrich, Prof. Dr. Mattias	Institute of Medical Informatics, Universität zu Lübeck
Huber, Prof. Dr. Robert	Institute of Biomedical Optics, Universität zu Lübeck
Hübner, Prof. Dr. Christian	Institute of Physics, Universität zu Lübeck
Husstedt, Dr. Hendrik	German Institute of Hearing Aids, Lübeck
Hüttmann, Prof. Dr. Gereon	Institute of Biomedical Optics, Universität zu Lübeck
Ingenerf, Prof. Dr. Josef	Institute of Medical Informatics, IT Center for Clinical Research, Universität zu Lübeck
Jürgens, Prof. Dr. Tim	Department of Applied Natural Sciences, Lübeck University of Applied Sciences
Kallinger, Prof. Dr.-Ing. Markus	Department of Applied Natural Sciences, Lübeck University of Applied Sciences
Karpf, Prof. Dr. Sebastian	Institute of Biomedical Optics, Universität zu Lübeck
Klein, Prof. Dr. Stephan	Medical Sensors and Devices Laboratory, Lübeck University of Applied Sciences
Leucker, Prof. Dr. Martin	Institute for Software Engineering and Programming Languages, Universität zu Lübeck
Linz, Dr. Norbert	Institute of Biomedical Optics, Universität zu Lübeck
Madany Mamlouk, PD Dr. Amir	Institute for Neuro- and Bioinformatics, Universität zu Lübeck
Meier, Sigrid	Academy of Hearing Aid Acoustics, Lübeck
Mertins, Prof. Dr. Alfred	Institute for Signal Processing, Universität zu Lübeck
Mohammadi, Prof. Dr. Esfandiar	Institute for IT Security, Universität zu Lübeck
Moll, Dr. Ralf	Department of Applied Natural Sciences, Lübeck University of Applied Sciences
Müller, Prof. Dr. Stefan	Medical Sensors and Devices Laboratory, Lübeck University of Applied Sciences
Neumann, Dr. Alexander	Institute of Medical Engineering, Universität zu Lübeck
Paulsen, PD Dr. Hauke	Institute of Physics, Universität zu Lübeck
Rafecas, Prof. Dr. Magdalena	Institute of Medical Engineering, Universität zu Lübeck
Rahmanzadeh, PD Dr. Ramtin	Institute of Biomedical Optics, Universität zu Lübeck
Reinholz, Dr. Fred	Institute of Biomedical Optics, Universität zu Lübeck
Rostalski, Prof. Dr. Philipp	Institute for Electrical Engineering in Medicine, Universität zu Lübeck
Rückert, Prof. Dr. Elmar	Institute for Robotics and Cognitive Systems, Universität zu Lübeck
Schildbach, Prof. Dr. Georg	Institute for Electrical Engineering in Medicine, Universität zu Lübeck
Schrader, Prof. Dr. Andreas	Institute of Telematics, Universität zu Lübeck
Schweikard, Prof. Dr.-Ing. Achim	Institute for Robotics and Cognitive Systems, Universität zu Lübeck
Song, Dr. Young-Hwa	Institute of Physics, Universität zu Lübeck
Spitzenberger, Prof. Dr. Folker	Centre for Regulatory Affairs in Biomedical Sciences, Lübeck University of Applied Sciences
Stille, Dr. Maik	Institute of Medical Engineering, Universität zu Lübeck
Tchorz, Prof. Dr. Jürgen	Department of Applied Natural Sciences, Lübeck University of Applied Sciences
Urban, Prof. Dr. Max,	Department of Applied Natural Sciences, Lübeck University of Applied Sciences
Wang, Prof. Dr.-Ing. Wen-Huan	Department of Applied Natural Sciences, Lübeck University of Applied Sciences
Warnack, Prof. Dr.-Ing. Dieter	Department of Mechanical Engineering and Business Administration, Lübeck University of Applied Sciences
Wendlandt, Dr. Robert	Clinic for Orthopedic and Trauma Surgery, Biomechanics Laboratory, University Medical Center Schleswig-Holstein, Lübeck
Willkomm, Prof. Dr. Dagmar	Department of Applied Natural Sciences, Lübeck University of Applied Sciences
Zechel, PD Dr. Christina	Neuro-Oncology, Department of Neurosurgery, University Medical Center Schleswig-Holstein, Lübeck
Zille, Dr. Marietta	Institute for Experimental and Clinical Pharmacology and Toxicology, Universität zu Lübeck

Preface and Acknowledgements

After the great success of the previous meetings from 2012 to 2020, the Student Conference 2021 shows continuing growth both in quality and quantity of scientific contributions. In this year, the 10th Student Conference on Medical Engineering Science is held together with the 6th Student Conference on Medical Informatics, the 4th Student Conference on Biomedical Engineering,the 3rd Student Conference on Auditory Technology, the 1st Student Conference on Biophysics and the 1st Student Conference on Robotics and Autonomous Systems.

The organization team in cooperation with the Chamber of Industry and Commerce (IHK) Lübeck has worked to provide an excellent conference, where master students of the campus present their recent research results to a broad public of academics and industry.

The contributions show how new approaches and methods in medical engineering and medical informatics can advance medicine, health, and health care. Moreover, this conference offers a good opportunity for both students and companies to get in touch at the Recruiticon, i.e. a satellite recruiting fair with industrial exhibition. Students from the Life Sciences programs present their results from projects carried out at the laboratories, clinics, and institutes of Lübeck's Universities, in international research facilities, or research-oriented industrial companies. The conference focus has been placed on topics ranging from medical engineering to medical informatics. The interdisciplinary field of medical engineering has been established at the Lübeck University of Applied Sciences for decades, and Medical Engineering Science (Medizinische Ingenieurwissenschaft – MIW) is an important bachelor and master program at the Universität zu Lübeck as well. Both universities jointly offer the international master degree programs Biomedical Engineering (BME) and Auditory Technology (Hörakustik und Audiologische Technik – HAT). Furthermore, in the master program Medical Informatics (Medizinische Informatik – MI) the 5th Student Conference on Medical Informatics is integrated as an important element where project results in the emerging field of digital medicine are presented by the students. These subject areas are widened by the master's programs Robotics and Autonomous Systems (Robotik und Autonome Systeme – RAS) and Biophysics (Biophysik – BP), which were added this year.

As Conference Chairs, we want to thank everybody who worked with enthusiasm and dedication to make the conference a successful event. We want to thank the companies who support the meeting. Moreover, our thanks go to Infinite Science for producing these proceedings and organizing the Recruiticon meeting supporting the Student Conference. Personally and on behalf of all colleagues of the Student Conference Committee, we especially want to thank Christina Debbeler and Ksenija Gräfe, they have been the central contact points for all questions of students and the program committee members, as well as Jan-Hinrich Wrage for editing the proceedings and furthermore Christine Droigk, Kristian Ehlers, Young-Hwa Song and Silke Venker. Their in-depth overview of all details of this event is the key to the success of the Student Conference 2021.

Lübeck, March 10-12, 2021

Prof. Dr. Thorsten M. Buzug
Chair of the 10th Student Conference on Medical Engineering Science

Prof. Dr. Heinz Handels
Chair of the 6th Student Conference on Medical Informatics

Prof. Dr.-Ing. Stephan Klein
Chair of the 4th Student Conference on Biomedical Engineering

Prof. Dr.-Ing. Alfred Mertins
Chair of the 3rd Student Conference on Auditory Technology

Prof. Dr. Christian Hübner
Chair of the 1st Student Conference on Biophysics

Prof. Dr.-Ing. Philipp Rostalski
Chair of the 1st Student Conference on Robotics and Autonomous Systems

Exhibitors

Dräger

B | BRAUN
SHARING EXPERTISE

PHILIPS

Sponsors

Infinite Science

VKK® Patentanwälte
Patents | Trademarks | Designs

IHK Lübeck

Contents

Biomedical Engineering

Biomechanics

Biomedical Optics

Biophysics

Medical Electronics

Safety and Quality

Sensor Data Analysis

Auditory Technology

Signal Processing

Image Processing

Medical Imaging

Machine Learning / AI

eHealth

1

Biomedical Engineering

Development of an User Interface for a Miniaturized and Automated Anaesthesia Device

Birger Köhne [1], Hendrik Fischer [2] and Tim Schrills [3]

[1] Medical Engineering Science, Universität zu Lübeck, birger.koehne@student.uni-luebeck.de

[2] Corporate Technology & Innovation, Drägerwerk AG & Co. KG, hendrik.fischer@draeger.com

[3] Institute for Multimedia and Interactive Systems, Universität zu Lübeck, schrills@imis.uni-luebeck.de

Abstract

Anaesthetic devices perform vital anaesthetic and ventilation functions, commonly used during operations. Most of these devices contain a monitoring system as well. To ensure an ideal course of treatment, a safe interaction, clearly stating the accurate operation of the device, is required. This paper deals with the design and development of a new, intuitive and well-arranged user interface (UI). The focus is placed on the visualisation and miniaturization of data, aiming to gain more space for additional patient information. Therefore, data is summed up and reduced to achieve more salient information, theoretically decreasing the mental workload of the operators. Finally, the UI was evaluated by several medical professionals, discussing the effects caused by novel design features.

1 Introduction

Anaesthesia devices support the operators to perform painless and ventilated surgical interventions on unconscious patients. In case of inhalation anaesthesia, the drugs are absorbed by the body through the lungs. Thereby, the patient is ventilated with a gas mixture, which leads to unconsciousness, muscle relaxation and analgesia. This gas mixture consists of the carrier gas oxygen, nitrous oxide or air, enriched with the anaesthetics isofluran, sevofluran or desfluran [1].

Due to the muscle relaxation of the patient, the anaestesia device needs to perform the patients ventilation. Therefore, the device provides pressure or flow controlled, automated ventilation. It also contains a monitoring system, to ensure a safe and transparent operation. The device monitors its own functionality as well as the vital signs of the patient and the depth of anaesthesia [1].

The anaesthesia device which is considered in this article, demonstrates technical improvements. The main innovations include an automation and a miniaturisation of the device. The mentioned automation, already known as "Target Controlled Anaesthesia" (TCA) from previous developed devices [2], is based on an electrical gasmixer and an electric anaesthetic gas dosage. The device also contains a battery, to ensure a portable use.

For this anaesthesia device, a UI-proposal is designed. The main goals of the design concept were to increase usability and to reduce the mental workload of the operators. To this end, the design elements were redesigned and rearranged to create an intuitive UI. Displayed data was merged, leading to additional display space. Therefore, the presentation of further supporting information was possible such as the medical records of the patient and an overview of further treated patients. Additional information, including the body-mass-index (BMI) and the end-of-charge time of the battery, were also presented to make them easily accessible. Furthermore, the most important information were highlighted.

Finally, the concept of the UI design is presented to some medical professionals to evaluate its appropriateness.

2 Theoretical Background

2.1 Automation

Automation is known as the transfer of tasks and functions of a process that were previously, or possible could be, executed by an operator, to an artificial system [3]. To classify the different systems, Raja Parasuraman et al. introduced several automation levels in their paper "A Model for Types and Levels of Human Interaction with Automation" [3]. They defined ten different levels of automation. A system with a very low level of automation is neither able to execute on its own nor is it able to offer any assistant to the operators whereas a system with a higher level of automation does. Very high levels behave to work more and more autonomous and even begin to ignore the operators completely at the highest level of automation.

They also introduced the way how humans process information and clarified the consequences of automation. For example, low levels of automation are dependent on the operators knowledge which can be hazardous in the case of a mistake made by the operators. They do not provide any assistance and display the whole information unfiltered which might lead to a high mental workload, too. Due to the fact that the operators do not need to make the decisions by themselves, high levels of automation often lead to a reduced situation awareness. This may also lead to an effect called complacency, better described as "over-trust" in automation, which can be dangerous because there might always be a system that fails under certain, unexpected conditions [3].

3 Material and Methods

3.1 Wizard of Oz Experiment

The development process of a modern anaesthetic device contains the test and validation of new processes and technologies. Therefore, a continuous evaluation during the development process is required. To do so, an early user feedback is also desirable.

To make sure the development process is goal orientated and to avoid redundant programming, the development of the UI design is realized as so-called wizard of oz experiment. This research experiment simulates the interaction with an interface of a computer system which seems to act automatically but is (partially) operated by external operators. In fact, the device does not act automatically but its tasks are controlled by the external operators in the background. Hence, it is possible to test the newly designed interface in an early state of the development-process [4]. The main advantage of this approach is the possibility to adapt changes quickly and to stay more flexible during the design-process of the UI. The implementation of the interface in the anaesthetic device will follow after having completed the recent design.

3.2 Evaluation Criteria

For evaluation purposes, several medical professionals (hereafter titled as experts) were invited to assess the UI design. Therefore, structured interviews were organised to revise the appropriateness of the design concept. Open questions were used to initialise a guideline, which allows the experts to discuss their opinion of the UI [5].

The interview was held personally and was structured in three parts. First, preliminary questions are asked to attune the interviewee to the UI design. Hereby, the interviewees are inspired to think about the main ideas of the design concepts before the presentation of the UI. Second, the UI is presented and the newly designed concepts are rated by the interviewee. Third, some questions regarding the automation level are asked to evaluate the acceptance of the TCA. To value the concepts, they are rated between 1 (very good idea) to 6 (bad, insufficient idea). The results of the evaluation are presented in section 5.

The evaluation process of the UI design is executed in an early state of the development. Therefore, changes can be applied quickly and the design can be optimized iteratively.

4 User Interface-Design

In the UI design itself, modules are used to display the data. They are chosen to stand out the data against the background and therefore make it easier to distinguish between the different parameters. As known from previous UIs, the headline presents basic information. In this case, Patient data, the current time, battery charge, state of the system and the volume are pictured. Some *additional information* were added, to display the important information directly. For example, the patient data got extended by the BMI of the patient, which should be calculated before every treatment [6]. Furthermore, the battery charge got extended by the actual end-of-charge value. From now on, the operators do not have to calculate it by themselves anymore, which makes it easier to check the remaining battery time and therefore reduces the error rate.

One of the main goals of the design concept was the reduction of the displayed data to reduce the mental workload and achieve display space. To this end, the displayed waveforms, picturing the ventilation parameters, were rearranged. The former concept displayed the waveforms of the ventilation parameters over time, showing several ventilation cycles one after another. The new concept, titled as *overlaid waveforms*, overlaps the ventilation cycles, always triggered by the increasing slope. In total, three waveform cycles are overlapped. The older ventilation cycles are displayed transparent behind the current cycle, as shown in Fig. 1. Therefore, differences between the varying cycles can be displayed very well, because they are compared with each other visually. The merging of the waveforms leads to free space in the UI, previously filled by the larger displayed waveform cycles. This space is used for further patient data, which will be described in detail afterwards.

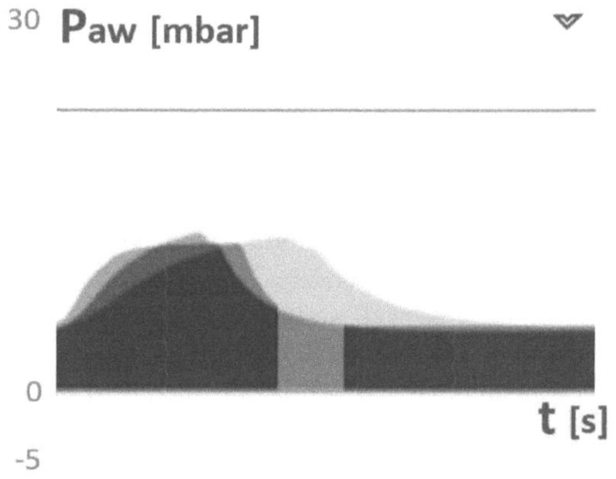

Figure 1: Overlaid Waveforms

To keep the possibility to display the whole ventilation-waveform, the design provides the option to expand the waveform. According to the direct manipulation, which allows a user to manipulate presented objects [7], the module including the overlaid waveform needs to be touched to expand it. To increase the affordance, this is supported by an arrow on the top right corner of the waveform, which can also be seen in Fig. 1. The affordance is known as the ca-

pability of the object, to describe itself [8]. In this case, the arrow clarifies the possibility to expand the waveform.
Another idea was the reduction of unnecessary information. Therefore, the displayed data is rated and classified in two classes, titled as *classification of measurements*. Measurements within the tolerated range are displayed green. Additionally, the values of the "green"-classificated values are not displayed as long as the measurements satisfy the criteria. Measurements exceeding the tolerated range are displayed red, including their values. The idea behind this presentation of the data is a reduction of the mental workload and an increase of the salience, because the operators directly notice whether the measurements are arranged in the tolerated range or not.
Due to the additional space which is achieved by merging the waveforms, further patient information are added. On the one hand further patient data is displayed, such as the medical records of the patient. This enables the operators to check the medical history of the patient on the UI. On the other hand, patient data of further treated patients, including for example patients which are currently inducted into the narcosis, are displayed. This enables the operators to keep track of these patients. Therefore, the operators keep the overview and quickly recognise when to intervene. To present the anaesthesia-status of these patients, they are classified and coloured either green, yellow or red. Similar to the classification of the measurements, green-displayed patients fit in the tolerated range, meaning everything is fine. Compared to a warning, yellow displayed patients need extra attention, being located in a critical boundary area. Finally, red displayed ones need to be focused immediately because they exceed the tolerated range.
An exemplary status of the UI, displaying "green"-classificated data, is shown in Fig. 2. Here, the considered patient fits the classification criterium and the anaesthetic treatment is performed without complications.

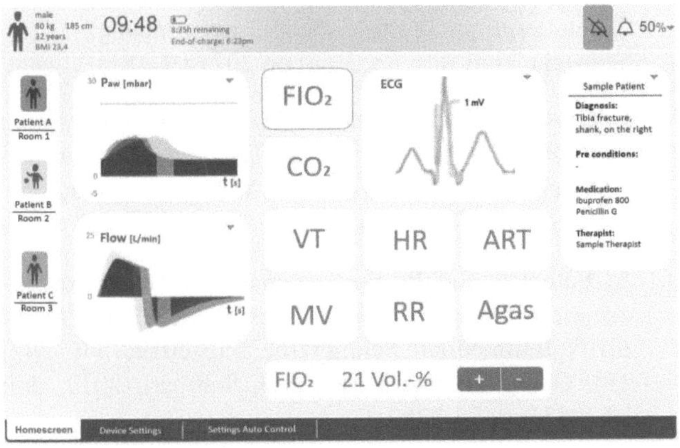

Figure 2: User Interface

5 Results and Discussion

For a first evaluation, experts were interviewed and asked to rate the UI design on a six-point likert scale.

During the first part of the interview, the experts were asked to define the most important measurements of the anaesthetic treatment. They were also asked to discuss the classification of the measurements, especially if some measurements are not quantified as long as they do not exceed a certain range. Besides, the history of the ventilation waveforms was mentioned. The experts were asked about the significance of the history, picturing not only the actual but also the elapsed ventilation cycles. In the second part of the interview, the design-concepts were discussed. The experts were asked to rate the main concepts, consisting of the overlaid waveforms, classification of measurements and additional information. In the third part of the interview, the experts were asked to discuss the usage of TCA and to mention the confidence in higher automation levels.
The results of the interviews are shown in table 1.

Table 1: Evaluation Results

	Design Concept	Average Rating
1.	Overlaid Waveforms	2,0
2.	Classification of Measurements	4,0
3.	Additional Information	2,3
4.	Usage of TCA	2,3

Due to the experts, the history of the ventilation waveforms which presents several ventilation cycles over time, is important. Especially the last two cycles are needed to monitor arising differences. The concept of the overlaid waveforms explicitly visualises the differences between the particular ventilation cycles. It also generates additional space in the UI due to the overlap. Therefore, referred to table 1, it was evaluated with an average rating of 2,0. Although one of the interviewees described them as confusing at first, it was intuitively clear that the elapsed ventilation cycles are displayed transparent over time and the most intense one is the most recent cycle.
The classification of measurements are overall rated with a 4. Generally, the idea of a classification of the measurements was evaluated as a good idea, giving the operators a feedback of the measurements significance. In contrast, the idea not to display the green-classified measurements was discussed critically, causing a reduction of the situation awareness of the operators. The main disadvantages are seen in the huge differences between different patients. Therefore, the measurements need to be estimated individually for every single treatment and cannot be classified. Another problem is seen in a slow drift of the measurements, which can not be seen as long as the measurements are located within the tolerated range. To relief this problem in the future development, a trend notification can be added to the measured parameters.
The additional information, displayed in the headline of the UI, are commended as very useful. Both, the calculation of the BMI and the end-of-charge are needed during the operation and do not need to be calculated manually by the operators anymore. To extend the notification, the time management should be implemented, comparing the end-of-charge

time with the calculated time for the treatment. Thus, the operators know whether the battery capacity is sufficient for the treatment.
Due to an electrical gasmixer and an electric anaesthetic gas dosage, the anaesthetic device is able to act automated, previously introduced as TCA. Referred to table 1, the usage of TCA is appropriated. The advantage is seen in savings in time. Due to the TCA, the operators do not have to monitor the whole set of parameters by himself and is able to focus on the patient more intense. Nonetheless, higher automation levels are highly controversial. While some of the experts support additional automation to decrease mistakes made by the operators and simultaneously increase the time spent with the patient, others do not. They have doubts about the doctors to use the automated functions.
During the evaluation process, the medical experts suggested some additional improvement for the UI, which should be discussed in the following. One idea is the implementation of a digital anaesthesia protocol in the UI instead of the additional patient information. Nowadays, it is mandatory to record the process of anaethesia, which is often done manually. Due to a digital anaesthesia protocol, the operators safe time and are able to concentrate on the treatment. Another idea was to request the most common error sources instead of displaying additional patient information. This remind the operators to check if everything is adjusted correctly and minimizes the risk of an error.
Both ideas have not been evaluated yet. But, since these suggestions were made by the medical experts as an alternative to the intended additional patient information, they should be discussed in the further development process. Because the patient information were rated highly during the evaluation, all three suggestions (additional patient information, digital anaesthesia protocol and displayed error sources) are going to be implemented and tested in different UIs. The realisation of all three suggestions is impossible, due to a lack of space.

6 Conclusion

This work reflects the early stage of the development of an UI design for an anaesthetic device. Different design-proposals, including the overlaid waveforms, the classification of measurements and additional information, were presented. Furthermore, the design-proposals were discussed and evaluated by a group of experts to check the proposals intuitive, safe and easy application in practice.
The classification of measurements was discussed critically, since it is causing a reduction of the operators confidence in the "green"-classified measurements. Therefore, this design-proposal will not be pursued in the furhter development process anymore. But the overlaid waveforms as well as the additional information in the headline and the feedback of the measurements significance due to coloration are claimed as good ideas and will therefore be considered in the future development process.
For future systems, the UI will be programmed on base of the evaluated findings and further implemented and tested in the anaesthetic device.
Finally, legally and standard conforming aspects have not yet been considered in this work.

Acknowledgement

This work has been carried out at the department Corporate Technology & Innovation at Drägerwerk AG & Co. KGaA in Lübeck and supervised by Thomas Franke, Institute for Multimedia and Interactive Systems, Universität zu Lübeck.

Author's Statement

Conflict of interest: Authors state no conflict of interest. All authors discussed the results and contributed to the final manuscript.

7 References

[1] E. Siegel, *Anästhesiegeräte*. In: R. Kramme (ed.) Medizintechnik, Springer, Berlin, Heidelberg, pp. 427-442, doi: 10.1007/978-3-540-34103-1_24.

[2] V. P. Patil, M. G. Shetmahajan and J. V. Divatia, *The modern integrated anaesthesia workstation*. In: Indian journal of anaesthesia, vol. 57(5), pp. 446-454, 2013, doi: 10.4103/0019-5049.120139.

[3] R. Parasuraman, T. B. Sheridan and C. D. Wickens, *A Model for Types and Levels of Human Interaction with Automation*. In: IEEE Transactions on Systems, Man, and Cybernetics - Part A: Systems and Humans, vol. 30, no. 3, pp. 286-297, 2000, doi: 10.1109/3468.844354.

[4] F. Hennecke, *"Wizard of Oz" as an method in UI design*. Available: http://www.medien.ifi.lmu.de/fileadmin/mimuc/mmi_ws0506/essays/uebung2-hennecke.html [last accessed on 2021-01-18].

[5] J. Gläser and G. Laudel, *Experteninterviews und qualitative Inhaltsanalyse: als Instrumente rekonstruierender Untersuchungen*. VS Verlag für Sozialwissenschaften, Wiesbaden, 2009.

[6] A. Fudickar and B. Bein, *Anästhesie bei Erwachsenen mit Adipositas*. In: Anästhesiologie Intensivmedizin Notfallmedizin Schmerztherapie 2019; 54: 242-254, Georg Thieme Verlag KG, Stuttgart, 2019, doi: 10.1055/a-0636-2782.

[7] B. Shneiderman, *Direct Manipulation: A Step Beyond Programming Languages*. In: Computer, vol. 16, no. 8, pp. 57-69, 1983, doi: 10.1109/MC.1983.1654471.

[8] D. Norman, *The Design of Everyday Things*. Basic Books, New York, 2013.

Evaluation of a Stopped-Flow Apparatus for Rapid Mixing of Small Fluid Volumes in Reaction Kinetic Studies

Elena-Thérèse Egerer [1], Janosch Kappel [2], and Christian Hübner [2],

[1] Medical Engineering Science, Universität zu Lübeck, elenatherese.egerer@student.uni-luebeck.de

[2] Institute of Physics, Universität zu Lübeck, {kappel,huebner}@physik.uni-luebeck.de

Abstract

The investigation of dynamic interactions of biomolecules provides important information about molecular processes, e.g. binding mechanisms and protein folding. These insights can contribute significantly to advances in the field of biophysics, the medical and pharmaceutical industry. The stopped-flow method is one of several techniques to observe the dynamic processes. Small fluid volumes are rapidly mixed and the utilized confocal fluorescent microscope is capable of displaying the kinetic processes. In this work a series of measurements were carried out to evaluate the functionality of a custom-built stopped-flow system in combination with a confocal fluorescence microscope. In order to examine the system in terms of reproductive measurement results, the acquired data is analyzed. A herringbone mixer was utilized to prepare the stopped-flow system for the use of a recently developed helical micromixer, that is designed to allow for even lower sample consumption and a shorter dead-time.

1 Introduction

The investigation of dynamic interactions of biomolecules provides important information about molecular processes, e.g. binding mechanisms and protein folding. These insights can contribute significantly to advances in the field of biophysics, the medical and pharmaceutical industry.

In real time, reaction rates among distinct states, conformational conversions in the molecule's structure and intermediate states can be detected.

The process of protein unfolding can be characterized as a first order reaction, which can be described as follows:

$$\mathrm{N} \underset{\mathrm{k_f}}{\overset{\mathrm{k_u}}{\rightleftharpoons}} \mathrm{U}. \tag{1}$$

The conversion from the native state of the protein (N) to the unfolded state (U) is defined including the rate constant k_{u}. Here, this is invoked by mixing of two reactants.

The velocity of a first order reaction, as it is described in (1), can be defined as:

$$v = -\frac{d[N]}{dt} = k_{\mathrm{u}}[N], \tag{2}$$

where [N] is the concentration of the native state and k_{u} is the unfolding rate constant in s^{-1}. This differential equation leads to an exponentially decaying concentration of the folded state's concentration:

$$N(t) = N_0 e^{-k_{\mathrm{u}} t}. \tag{3}$$

If a signal N is detected, which is proportional to the concentration of the native state, this signal follows an identical decay law.

The inverse of the rate constant k_{u} is called the decay time constant τ_{u} [1].

$$k_{\mathrm{u}} = \frac{1}{\tau_{\mathrm{u}}} \tag{4}$$

Three commonly used methods for the investigation of fast reaction kinetics are continuous-flow (CF), quenched-flow (QF), and stopped-flow (SF). The reaction kinetics can be assessed with optical measurement methods, e.g. the detection of emitted fluorescence, or by means of electrochemistry, e.g. determination of conductivity [2].

The suitable method for the reaction of interest varies because every technique shows its advantages and disadvantages. For instance, the most important advantages of the stopped-flow method are the short dead-time and the low sample consumption. This is an advantage in the case of time-consuming sample preparation.

In this work a series of measurements were carried out to evaluate the functionality of a custom-built stopped-flow system in combination with a confocal fluorescence microscope. In order to examine the system in terms of reproductive measurement results, the acquired data is analyzed using IGOR Pro 8. A commercially available herringbone mixer was utilized to prepare the stopped-flow system for the use of a recently developed helical micromixer that is designed to allow for even lower sample consumption and a shorter dead-time.

2 Material and Methods

In the following the stopped-flow method including the different microfluidic mixers is described. Additionally, the confocal fluorescence microscope used for detection is explained. Also the test reaction used for the evaluation of the system is presented.

2.1 The Stopped-Flow Method

Fast biochemical reactions can be detected and observed by using the stopped-flow method. After rapid mixing of the fluids, these reactions, e.g. protein dynamics like structural changes, can be investigated with the desired observation setup. The first stopped-flow apparatus was developed by Britton Chance in 1937 [3]. Afterwards it has been revised and adapted several times with the emergence of new applications and technological advances.

Before reaching the observation chamber the two or more used reactants are mixed together at high velocities. As the name of the method suggests, the flow is stopped as soon as the observation chamber is filled with the mixed reactants [4]. Using a data acquisition system with high temporal resolution, the reaction between the reactants can be detected as a change in signal over time. Different detection methods can be optical absorbance, fluorescence, or circular dichroism (CD) [5].

An important limiting factor in such a stopped-flow experiment is the dead-time. It is the time between the first encounter of the two reactants and the mixture of both getting stopped in the observation chamber for data acquisition. Decisive factors that influence the dead-time are the mixing time, the flow rate and the general mixer geometry. The investigation of the dead-time can be achieved by detection of the fluorescence and the absorption signals.

A crucial characteristic of the stopped-flow method is the low sample consumption. The detection device can be focused on a single area, therefore no scanning is necessary.

2.2 Microfluidic Mixing

In order to observe the reaction between two samples, e.g. the inspection of protein unfolding by adding a denaturant to a protein solution, both substances must come into contact with each other. Afterwards they have to reach the observation chamber so the expected change in signal can be detected. As the mixing and detection process need to be very fast for such reactions, a slow mixing by diffusion is not feasible.

A passive mixer is used to create a chaotic flow pattern, so no external energy source needs to be connected. Due to the unique channel geometry the boundary layer of the fluids is increased, as the fluids are pushed through the channels of the mixer leading to an effective mixing process. The mixing unit and the observation chamber are placed in one element to achieve a short distance between both. The used stopped-flow system is custom-built and designed for the use of a particular customized micromixer with a helical mixing structure that is shown in Fig. 5, and for a very small interval volume to allow for dead-times in the sub-millisecond regime and a sample consumption of just a few microlitres.

In a first approach, a commercially available herringbone mixer was used first to evaluate the functionality of the described measurement configuration, before the more fragile helical micromixer is used. This herringbone mixer shows a certain number of grooves resembling fish bones. These grooves are alternating with a complementary set mirrored at the centerline, as illustrated in Fig. 1. In addition to that the mixer's channels are rectangular. Therefore the mixing unit is characterized by low flow resistance and a generated cross flow due to its geometry [6].

2.3 Stopped-Flow Apparatus with Confocal Fluorescence Detection

The SF method can also be combined with a setup for the detection of fluorescence. A confocal fluorescence microscope (CFM) has proven to be particularily suitable for measurements including small sample volumes and low concentrations of reactant. A syringe drive, controlled by a computer, pushes a certain amount of both reactants into the mixing chip. The fluids come together in the herringbone mixing unit. After the mixture of both reactants is guided into the observation chamber it is excited by the light source of the system, a 488 nm laser. In order to detect the emitted fluorescence, a dichroic mirror is used to separate the excitation light from the emission light. An emission filter is followed by a lense that focuses the fluorescent light on the detection system, an avalanche photodiode. A simplified representation of the confocal fluorescence microscope used for this work can be seen in Fig. 1. The microfluidic elements of the stopped-flow setup are shown in Fig. 2.

2.4 Test Reaction for Evaluation

The green fluorescent protein (GFP), originally discovered in the jellyfish Aequorea victoria in 1962 by Shimomura et al. [7], is widely used in biochemistry and cell biology. The utilized version of GFP used for this work is called eGFP, which can be excited with a 488 nm laser and whose emission peak is at 511 nm. The extremely stable autofluorescent protein can be denaturated by using sodium dodecyl sulfate (SDS) at a pH of 6.5 [8]. The unfolding reaction leading to the loss of fluorescence occurs on a timescale of about one minute. The fluorescence diminishes from the maximum value N_0 to a value in dependence of time, N_t.

3 Results and Discussion

In the following section the data acquisition using the stopped-flow setup will be explained. Afterwards the data evaluation with IGOR Pro 8 (Wavemetrics, USA) will be shown. In addition, the evaluated results are illustrated in two figures.

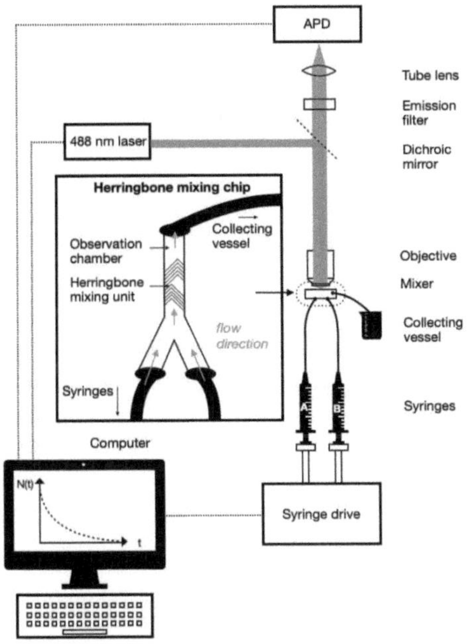

Figure 1: The used confocal fluorescence microscopy setup including the syringe drive and the herringbone mixing chip. The fluids, included in syringes A and B, are pushed into the mixing chip by the syringe drive. A 488 nm laser excites the fluorescent dye in the observation chamber after it has been mixed in the herringbone mixing unit. The fluorescence emission is separated from the excitation light using a dichroic mirror. Emission filter and a lense guides the fluorescent light to the avalanche photodiode (APD) for detection purposes.

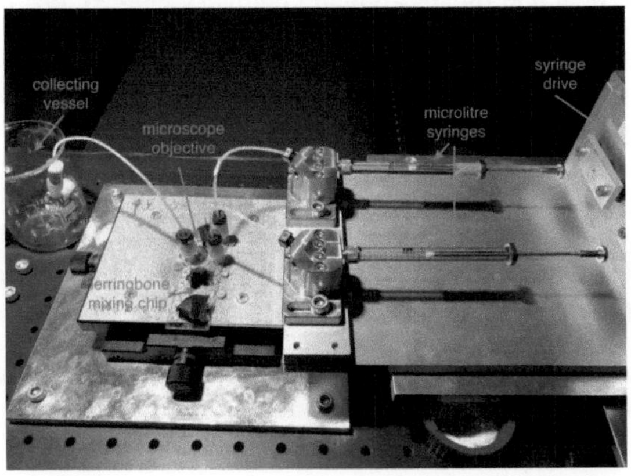

Figure 2: The filled syringes are fixed in the syringe drive. Small hoses lead from the syringes into the herringbone mixing chip. The blue laser light is focussed on the observation chamber from the bottom. The fluids are guided from the mixing chip into a collecting vessel.

3.1 Data Acquisition

The microfluidic system was rinsed with buffer solution before the syringes were filled with the two reactants. The GFP-syringe contained 0.5 µM eGFP in 100 mM sodium phosphate with a pH of 6.5 and the SDS syringe contained 1% SDS in 100 mM sodium phosphate with a pH of 6.5 as well. Several single shots of 10 µl each are made using the syringe drive. One mixing detection cycle was done using a multi shot sequence of 10 shots in total. After a pause time of 2.5 minutes the next shot is executed. Not every shot was usable as some restrictions, e.g. air bubbles in the microfluidic system, resulted in a rather atypical curve progression.

3.2 Data Evaluation

A typical stopped-flow shot measurement of the test reaction decribed in section 2.4 shows a steep increase in fluorescence signal and a slow exponential decrease. For the data evaluation in this work a measuremt with three shots was utilized. A commercially available herringbone mixer was installed as the microfluidic mixer to prepare the stopped-flow system for a recently developed helical micromixer. It was necessary to make sure that the system was working properly before using a new element. Hence an analysis of the stopped-flow time trace is acquired to identify possible sources of error.

3.2.1 Comparison of Shots

In Fig. 3 three shots are displayed for comparison. By using the IGOR Pro 8 software the shots were selected from the overall fluorescence timetrace of a shot sequence. The shots are normalized and the background is substracted. After an overlay of all the shots the average is calculated and plotted in Fig. 4. The execution of a shot performed by the syringe drive can be seen as the rapid increase of fluorescence signal in Fig. 3 at t = 0 s.

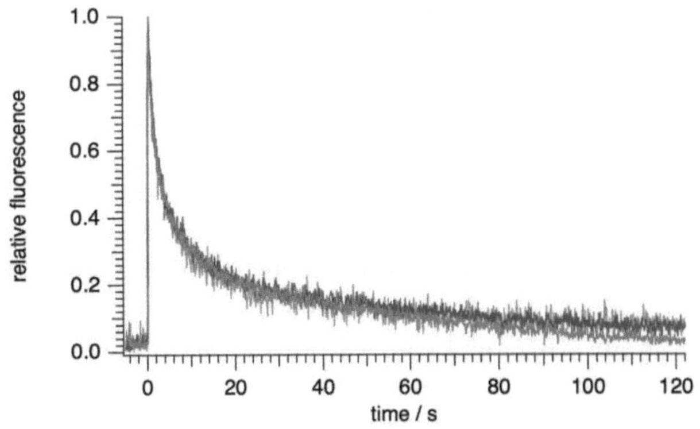

Figure 3: Three different shots, in blue, green and red, are shown. The relative fluorescence is plotted against the time in seconds.

The software enabled fitting of a double exponential model to the experimentally obtained decays. In Fig. 4 the double exponential curve is fitted to the average of the shots. Furthermore, the residual values are calculated. The residues show the difference between the measured value and the double exponential fit. After fitting the double exponential curve the software computes coefficient and constant values. The values of τ can be seen in the box. As shown in (4) the rate constant k_u can be determined. The calculated value of $k_{u,1}$ is 0.324 s^{-1} and the value of $k_{u,2}$ is 0.026 s^{-1}.

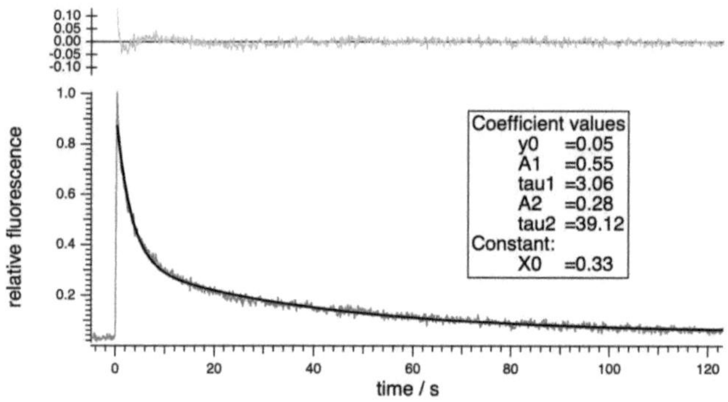

Figure 4: In the lower graph the relative fluorescence is plotted against the time in seconds.The average of all three shots is illustrated in red. A double exponential fit is shown in black. On top the residuals are displayed in orange. The values of τ can be seen in the box. The calculated value of $k_{u,1}$ is 0.324 s^{-1} and the value of $k_{u,2}$ is 0.026 s^{-1}.

4 Conclusion and Outlook

In this work a series of stopped-flow measurements has been carried out, utilizing a custom-built stopped-flow system and a herringbone mixing chip. The change in fluorescence of eGFP during the chosen test reaction has been detected with a confocal fluorescence microscope. The measured data were analyzed using IGOR Pro 8.
The occurance of air bubbles inside the microfluidic system is a major obstacle during the acquisition of reliable data. The interaction of the entire setup shows the fully desired functionality. A helical micromixer has been developed recently, which will allow for even lower sample consumption and a further reduced dead-time than for the utilized herringbone mixer. The special helical micromixer has been fabricated in quartz glass by using in-volume selective laser etching (ISLE) [9]. The helical micromixer offers the main characteristics of a chaotic micromixer. The mixing unit is in a helical shape to ensure chaotic mixing of the fluids. The measurement and the following data evaluation show that the whole setup can be used with all its desired functions. The insertion of a helical micromixer instead of the commercially available herringbone mixer prospectively leads to a drastic shortening of the dead-time and the reduction of the sample volume.

Acknowledgement

The work has been carried out at the Institute of Physics, Universität zu Lübeck and supervised by Janosch Kappel.

Author's Statement

Authors state no conflict of interest.

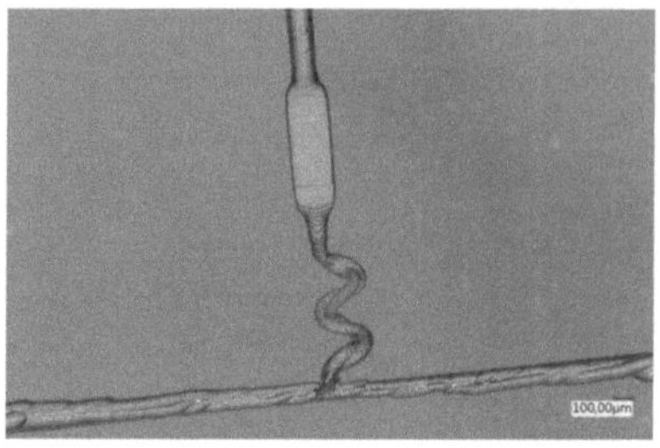

Figure 5: The helical micromixer offers the main characteristics of a chaotic micromixer. The mixing unit is in a helical shape to ensure chaotic mixing of the fluids. Above the mixing channels the observation chamber can be seen.

5 References

[1] M. Binnewies, M. Finze, M. Jäckel, P. Schmidt, H. Willner, G. Rayner-Canham, *Allgemeine und Anorganische Chemie.* Springer Spektrum, pp. 355-362, 2016.

[2] S. M. H. Khorhassani, A. Ebrahimi, M. T. Maghsoodlou, M. Shahraki, D.Price, *Establishing a new conductance stopped-flow apparatus to investigate the initial fast step of reaction between 1, 1, 1-trichloro-3-methyl-3-phospholene and methanol under a dry inert atmosphere.* Analyst, 136(8), pp. 1713-1721, 2011.

[3] R. Bleul, M. Ritzi-Lehnert, J. Höth, N. Scharpfenecker, I. Frese, D. Düchs, et al., *Compact, cost-efficient microfluidics- based stopped-flow device.* Analytical and bioan- alytical chemistry, 399(3), pp. 1117-1125, 2011.

[4] R. A. Harvey, *A simple stopped-flow photometer.* Analytical biochemistry, 29(1), pp. 58-67, 1968.

[5] S. M. Hargrove, *Ligand binding with stopped-flow rapid mixing.* Protein-Ligand Interactions: Methods and Applications, Humana Press, Totowa, New Jersey, pp. 323-341, 2005.

[6] A. D. Stroock, S. K. W. Dertinger, A. Ajdari, I. Mezić, H. A. Stone, G. M. Whitesides, *Chaotic Mixer for Microchannels.* Science, 295, pp. 647-651, 2002.

[7] R. Y. Tsien, *The Green Fluorescent Protein.* Annual Review of Biochemistry, 67:1, pp. 509–544, 1998.

[8] K. M. Alkaabi, A. Yafea, S. S. Ashraf, *Effect of pH on thermal- and chemical-induced denaturation of GFP.* Applied biochemistry and biotechnology, 126(2), pp. 149-156, 2005.

[9] J. Kappel, *Development of a stopped-flow apparatus for the rapid mixing of small fluid volumes in reaction kinetic studies.* Master Thesis, Universität zu Lübeck, 2018.

Development of a Safety Mechanism for the Patient Compartment Hood of an MR-Compatible Incubator

David Pysik [1], Judith Müller [2], Marian Taube [2], and Georg Schildbach [3]

[1] Medical Engineering Science, Universität zu Lübeck, david.pysik@student.uni-luebeck.de
[2] LMT Medical Systems GmbH, Lübeck, {j.mueller, taube}@lmt-medicalsystems.com
[3] Institute for Electrical Engineering in Medicine, Universität zu Lübeck, georg.schildbach@uni-luebeck.de

Abstract

An unintentional impact on the patient compartment hood of the incubator system nomag® IC Advanced during patient preparation can cause injuries due to the hood dropping onto the medical staff. In this paper, we discuss the development of a snap-fit like safety mechanism to prevent this case. The mechanism locks passively and can be released actively. We present the mechanism design process, which includes determining the occurring forces onto the hood and selected material as well as the manufacturing process. Furthermore, we show the assembling method on the incubator and point out the relevant mechanism properties. The safety mechanism can resist forces over 180 Newton without breaking and can be easily released with a force of about 20 Newton.

1 Introduction

The nomag® IC Advanced is a magnetic resonance (MR)-compatible incubator system of the company LMT Medical Systems GmbH, which is used to examine premature infants of the intensive care with the non-invasive imaging technique of magnetic resonance imaging (MRI). This modality is nowadays an established diagnostic imaging technique in a clinical routine [1]. Acceleration of the acquisition time and the increase of the spatial resolution greatly impacted the technology [2]. One advantage of MRI is that it allows functional and morphological information from the patient scan. Moreover, there is no ionizing radiation used in MRI [2], which is a great advantage in terms of the vulnerable patient group of premature infants. MRI of the brain allows early detection and prediction of later diseases or developmental disorders in premature infant's early life stages [3]. This information can be used for individual therapies. During transport to the MR-device and throughout the entire imaging, the premature infant has access to life-supporting systems inside like constant temperature and humidity. This way, the patient experiences less stress and stays calmer. This allows an examination without sedation.
The incubator's patient compartment hood enables access to the infant and can be fully opened to the end position without the possibility of locking the hood. The developed safety mechanism should protect the medical staff from injuries caused by the hood falling due to an unintentional impact. Due to usage in a MR-device and the fact of the incubator as a medical product, the mechanism needs to fulfill special requirements. The material used for the mechanism shall not cause any image artifacts that can lead to misinterpretation of the scans [4]. This and the low quantity needed, restrict the selection of materials and manufacturing processes. This paper presents the used design, development and manufacturing as well as their methods for an MR-compatible safety mechanism suitable for series production of the incubator system nomag® IC Advanced.

2 Material and Methods

In this section, the methods and the design process for the development of the safety mechanism are presented. The force that has to be withstood and the force for releasing is determined with a force sensor wherefrom the corresponding force on the mechanism is calculated. With these values, the geometry of the design is adjusted with the support of a finite element method (FEM)-simulation to determine the thickness of the part that can be actively pushed. Following, the mechanism is tested regarding the forces and its closing and releasing behaviour.

2.1 Determination of Impact Force

The Medical Device Regulation from the year 2020 [5] does not provide any exact information regarding the maximum force of an impact that the mechanism must withstand. To design the safety mechanism, the mechanical force on the hood must be determined first. For this, we use the measurement device ALMEMO® 2390-3 of the company Ahlborn GmbH and the suitable force sensor K25 for pressure and traction measurement. The sensor is based on a cantilever with strain gauges to measure a force. The sensor and the connected measurement device are shown in Fig. 1.

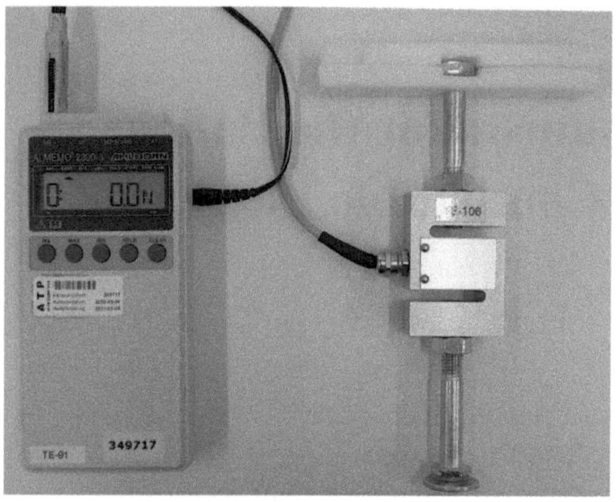

Figure 1: The force sensor K25 and the connected measurement device from the company Ahlborn Gmbh are used to determine the impact force.

We simulate an impact with a shoulder on the upper edge of the patient compartment hood and measure an average corresponding force of about F_{impact} = 50 Newton. The incubator is shown in the following Fig. 2 with the point of force application of F_{impact}.

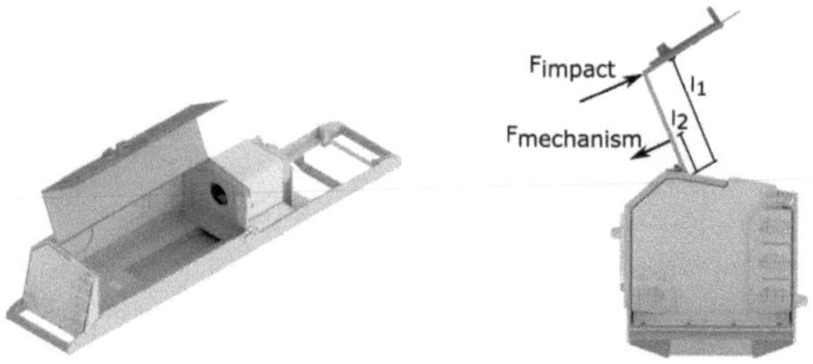

2.1 Front view 2.2 Side view

Figure 2: Model of the opened incubator from two different views with the points of force applications and co responding lever arms. Currently, the incubator is determined in its end position through an end stop only, which has an angular surface.

The force the mechanism has to resist will be different from this measured force because the momentum depends on the subsequent relative position of the incubator's mechanism concerning the force application. Both lever arms can be seen in Fig. 2.2. The lever l_2 determines the induced force $F_{mechanism}$ on the mechanism.

2.2 Product Development

We choose to develop the safety mechanism according to the VDI 2221 Guideline. Accordingly to the method, product design and development can be separated into four main phases. These are the planning-, concept-, design- and elaboration phase [6]. Thereby the individual phases are often characterized by an iterative process between them [6].
The first step for designing the mechanism is to formulate a list of requirements. There are some special requirements about the material that can be used within the MR-environment. The highest priority is to select MR-safe and -compatible materials for the mechanism. To guarantee a safe operation of the mechanism, it has to lock passively and can only be released actively. Furthermore, the connection to the existing system shall be without significant changes. Maintainability and ergonomics as well as low manufacturing costs are secondary objectives.
The next step of the design process is the development of simple concept ideas and operating principles, which are outlined by sketches or just formulated with words. A three-point scoring system is used to choose the best concept regarding the requirements for further improvement.
In the design phase, we create the first simple computer-aided design (CAD)-models of the concept. It is based on a two-part snap-fit like mechanism. Furthermore, there are snap-in points on both parts. This geometry additionally creates a form fit, which allows enduring a higher force against an impact. The mechanism can be released by bending through pushing on the lever of one of the parts. After the first evaluation of the concept design, the need for further improvements has become apparent to better fulfill the requirements. Therefore, we iterate through the design phase again. We adjust the geometry, which leads to a mechanism with just a single but larger snap-in point geometry on both parts. Moreover, both parts receive two holes for assembling on the incubator. The base of part 1 becomes larger than before. This allows the usage of the already existing holes on the incubator's frame for the assembling of part 1. The rounding of all edges on both parts enables an easier cleaning of the mechanism and a lower risk of injuries in later use. These adjustments lead to the final design of the safety mechanism which is shown in Fig. 3.

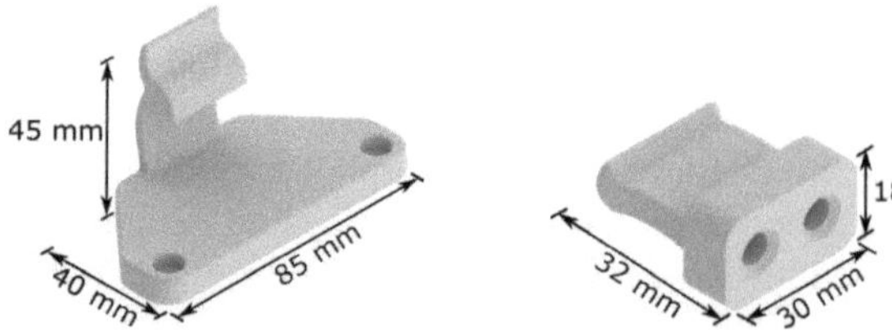

3.1 Part 1 3.2 Part 2

Figure 3: Model of both parts of the final safety mechanism containing the overall final dimensions.

In this last phase of the design process, we work out the details of the design. The additive manufacturing technology of selective laser sintering (SLS) is chosen for manufacturing. The technology is predestined for this design because of the more complex geometry and the smooth edges. It also provides a possibility for cheap manufacturing if just a low quantity is needed. We select polyamide 12 (PA12) as material for the following reasons: It is the most used material in SLS processes [7]. It also generates no significant signal in the MR-scans following existing internal LMT measurements, subsequent there is no influence on the image quality.

2.3 Force Calculation and FEM-Simulation

To get a good ratio between strength and flexibility of part 1, we use the FEM tool SimulationXpress from SolidWorks®. This allows us to evaluate and adjust a minimum thickness of the functional section of part 1. Table 1 shows the mechanical properties for the simulation of PA12 similar chosen to [8] but with the assumption of isotropic behaviour because the FEM-tool does not offer the simulation of anisotropic material.

Table 1: Mechanical properties of PA12 according to [8], where R_m is the tensile strength, E the Young's modulus, R_e the yield strength and γ the Poisson's ratio.

$R_m\ [MPa]$	$E\ [MPa]$	$R_e\ [MPa]$	γ
30	1500	21	0,39

The force $F_{release}$ required for easy release is determined with the same force sensor out of section 2.1 by pushing on it until it becomes too heavy and is about 20 Newton. For the simulation, we calculate the force on the mechanism, which is induced through an impact. Therefore, we use the force F_{impact} and determine the related lever arms of the force application points l_1 and l_2 out of Fig. 2.2 to the hood's pivot point. As a result, we calculate the force that occurs on the mechanism to about 140 Newton. Fig. 4 shows the occurring stress on part 1 for the impact force and the force for releasing the mechanism. The thickness of part 1 in this figure is adjusted in such a way that the safety factor is near above 1 for the force of 140 Newton.

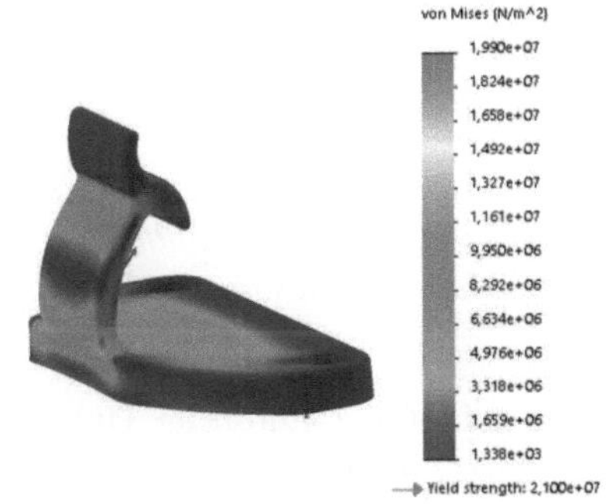

4.1 Mechanical stress during an impact

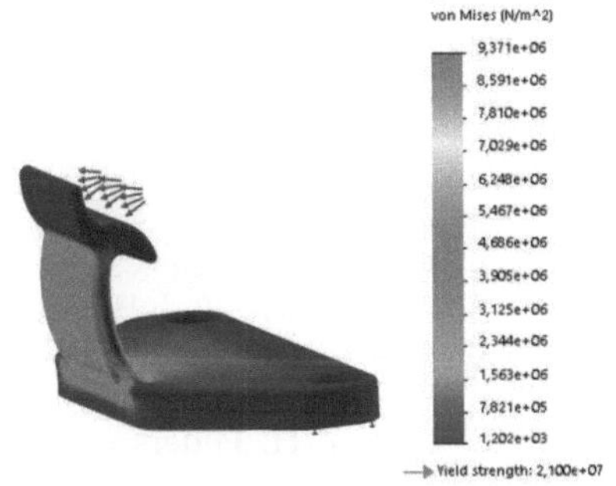

4.2 Mechanical stress during releasing

Figure 4: Simulated stress on part 1 with the force that occurs during an impact and the force which is needed for releasing. The purple arrows indicate the occurring forces.

The average element size of the mesh is set to 1,5 mm with the FEM-tool. The highest occurring stress is under the yield strength R_e of the material. Therefore, it appears primary elastic deformation of the material. The final thickness of part 1 is slightly adjusted larger to guarantee a higher safety factor. Part 2 needs no simulation to prove the stress it can resist because the thickness is much higher than of part 1, which can be seen in Fig. 5.

2.4 Assembling of the Safety Mechanism

Two holes with a diameter of five millimeters are needed in the hood for the mechanism's assembly of part 2. The two holes of part 2 are provided with thread inserts because they enlarge the stability of the screw connection and resist a higher mechanical stress. We assemble both parts with M4 screws and suitable washers made of polyether ether ketone (PEEK). We choose PEEK screws because of their good mechanical properties and the fact, that PEEK generates no significant signal in MRI. During the screwing of the parts,

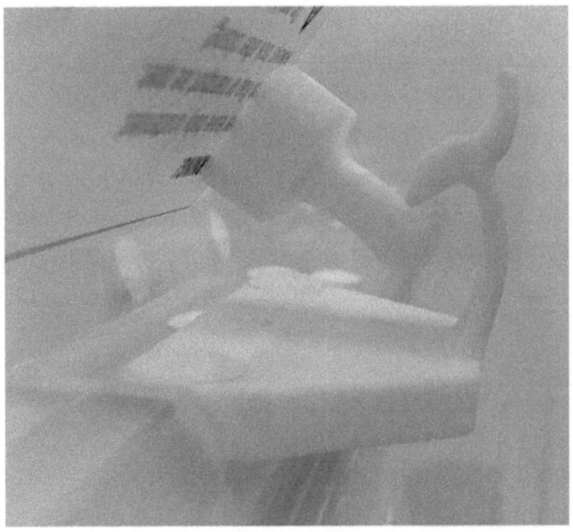

Figure 5: Assembled safety mechanism on the incubator.

we align them to each other so that the components have enough overlapping area. This can be seen in Fig. 5. The needed alignment is possible due to the big through-holes compared to the used screws. The holes are covered with caps to avoid fluids from seeping into them. The caps also simplify the cleaning of the mechanism.

2.5 Testing of the Safety Mechanism

The mechanism is tested in terms of the force needed to release it and the force it can withstand. We use the same force sensor as described in section 2.1. First, the force to bend part 1 for releasing the mechanism is determined. To this end, we pull on the surface of part 1 with the sensor and measure the force until part 2 can be released. Second, we push with the sensor against the hood's upper edge and measure the occurring force. We use the same point of force application that we used for the measurement of the impact in section 2.1. Furthermore, we evaluate the passive locking and the position of the parts to each other during assembling.

3 Results and Discussion

The force for releasing the mechanism $F_{release, real} = 20 \pm 2$ Newton is close to the desired force $F_{release}$. This allows the user to release the mechanism comfortably. In the second measurement, the force $F_{impact, real} = 65$ Newton can be resisted. We had to stop the measurement at this value because the end stop for the incubator's hood gets quite fragile and begins to deform slightly and hence there is the risk of damaging it. However, this result is greater than the value for F_{impact} we set in section 2.1, which should be withstood. The force $F_{impact, real}$ on the hood corresponds to about $F_{mechanism, real} = 180$ Newton that the mechanism can resist in any case. Both parts need alignment. This fact shows that the function of the mechanism is quite sensitive to minor deviations in its position, due to less overlapping of both parts. In this case, the mechanism could not resist the measured high force and parts slide off each other at lower forces. The passive locking of the safety mechanism works and depends slightly on the users closing behaviour. Seldom, when the hood is opened with a meager amount of force to its end position, the parts of the mechanism lay on each other without snapping in. It snaps into place when a small force of a few Newtons is subsequently applied to the hood handle. The shape of the mechanism's geometry allows a good cleaning and a low risk of injury during use. But the SLS surface is quite rough due to the selected manufacturing method, which leads to a needed varnish for using the mechanism on the incubator as a standard part.

4 Conclusion

The developed safety mechanism provides a comfortable and ergonomic way to secure the patient compartment hood from falling down due to an unintentional impact. A further advantage of the mechanism is that the required holes for fixation of part 1 already exist on the incubator. This allows just a minimal change of the existing system and consequently lowers costs. For the introduction as a series part, the mechanism needs some slight adjustments on the geometry for enhanced closing behaviour and a less vulnerable alignment of both parts. Furthermore, the position may shift slightly due to frequent use of the mechanism. This would cause a potential failure. For preventing this failure, the screw connections must be evaluated frequently in more detail. This may help to find a less sensitive method for position shifts when assembling the safety mechanism. In later use, the mechanism will be used each day and the regular service cycle for the incubator is about two years. Therefore, the mechanism must endure many load cycles before it is scheduled to be exchanged. A prediction of the life cycle with a suitable simulation is desired.
Another aim is to change the used manufacturing method because varnishing of the parts can change the obtained results, causes higher costs and increases the manufacturing time. Flaking of the varnish could also occur after repeated use. Therefore, the vacuum casting method could be an alternative that provides a better surface roughness of the manufactured parts. For a better simulation, the anisotropic behaviour of the SLS-printed PA12 should also be observed.

Acknowledgement

The work has been carried out at the development and construction department at LMT Medical Systems GmbH and supervised by the Institute for Electrical Engineering in Medicine, Universität zu Lübeck.

Author's Statement

Conflict of interest: Authors state no conflict of interest. All authors read and approved the final version of this manuscript.

5 References

[1] W. R. Nitz, *Magnetresonanztomographie (MRT)*. In: R. Kramme, *Medizintechnik Verfahren - Systeme - Informationsverarbeitung*. Springer Verlag Berlin Heidelberg, pp. 338-356, 2011.

[2] O. Dietrich, M. F. Reiser, S. O. Schoenberg, *Parallel Imaging in Clinical MR Applications*. Springer Verlag Berlin Heidelberg, 2007.

[3] L. J. Woodward, P. J. Anderson et al., *Neonatal MRI to Predict Neurodevelopmental Outcomes in Preterm Infants*. Massachusetts Medical Society, The New England Journal of Medicine, vol. 355, no.7, pp. 685-694, 2006.

[4] U. S. Department of Health and Human Services, FDA, *Establishing Safety and Compatibility of Passive Implants in the Magnetic Resonance (MR) Environment*. 2014.

[5] Official Journal of the European Union, *Regulation (EU) 2020/561 of the European Parliament and of the Council of 23 April 2020 amending Regulation (EU) 2014/745 on medical devices, as regards the date of application of certain of its provisions* 2020.

[6] VDI, *Design of technical products and systems - Model of product design*. Beuth Verlag, 2019.

[7] M. Schmid, *Additive Fertigung mit Selektivem Lasersintern (SLS) Prozess- und Werkstoffüberblick*. Springer Vieweg, Wiesbaden, 2015.

[8] A. Lindberg, J. Alfthan, H. Peterssonb G. Flodberg, L. Yang, *Mechanical performance of polymer powder bed fused objects–FEM simulation and verification*. Elsevier, Additive Manufacturing, vol.24, pp. 577-586, 2018.

Gaussian Process Optimized Model Predictive Control of Ventilation Pressure for Spontaneously Breathing Patients

Kerrin Tessars [1], Georg Maennel [2], and Jan Graßhoff [2]
[1] Medical Engineering Science, Universität zu Lübeck, kerrin.tessars@student.uni-luebeck.de
[2] Institute for Electrical Engineering in Medicine, Universität zu Lübeck, j.graßhoff, ge.maennel@uni-luebeck.de

Abstract

In modern medicine, mechanical ventilation is essential. One important goal is to support spontaneous breathing with an optimal level of ventilation. To ensure there is no harm due to i.e., high pressure, the ventilation parameters must be adjusted precisely. In this work, an existing model of the dynamics of the pneumatic system of an anaesthesia workstation ventilation unit is to be extended by a latent-force model, with the help of which disturbances occurring in the system as well as the patient's respiratory effort are to be estimated. For this purpose, Gaussian process (GP) approaches for respiratory activity estimation must be converted into state-space form and integrated into a state-space model used for control. Furthermore, the model is to be extended in such a way that other disturbance processes can also be learned by the extended latent-force model. The found model is to be evaluated on a simulation model.

1 Introduction

Mechanical ventilation enables gas exchange to be maintained in the event that the patient's own breathing is limited due to either medication or illness. Ventilation with positive pressure and increased oxygen concentrations, in turn, is non-physiological and carries an increased risk of harming the patient. Furthermore, the patient should still be able to breathe spontaneously, so the device should be able to adapt to the patient's respiratory effort to prevent degeneration of the respiratory muscles. Ideally, the patient's respiratory effort could be determined from the flow and pressure data at the patient's airways, but this is often only possible to a limited extent due to the uncertain mechanical lung properties. Within this paper we propose to use Gaussian process (GP) regression in combination with a first principle modeling to estimate the breathing effort of the patient and consider it in the control scheme. Therefore we augment a dynamics model of the pneumatic ventilation system with a latent force for the pressure generated by the breathing muscles. The latent force is described by a GP. GP Priors can be transformed by representing their spectral density as rational functions and using spectral factorization [1]. In contrast to other, highly parameterized regression methods, GP regression exclusively requires a mean and a covariance function for modeling. When choosing an appropriate covariance function, the latent force can be described in state-space representation and thus overcome the practical limitation on large data sets. Further on, the model is to be extended in such a way that other disturbance processes can also be learned by the extended latent-force model. Additionally, different control designs are presented.

2 Material and Methods

In this section we introduce the system model, which is adopted from [2], as well as the proposed GP in latent force model. Furthermore, the applied methods for disturbance prediction and pressure control are established.

2.1 The system model

It is important not to damage the patient's lungs over the course of mechanical ventilation. During spontaneous breathing, a negative pressure is generated around the lungs by contraction of the respiratory muscles. This creates a flow of oxygen through the pulmonary airways in the direction of the descending pressure gradient [3]. Within this paper, the lungs are assumed to behave as a single linear system governed by two parameters. First, a parameter E related to the restoring force of the lung. The resulting pressure $P_{el} = EV$ counteracts the increasing volume V. The second parameter is the resistance of the airway R, and the resulting pressure drop with the equation $P_{res} = R\dot{V}$. The differential equation describing the flows in and out of the lungs is given by eq. (1), where P_{mus} represents the pressure proportional to the force generated by the patient's muscles and P_{aw} is the pressure at the airway

$$P_{aw} = R\dot{V} + EV - P_{mus} + P_0. \tag{1}$$

In this equation the parameter P_0 is the so-called PEEP (positive end-expiratory pressure) and $\dot{V}$ the flow. The positive offset pressure within the lungs at the end of expiration protects the alveoly from collapsing. For simplicity, it can assumed to be zero in this work, since it will not be changed during the course of the paper and only dynamical

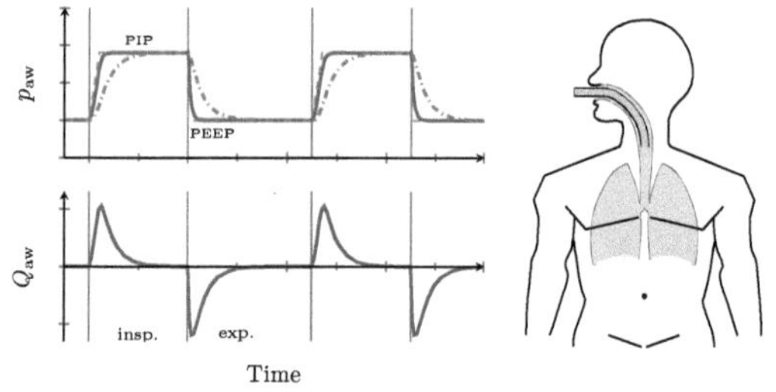

Figure 1: Pressure-time and flow-time diagram for pressure controlled ventilation [2].

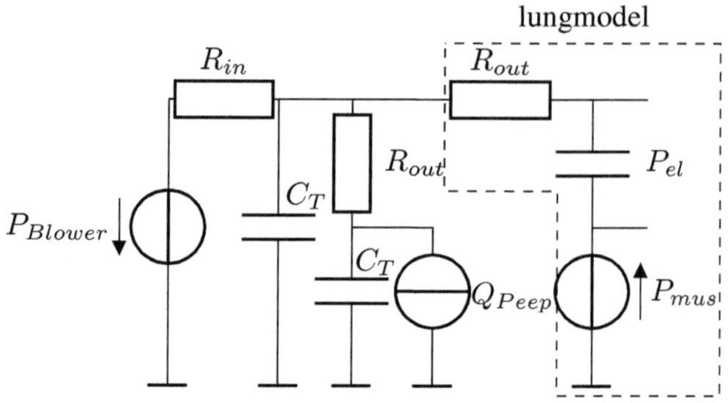

Figure 2: Scheme of the electrical equivalent circuit for the ventilation system. The lung model is contained by the dashed box.

factors are of relevance for the presented results. In Fig. 1, the trajectory of the airway pressure (AP) during pressure controlled ventilation is depicted in the upper diagram, with the blue solid line representing an ideal controlled and the red dashed dotted the resulting pressure in the aveoly of the patient. The lower diagram depicts the resulting flow Q_{aw} into the patient [2]. The single compartment model of the lung can be represented as an electrical equivalent circuit (dashed box in Fig. 2). The equivalent circuit for the entire ventilation system of an anaesthesia workstation consisting of a tube model and the actuators of the mechanical ventilator can be seen in Fig. 2. Here, the model of the lung and tubes is assumed to be a series connection of a resistor and a capacitor [3]. The blower is equivalent to the pressure source (P_{blower}) and the PEEP valve is the flow source (Q_{PEEP}). Based on this, the differential equation describing the dynamics of the physical system can be transformed into the following state space representation:

$$\begin{aligned}\frac{\mathrm{d}x(t)}{\mathrm{d}t} &= A_p x(t) + B_p u(t) + B_w w(t) \\ y_k &= C_p x(t_k) + \epsilon_k.\end{aligned} \tag{2}$$

A_p, B_p and C_p are the system matrices and $x(t)$ the states of the physical system i.e., the pressure at the airway, alveolies, expiration tube and blower and the flow, which were derived in [2], with a system complexity of five states and two inputs and outputs each. Moreover, $u(t)$ is the control input, y_k are the systems measurements, $w(t)$ with the matrix B_w is the latent force acting on the system and $\epsilon_k \sim \mathcal{N}(0, Q_\epsilon)$ is the Gaussian measurement noise.

2.2 Gaussian process in latent force model

Gaussian processes are stochastic processes, which results in a normal distribution when evaluated over any finite set of inputs. The GP can be used to create a distribution over functions and assign probabilities to them. When controlled systems are confronted with unknown disturbance structures, one way to describe them is with a non-parametric GP prior. These models are called latent force models (LFMs) and belong to the category of grey box models, where part of the model is derived by first-principles methods and other parts are adapted to fit the observed data. In several papers, e.g., [1] and [4], it has been shown that GP Priors can be brought into the state-space representation. With an appropriately chosen covariance function, to define a suitable model for the GP, the latent force $w(t)$ can be described by a multivariant stochastic differential equation

$$\begin{aligned}\frac{\mathrm{d}z(t)}{\mathrm{d}t} &= A_g z(t) + B_g e(t) \\ w(t) &= C_g z(t).\end{aligned} \tag{3}$$

Hereby A_g, B_g and C_g are the system matrices of the GP and $e(t)$ corresponds to Gaussian white noise with the spectral density Q_e.
By combining the GP model in eq. (3) with the physical lung model in eq. (2), the augmented state-space representation of the LFM can be achieved

$$\begin{aligned}\frac{\mathrm{d}g(t)}{\mathrm{d}t} &= Ag(t) + Bu(t) + B_e e(t) \\ y_k &= Cg(t_k) + \epsilon_k.\end{aligned} \tag{4}$$

Similarly, in eq. (4) $e(t)$ corresponds to the white noise. The vector g and matrices A, B, B_e and C are defined as follows:

$$\begin{aligned} g = \begin{pmatrix} x \\ z \end{pmatrix}, A = \begin{pmatrix} A_p & B_w C_g \\ 0 & A_g \end{pmatrix}, B = \begin{pmatrix} B_p \\ 0 \end{pmatrix}, \\ B_e = \begin{pmatrix} 0 \\ B_g \end{pmatrix}, C = \begin{pmatrix} C_p & 0 \end{pmatrix}. \end{aligned} \tag{5}$$

Measurement data is usually available at discrete time points, so the continuous model for discrete time intervals t_k can be converted to a discrete dynamic model

$$\begin{aligned} g_{k+1} &= A_d g_k + B_d u_k + q_k \\ y_k &= C g_k + \epsilon_k \end{aligned} \tag{6}$$

with $q_k \sim \mathcal{N}(0, Q_d)$.

2.3 Disturbance prediction

For the estimation of the states of the model and non-modeled disturbances, a Kalman filter and Kalman smoother [5] is integrated. Further, the time-discrete dynamic model in eq. (6) can be used in standard Bayesian state estimation. Classically, this would be solved by using

GP regression, but this has significant limitations in practical implementation [1]. This can be avoided by using the equivalent state-space representation for the GP prior and solving the inference problem with Kalman filtering and smoothing, which enables linear time complexity [6]. In this work the Rauch, Tung, and Striebel smoother (RTS smoother) was used to calculate the estimation and covariance of the GP. It is a stochastic process where the state x is a random variable with a normal distribution of mean m and variance P. The forward filter is executed with the standard forward Kalman filter. For time points $k = 1, \cdots, N$ (where N is the final time) execute [5]:

$$\begin{aligned} \text{Prediction step: } m_k^- &= A_{k-1}m_{k-1}^+ + B_{k-1}u_{k-1} \\ P_k^- &= A_{k-1}P_{k-1}^+A_{k-1}^T + Q_{k-1} \\ \text{Update step: } K_k &= P_k^- H_k^T (H_k P_k^- H_k^T + R_k)^{-1} \\ m_k^+ &= m_k^- + K_k(y_k - H_k m_k^-) \\ P_k^+ &= P_k^- - K_k H_k P_k^- \end{aligned} \quad (7)$$

The variable K corresponds to the Kalman gain, Q is the covariance of the process noise and the matrices A and H are being provided from the discrete model. Subsequently execute the smoothing step for Kalman smoother with $k = N-1, \cdots, 1, 0$ [5]:

$$\begin{aligned} K_k &= P_k^+ A_k^T (A_k P_k^+ A_k^T + Q_k) \\ m_k &= m_k^+ + K_k(m_{k+1} - (A_k m_k^+ + B_k u_k)) \\ P_k &= P_k^+ + K_k(P_{k+1} - (A_k P_k^+ A_k^T - Q_k))K_k^T. \end{aligned} \quad (8)$$

2.4 Control design

In order to determine the input signal for the actuators, to track the given reference a feedforward controller is designed [7]. The feedforward gains can be calculated by solving:

$$\begin{bmatrix} 0 \\ 1 \end{bmatrix} = \begin{bmatrix} A & B \\ C & D \end{bmatrix} \begin{bmatrix} N_x \\ N_u \end{bmatrix} \quad (9)$$

To calculate the inputs from the reference signals, it is possible to calculate a Matrix $\bar{N}$ by eq. (10), given by the solution for N_x and N_u of eq. (9) and the state-feedback gain matrix K.

$$\bar{N} = N_u + KN_x. \quad (10)$$

$\bar{N}$ multiplied by the reference point, gives the System inputs that correspond to a stable point in the state space.
For closing the control loop a linear quadratic regulator (lqr) was implemented for the physical plant model, where the weighting matrices Q_{lqr} and R_{lqr} are chosen to be diagonal matrices to achieve the ideal pressure trajectory given in Fig. 1. Q_{lqr} is a zero matrix, except for the second diagonal entry corresponding to the P_{aw} being 0.0001, and R_{lqr} being the identity matrix.

3 Results and Discussion

In the following, the results of the simulation and estimation of the LFM are presented and discussed.

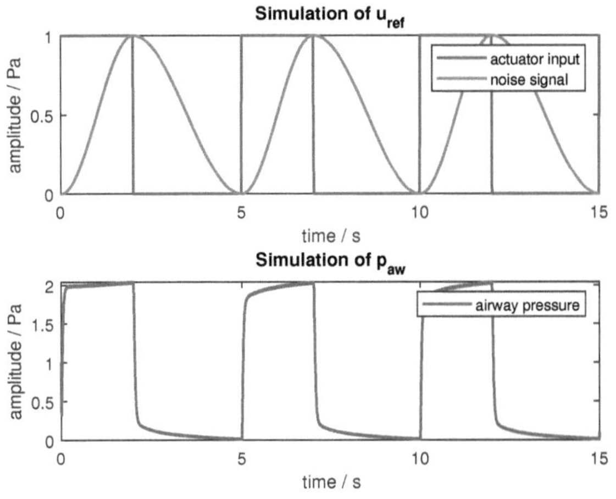

Figure 3: Simulation of the augmented steady-state representation. The reference is a rectpuls signal, while the second input, the spontaneous breathing representing the noise, has a sinusoidal form. The lower plot shows the simulation of the airway pressure.

Combining the existing physical lung model with an equivalent state-space model of a GP representing the unknown latent force, yields an augmented model as introduced in eq. (5). In simulations of this augmented model, a rectpuls signal is chosen as reference signal and a sinusoidal shaped signal as disturbance input, which corresponds to the patient's spontaneous respiration, with an inspiration time of two and an expiration time of three seconds for each breathing cycle. The result of the simulation can be seen in Fig. 3, where the upper plot shows the input signals and the lower plot the simulation of the AP p_{aw}. When comparing the simulation of the AP in Fig. 3 with the expected pressure curve in Fig. 1, they look very similar. It can be concluded that AP simulation provides good results for the inclusion of GP priors as a disturbance input. The simulation of the augmented system is followed by an implementation of a Kalman filter and smoother, as discussed earlier in section 2.3, estimating the systems states and disturbances. Therefore, a discrete-time model is implemented with two rectpuls signals as reference inputs for the blower and PEEP valve, which are derived using the feedforward controller. In Fig. 4 the estimation of the AP is shown. Comparing the result of the estimated AP with the expected and simulated AP, no significant differences occur. To analyze the differences between simulation and estimation more precisely, the states and the latent force p_{mus} were extracted and compared. Fig. 5 shows the results for the simulation and estimation in the top two plots. The calculated difference between those two is shown in the lower plot. Looking at the restoring force pressure p_{el} in the simulation it increases and decreases slower, than in the estimation. The AP (p_{aw}) and expiration pressure (p_{exsp}) only show peaks, when the breathing cycle changes from inspiration to expiration and vice versa. In addition, the differences of the blower pressure and Q_{PEEP} are very small. The estimated signal is very smooth and displays a larger signal variance

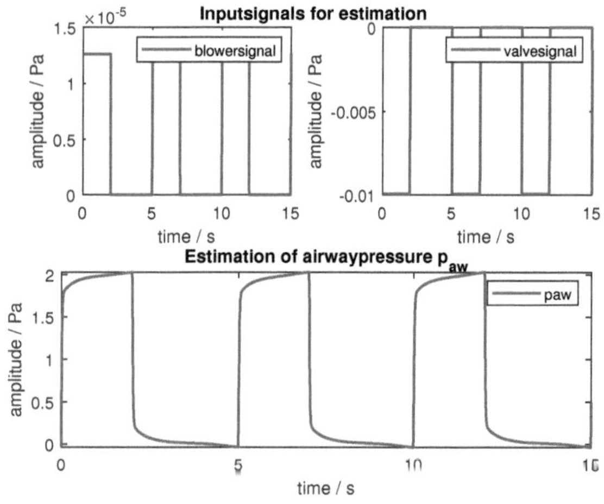

Figure 4: State estimation of the AP (p_{aw}) using Kalman filter and smoother. The top two graphics show the reference signals and the bottom one the result of the AP estimation.

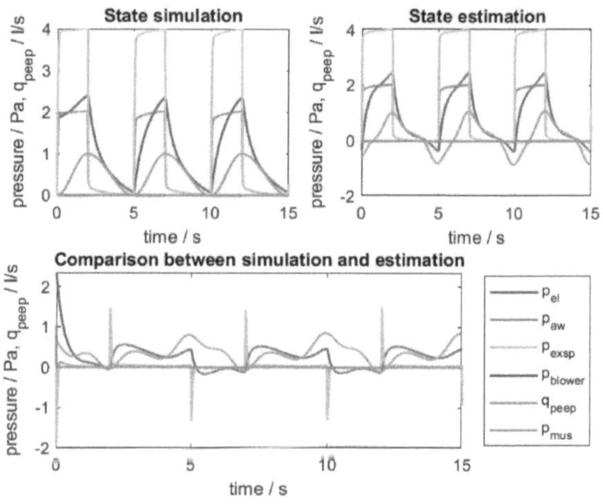

Figure 5: The top two graphics show the states simulation and estimation of the states and the spontaneous breathing p_{mus} as GP. In the bottom graphic a subtraction between those is shown.

then the simulated input. The mismatch between simulated and estimated p_{mus} probably also causes the increased error in the p_{el}, since the latent force directly acts on this system state. These initial results are promising regarding the detection and estimation of patient activity, allowing to adapt the controller accordingly. Thus, increasing the patients safety, e.g., by preventing over extension of the lung.

4 Conclusion

In this paper LFM framework, which augment first-principle (physical) models with non-parametric GP priors as latent force, have been studied. This framework used GPs in an equivalent state-space representation for controlling the pressure of mechanical ventilation and provides the advantage of efficient disturbance prediction by means of Kalman filtering and smoothing methods. Thus, the patient's spontaneous breathing as disturbance could be included, adapting to better pressure control. The LFM method on pressure controlled ventilation is simulated and estimated based on an existing physical lung model. In simulation promising first results have been achieved, even when only including feedforward control as input to the model. The estimation of the states using the Kalman filter showed a good fit for the technical parameters, but a mismatch in the physiological part of the system. Yet the results are promising, such that patient activity can be estimated and with a better tuning satisfyingly estimated. Thus providing useful information to increase the patients safety, e.g. by improving the closed loop control concept.

Acknowledgement

The work has been carried out and supervised by the Institute for Electrical Engineering in Medicine, Universität zu Lübeck and Fraunhofer-Institut für Individualisierte und Zellbasierte Medizintechnik IMTE.

Author's Statement

Conflict of interest: Authors state no conflict of interest.

5 References

[1] J. Grasshoff, G. Männel, H. S. Abbas and P. Rostalski *Model Predictive Control using Efficient Gaussian Process for Unknown Disturbance Inputs.* IEEE 58th Conference on Decision and Control (CDC), Nice, France, 2019, pp. 2708-2713, 2019.

[2] G. Männel, M. Siebert, C. Brendle, and P. Rostalski, *Robust Model Predictive Control of an Anaesthesia Workstation Ventilation Unit, Robuste Modellprädiktive Regelung der Beatmungseinheit eines Anästhesiearbeitsplatzes.* at - Automatisierungstechnik, vol. 68, issue 11, pp. 941–952, October 2020.

[3] J. H. T. Bates, *Lung Mechanics: An Inverse Modeling Approach.* Cambridge: Cambridge University Press., 2009.

[4] S. Säkä, M. A. Álvarez and N. D. Lawrence, *Gaussian Process Latent Force Models for Learning and Stochastic Control of Physical Systems.* IEEE Transactions on Automatic Control, vol. 64, no. 7, pp. 2953-2960, July 2019.

[5] D. Simon, *Optimal State Estimation: Kalman, H_∞, and Nonlinear Approaches.* John Wiley & Sons, 2006.

[6] H. Rauch, F. Tung, and C. Striebel, *Maximum likelihood estimates of linear dynamic systems.* AIAA Journal, 3(8), pp. 1445-1450, August 1965.

[7] B. Messner, D. Tilbury, R. Hill, *Control Tutorials for Matlab and Simulink.* Carnegie Mellon University, University of Michigan, University of Detroit Mercy, 1996.

Continuous delivery to integrate a flow sensor

Cole Saunders [1], Georg Männel [2]

[1] Robotics and Autonomous Systems, Universität zu Lübeck, c.saunders@student.uni-luebeck.de
[2] Institute for Electrical Engineering in Medicine, Universität zu Lübeck, ge.maennel@uni-luebeck.de

Abstract

When developing a controller for a physical system, automation can improve productivity and efficiency. This includes automating the controller deployment, testing and optimization. One approach to process automation is continuous delivery (CD). This paper demonstrates how CD is used to automatically build, deploy and test the controller software on the actual system hardware by developing a CD pipeline using Jenkins. To show its capabilities, the pipeline is used to integrate a sensor into a previously developed controller and hardware. The CD pipeline was successfully built using Jenkins. The sensor communication via controller area network (CAN) bus was integrated into the existing hardware and the measurements from the sensor were successfully integrated into the existing controller. The CD pipeline can be used in further controller optimization and can be adapted for use in other systems and controllers.

1 Introduction

Implementing a controller for a physical system requires time and effort. The system dynamics must be considered, as well as the sensors, other hardware and the closed loop controller for the actuator [1]. To fit a controller to a system, models of the system are commonly used for development. Unfortunately, a model does not contain all the nuances of the physical system since it is not an exact representation of the actual system [1]. Uncertainties in the system, and fluctuations in the actuator and measurements from the sensors, can be modelled well, but never perfectly. For these reasons, a controller for a system should not only be tested on a model, but also on the physical system. This way, the controller can be optimally calibrated to the physical system. Since advanced control techniques has led to the need for digital and software controllers rather than analogue circuits, any changes to the software should optimally result in a test of the control or control loop performance on the system. Testing so often on the physical system cannot be feasibly implemented when done manually. Instead, continuous delivery (CD), in combination with a test environment, can automate the testing process to save time and make the development process easier and more efficient [2].

CD is the automatic building of the changed code, followed by the automatic deployment to a test environment and testing of the code [3]. Throughout this paper, the test environment is an actual system with its hardware. CD is required for the automatic testing of the correct operation of the software on the target hardware after software changes. When the software changes are detected, the changed code can be built, deployed to the hardware and tested by using an automation tool [3], such as Jenkins. Some perceived benefits of using automation, such as CD, are the increase in quality of the product and the increase in efficiency and productivity of the developer [2].

This paper will present the development of a CD pipeline and its benefits. To show the use of CD for system development and prove that the pipeline works, a pipeline will be created for a simple fluid flow system. The CD pipeline will then be used to integrate a new flow sensor into the already built controller.

2 Material and Methods

2.1 Fluid System Setup

The initial fluidic system setup consists of two XMC4800 microcontrollers from Infineon connected over an EtherCAT (ECAT) fieldbus run at 1 ms on a Raspberry Pi. One microcontroller provides a user interface (UI), which enables the input of set values to the system and displays data for the user. The UI-microcontroller sends a set value to the second controller, which controls the actuator, a pump, of the fluidic system. The goal is to implement a control loop for the fluid flow through the system generated by the pump. Therefore, a flow sensor has to be integrated into the system. Fig. 1 shows this system with hardware.

The flow sensor being integrated is an original equipment manufacturer (OEM) system, which measures the flow rate every 500 µs and sends the measurements using a controller area network (CAN) communication protocol every 1 ms. The measurements are averaged over the last 10 samples, ie. the last 5 ms.

The differences between this sensor and the previous sensor, a OEM laboratory device, is the communication interface and the sampling rate. Whereas the previous flow sensor uses universal asynchronous receiver transmitter (UART) communication, the new sensor uses CAN bus communi-

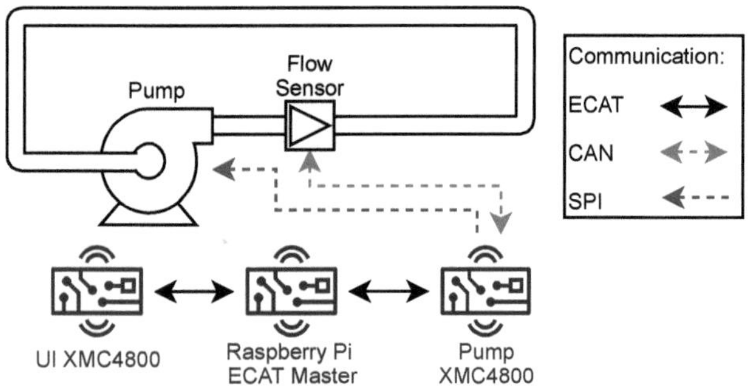

Figure 1: A diagram of the fluid flow system with hardware.

cation. The communication over CAN bus is an improvement, as it allows for the coordination of multiple sensors with the microcontroller much easier than UART communication. The new sensor also has an increased sampling rate of 1 ms, compared to the old sampling rate of 100 ms.
The controller used with the system was already developed and optimized for the old sensor. It is a PI-Controller with an additional feed forward controller. When a set flow rate is given, the feed forward controller will determine the electrical current to be sent to the pump in milliampere. If the measured and set flow rates deviate from one another, the current proportional to the difference will be increased. Likewise, the difference between set and measured flow rate is added every control step and the current is increased proportional to the integrated difference. In this way, the controller should be able to reach the desired flow rate.

2.2 Continuous Delivery via Jenkins

CD is defined as the automated deployment of software to a test environment, where tests are executed [3]. In this paper, the testing system is the hardware of the simple flow system, described in Section 2.1.
To implement CD with the flow system, the source code for the microcontrollers and ECAT master needs to be automatically built and deployed on the respective hardware. The software Jenkins, an automation server with open source code [4], is used to do this. It uses pipelines to automate multiple tasks, such as building, testing and documenting code. A Jenkins pipeline can be automatically started by a new source code commit and will notify users of the results of the pipeline. It also contains an archive, where the pipeline can store files or results. In our CD implementation, the two main tasks are building the source code for the individual modules and deploying the built files onto the corresponding devices for testing. The CD implementation uses two different pipelines to correspond with these tasks.
The first pipeline, the module pipeline in Fig. 2, builds the source code of the different modules used, creates the documentation and stores the resulting built binary files, as hex or executable files, in an artifactory, a repository manager for binary files. The pipeline begins when a source code change is pushed to the source code management (SCM). When a module pipeline is successful, it triggers the second pipeline to start. Each separate module pipeline for

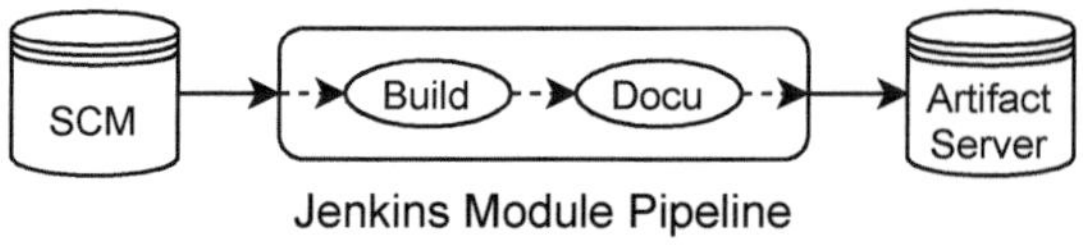

Figure 2: A representation of the module pipeline in Jenkins.

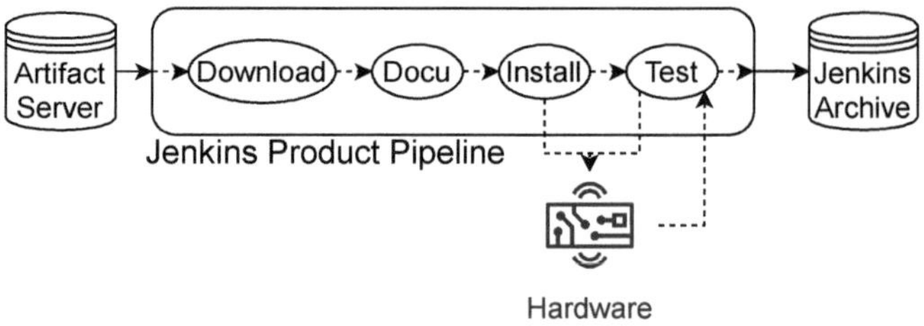

Figure 3: A representation of the product pipeline in Jenkins.

each module will notify the collective second pipeline after a successful execution. The module pipeline is used for the pump control module, the test UI module and the ECAT master module.
The second pipeline, the product pipeline in Fig. 3, retrieves the necessary built binary files and deploys it to the corresponding hardware. The retrieved binary files for this CD implementation are the hex-files for the microcontrollers and the executable for the ECAT master module. After deployment, the pipeline executes any tests that are necessary, and then evaluates the results. The results are also stored in the Jenkins archive to be analyzed further later. The product pipeline can use multiple modules, so it can be triggered by each module pipeline. The product pipeline is shown in more detail in Fig. 4.
The pipelines created in Jenkins are based on the templates supplied by [5]. Hamann [5] already built the connection between the Jenkins server and the hardware to allow the CD pipeline to deploy the executables.
The CD pipeline should also be compared to a manual implementation to show that it is faster and more efficient for the user. The manual implementation will include the following steps of code building, code deployment, system testing and data processing. We will measure the number of manual steps and the duration five times for each implementation, then compare the results.

2.3 Sensor Integration

To show how the CD pipeline can be used, we will integrate the new flow sensor into the fluidic system. The integration of the new sensor occurs in two steps.
Firstly, we must test the communication protocol between the sensor and the microcontroller. For this step, a set electrical current is sent from the test UI to the microcontroller and then to the pump. The set current increases in steps of 2 mA from 4 mA to 20 mA and then decreases back to 4 mA. Each step lasts 10 s. For the communication to be complete, the measured value should show the increasing

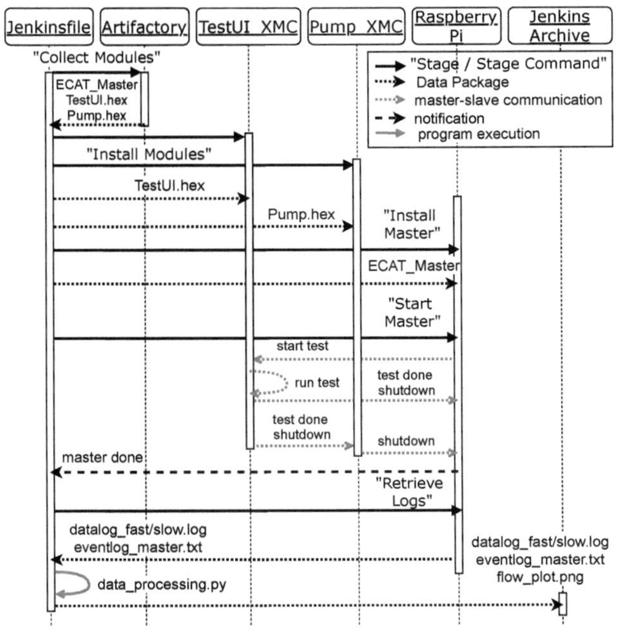

Figure 4: Step by step presentation of the Jenkins product pipeline for testing of the flow system.

and decreasing fluid flow rate corresponding with the increasing and decreasing set current. These measurements must also be sent to the ECAT master to be recorded, otherwise the exact location of any problems in the operation of the software cannot be verified. Proving the functionality of the ECAT master also shows that building and deploying the ECAT master functions correctly on the CD pipeline. This is important for future CD pipelines, since future systems using the CD pipeline will frequently use ECAT communication. If this occurs, the communication protocol has been integrated.

Secondly, we must update the control of the pump to use the measurement values from the new sensor. For this step, a set fluid flow is sent from the test UI to the microcontroller in steps of 250 mL/min from 500 mL/min to 2500 mL/min and then back to 500 mL/min. Each step lasts 10 s. For this test to be successful, the control of the pump does not have to be optimal, but the measured values should approach the set values during the step stage. This would mean that the controller is using the measurement values to update the fluid flow.

3 Results and Discussion

3.1 Continuous Deployment Pipeline

The CD pipeline is set up using the Jenkins server. The duration of the CD pipeline and manual pipeline were both tested. The average results of the duration testing of both implementations are shown in Table 1. The CD pipeline is shorter than the manual implementation by 42 s on average. This is due to the reduced amount of time spent on deploying the code and processing the results of the test. We deployed the code manually via the Dave code generating tool from Infineon, which took longer than the automatic pipeline deployment tool, the J-Link Commander from SEGGER. On the other hand, building and testing the code on the system manually took less time than with the CD pipeline. This is due to the extra steps done in Jenkins. This includes collecting the files from the SCM and notifying the SCM if a build is successful or not; collecting the modules to be deployed from the artifactory; and, triggering the second pipeline when the build was successful. These extra steps did not occur in the manual implementation.

The CD pipeline is not only efficient because it is faster, but also because it requires less manual interaction. As shown in Table 1, the user must perform a total of one manual step for the CD implementation. This is the initial commit of the software changes. In contrast, the user must perform 14 manual steps over the duration of the manual implementation. These steps include manually starting the building, the deployment, the testing and the data processing, as well as manually resetting the microcontrollers and transferring the results of the data from the raspberry pi master. The absence of manual steps in the CD implementation allows the user to efficiently focus on other tasks while the pipeline is running. It also makes the process more convenient for the user. When using the manual implementation, the user always has to be ready to start the next step in the process and cannot focus on other tasks during the process.

3.2 Evaluation of Test Case

The first step of the integration of the sensor was successful. As shown in Fig. 5, the measurements of the flow rate increase at the same point in time as the increase in current sent to the pump. In Fig. 5 and Fig. 6, the ultrafast flow is the measured flow rate averaged over 5 ms, the fast flow over 50 ms and the moderate flow over 500 ms. The timing of the flow rate increase means that the measurements are being sent to and read by the microcontroller. Therefore, the CAN communication is successful.

The second step of the sensor integration was also successful. As shown in Fig. 6, the controller attempts to regulate the flow rate within a step to match the set flow rate. This can be seen especially well between 35 and 75 s. The flow rate decreases or increases over time in the step stages to approach the set flow rate.

4 Conclusion

This paper presents the development of a CD pipeline for the flow system using Jenkins. The pipeline automatically builds the source code into executables when a change has been committed and automatically deploys and tests the code on the hardware. The system tests are automatically executed and results from the test are automatically evaluated. The CD pipeline is faster and more efficient than an equivalent manual implementation of the pipeline processes. It is also easier and more convenient for the user.

The principle function of the CD pipeline is shown by integrating a new sensor in a flow system. The change in the

Table 1: Step Duration for CD vs. Manual Implementation Tests

Step	Continuous Delivery			Manual		
	Average Duration, s	Standard Deviation, s	Manual Steps	Average Duration, s	Standard Deviation, s	Manual Steps
Build Code	86.0	17.7	1	62.2	6.3	1
Deploy Code	20.6	1.9	0	43.8	4.5	4
Test System	191.4	1.4	0	181.0	1.4	1
Data Processing	28.4	4.8	0	81.4	12.7	8
Overall	326.4	16.3	1	368.4	21.0	14

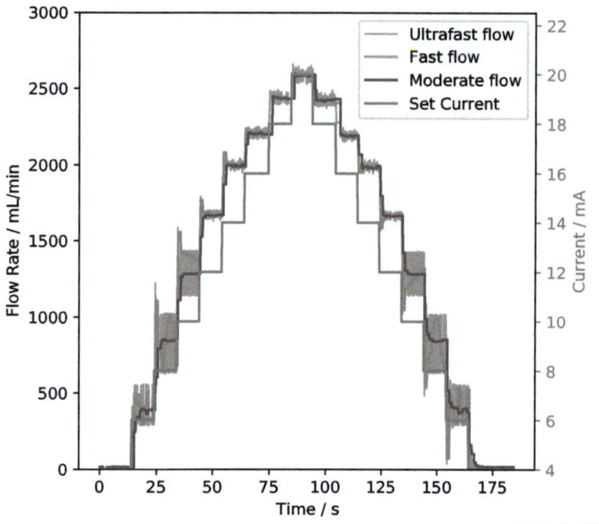

Figure 5: The flow rate measurements and current sent to the pump as a function of time. CAN communication is shown to be successful by the increase and decrease in flow rate corresponding to the increase and decrease in current.

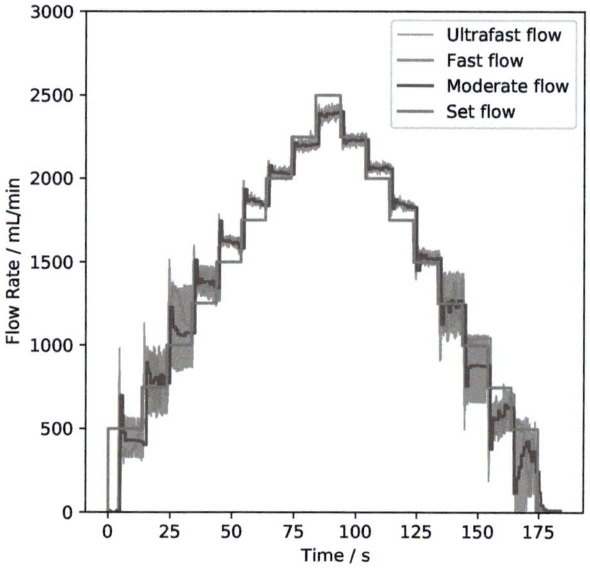

Figure 6: The flow rate measurements and set flow rate as a function of the time. Sensor integration in the controller is shown to be successful by the change in flow rate over time in a single step stage.

sensor communication to CAN bus on the microcontroller is implemented and the sensor measurements are integrated into the existing controller. By using the CD pipeline, the integration was tested. The process was faster and more efficient than using a manual implementation.
Further work on the CD pipeline and the sensor integration can be done. The data processing for the CD pipeline can still be improved and expanded by automatically evaluating the controller properties. Also, the controller for the flow system can also be further optimized with regards to the new sensor.

Acknowledgement

The work has been carried out at Dräger AG & Co. KGaA, Lübeck and supervised by Prof. P. Rostalski, Institute for Electrical Engineering in Medicine, Universität zu Lübeck.

Author's Statement

Conflict of interest: Authors state no conflict of interest.

5 References

[1] J. van Amerongen and P. Breedveld, *Modelling of physical systems for the design and control of mechatronic systems*. Annual Reviews in Control, vol. 27, no. 1, pp. 87–117, 2003.

[2] L. Chen, *Continuous Delivery: Huge Benefits, but Challenges Too*. IEEE Software, vol. 32, no. 2, pp.50-54, 2015.

[3] Atlassian, *Continuous integration vs. continuous delivery vs. continuous deployment*. Available: https://www.atlassian.com/continuous-delivery/principles/continuous-integration-vs-delivery-vs-deployment [last accessed on 2021-01-07]

[4] Jenkins, *Jenkins User Documentation*. Available: https://www.jenkins.io/doc/ [last accessed on 2021-01-05].

[5] P. J. Hamann, *Continuous Deployment for a medical device demonstrator of intelligent modules*. Bachelorthesis, Hamburg University of Applied Sciences, 2020.

Designing a Disposable and Magnetically Suspended Centrifugal Pump

Noah Radtke [1]
[1] Biomedical Engineering, Luebeck University of Applied Sciences, noah.radtke@stud.th-luebeck.de

Abstract

A centrifugal pump is used to supply energy to the fluid in order to increase the pressure. The energy transmission is done indirectly by increasing the pressure of the fluid by obtaining the energy from the runner of the pump. In medicine, centrifugal pumps are gaining importance because of their compact and simple build-up. Thus, it is predetermined to be used as a disposable turbo machine inside a hygienic treatment. Moreover, the presented design bases on predefined requirements. This article will focus on the calculation of the pump to check the feasibility of a magnetically suspended centrifugal pump. During the calculation, the focus will also lie on finding the optimal blade design in order to get the best streamflow. In the end, the calculation of the disposable pump proves theoretical feasibility, since the pump can generate a volume flow rate of 5 l/min at 120 mmHg.

1 Introduction

The group of centrifugal pumps consists of four types: axial pump, radial pump, diagonal pump, and side-channel pump. This study will focus on the radial-pump where the working principle is summarized by a few steps. The fluid enters the impeller at the center, is then accelerated due to the spinning of the blades, and is pushed by centrifugal forces to the outlet at the blade tips. At the moment, displacement pumps are frequently used in medicine. Here, the fluid is transported by squeezing the peristaltic pump tubing between the pump head rollers and the tubing bed. This squeezing can be problematic for delicate fluids. Due to this compact and simple build-up, centrifugal pumps are suitable for the described use if some problems are handled. A major problem is the heat transmission of the pump to the fluid. An approach to solve this problem is to construct a contactless centrifugal pump. Using the magnetic levitation principle to provide a bearingless system not only reduces the problem of heat transmission but also supports the hygienic design tremendously [2], [3], [4], [6]. The following calculation uses the equations from the book [1] of Klaus Menny to develop the pump dimensions.

2 Material and Methods

2.1 Mathematical Model

The parameters for the calculation are a flow rate of 5 l/min, a pressure of 120 mmHg, a fluid density of 1060 kg/m³ and a rotational speed of 3000 rpm [2], [5]. Moreover, a safety factor of 3 is defined to provide some buffer which sets the demanded volume flow rate to 15 l/min and fluid pressure to 360 mmHg.
"H" is the pump head which is defined by the quotient of pressure, the gravitational constant, and the fluid density (1)[1].

$$H = \frac{p}{g\varrho} \tag{1}$$

With (2) [1] the type of runner is discerned using the defined rotational speed and volume flow rate. Here the type number σ is defined by:

$$\sigma = \frac{2n\sqrt{\pi\dot{V}}}{(2gH)^{3/4}} = 0.096 \tag{2}$$

The book [1] sets a good range for single bent vanes at $\sigma = 0.08$ and the spatially curved vanes at $\sigma = 0.16$. Thus, the single bent vanes are selected because the σ is the closest to the calculated result. The Cordier diagram is used to design the pump because it displays the relation between the specific revolutions δ and the specific diameter δ for highly efficient turbomachinery. Hence from Fig.1 a) the ratio b_2/D_{2a} is determined.
In Fig.1 b) a sketch of the runner cross-section with the variables is presented.
In order to obtain b_2, D_{2a} is computed by (3) [1] and the rounded result of this is $D_2 = 0.05m$.

$$D_{2a} = \frac{2\delta}{\sqrt{\pi}} \sqrt[4]{\frac{\dot{V}^2}{2gH}} \tag{3}$$

Based on the impeller dimensions including b_1,b_2, D_1 and D_2 the rest of the pump dimensions are adjusted, regarding the volute casing and the blade size.

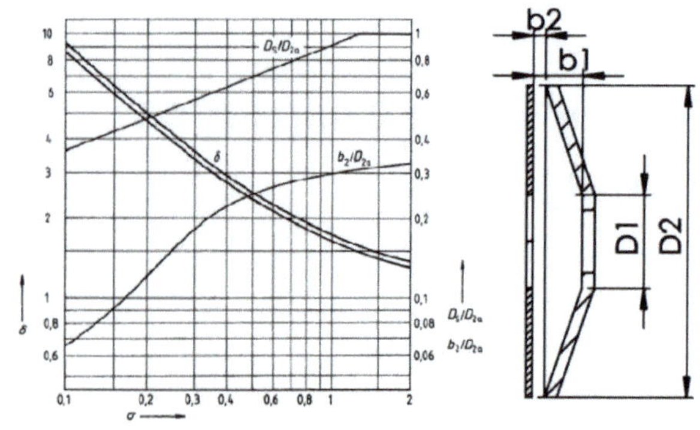

Figure 1: a) Cordier-Diagram b) Impeller

2.2 Optimized Vane Shape

The specific blade work "Y" of a turbomachine is defined by the Euler formula (4)[1].

$$Y = (u_1 c_{1u} - u_2 c_{2u}) \approx 45m^2/s^2 \quad (4)$$

The movement of the fluid particles inside the runner is distinguished between absolute "c",circumferential "u" and relative stream velocity "w". Thus, the absolute velocity is described by an outer observer seeing the spinning runner and the movement of the streamflow particles from the inlet to the outlet. The same perspective is used to characterize the circumferential speed where a certain point on the blade of the rotating runner moves with a certain velocity. Contrary to that, is the definition of the relative velocity where the observer theoretically rests inside the blade channel and regards the in- and outflow. In calculation, the relative and absolute velocity is divided into components parallel and vertical to the circumferential speed. In doing so, the parallel component is described by the circumferential index "u" and the vertical component by meridian index "m". Hence, u_1 and u_2 describe the circumferential speed of the inner and outer diameter and c_1u and c_2u the absolute velocity parallel to the circumferential speed. To determine the optimal shape of the blade, the inflow and outflow angle β_1 and β_2 of the bend vanes are calculated by iteration with (5) and (6)[1].

$$\beta_1 = arctan\left(\frac{c_1}{-u_1}\right) + 180° = 153° \quad (5)$$

$$\beta_2 = arctan\left(\frac{c_{2m}}{c_{2u} - u_2}\right) + 180° = 122° \quad (6)$$

To obtain the mean lines of the circular arc of the blade, the radius in (7) and the eccentricity in (8) are computed [1]. Here "R" represents the diameter of the circle forming the shape of the bent blade.

$$R = \frac{D_2^2 - D_1^2}{4(D_1 cos\beta_1 - D_2 cos\beta_2)} \quad (7)$$

$$e = \sqrt{\frac{D_2^2}{4} + R^2 + D_2 R cos\beta_2} \quad (8)$$

2.3 Magnetic Levitation

To reduce heat transmission from the pump to the fluid and provide a hygienic and disposable design, a contactless magnetic bearing is chosen. The pump is passively levitated by permanent magnets which are included in the bottom of the impeller as can be seen in Fig.7. Furthermore, to center and drive the pump, electric coils are included in the brushless DC motor which change their magnetic field strength dynamically. Thus, the rotation of the rotor is generated by the impeller following the dynamic magnetic field of the stator. In this study, a gap of 0.3 mm between the pump casing and the vane tips is assumed [2], [3], [4], [5]. Additionally, distance sensors are used to control the clearance. In case the air gap becomes smaller or bigger, the control system changes the strength of the specific coil to keep a gap of 0.3mm. When inserting the pump head into the driving part, the pump head snaps into the driver and is fixed due to the magnetic force of the permanent magnets. To decouple and dispose the pump the attraction force of the magnets has to be surpassed. In Fig. 2 a cross-section of the electric drive is demonstrated. The rotor holds 6 permanent, which are put together into 3 pole pairs. Likewise, the stator has 3 coil pairs which are combined into 9 slots. Changing the magnetic field forces the permanent magnets in the rotor to follow the dynamic magnetic field of the coils and thus generates the rotor spin.

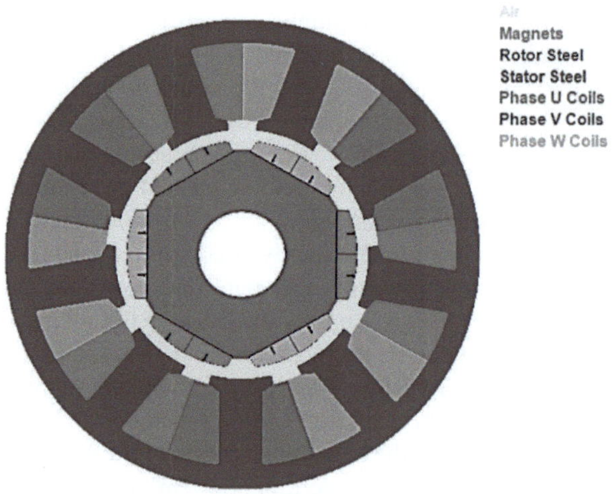

Figure 2: Cross-section of the driver illustrates the 6 magnets of the stator and 9 slots of the rotor and was created in smartFEM. The area between the magnets and the slots shows the air in between

2.4 Theoretical pump curve

Generally, the specific pump head of a centrifugal pump is distinctively dependent on the volume flow at a constant rotational speed. Besides, the characteristic pump curve can be only correctly obtained by experiments. Nevertheless, the theoretical pump curve helps to understand the working principle of the centrifugal pump. The characteristic curve is estimated by the assumption of a blade congruent flow and subtracting the losses from it. Hence, the loss-free and blade congruent flow is defined by

$$Y_{th} = u_2^2 + \frac{\dot{V}}{\dot{V}_N} \frac{u_2 w_{2mN}}{tan\beta_{2\infty}} / (1+p) \tag{9}$$

Besides that, the index "N" describes the values the calculation was run with. In other words, $\dot{V}$ can be changed and $\dot{V}_N$ stays 15 l/min. Here "p" represents the correction factor which is set to 0.3 and $tan\beta_{2\infty}$ the outflow angle of the streamflow in case of an infinite number of blades. To obtain the theoretical pump curve the impact loss (10) and the friction loss (12) are subtracted from (9)[1]. In [1] the hydraulic efficiency η_h=0.82 is used to calculate the losses of a radial pump. Thus, η_h is assumed to be 0.8 here.

$$\Delta_{lossfric} = (1-\eta_{hN})\, Y_{th}\, (1+p) \left(\frac{\dot{V}}{\dot{V}_N}\right)^2 \tag{10}$$

$$\Delta_{lossimp} = \left(\frac{0.25}{0.35}\right) \left[u_1^2 + \left(\frac{u_2}{1+p}\frac{D_2}{D_4}\right)^2\right] \left(\frac{\dot{V}_N - \dot{V}}{\dot{V}_N}\right)^2 \tag{11}$$

3 Results

Velocity Triangles represent the kinematic movement of vectors. Usually, the inflow for centrifugal pumps is swirl-free. Based on the velocities from section 2.2 a right-angled triangle is formed for the inflow as shown in Fig. 3. The velocity triangle for the outflow is displayed in Fig. 4. In the outflow, the relative velocity part is in comparison to the absolute velocity small because at the tip of the blade the absolute velocity plays the major role. Comparing these triangles to other velocity triangles from applied pumps, many similarities are shown. The angles and velocities are in the range of pumps with similar parameters.

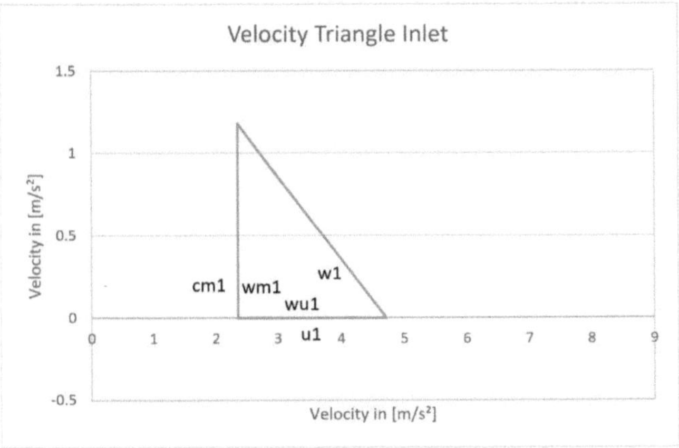

Figure 3: Velocity triangles for the inlet of the pump

In Fig. 5 the theoretical pump curve is displayed. This volume-flow-pressure diagram presents the six assumed pump curves, in the range of 500 rpm to 3000 rpm. They are

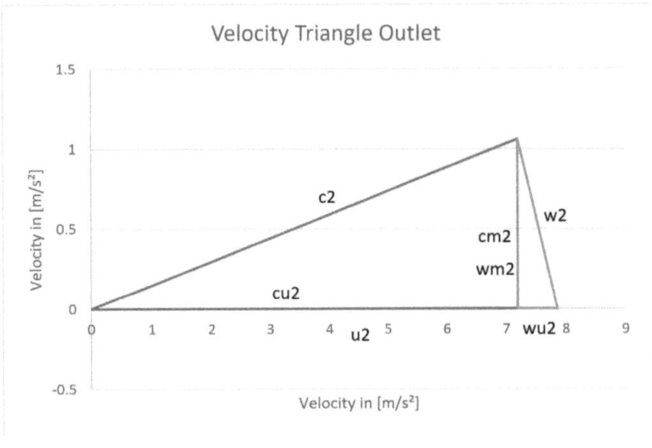

Figure 4: Velocity triangle for the outlet of the pump

obtained by changing the rotational speed at constant volume flow in equations (9), (10), and (12). On the x-axis, the volume flow rate in l/min, and on the y-axis, the pressure in mmHg is displayed. Given the diagram, the total pressure range of the pump is from 0 to around 400 mmHg. In the interest of the given parameters, the diagram has the volume flow rate range of 0 to 15 l/min. In the low RPM region of the grey curve representing the calculation with 500 rpm and the yellow curve of 1000 rpm, the functions are relatively straight. The higher the rotational speed is the bigger the slope becomes. For the demanded volume flow rate of 5 l/min, the pressure range lies between 25 mmHg and 355 mmHg. Considering the diagram, the pump can generate a maximum rotational speed of 3000 rpm, a volume flow of 15 l/min at around 175 mmHg.

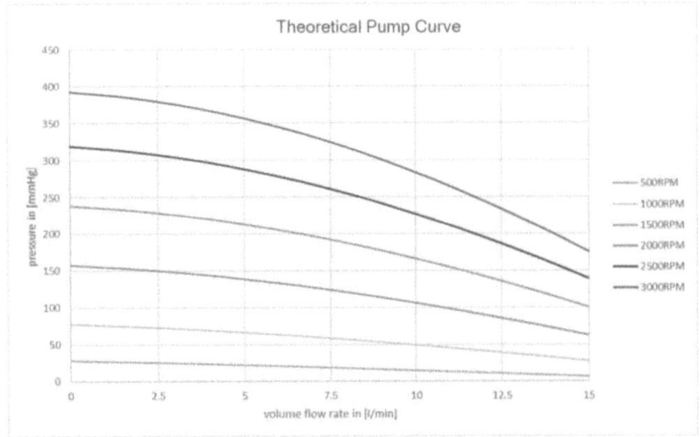

Figure 5: Volume-flow-Pressure-Diagram showing six curves in the range of 500RPM to 3000RPM

Besides that, using the principle of angular momentum the torque is defined by

$$M = \frac{\dot{V}}{\varrho}(c_{u2}r_2 - c_{u1}r_1) \approx 0.05\ Nm \tag{12}$$

and gives the result of around M=0.05 Nm. The loss-free power output is obtained by the multiplication of the torque and the angular velocity:

$$P = \omega M \approx 15\,W. \tag{13}$$

Based on these calculations a 3D-CAD-model is developed as laid out in Fig. 6 and Fig.7. In Fig. 6 the top view shows the five blades and the volute casing. Fig. 7 delineates the air clearance and the magnetic part on the bottom of the impeller.

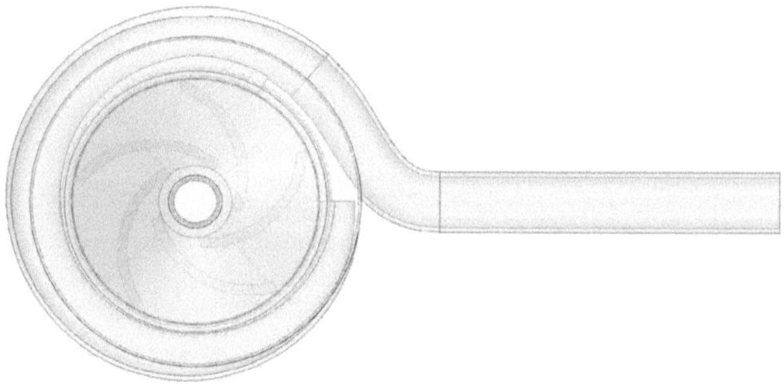

Figure 6: Top view of the 3D-model

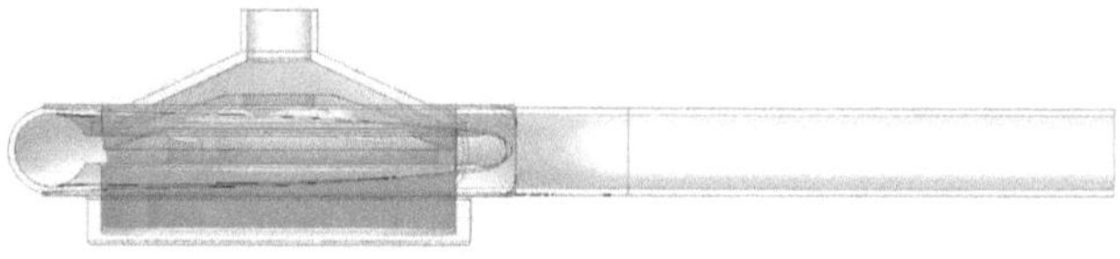

Figure 7: Side view of the 3D-model

Comparing the outcome of (12) and (13)[1] to the studies [2], [3] and [6] shows that the obtained results are realistic and feasible.

4 Conclusion

The calculation results prove the feasibility of a disposable centrifugal pump at a volume flow rate of 5 l/min and a pressure of 120 mmHg. Furthermore, the developed design provides the desired volume flow rate and pressure at a minimal dimensional size compared to the size and weight of displacement pumps. Owing to Fig.5 the assumption is made that between 1500 RPM and 2000RPM a volume flow rate of 5 l/min at a pressure of 120 mmHg can be provided. Other than that, the pump can provide a maximum volume flow rate of 15 l/min exceeding the desired pressure of 120 mmHg. Besides, the diagram shows the limits of the theoretic pump curves. Looking into this diagram shows that all the lines touch the x-axis at a volume flow rate bigger than 15 l/min. In real-life experiments, it is expected that the low RPM curves will not reach the volume flow of 15 l/min. In reality, it is expected that the lower curves will not reach a volume flow rate of 15 l/min in the functional system, as more losses are prevailing there. The realized 3D-CAD-model exposes the results of the calculation. In the next step, the 3D-model is simulated in CFD. A major focus will lie on the streamflow at the blades as well as the pressure and velocity distribution. The pump will be simulated with different rotational speeds of the impeller and distinct volume flow rates similar to [7]. With these results, the pump design will be refined regarding the blades. Subsequently, a prototype will be 3D-printed to do experiments and determine the correct characteristic pump curve.

5 Acknowledgement

The work has been carried out at the Drägerwerk AG Co. KGaA in Lübeck, Moislinger Allee 53 – 55, and supervised by the Technische Hochschule Lübeck.

6 Author's Statement

Conflict of interest: Authors state no conflict of interest.

7 References

[1] Strömungsmaschinen. (2006). Teubner. https://doi.org/10.1007/978-3-8351-9035-1

[2] Hoshi, H., Katakoa, K., Ohuchi, K., Asama, J., Shinshi, T., Shimokohbe, A., Takatani, S. (2005). Magnetically Suspended Centrifugal Blood Pump With a Radial Magnetic Driver. ASAIO Journal, 51(1).

[3] Püntener, P., Schuck, M., Kolar, J. (2020). The Influence of Impeller Geometries on Hemolysis in Bearingless Centrifugal Pumps. IEEE Open Journal of Engineering in Medicine and Biology, PP, 1. https://doi.org/10.1109/OJEMB.2020.3037507

[4] Akamatsu, T., Tsukiya, T. (1998). Development of a centrifugal blood pump with magnetically suspended impeller and the related fluid mechanical problems. Sadhana, 23(5), 597–603. https://doi.org/10.1007/BF02744582

[5] Chernyavskii, A. Medvedev, Alexey Prikhod'ko, Yu Fomin, V. Vladislav, Fomichev Fomichev, A. Lomanovich, K. Ruzmatov, T. Karaskov, A.. (2017). Flow-Rate–Pressure Characteristics of a Disk Blood Pump. Journal of Engineering Physics and Thermophysics. 90. 10.1007/s10891-017-1708-5.

[6] Chun, S., Jin, J. (2012). Output power measurement of a blood pump considering pulsating flows. Journal of Mechanical Science and Technology, 26(3), 793–798. https://doi.org/10.1007/s12206-011-1239-5

[7] Malinauskas, R. A., Hariharan, P., Day, S. W., Herbertson, L. H., Buesen, M., Steinseifer, U., Aycock, K. I., Good, B. C., Deutsch, S., Manning, K. B., Craven, B. A. (2017). FDA Benchmark Medical Device Flow Models for CFD Validation. ASAIO Journal, 63(2).

Finger blood pressure measurement – Development of a finger cuff prototype –

Raffaela Wegner [1], Heidi Fröhlich [2], Ulrich Timm [2], Bernd Lindner [2], and Ksenija Gräfe [3]

[1] Medical Engineering Science, Universität zu Lübeck, raffaela.wegner@student.uni-luebeck.de
[2] Bluepiont Medical, {h.froehlich, u.timm, b.lindner}@bluepoint-medical.com
[3] Institute of Medical Engineering, Universität zu Lübeck, graefe@imt.uni-luebeck.de

Abstract

Due to the demographic change, it is becoming increasingly difficult to maintain good medical care for the elderly, especially in rural areas. Medical support for this patient group is often further complicated by immobility and the absence of other household members that can support the daily medical routine. Especially in this target group, it is important to check the blood pressure (BP) regularly in order to detect and monitor existing diseases at an early stage. The existing BP monitors with upper arm cuffs are uncomfortable and difficult to use with one hand. To address these shortcomings, bluepoint Medical is developing a new finger BP monitor. A novel finger cuff was constructed and evaluated. It was shown that this method combines accurate and reliable BP measurement with promising user-friendliness and simplicity.

1 Introduction

Poor medical care in rural areas, especially for the elderly, is a major problem. Regular monitoring of vital parameters, such as the BP, is particularly difficult in this patient group. More than half of the over-60s in Germany suffer from hypertension [1]. During the last decade, scientists have emphasized that innovative solutions must be developed to monitor the BP conveniently from home [2]. Stress and anxiety of patients could be reduced, by facilitating easy and regular monitoring of vital parameters into the daily life [3]. Currently, the most popular non-invasive BP monitoring devices use an upper arm cuff. When using upper arm cuffs, changes in the compliance of the main arteries can lead to a pulse time delay [4], or venous compression [5]. Also, a larger bone-to-volume ratio compared to the finger may result in lower pressure transmission efficiency [6]. Ease of use suffers from the difficulty of applying the cuff correctly and finding the right position, as well as from the bulky size of the cuff [6]. Therefore, laypersons often have problems applying the device to the upper arm [7], necessitating a second person to apply the cuff. The aim of the project was to develop a small and handy finger cuff for the finger phalanx proximalis (FP) for BP measurement that meets all medical requirements, such as accurate measurement values, short measurement duration, comfortable to wear, easy and quick to use, and user-friendly for our target group. Since the vessels and the surrounding tissue of the index finger vary at the level of the phalanx proximalis compared to the upper arm, the accuracy and reliability of the oscillometric BP measurement method at this position must be evaluated. In this project, the feasibility of measuring BP at the FP was examined. Based on the results, a prototype cuff for the finger was developed to improve and optimize the application and handling of the BP cuff.

2 Material and Methods

2.1 Oscillometric BP Monitor

The oscillometric BP monitor applies a cuff to pressurize the finger by inflating and deflating the cuff. The cuff pressure and the pressure oscillation caused by arterial pulsation in the tissue are recorded by a pressure sensor connected to the cuff. The sequence of the oscillometric measurement is shown in Fig. 1. When the cuff is inflated or deflated, the cuff pressure is transmitted to the arterial wall via in our case the finger tissue and exerts extravascular pressure on the arterial wall. The amplitude of the blood volume pulsation changes with the varying transmural pressure regulated by the cuff. The changes in blood volume are transmitted back to modify the cuff volume and cause cuff pressure variations in heart rate. When the artery is not under transmural pressure and is at its greatest compliance, blood volume pulsation reaches its maximum. Assuming that the extravascular pressure is equal to the cuff pressure, it was found that the cuff pressure corresponding to the maximum cuff pressure oscillation is equal to the mean blood pressure (MBP). It should be noted that systolic blood pressure (SBP) and diastolic blood pressure (DBP) are traditionally determined empirically using specific portions of the maximal oscillation amplitude [6]. The point during the deflation phase at which pulsations recover is equal to SBP. A cuff pressure between DBP and SBP results in a narrowing of

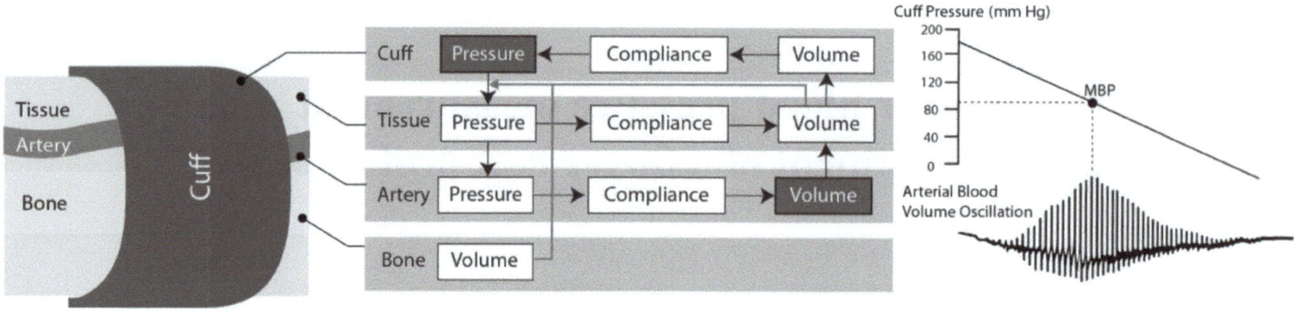

Figure 1: Work principle and chain of event of the oscillometric blood pressure measurement with cuff. The gray shaded boxes for arterial volume and cuff pressure represent the sources of oscillation and the resulting oscillation for observation, respectively. The red lines indicate that pressure transmission from the cuff to the tissue is affected by tissue and bone volume. Taken from [6]

the artery under the cuff when the arterial blood pressure is less than the cuff pressure. When arterial BP is greater than cuff pressure, blood can flow through the artery [4]. One way to calculate MBP is usually with the standard formula:

$$MBP = DBP + 1/3(SBP - DBP)[8]. \quad (1)$$

The key factor which affects measurement accuracy of the oscillometric BP measurement method is the efficiency of pressure transmission from the cuff to the artery. When performing oscillometric blood pressure measurements on the finger, the influence of specific physiological body structures, for example, the tissue and the ratio of bone-to-volume, have to be taken into account by the efficiency of pressure transmission [6].

2.2 Protocol

A female subject aged 22 years, with no known cardiovascular abnormalities, was recruited for the experiment. During the experiment, the subject was in a sitting position without speaking or making excessive body movements, with her hand resting on a table. Eleven consecutive measurements were taken over a period of 20 min, using oscillometric BP module (NIBP2020 UP, PAR Medizintechnik GmbH & Co. KG with accuracy specification $\pm$ 3 mmHg or 3 % of the measurement value, whichever is greater and a disposable neonatal cuff (prototype 1). Measurement is performed in neonatal mode (measurement range of the NIBP module: systolic pressure 20 to 150 mmHg; diastolic pressure 10 to 130 mmHg) The neonatal cuff was wrapped around the middle finger. The results are presented in Fig. 3. One oscillometric measurement lasted for two minutes. There was a pause of five seconds between each measurement. Subsequently, the measurement accuracy was tested using a calibrated patient simulator (ProSim 8, Fluke). A neonatal BP cuff (prototype 1) was wrapped around the Fluke finger phantom, previously specified systoles and diastoles were simulated. Ten measurements were performed per specified value. In total, a measurement range of 35 to 150 mmHg as systole and 15 to 110 mmHg as diastole was tested. There was a pause interval of five seconds between each measurement. The results are presented in Fig. 4.

2.3 Construction finger cuff prototype 2

Based on the results of the measurement with prototype 1, a finger cuff (prototype 2) was developed. It consists of an elliptic solid outer metal ellipsoidal ring with dimensions of 33 x 30 mm. The flexible inner silicone ring is divided into eight compartments, which can be filled with air and expanded towards the center. Since the outer cuff ring is rigid, the silicone membrane of the inner cuff ring can apply sufficient pressure to the tissue. As shown in Fig. 2, only the inner silicone ring comes into contact with the skin. The pressure inside the cuff can be recorded at any time during BP measurement. A flexible tube is attached to the outside of the ring cuff where an air pump and the electropneumatic transducer can be connected. The pressure in the cuff can be controlled by applying and removing air.

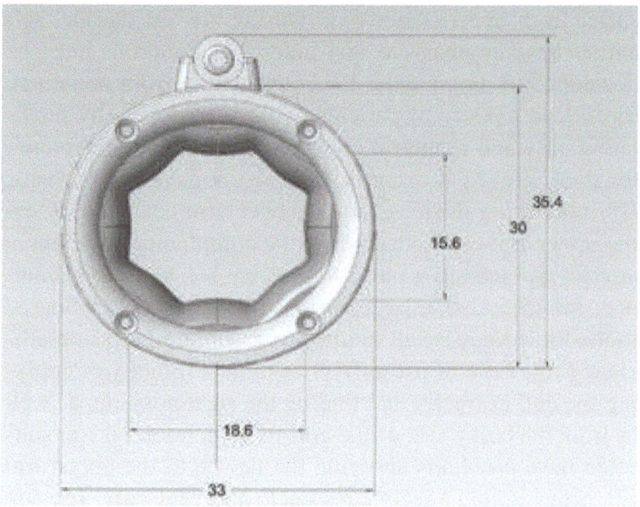

Figure 2: Prototype 2 with dimensions in mm

3 Results

All measurement results were captured with prototype 1. Stable measurement results were obtained during the continuous sampling measurement on the finger over a period of 20 min (see Fig. 3 and Tab. 1).

Table 1: Feasibility test

Value	Mean /mmHg	Standard Deviation /mmHg
Systole	121,64	7,26
Diastole	73,36	4,20

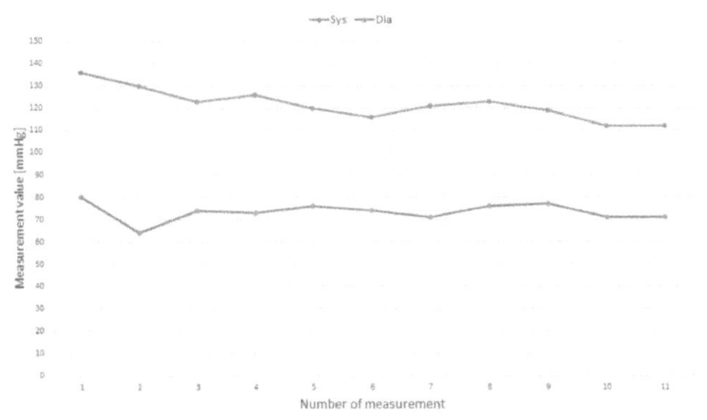

Figure 3: Blood pressure measurement on the human finger. Using a neonatal cuff (prototype 1) with an oscillometric blood pressure module (NIBP OEM module S757, PAR Medizintechnik GmbH & Co. KG), systolic and diastolic blood pressure was measured eleven times on the human middle finger.

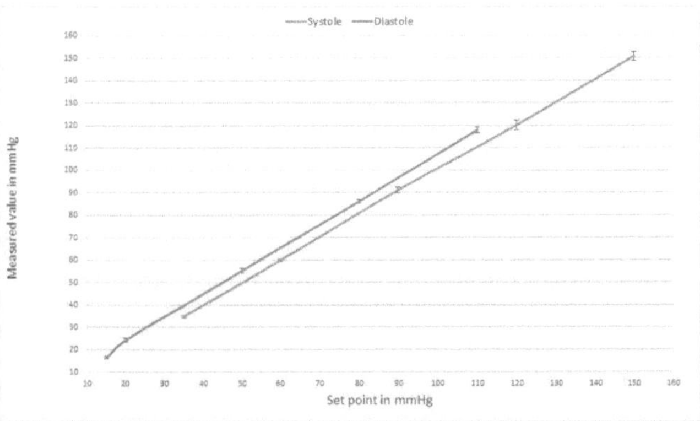

Figure 4: The measured value of systole plotted against the set value of systole of the ProSim 8 patient simulator with standard deviation.

Fig. 4 and Fig. 5 present the results of the calibration measurement with the ProSim 8 patient simulator. The deviation between systolic set point and systolic mean measurement value is less than 1 mmHg. Relevant deviations were not observed; the standard deviation is less than 2,2 mmHg. All systolic results are within the specification of the oscillometric BP module specification ($\pm$ 3 mmHg or 3 %, whichever is greater). In case of the diastolic measurement, the results are not in specification of the oscillometric BP module. A positive offset is found with largest deviation in the higher range of the scale. The maximal deviation between set point and mean value is 8 mmHg. The standard deviation however is small (below 1,4 mmHg) and the values are therefore comparatively constant.

4 Discussion

The aim of the project was to test the feasibility, accuracy and reliability of oscillometric finger BP measurement. Consistent with the literature [6, 9], this study demonstrated that BP measurements on the finger can be performed reliably and without discomfort for the subject. During the first experiment using prototype 1, a few problems were noticed, such as wear of the fastener, material used deteriorated over time, position slipped and neighbouring fingers could exert pressure on the cuff and falsify the values. All this necessitated the development of a finger-customized prototype (prototype 2). Especially elderly people often find it difficult to suppress movements of the fingers during the measurement. A rigid outer ring is required for a finger cuff to avoid falsification of the measured values due to pressure exerted by other fingers. The ring shape has the advantage that the cuff can be easily applied on the finger and only one hand is needed, unlike cuff types that work with velcro. Compartmentalization of the inner silicone ring allows an optimal fit for the finger without the formation of cavities or bruises. The assumption was made that especially for elderly people, it is easier to apply a ring over the finger correctly, compared to attaching to the FD, which can slip. The reason for the offset in the diastolic measurement, see Fig. 5, requires further investigation. The current BP module was developed and calibrated for upper arm measurement. The offset found can be corrected by adjusting the algorithms and calibration to the sensor signal for finger measurement. Liu et al. [6] and Lee et al. [9] provides possible approaches to this task.

5 Conclusion

This work confirms previous studies (see [6] and [9]) that the oscillometric MBP measurements at the finger (FP) is possible. It has been found, that the presented prototype 2 provides optimal user comfort, which is advantageous for home care applications. According to the experimental results, measurement at FP is an optimal alternative to oscillometric BP measurement at the upper arm. Moreover, oscillometric BP measurement at the FP makes miniaturization of the device easier, as a smaller cuff size is used compared to devices for other extremities. Further development of the oscillometric finger BP cuffs through software optimization and implementation of measurement and calibration parameters, such as tissue-to-bone ratio, is a promising approach to correct the offset in diastolic measurement. In addition, conditions that may negatively affect accuracy must be analyzed and taken into account during calibration (e.g. low perfusion, different finger diameters). For this, more measurements are required which consider a larger number of subjects with different finger parameters. In addition, the cuff geometry and materials used may be opti-

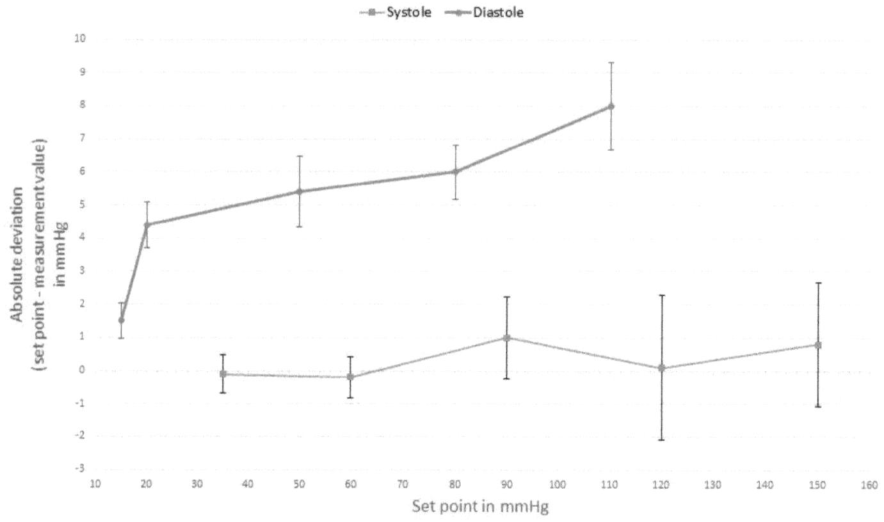

Figure 5: The absolute deviation from the systolic and diastolic set point versus the systolic and diastolic set point of the ProSim 8 patient simulator plotted with standard deviation.

mized for different finger types and user groups for optimal use in a home care environment.

Acknowledgement

The work has been carried out at bluepoint MEDICAL GmbH & Co. KG, Selmsdorf and supervised by the Institute of Medical Engineering, Universität zu Lübeck. At this point I would like to thank everyone who supported and motivated me in the preparation of this paper. Special thanks goes to the management 'bluepoint MEDICAL GmbH & Co. KG', Mr. Bernd Lindner, for the constructive ideas and discussions, the financial support/ provision of all materials and making the internship possible and to PAR Medizintechnik GmbH & Co. KG for providing the blood pressure modules.

Author's Statement

Conflict of interest: Authors state no conflict of interest.

6 References

[1] H. Neuhauser, M. Thamm, and U. Ellert, "Blood pressure in germany 2008-2011," *Bundesgesundheitsblatt - Gesundheitsforschung - Gesundheitsschutz*, 2013.

[2] A. C. Ilie, A. I. Pîslaru, I. Crăcană, R. Ştefăniu, and I. Dana Alexa, "Home blood pressure monitoring — one step towards reducing defensive medicine," *2015 E-Health and Bioengineering Conference (EHB)*, pp. 1–4, 2015.

[3] X. He, R. A. Goubran, and X. P. Liu, "Evaluation of the correlation between blood pressure and pulse transit time," *2013 IEEE International Symposium on Medical Measurements and Applications (MeMeA)*, pp. 17–20, 2013.

[4] M. Nitzan, C. Rosenfeld, A. Weiss, E. Grossman, A. Patron, and A. Murray, "Effects of external pressure on arteries distal to the cuff during sphygmomanometry," *IEEE Transactions on Biomedical Engineering*, pp. 1120–1127, 2005.

[5] Y. Song, S. Gao, A. Ikarashi, and K. Yamakoshi, "A new cuff unit for measuring instantaneous blood pressure at the finger artery by local pressurization," *2009 3rd International Conference on Bioinformatics and Biomedical Engineering*, pp. 1–4, 2009.

[6] J. Liu, C. G. Sodini, Y. Ou, B. Yan, Y. T. Zhang, and N. Zhao, "Feasibility of fingertip oscillometric blood pressure measurement: Model-based analysis and experimental validation," *IEEE Journal of Biomedical and Health Informatics*, pp. 533–542, 2020.

[7] E. Bresch, L. Schmitt, D. De Matteis, and J. Muehlsteff, "Cuff-pressure induced pat changes — modelling and experimental verification towards calibration of blood pressure surrogates," *2016 38th Annual International Conference of the IEEE Engineering in Medicine and Biology Society (EMBC)*, pp. 4252–4255, 2016.

[8] G. Sainas, R. Milia, G. Palazzolo, G. Ibba, E. Marongiu, S. Roberto, V. Pinna, G. Ghiani, F. Tocco, and A. Crisafulli, "Mean blood pressure assessment during post-exercise: Result from two different methods of calculation," *J Sports Sci Med*, p. 4974855, 2016.

[9] J. Y. Lee, E. Y. Choi, H. J. Jeong, K. H. Kim, and J. C. Park, "Blood pressure measurement using finger cuff," *2005 IEEE Engineering in Medicine and Biology 27th Annual Conference*, pp. 3575–3577, 2005.

Development of an in-vitro Model for Validation of Pulse Wave Velocity Measurements of Blood Vessels Under MRI

Mohammed Rasheed [1], Christian Damiani [2],
[1] Biomedical Engineering Science, Technische Hochschule Lübeck, mohammed.rasheed@stud.th-luebeck.de
[2] Medical MDGT Lab, Technische Hochschule Lübeck, christian.damiani@th-luebeck.de

Abstract

Measuring pulse wave velocity (PWV) in clinical practice is relevant for estimating arterial stiffness. Different methodologies and procedures exist that utilize invasive and non-invasive techniques to assess the PWV. However, the elaboration and evaluation of such methodologies are complicated. Indirect methods like MRI can also be used to determine PWV on vessel sections, but need to be validated at least on in-vitro models. In this work, an experimental in-vitro setup to determine the PWV in silicone vascular models was built and tested. These results should be used later for validation of MRI data using the same models. The measurements were done by sensing the pressure pulses between two points separated by a known distance along the vessels. Water was used as a testing fluid. The elasticity of the wall has a significant influence on the PWV, the lower the elasticity the higher PWV. The PWV in the straight model, which has the lowest elasticity, was 27.5 m/s with multiple pulse reflections. In the aorta model , the PWV was 11.3 m/s with less pulse reflections and oscillations. The pulse duration and magnitude have influenced the appearance and the geometry of the reflected waves. The shorter the pulse duration, the less noticeable reflected wave, but the easier peaks identification.

1 Introduction

The viscoelasticity of arteries is relevant for understanding clinical pathologies related to the hemodynamics of blood vessels. Loss of vessels compliance can be caused by high blood pressure, aging, or diabetes. To assess the compliance of blood vessels, different approaches are being investigated [1]. These can be non-invasive, such as tonometry or doppler, where the probes are placed on specific places on the body and the distance between the probing sites is determined [2]. (Fig. 1)

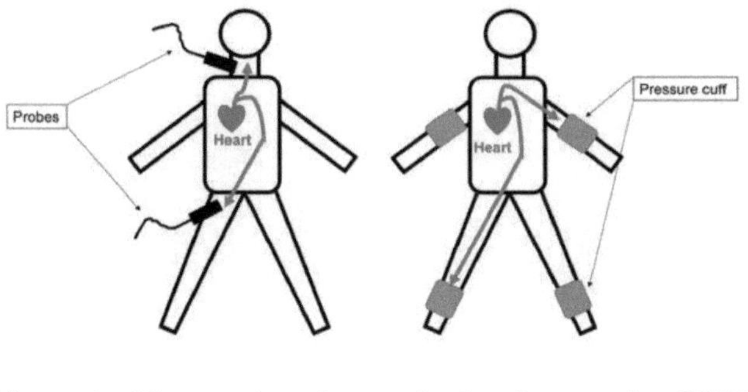

Figure 1: The non-invasive methods of measuring PWV. The obtained results in this way are not accurate due to the uncertainty in the estimation of wave path length [2].

Alternatively, PWV can be measured in an invasive way using a catheter connected to pressure sensors directly or through fiber optics. Normally, two catheters are placed inside the artery in different positions with a known distance between them. This is the most accurate method so far, but it requires catheterization. Due to its high costs and complexity, in addition to ethical limitations, this method can only be used for technical evaluation of newer approaches, such as the magnetic resonance imaging (MRI). Both MRI and Ultrasound are non-invasive methods which can be used to estimate the PWV by tracking the motion of the pressure wave. Using 4D MRI, for example, both the length and the transmit time of pulses can be determined, from which the PWV can be easily calculated. The arterial stiffness is estimated by the increase in the PWV value. Although this seems simple in theory, pulse reflections, non-uniform thickness of the vessels, and non-homogeneous vessel structure introduce complexity in assessing the arterial stiffness. This comes in addition to technical limitations, like temporal resolution and sampling error in 4D MRI [1]-[3].
In biomechanics, the factors affecting the PWV are described by the Moens–Korteweg equation [2]:

$$PWV^2 = (E \cdot h)/(r \cdot \rho) \quad (1)$$

Where E is the elastic modulus of the vessel, h is the wall thickness, r is the vessel radius, and ρ is density of blood. Larger h and smaller r lead to an increase of the measured PWV. Thus, by measuring the PWV, the stiffness of the vessels can be determined (modulus of elasticity) from equation (1), provided the other parameters can be estimated or measured, as shown in Fig. 2.

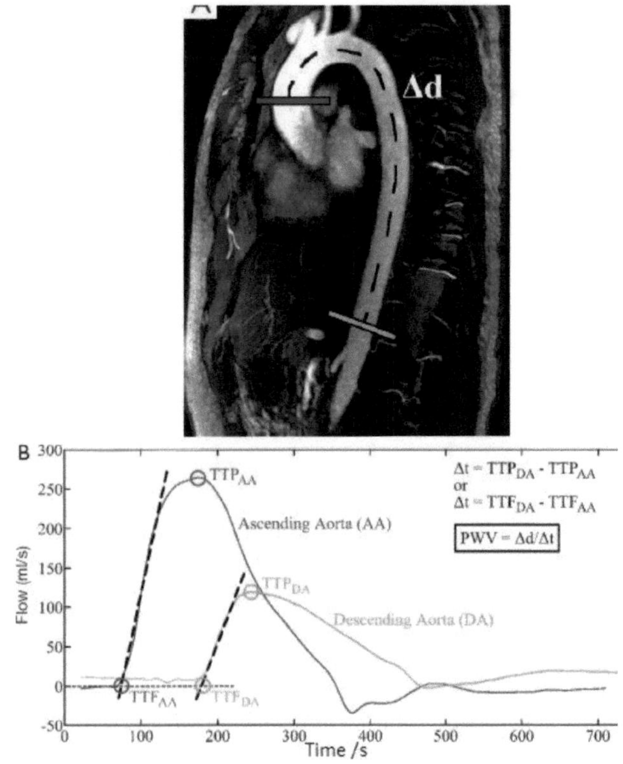

Figure 2: A) The thoracic aorta from MRI diagnosis for pulse wave. B) The time to foot (TTF) and the time to peak (TTP) approaches were used here to estimate the time difference between the pulse wave speed at the two different positions (Blue and Green) [3].

The increase of arterial stiffness impacts the cardiac afterload. The reason behind this is that the contractile pressure of the heart needs to be increased to maintain enough ejection of blood into the aorta. Part of the travelling pulse will be also reflected, this happens at sites where there is a significant increase of wall resistance, e.g. arterial branching. The increase in the stiffness can lead to pulse reflections as well, as shown in Fig 3. This can be seen by analyzing the recorded traveling waves [2]-[4].

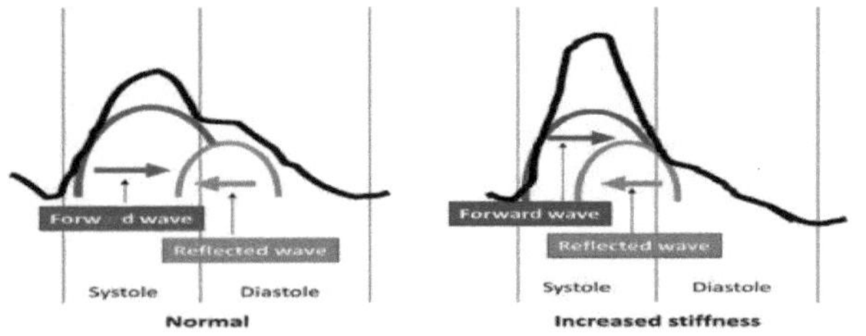

Figure 3: A measured travelling wave inside a healthy vessel (left) where the travelling and reflected waves have no sharp slopes. On the right, the large slope is an indication of increased stiffness [2].

To better understand how waves travel inside blood vessels, this work presents a simple in-vitro environment to assess PWV using two different approaches. This will be later used to validate 4D MRI measurements of the same in-vitro model.

2 Material and Methods

To simulate a native blood vessel, two silicon models of known dimensions were used in a similar setup. One of the models, a straight homogeneous silicon hose of 20 mm inner diameter, allowed for better control of the measurements parameters, in terms of easier interpretation of the results. The second model had a simplified aorta-like geometry with an average internal diameter of 35 mm, and was manufactured using rapid prototyping and silicone casting as shown in Fig 4. Two pressure sensors (S-11, WIKA industry, 0-6 bars) were used to detect the passing of the pulses at the beginning and the end of the model.

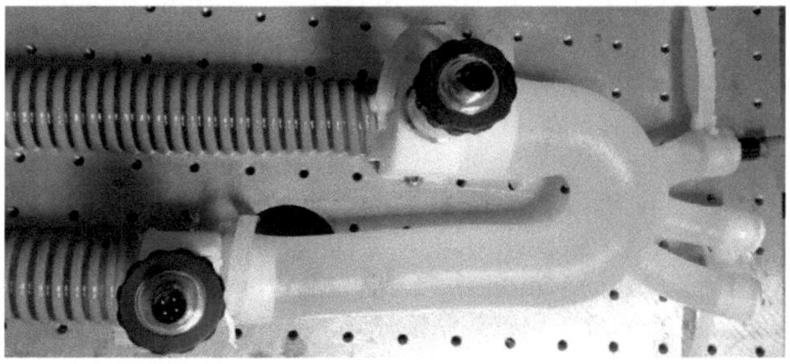

Figure 4: The Aorta model manufactured using rapid prototyping and silicone casting .

The connection between the silicon models and the sensors was achieved by designing a holder for the two sensors. The design was manufactured by 3D printing using a high impact polystyrene (HIPS), followed by post processing to seal the model surface (Fig. 5). The system was filled with water and air bubbles were eliminated to prevent any artifacts caused by the high compressibility of the air. A water tank was installed at a height of 60 cm over the silicon model to simulate a static back pressure similar to physiological conditions. The reservoir was connected to the model using a stiff tube segment to reduce possible compliance artifacts during the measurements.

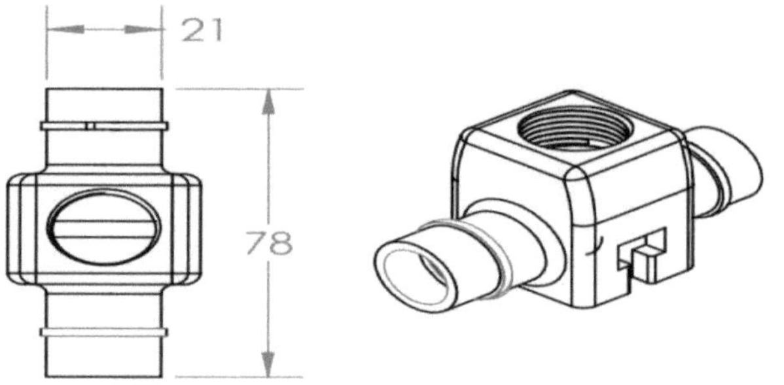

Figure 5: Holder for a pressure sensor, made of high impact polystyrene, to connect the sensor directly to the fluid. (Dimensions in millimeters).

The two pressure sensors, in Fig 6 and 7, were mounted into the holders and had direct contact with the fluid. The distances between the sensors were 55 cm and 34 cm for model 1 and model 2 respectively. The reading from the sensors were recorded by a analog to digital converter (SENSOR-CASSY 2, LD Didactic group), with time resolution of 20 ns.

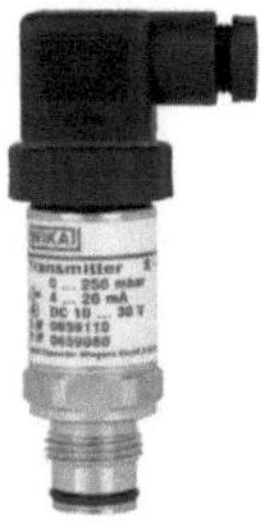

Figure 6: Analog pressure sensor with 0 to 6 bar measurement range [5].

Two approaches are used normally to detect the time difference of the wave at the two Pressure sensors. The time to foot (TTF) approach depends on the start of the wave (the foot of the wave). Since in some cases it is not clear where the wave starts; another approach called "The time to peak(TTP)" was used. The TTP measures the time difference between the pulse peaks at the two sensors [3]. Pulses were generated by a direct hit on a syringe plunger connected to the system. The readings were recorded with the help of a trigger set in the CASSY at approximately 10% of the maximum pulse signal. A special function of the software also allowed to register the 30 ms before the actual trigger, preventing cropping the measured signal. The complete setup is shown in Fig 7, and was mounted on a heavy metal block to prevent the system movement during pulse application.

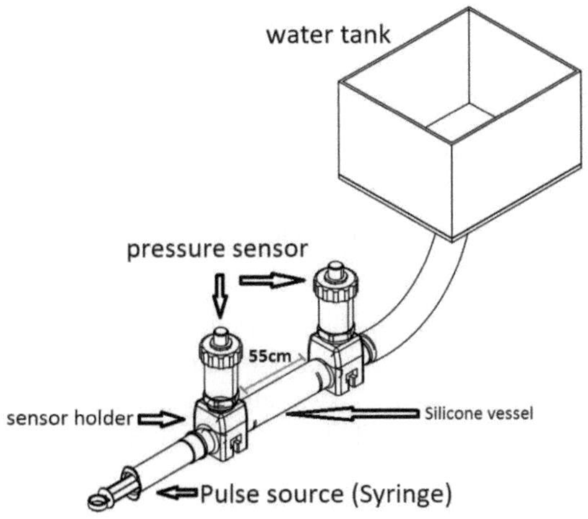

Figure 7: A complete experimental setup. The water tank acts as a damper to reduce oscillations.

Two different pulse generating methods were conducted. Ten direct high-speed pulses on the syringe plunger and another ten slow accelerating pulses. In total, 20 measurements were conducted in each setup. The results were exported as discrete samples and processed later by a python script to find the time difference and the PWV by implementing the TTP approach.

3 Results and Discussion

The way the pulse was generated affected the wave shape significantly. With the straight silicone vessel, the average time difference of the wave travel was 0.02 s and the PWV was 27.5 m/s. The PWV was higher and showed more pulse reflections and post-pulse oscillations in the system; although they were damped quickly. as shown in Fig. 8 and 9. The reason the wave damped in short time is due to the stiffness of the hose and the large surface area of the static pressure tank.

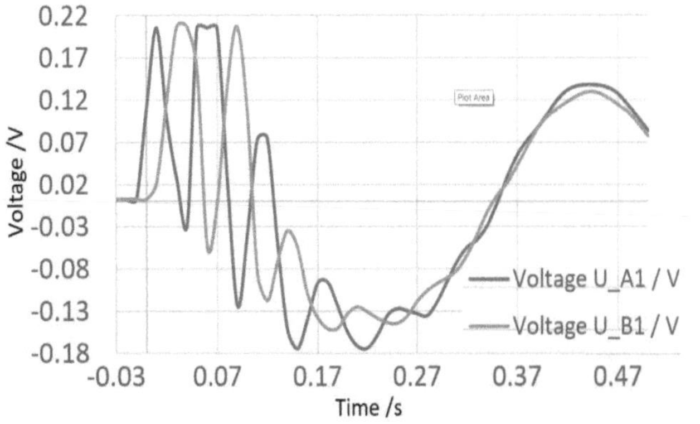

Figure 8: The PWV of the straight silicon model, showing multiple pulse reflections.

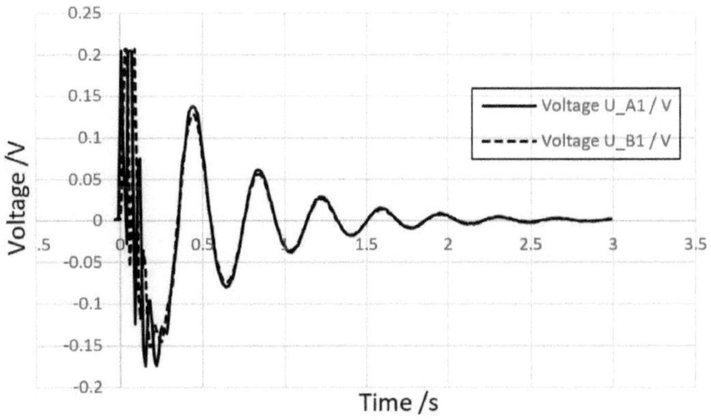

Figure 9: The PWV of the straight silicon model. The wave showed strong oscillations, but damped shortly after.

In the Aorta model, the results were different as for the straight model, as shown in Fig 10. The travel time of the pulse between the two sensors was longer than for the straight model (Δt= 0.03 s); although the travel path was shorter. The PWV was 11.3 m/s. Also, several pulse reflections were detected during the measurements.
The difference in speed between the two models is due to the difference in diameter, wall thickness, and the shore A hardness. As the inner diameter and the wall thickness

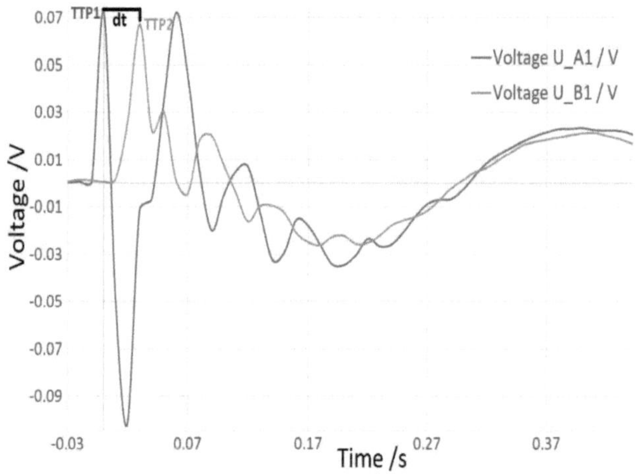

Figure 10: The PWV of the aorta model. With a high time resolution, the TTP at both sensors were identified and the PWV was calculated.

of the straight model are smaller than the aorta model, the speed was higher in the straight vessel. Besides that, the shore A hardness of the straight model was tested using Shore durometer, and resulted in 50. Compared to the one of aorta model which was 20. The larger shore hardness is an indication of higher Elastic modulus. Those results agree with Moens–Korteweg equation.
The pulse duration and sharpness affected the visibility of the pulse reflections. The shorter the pulse duration, the easier it was to detect the peak of the signal to carry out the TTP approach (Fig. 8 and 10). With Slow pulses, sensor 2 record higher readings than sensor one by 0.00165 V. Although pulse reflections were clearly visibly, the pulse peak was hard to recognize, as shown in Fig. 11.

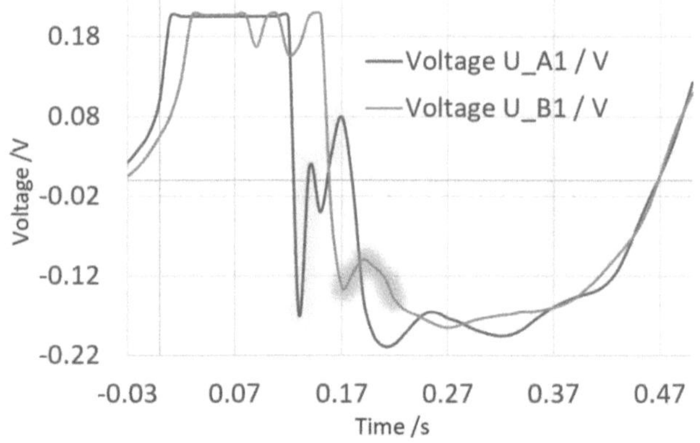

Figure 11: The slow pulse caused the water to accelerate toward sensor 2. The yellow shaded part of the signal is the pulse reflections at sensor 1. The green shaded part of the signal is the reflections at sensor 2.

4 Conclusion

In this work, the pulse wave velocity has been measured for two silicone vessel models by detecting the delay of the pressure wave. The method is a promising way for validating PWV measurement using 4D MRI. The pulse generating mechanism should be further developed to improve the overall reproducibilty and to better control the pulse shape. The work can be developed to implement more analysis mechanism and to compare the results to the 4D MRI measurements.

Acknowledgement

The work has been carried out at Technische hochschule and supervised by Dr. Christian Damiani.
Special thanks to Dr. Maren Balks, Dr. Thekla Oechtering Dr. Tim Schaller, Dr. Michael Scharfschwerdt and , Constantin Scharek of the UKSH Lübeck for motivating and providing valuable information for this work.

Author's Statement

Conflict of interest: Authors state no conflict of interest.

5 References

[1] Salvi, P., Magnani, E., Valbusa, F. et al., *Comparative study of methodologies for pulse wave velocity estimation*. Journal of Human Hypertension,2008.

[2] H. Tomiyama, A. Yamashina, *Encyclopedia of Cardiovascular Research and Medicine*.2018.

[3] Wentland AL, Grist TM, Wieben O. , *Review of MRI-based measurements of pulse wave velocity: a biomarker of arterial stiffness*.Cardiovasc Diagn Ther. 2014.

[4] Patrick Segers, Ernst R. Rietzschel, Julio A. Chirinos, *How to Measure Arterial Stiffness in Humans* .Arteriosclerosis, Thrombosis, and Vascular Biology. 2020.

[5] WIKA industry, *Flush pressure transmitter For viscous and solids-containing media*. Available: "https://www.wika.com/en-en/s11.WIKA" [last accessed on 2021-1-26].

[6] Ld-didactic industry, *measuring instrument is ideal for the acquisition of measurement data in complex demonstration experiments*. Available: "https://www.ld-didactic.de/software/524221en.pdf" , [last accessed on 2021-1-26].

Development of a Micro-Force-Spectroscope for measuring the deformation energy of softpellets

Leonora Meier [1], Christian Pottkämper [2], Thomas Gutsmann [3], and Christian Nehls [3]
[1] Biophysics, Universität zu Lübeck, leonora.meier@student.uni-luebeck.de
[2] Medical Engineering Science, Universität zu Lübeck, christian.pottkaemper@student.uni-luebeck.de
[3] Biophysics Group, Research Center Borstel, {tgutsmann, cnehls}@fz-borstel.de

Abstract

For treatment of tuberculosis, there are several options available most of which are oral administrations. In case of most lung diseases however, it could be advisable to have an inhalative alternative, because active agents of the medication could reach their destination, i.e. the lung, faster and more efficiently and accumulate there more easily. For storage, the medication is aggregated into softpellets which then have to be nebulized for inhalative application. To nebulize these pellets their deformation energy has to be known, so a suitable device can crush the pellets into an inhalable powder. Measurements with an Atomic Force Microscope (AFM) were not possible and thus a Micro-Force-Spectroscope was designed and developed. The device was tested and used to measure several different samples of softpellets and in first tests it seemed sensitive enough to measure the force required to crush the sample.

1 Introduction

Diseases of the airways can be treated with different methods; they can be treated systematically (meaning potentially affecting the whole body) or locally. The use of oral medicine normally leads to systematic treatment as the medication is broken down via the digestive tract and transported through the blood stream to all organs, so the affected organ can be treated.
Locally administered drugs are only directed at the area of the treatable disease, in this case the lung. This comes with several advantages, the main ones being no agglomeration in non-target organs and that treatment can be carried out with smaller doses of active agent and thus fewer side effects [1].
There are different devices that can be used for inhalative treatment like nebulizers, metered-dose inhalers or dry powder inhalers (DPI). DPIs are increasingly used because they don't use any further propellants, carriers or other drug additives; instead they use agglomerated micronized powder which forms so-called softpellets (see Fig. 1). These softpellets are hard enough to be handled well but soft enough to get deagglomerated and dispersed during inhalation utilising a suitable inhaler like a Turbohaler® [1].
The softpellets are agglomerations of active component and can therefore build large structures in the micrometer range. To crush these pellets (i.e. disaggregate them) and release them properly, the deformation energy of the pellets has to be known.
Tuberculosis is a lung disease which is often treated by oral medication and lasts at least six months [2], [3]. Christian Etschmann from the Department of Pharmaceutics and Biopharmaceutics of the CAU Kiel developed a method in which the active agent Rifampicin is agglomerated into softpellets and can later be inhaled.

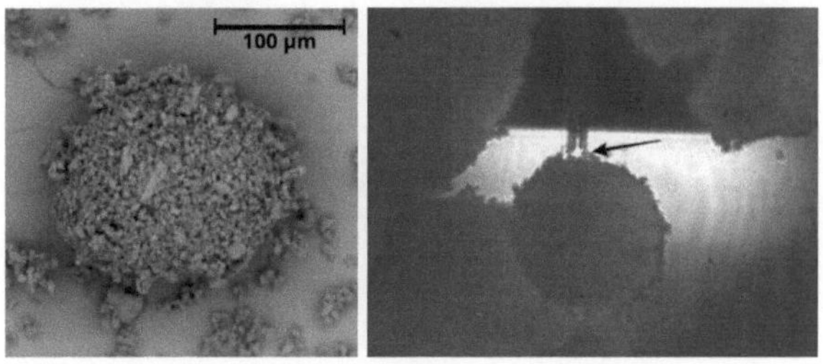

Figure 1: Left: SEM-Picture (Scanning Electron Microscopy) of a Lactose softpellet that was sifted through a 180 µm sieve with 1000x magnification [4].
Right: Softpellet being measured with an AFM; the arrow indicates where the cantilever tip presses into the pellet [5].

For inhalation the softpellets have to be pulverized beforehand and therefore the deformation energy of the pellets has to be known. Measurement with an Atomic-Force-Microscope (AFM) is possible, but the largest cantilever tip is still so small that only a local area of the softpellet is dented and not the pellet as a whole as can be seen in Fig. 1. Therefore, a device has to be developed to measure the deformation energy of a whole softpellet.

2 Material and Methods

For this device to be constructed, some considerations had to be made for example the mobility of the device; it should be easily accessible and preferably mobile for practicality. Also fitting components and materials had to be chosen that are suitable for its purposes; for example the materials and components have to be stable enough to withstand the vibrations of the stepper motor and the components should not overheat.

2.1 Materials and Construction

There have to be several components, the most important being a physical sensor - in this case a cantilever similar to cantilevers of an AFM that pushes into the pellets - and a digital sensor that converts the physical movement into digital data that can be measured and subsequently interpreted. Here, a Linear Variable Differential Transformer (LVDT, Series 200 DC-DC by Transtek) was used for this purpose because it can convert axial movement into change in voltage which can be measured.

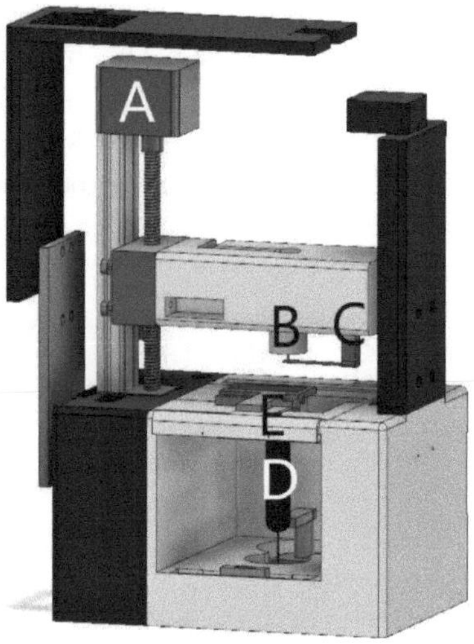

Figure 2: CAD-Drawing of the Micro-Force-Spectroscope done in Autodesk Fusion 360 by Christian Pottkämper [5]. **A** marks the stepper motor that is connected to a rail guide where one of the main components - the mount - can exert a vertical movement (up and down). **B** is the retainer for the LVDT where the iron core of the LVDT will slide into the LVDT. **C** is the attachment for the cantilever which will press onto the softpellet. **D** is the microscope camera. **E** shows the clamp for the object slide on which the softpellets will be placed.

Except for these components (i.e. the cantilever and the electrical components seen in the circuit diagram in Fig. 4), most of the components were constructed using Autodesk Fusion 360 and subsequently 3D-printed (model i3 MK3, manufacturer Prusa3D). These can be seen in Fig. 2. The components are not shown assembled but with spaces in between, so each component is visually accessible.
The components of Fig. 2 are numbered: **A** is where the stepper motor is connected to a rail guide. On the rail guide a major component is mounted that holds the LVDT (**B**) and the cantilever (**C**). This mount can move vertically up and down the rail when the motor is on, the main principle being that the cantilever is pushed onto the softpellet and the attached iron core on the cantilever can slide further into the LVDT so that a signal change can be measured. **D** is the microscope camera (PX-8209-919 by Somikon with 500x magnification) which is used to position the softpellet into place under the cantilever tip. **E** shows the clamp for the object slide on which the softpellets are placed. This clamp table can be moved back and forth or left and right.

2.2 Measurement principles

To measure the deformation energy of the softpellets, a cantilever with a rounded tip presses onto the pellet until it breaks (Fig. 3). The cantilever measures 6 mm (or 2 mm in a second experiment), 42 mm, 0,1 mm in width, length and thickness, respectively and is cut from a copper sheet. At the tip of the cantilever, a small ball is fastened that exerts pressure onto the softpellet until it is crushed but without puncturing it. An iron (ferromagnetic) core is attached to the top of the cantilever which is part of an LVDT to measure displacement of the cantilever tip.

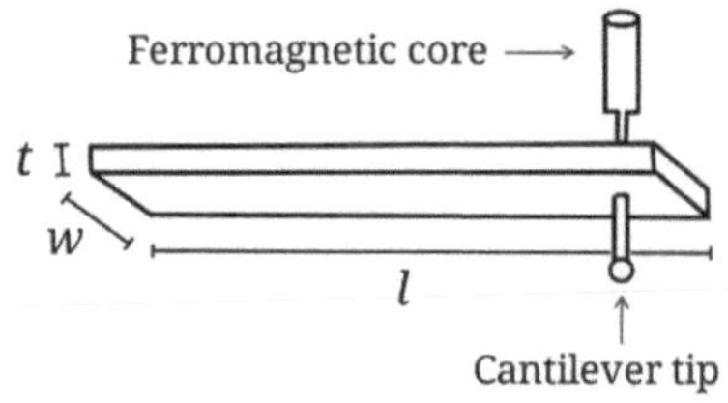

Figure 3: Schematic drawing of the cantilever which measures height $h = 0{,}1\,\mathrm{mm}$, width $w = 6\,\mathrm{mm}$ (or $2\,\mathrm{mm}$) and length $l = 42\,\mathrm{mm}$. Fastened on top of the cantilever is the ferromagnetic core of the LVDT and beneath it is the cantilever tip with a small sphere with a diameter d of 3,5 mm.

When the cantilever is lowered onto the sample, the core on top will be pushed back which in turn then slides farther into the opening of the LVDT and a signal can be seen. When the tip crushes the sample, the core slides back out and the subsequent signal change can be analyzed to reveal the deformation energy of the sample.

2.3 Implementation

The vertical movement of the cantilever onto the softpellet sample is accomplished by a stepper motor (NEMA17) that is attached to a rail guide. Fastened to the rail guide is the mount which contains the cantilever and the LVDT.
The motor has a step angle resolution of 1,8°. One winding of the rail (i.e. 360°) amounts to 5 mm. So one step of the motor would move the mount 0,025 mm up or down. A better resolution can be achieved by wiring the motor to a motor driver. Here, the motor was wired to a DRV8825 motor driver (see Fig. 4) that enables 1/32 steps per motion unit which translates to a vertical movement of 0,7812 µm per step.
All electrical components are wired to a microcontroller -

an Arduino Mega 2560 - which is controlled with the programming software Arduino. The ATmega 2560 has connections to the LEDs which specify the state of the device, to the joystick with which the motor can be controlled manually, to the Start- and MAX-buttons which are crucial for the measurement states and to the motor driver which in turn connects to the stepper motor. The LVDT is not read by the microcontroller; instead it uses a separate device, a Multifunction I/O Device by National Instruments (NI USB-6212 Screw-Terminal).

These connections can be seen in the circuit diagram in

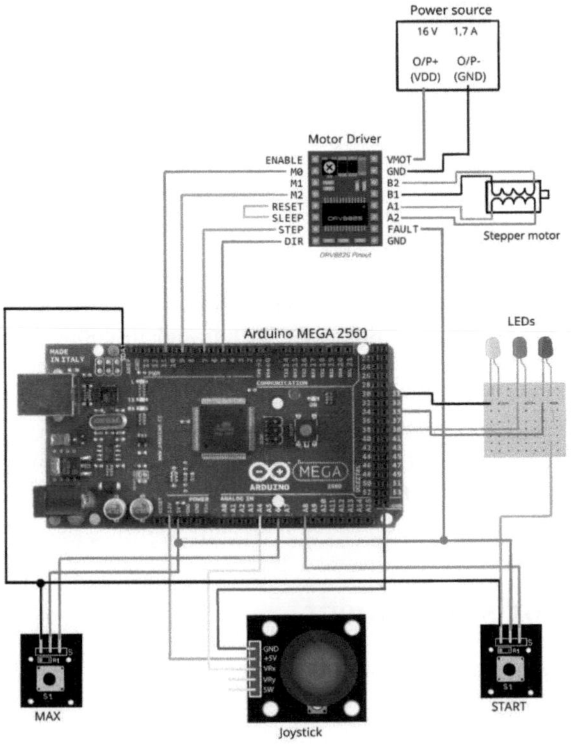

Figure 4: Circuit diagram of all electrical components of the device. At the center of this diagram lies the Arduino micro controller, which is controlled via the Arduino software with fitting code. The LEDs are yellow, red and blue, respectively, from left to right.

Fig. 4. It shows how the wires are connected to the microcontroller pins, with the top and right rows of pins of the ATmega 2560 being the digital pins, and the bottom pins being analog and power pins.

2.4 Operating modes

The device is turned on when the microcontroller is plugged in and the external power source (Voltcraft LSP-1403) is turned on. The blue LED is glowing. There are two modes of operation: either cycling through a protocol or operating freely with the joystick. The automated measurement protocol is used for controlled tests whereas in manual mode the joystick can be used to coarsely position the softpellet underneath the cantilever before starting a protocol measurement.

The protocol starts when the Start button is pushed. The motor moves toward the sample until an extended arm on the backside of the mount pushes onto the Max button and thereby the cantilever tip is crushing the sample. As soon as the Max button is pushed the motor stops and then moves 4000 steps up (approximately 50 mm). It remains there for 10 seconds; the time in between should be used to clean the cantilever tip and the sample slide of the crushed softpellet. After the waiting period, the motor moves 4000 steps towards the slide and pushes against the glass slide. After that, the motor moves 4000 steps upwards again and the initial state has been reached.

The first measurement is therefore to be seen as interpretable data and the second as reference.

3 Results and Discussion

3.1 Measurement of the spring constants

The spring constant of the cantilever is an integral part of calculating the force that is exerted on the sample. The spring constant D was calculated by measuring the displacement x of the cantilever with increasing weight m, plotting those against each other and calculating the slope. Hooke's law and Newton's second law equated and solved for D yields

$$D = \frac{m \cdot g}{x}. \quad (1)$$

Thus, the slope has to be inversed and multiplied with the gravitational acceleration g as shown in (1). The measured data, the resulting best-fit lines and the slope of the curves for each cantilever are shown is Fig. 5. The green markers

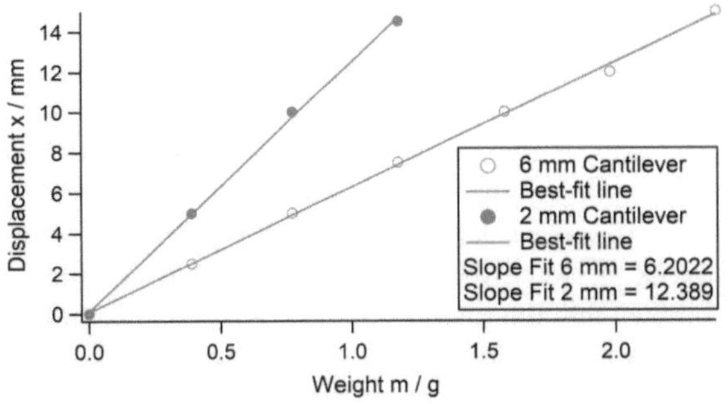

Figure 5: Displacement of the cantilever plotted against applied weight. The marker indicate the measured data which is fitted with a best-fit line that yield the respective slopes. The green markers represent the data for the 2 mm cantilever, the red ones for the 6 mm cantilever.

and the fit curve represent the 2 mm cantilever and the red ones the 6 mm cantilever.

The resulting spring constants for the 6 mm and the 2 mm cantilever are $1{,}58\,\mathrm{N\,m^{-1}}$ and $0{,}79\,\mathrm{N\,m^{-1}}$, respectively.

3.2 Sample measurements

Several samples (14 overall) of both active agent (rifampicin and isoniazid) and lactose placebos with different softpellet sizes were measured (each sample was measured 10 times with new softpellets, respectively). A measurement of a rifampicin softpellet with the 6 mm cantilever is shown in Fig. 6; the voltage measured by the LVDT is plotted against the time (the time will later be converted into distance and the voltage into force). When the cantilever tip pushes on the softpellet the voltage increases, stagnates when the MAX-button is pushed and decreases when the motor drives back up. This can be seen in the first peak of the graph. After that the motor stands still and the cantilever and slide can be cleaned which also causes change in the voltage. Then the motor drives toward the slide again and pushes against it, causing the second reference peak. The

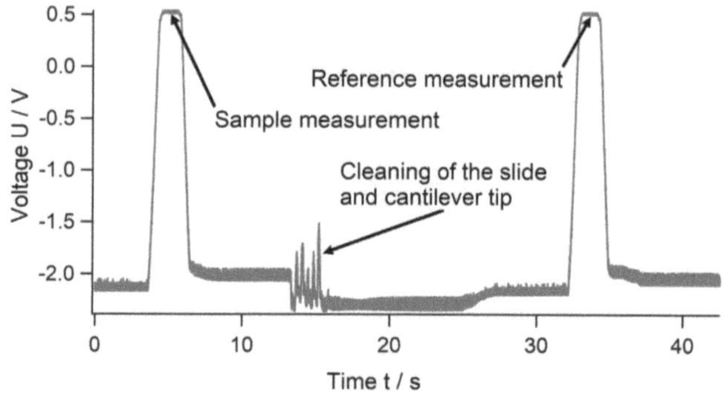

Figure 6: Measurement of a Rifampicin softpellet, sifted through a 500 µm sieve and prepared 6 times on a vibrational rail. The graph plots the measured voltage of the LVDT against the time. The first peak indicates when the cantilever crushed the softpellet, the second big peak shows the reference. The noise in between the peaks shows when the cantilever was cleaned of the crushed sample.

two relevant peaks should show a difference in the rising slope when the cantilever tip presses on the sample because the crushing of the softpellet should require a little more time. To compare the respective slopes, the two peaks can be isolated and be depicted overlapping thus showing the difference between the two. This is shown in Fig. 7. It can be seen that the reference peak (blue) is slightly steeper than the sample peak slope (as could be seen in several other measurements). This suggests that the sensitivity of the device is sufficient to measure the force used to crush the softpellets. Further evaluation of the data of the different softpellets with both cantilevers has yet to be done.

4 Conclusion

In summary, the device is functional and works steadily. For the several measurements that have been performed it worked sufficiently, but it still remains to be seen if the sensitivity is good enough to measure the force of the various softpellets. If the sensitivity is not sufficient, adjustments have to be made; for example the material of the cantilever can be modulated, another stepper motor with a smaller step angle could be used or suitable filtering could be applied to measured data.

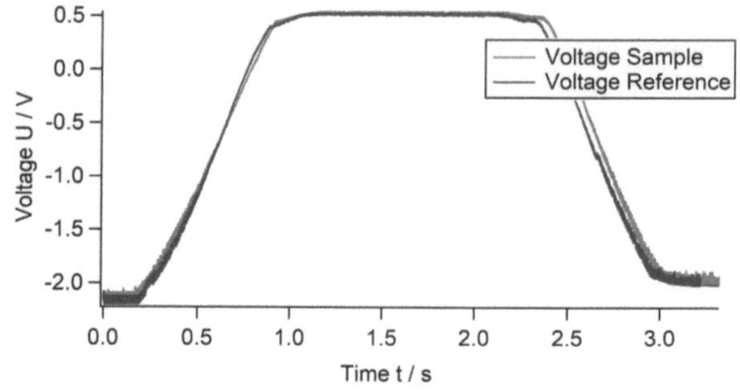

Figure 7: The same sample and axis as in Fig. 6, but with the reference peak (blue) and sample peak (red) overlapping. A slightly different slope is discernible as was the case with all other measurements that have been evaluated so far which suggests that the device is sensitive enough to measure force changes in the desired range..

Acknowledgement

This work has been carried out at the Research Center Borstel in the Biophysics Research Group and in cooperation with the Department of Pharmaceutics and Biopharmaceutics of the Christian-Albrecht-Universität (CAU) Kiel. Special thanks to Christian Etschmann who researched, produced and provided the rifampicin softpellets. This work is a continuation of the work of Christian Pottkämper, who started this project and printed the components.

Author's Statement

Authors state no conflict of interest.

References

[1] K. Wetterlin, "Turbohaler: A New Powder Inhaler for Administration of Drugs to the Airway," *Pharmaceutical Research*, vol. 5, no. 8, pp. 506–508, 1988.

[2] W.H.O., *Treatment of Tuberculosis Guidelines*. World Health Organization, 4 ed., 2010. Chapter 3, ISBN 978 92 4 154783 3.

[3] C. R. Horsburgh, C. E. Barry, and C. Lange, "Treatment of tuberculosis," *The New England Journal of Medicine*, pp. 2149–2152, 2015.

[4] C. Etschmann, "Softpellets for high dose pulmonary delivery," in *Drug Delivery to the Lungs*, 2018.

[5] C. Pottkämper, T. Gutsmann, and C. Nehls, "Towards measurement of the deformation energy of softpellets: Design and Development of a Micro-Force-Spectroscope," *Student Conference Proceedings 2020*, 2020.

Feasibility Study of a Smart Device Controlled Single Use Infusion Pump

Jonas Reck [1], Philipp Kraus [2]
[1] Medical Engineering Science, Universität zu Lübeck, jonas.reck@student.uni-luebeck.de
[2] PROMECON GmbH, 20095 Hamburg Germany, kraus@promecon-medical.de

Abstract

Infusion pumps are commonly used medical devices in postoperative pain therapy for the administration of drugs. This study focuses on battery powered electronic infusion pumps which enable a free configuration of infusion protocols and battery-free single use elastomeric infusion pumps with predefined infusion protocols. The aim of this study is to investigate the feasibility of a smart controlled single use infusion pump which combines technical, patient and user benefits of both pump systems. In order to test the feasibility, a survey was created and sent to different hospitals. The survey is still ongoing, but preliminary results show that it is important for medical staff that infusion protocols can be adjusted during therapy. Furthermore, the menu navigation of the electronic pumps seems to be too complex and a system for the transfer from the event log to the PDMS is missing.

1 Introduction

Infusion pumps can supply the patient with fluids, medications or nutrients and are thus an indispensable part of daily hospital routine. Especially for the administration of pain medication in various areas of pain therapy the pumps play a major role. Infusion pumps can be distinguished between gravity systems, single use infusion pumps, syringe pumps and electronic infusion pumps [1]. In this study, only mobile single use infusion pumps and mobile electronic infusion pumps are considered. Mobile in this case refers to the mobility of the patient which is enabled by the design of the infusion pumps e.g. low weight and size or the independence from wired power supply. These pumps are used for various pain therapies, including PCA (patient-controlled analgesia). For the PCA it can be distinguished between continuous basal rate with bolus administration or bolus-only administration. Continuous basal rate means that the infusate is administered at a defined flow rate over time. In contrast, the bolus is defined as an amount of infusate defined by the physician that the patient can repeatedly administer to himself (in addition or exclusively). The lock-out time defines the intervals at which the patient can administer the bolus to avoid an overdose [2]. Single use infusion pumps are disposable pumps that are used for one patient and one application only, such as the elastomeric pumps [3]. Elastomeric pumps allow the infusion of medications without an external power source and the need for control technology. The pumping work in these devices is performed by a preloaded elastomeric balloon (e.g. silicone tube) filled with medication and the flow rate is defined by the restrictor's length and cross section which is inserted in the infusion line [4]. Elastomer pumps contain different advantages and disadvantages listed in Table 1.

Table 1: Advantages and disadvantages of elastomeric pumps [5].

advantages	**disadvantages**
no external power supply → light weight	lack of programming causing limited, inflexible setting options
very simple operation → low training effort	no data storage in digital form
non-kinking infusion lines and air-expelling filters reduce the need of alarms	limited settings for infusion protocol parameters such as flow rate, bolus volume and lock-out time
no need for programming → no programming errors	
low price and no maintenance costs	

In contrast to elastomeric pumps, electronic infusion pumps have a motor that drives a conveying unit. In these, the infusate is pushed through the hose by an external mechanical deformation of the hose and it is possible to clearly define how much infusate is conveyed per rotation for each pump [6,7]. Similar to the elastomeric pumps, the electronic pumps contain different advantages and disadvantages listed in Table 2. The aim of this study is to investigate the feasibility of a new pump system which combines as many advantages of the two pump systems as possible. This includes combining the easy handling of the elastomeric pumps with the electronics of the electronic pumps but without the complexity of programming, the heaviness and the high training costs. It should be possible to create and operate an infusion protocol with the new pump system without much programming effort but specifically designed for pain therapy. In addition, the new pump system should be less expensive than currently existing electronic pumps.

Table 2: Advantages and disadvantages of electronic pumps [1, 7].

advantages	disadvantages
controllability of the drive mechanism	require regular recharging
individually adjustable infusion protocols with high accuracy	relatively high level of training for the staff
infusion protocols with defined parameters that are pre-set in the device	significantly heavier as elastomeric pumps
changes during the infusion time are possible to respond directly to the patient's pain perception	high purchase price which leads to limited availability of the devices
event log to store information of the infusion therapy	very strict regulations must be observed
alarm functions are available	regular maintenance is necessary

The present study consists of a feasibility study to verify if a smart (electronical device with wireless protocol) device controlled single use infusion pump can be implemented. In order to test the feasibility, a survey is created that tries to determine the problems, application and relevant pump parameters of existing elastomeric and electronic pumps in pain therapy. With this information a concept should be created, which is able to combine the advantages of both pump systems in a new pump system in a meaningful way.

2 Material and methods

In order to be able to develop a possible concept for linking the advantages of the two pump systems, extensive research about the state of the art of pumps was necessarily followed by the creation of a survey to determine the feasibility of this pump system. For this purpose, a literature research was conducted in combination with interviews of medical staff. Here, information could be gained about the technical possibilities of the pump systems as well as various pain therapy options. Using this information, key aspects were elaborated which are important to know for the development of a new pump system. These key aspects are as followed: 1) pump system used, 2) inpatient or outpatient therapy, 3) infusion protocols, 4) medication bags, 5) questions about operation/application, 6) source of complications, 7) advantages/disadvantages, 8) alarm function and 9) digital patient file. At the beginning of the survey, an overview is first created of how the distribution between electronic and non-electronic pumps is in daily hospital routine and whether these are predominantly used in inpatient or outpatient therapy. This will give an impression of the need for a new pump system and for which application areas it should be adapted. By asking specific questions about the infusion protocol and the medication bag, important parameters can be marked out that must be considering for the definition of the specification sheet, e.g., which sizes of medication bags are frequently used and which settings the infusion protocols (basal rate, bolus volume, lock-outtime) must contain. Bearing these aspects into account, medical staff are asked which parameters are set and which are changed or adjusted during therapy. This makes it possible to distinguish between important and indispensable parameters and these are not used for everyday use and thus have no or limited benefit. Consequently, these parameters would not be necessarily taken account in a new pump system. Information about the operation and application of the infusion pumps makes it possible, for example, to draw conclusions about how many access restrictions must be implemented and how much training would be required. Essentially important operating elements can also be identified. By asking for sources of complications, an attempt can be made to prevent these errors from occurring in the new pump system. Direct feedback from the user makes it possible to analyse and prevent possible problems and user errors prior the development of a. If the disadvantages and advantages are described directly by the user, it can be analysed which functions can be improved and which should be implemented in any case in a new pump system. The query of the alarm functions shows which aspects are particularly important for a smooth process and which alarm functions are perceived by the personnel as disturbing. This information shall be used to design a pumps systems where commonly known errors are avoided or reduced to a minimum so alarms will occur less frequently. Another important part of the survey deals with the use of a digital patient record or PDMS (Patient Data Management System). Here, we will ask whether such a system is used and whether the event log is read out and entered into a corresponding data management system. This will allow consideration of whether an event log should be available and, if so, how to transfer it conveniently to an appropriate system. With the help of these key aspects, questions for the survey could be generated. Some exemplary questions with the corresponding key aspects can be seen in Table 3. The anonymous survey was created with the freely usable website www.LamaPoll.de and sent to different hospitals. The target group of this survey was physicians and medical staff working in pain therapy. By questioning this target group, an impression should be gained of how infusion pumps are used in the field of pain therapy in daily hospital routine. A total of 29 hospitals including a pain area have been contacted so far. An evaluation of the survey can take place as soon as sufficient responses are received.

Table 3: Key aspects with associated exemplary questions from the survey.

key aspects	exemplary questions
pumps system used	-what types of pumps are more commonly used in your clinic? electronical or non-electronical
inpatient or outpatient therapy	-what is the distribution between inpatient and outpatient use of pumps?
infusion protocols	-how often are infusion protocols changed/adjusted during the application period? -what is changed/adjusted?
medication bags	-what reservoir sizes are needed?
advantages/ disadvantages	-where do you see the greatest advantages/disadvantages in the pump(s) used?
alarm function	-which alarms occur particularly frequently? -which alarm functions are generally switched off?
digital patient file	-do you use a digital patient record or PDMS? -are event logs of the electronic pumps entered into the PDMS?

3 Results and discussion

At present, the survey is still ongoing and partial results and discussions can be presented. Due to the current COVID 19 situation, 5800 intensive care beds in Germany are occupied and anaesthetists are also intensively deployed in intensive care units. This could lead to a reduced number of completed surveys [8]. Nevertheless, a statement can be made about what results could be expected and which preliminary trends can be read out. When asked what type of pump is used in daily clinic routine, there is a clear trend that electronic infusion pumps (90%) are preferred to non-electronical infusion pumps and that these are mostly used in the inpatient area. To learn more about the infusion protocol and related parameters, questions were asked about use and adaptation of the infusion protocols. The preliminary results indicate that both nurses (43%) and physicians (50%) adjust the infusion protocols. This includes changing the protocols once a day (44%) to several times a day (33%) during the application time and tending to change both the basal rate and the bolus rate (75%). Furthermore, the preliminary results of the survey suggest that almost all of the available medication bag sizes are used, with the smaller sizes tending to be used more frequently. The distribution is as follows: 50-100 ml (36%), 150-200 ml (21%), 250-300 ml (29%), 350-400 ml (0%), 40-500 ml (14%). Since most participants indicated that they use electronic pumps, the advantages and disadvantages listed are predominantly related to electronic pumps. A recurring advantage of electronic pumps is the easy handling. From the context it can be concluded that this is probably about the handling of the device itself, something like connecting medication bags, and not about the programming. Other advantages are the accuracy and the compactness of the system. Disadvantages include battery consumption and costs, and the complicated menu navigation already mentioned. In the case of electronic pumps, there are several alarm functions, of which overpressure (71%), battery empty (29%) and reservoir empty (71%) were particularly mentioned in the survey. In addition, it was mentioned that all alarm functions tend to be used and none are switched off. Although the patient record tends to be used in the clinics (67%) and the internal memory of the electronic pumps is used (71%), the event logs tend not to be entered into the PDMS (86%). Among the reasons given was that this process is of little use, but at the same time requires a lot of work. If the results had been in favour of the non-electronic pumps, it would have been clear that there was no need for a combined pump system, as the disposable infusion pumps are sufficient for everyday use. The results reinforce the need for a combined pump system because, on the one hand, it could avoid the disadvantages of the electronic pumps such as high cost and complexity, and on the other hand, it could maintain the advantages such as individually adjustable infusion protocols and alarm functions. Since both physicians and nurses set the infusion protocols, both would need to be trained in the use of the electronic pumps. It must also be considered that the infusion protocol parameters could be changed several times a day and therefore easy access is important without being complicated by unnecessary restrictions. Since both bolus and basal rate changes occur in daily clinical routine, both options must also be available in a combined pump system. In addition, it would be unfavourable to impose a restriction on the size of the medication bags, since all sizes tend to be used. However, since the small sizes tend to be used even more frequently, there is no need to consider providing even larger bags to minimize the change rate. Unfortunately, the survey does not further specify what is meant by handling and this can only be inferred from the context. Should this still be the case, if there are sufficient returns, the conversation with medical staff should be sought to specify this more precisely. This is the only way to ensure that a combined pump system really has advantages over the current electronic pumps. The accuracy of the electronic pump systems has already been identified as an advantage of this pump type and is underlined by the survey again [1]. This aspect should be considered and guaranteed in a combined pump system likewise the compactness of the system. As disadvantages of the electronical pumps the high costs and the complexity of the programming were already specified and are supported by the survey [1]. In the design of a combined pump system, attention should be paid to reducing these costs and making the programming less complex, but still maintaining the important parameters. The survey could show so far that all alarm functions tend to be turned on and thus all are seen as important. Due to the fact that one of the most common alarms is the empty batteries, one could work on the power supply and consider how a combined system could ensure a longer battery life. Furthermore, while there is often an alarm regarding an empty reservoir, the responses regarding reservoir sizes indicated that the smaller bags are preferred and there does not seem to be a need for larger bags. The overpressure alarm could be addressed in the conceptual design and further consideration could be given to what causes this overpressure and how it can be prevented in future systems. There is a tendency to use the event log of the electronic pumps, but not to transfer it to the PDMS, because this taking time to the medical staff and also it was described by them, that it is a tedious task, due to the difficult navigation trough the menus. This makes clear that the event log is important and must continue to be used, but there is still work to be done to transfer the data adequately to a data management system. The preliminary results of the survey can already give an information of the problems, applications and relevant pump parameters of existing elastomeric and electronic pumps in pain therapy. In addition, these results show that there are interfaces between both pump systems and it seems to make sense to combine them. This means that the advantages of the electronic pumps, such as accuracy, alarm functions and individually adaptable infusion protocols (Table 2), should be used in combination with the advantages of the non-electronic pumps (Table 1). This would avoid the disadvantages of the electronic pumps such as the high cost and complicated programming. For an exact analysis we need more returns of the survey, which hopefully will give a final and even more comprehensive impression of the question, with which a combined pumping system can be conceptualized.

4 Conclusion

This study focuses on electronic and single use infusion pumps operated in the field of pain therapy. The aim was to investigate the feasibility of a new pump system which combines as many advantages of the two pump systems as possible. To assess this feasibility, first an anonymous survey was created to collect information on the use of infusion pumps in daily hospital routine. Although the survey is still ongoing preliminary trends can already be read out and give indications of which parameters and functions are important and need to be considered when designing a new combined pump system. Among others, the preliminary results show that electronic pumps are primarily used in hospitals. Furthermore, it should still be possible to flexible adapt infusion protocols in a new pump system and all alarm functions should be available. It is also desirable to transfer the event logs to a PDMS, which could be made possible by using wireless technology, for example. For definite results, it is necessary to wait until the end of the survey.

Acknowledgment

The work has been caried out at Promecon GmbH, 20095 Hamburg and supervised by Prof. Dr. M. Leucker, Institute for Software Engineering and Programming Languages, Universität zu Lübeck. We thank Dr. A. Calavrezos (Promecon GmbH) for the opportunity to realize this project and Prof. Dr. M. Leucker for supervising this work. Further thanks go to the entire Promecon GmbH team and the scientific staff of UniTransferKlinik Lübeck GmbH.

Author`s Statement

P.K. conceived of the presented idea. P.K. and J.R. planned the procedure. J.R. performed the research and designed the survey. J.R. wrote the manuscript with support from P.K. Conflict of interest: Authors state no conflict of interest.

5 References

[1] pfm medical *Infusionssysteme* [Online]. Available: https://www.pfmmedical.de/wissen/infusionssysteme/index.html. [Access: 20 January 2021]

[2] Stefan Grond, Karin Bornhövd, Hugo Van Aken, *Prinzipien der postoperativen Schmerztherapie: nicht-invasive PCA mit IONSYS,* Georg Thieme Verlag, pp. 24-34, 2008

[3] ISO Copyright office, *ISO 28620:2020 - Medical devices - non-electronically driven portable infusion devices*, Genf: ISO Copyright office, 2020

[4] M. L. (. S. A), *Elastomeric Pump.* Spanien Patent WO 02/22189 (A1), 21 März 2002.

[5] E. A. Skryabina und T. S. Dunn, *Disposable Infusion Pumps*, American Journal of Health-System Pharmacy, Nr. 63, pp. 1260-1268, 2006.

[6] Frank Wolter, *Untersuchungen zu neuartigen Infusionspumpen für die Medizintechnik,* Institut für Mikrointegration der Universität Stuttgart, 2013

[7] DIN EN 60601-2-24:2015 *Medizinische elektrische Geräte-Teil 2-24: Besondere Festlegungen für die Sicherheit einschließlich der wesentlichen Leistungsmerkmale von Infusionspumpen und Infusionsreglern*, VDE VERLAG GMBH, Berlin, 2016

[8] DKGev *Coronavirus: Infos und Fakten Derzeitige Corona-Situation in den Krankenhäusern* [Online]. Available: https://www.dkgev.de/dkg/coronavirus-fakten-und-infos/ [Access: 8 February 2021]

Electrical Impedance Tomography for Different Hand Gestures

Minshang Liang [1], Ole Thomsen [2] and Alfred Mertins [2]
[1] Medical Engineering Science, Universität zu Lübeck, minshang.liang@student.uni-luebeck.de
[2] Institute for Signal Processing, Universität zu Lübeck, {o.thomsen, alfred.mertins}@uni-luebeck.de

Abstract

Electrical Impedance Tomography (EIT) is a modern medical instrument. It can determine the bioimpedances of the body and reconstruct a tomographic image from it. The advantages are a compact and cheap design as well as a radiationless usage. In our research we try to build an EIT in order to investigate the usage for hand gesture recognition. A low-cost EIT will be designed and programmed for the project. Subsequently, different hand gestures will be examined in experiments in order to classify them on the basis of the signals.

1 Introduction

Electrical Impedance Tomography (EIT) is a non-invasive tomoimaging method. Eight electrodes should be placed around the arm. A defined current flows between two selected electrodes and the voltage drop across the others is measured to calculate the frequency depending bioimpedance, as shown in Fig. 1. Like other tomographic methods, for example CT, it also needs a reconstruction algorithm to get an image. The difference is that CT is based on absorption of X-ray in the body and EIT is based on different impedances in the body. EIT has been used in a wide range of applications. That is, not just in the medical field, but also in geography, environmental science, biology, and industrial monitoring [5]. Thought permuting the current stimulating points by simultaneously measuring the voltages, various transfer impedances can be determined, on the basis of which the two-dimensional conductance distribution of the test object can be approximately reconstructed and visualised with the aid of special reconstruction algorithms [7].

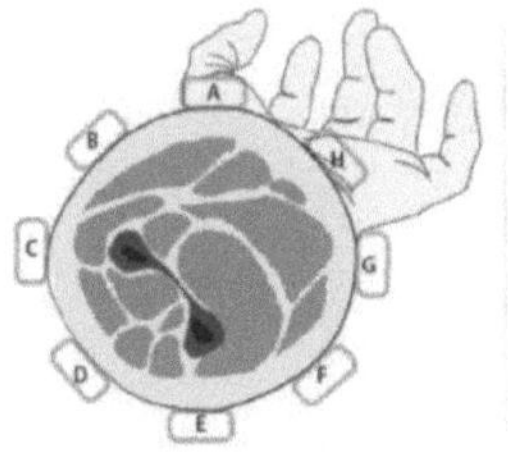

Figure 1: Principle of EIT from[6]. Electrodes A to H can be connected via multiplexers either to a current source or to a voltage measurement system.

For the classification of hand gestures, electromyography (EMG) signals are usually used [6]. However, these signals are susceptible to noise and could lead to missclassification. It could be shown that additional signal modalities like an inertial measurement unit could improve the classification results [8]. In addition, it could also be shown that EIT leads to good classifications [6]. Where EMG is based on biosignals and EIT on direct anatomical changes.

2 Material and Methods

The EIT consists of three main parts, the analog front end, the control software and the reconstruction algorithm. This means that not only the electrical circuit must be designed, but also a program for controlling and reconstruction for a microcontroller is needed.
The electrical circuit of EIT consist of a voltage controlled current source (VCCS), electrodes, amplifier and band-pass filter. VCCS can be used to provide required current. The band-pass filter has the function of filtering of noise such as noise from Wlan or EMG. The frequency band of the stimulus signal is 10 kHz to 50 kHz, so signals in the other bands will be filtered. INA 114, Texas Instruments, is used as instrumentation amplifier which is used to increase the measured signal. And LMC6482, Texas Instruments, is used for operational amplifier which is an indispensable component for VCCS. The circuit was designed and simulated in LTspice and then tested in the laboratory and compared with the simulation. The VCCS is shown in Fig. 2.
Considering the condition in Eq. (1), the output current of the circuit which depends only on the input voltage V_{in} and the resistor R1, as shown in Eq. (2). The bioimpedance is simulated by Z_L. The output current I_{out} generates a voltage drop across the load. This represents the signal to be measured, which can be used to calculate the impedance via Ohm's law. The power supply should also be noted, because to avoid a voltage inverter a virtual ground at 5 V is used. The other important thing is that many parameters should be tested, such as frequency and amplitude for V_{in} to deter-

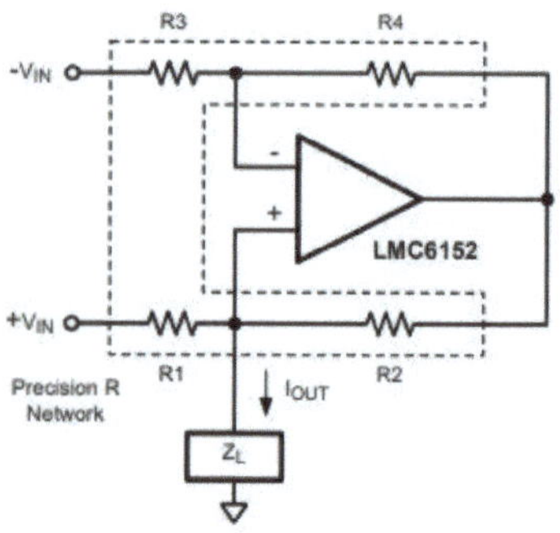

Figure 2: The figure shows the VCCS circuit from [1]. The current through a simulated load Z_L depends only on the input voltage and the resistance R1 according to Eq. (2), under the condition given in Eq. (1).

mine the best settings for measuring the bioimpedance.

$$R1/R2 = R3/R4 \tag{1}$$

$$I_{out} = V_{in}/R1 \tag{2}$$

There is also one microcontroller with an integrated analog-to-digital converter (ADC) and four multiplexers in the setup. The microcontroller should control the process, perform the ADC conversion and the reconstruction. Four multiplexers allow the measurement of different electrode combinations to cover the entire cross-section of the arm. Fig. 3 shows a block diagram of our EIT system.
A setup with four electrodes (four-pole) is more accurate than a setup with two electrodes (two-pole), because the four-pole measurement has two additional electrodes for measuring [2]. This prevents the disturbing influence of the voltage drop across the rather large impedance of the electrode skin contact. The two-pole and four-pole systems are shown in Fig. 4.
Assuming that the current through the voltage meter, which is the instrumentation amplifier, is approximated to zero, we see that in the two-pole measurement there is also a voltage drop across the skin impedances, while in the four-pole measurement this voltage drop is negligible. Thus the direct voltage across the bioimpedance can be measured in the four-pole system.
For the first setup an STM32 Nucleo Board from STMicroelectronics is used. It is similar to an adruino board, but based on an ARM architecture, which brings greater computational power and more functions like a more precise ADC and more GPIO pins. Moreover, the software for the microcontroller design involves control of the multiplexer and analysis of the data.
Multiplexers are used to control the different electrode combinations. This allows excitation and measurement with different electrode combinations. ADG1608, Analog Devices, is used for the multiplexer which can be used for analog signals. It contains three control signals, eight input and one output pin. It means, it can provide eight different input-output settings.

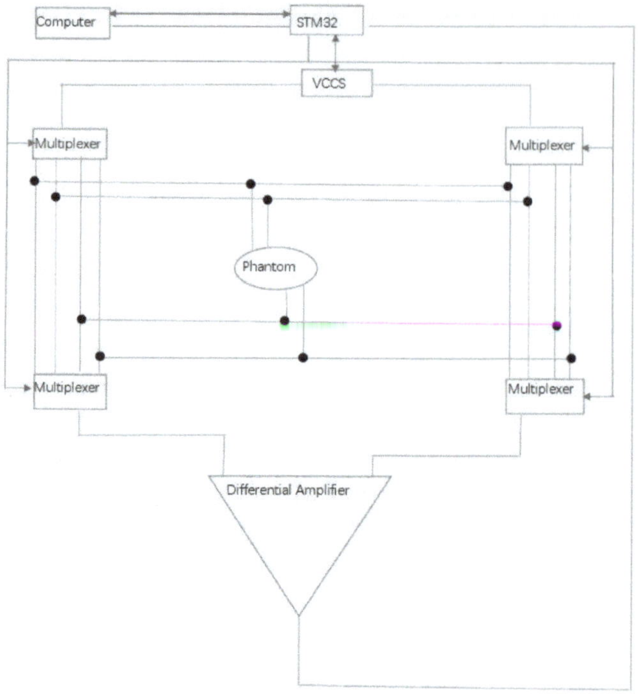

Figure 3: A schematic of our system. The line with double arrow describes the voltage signal. The line without arrow describes the current signal. The line with single arrow describes the control signal.

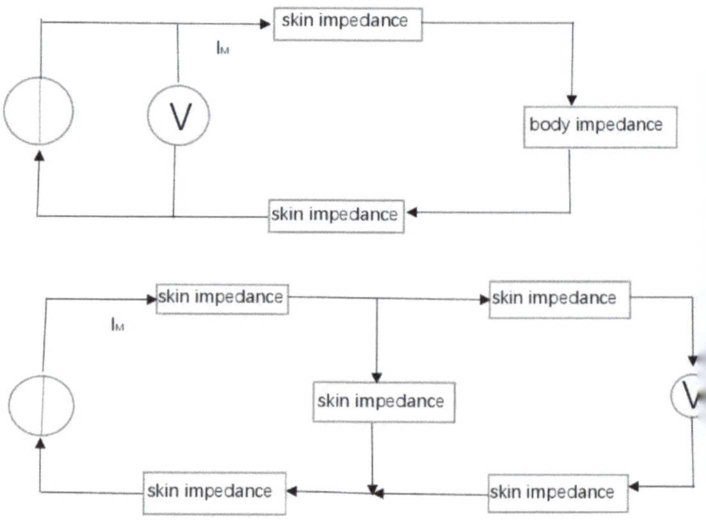

Figure 4: Basic measuring principle of four-pole and two-pole. The figure on the upper describes the two-pole system and the figure in the bottom describes the four-pole system.

Electrical generator and DC power supply are also necessary. Electrical generator provides reference signal with different frequency for the VCCS to generate AC current. A DC power supply is also needed as operating voltage for the VCCS and the multiplexer.

3 Results and Discussion

3.1 VCCS

A injected signal with 4 V and 100 Hz has been used in this experiment, the circuit is shown in Fig 2. The tested resistors is 500 Ω. With this example, it can be seen that the measured value is 3.99 mA with 100 Hz. The theoretical value of the experiment should be 4 mA with 100 Hz. Therefore, the relevant error can be calculated with the Eq. (3) which to be 0.25%.

$$f_{\%} = \frac{x - x_R}{x_R} * 100\% \tag{3}$$

The relevant error is $f_{\%}$, the measured value is x and the the theoretical value is x_R.

3.2 Simulation of Bioimpedance

Bioimpedance consist of not only resistance but also capacitance. To examine the circuit, it is simulated in LTspice. For this purpose, an equivalent circuit for the bio-impedance from [2, 3] is simulated.
Bioimpedance consist of the resistance of the skin and the capacitance of the skin as well as the inner resistance of the body. The resistance of the skin and the capacitance of the skin connect to each other in parallel. C1, R5 and C2, R6 are the skin impedance for the VCCS sources. R9 is the inner resistance of the body. C3, R7 and C4, R8 are the impedance of the skin for the measurement electrodes. Four electrodes are used, so there are four resistances of the skin and capacitances of the skin. The total resistance is about 1500 Ω and the total capacitance is approximately between 100 pF and 300 pF [3]. Among them, the inner resistance of the body is 500 Ω. The Signal from this simulated circuit is too weak for a direct analog digital conversion, therefore it has to be amplified by an instrumentation amplifier.
Two types of systems are simulated. The circuit with four-pole is shown in Fig. 5 and with two-pole is shown in Fig. 6. The same parameters have been used in the two systems.

The simulation results for these two systems are very different. The measured voltage of two-pole and four-pole system with different frequencies is shown in Table 1. The voltage of the two-pole system is higher, as expected, because the current also causes a voltage drop across the skin impedance. It is also to be expected that, the higher the injected frequency, the lower the simulated impedance, because the impedance in capacitor can be reduced with higher frequency. It is also ensured from the simulation that the injected signal with 10 kHz is best for the four-pole

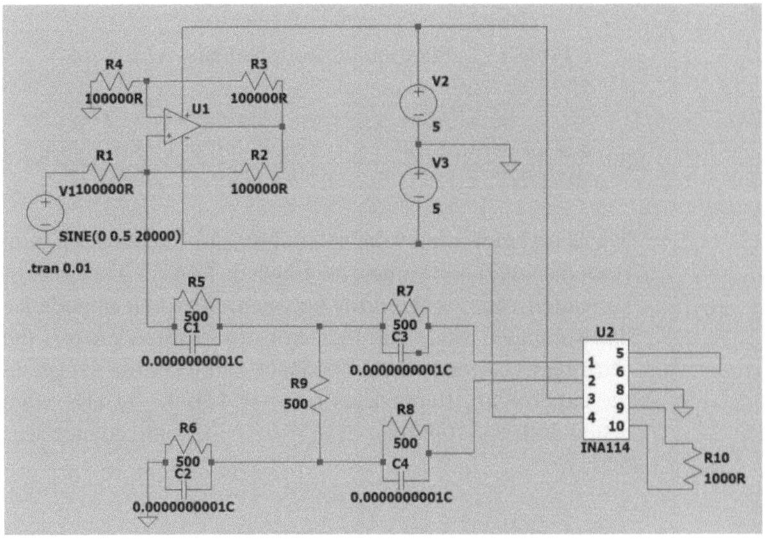

Figure 5: The simulated schematic of bioimpedance with two-pole. The injected voltage is 0.5 V and the resistors in VCCS are 100000 Ω, so the input current is 5 μA. The frequency is from 10 kHz to 40 kHz. The instrumentation amplifier has a magnification of 51.

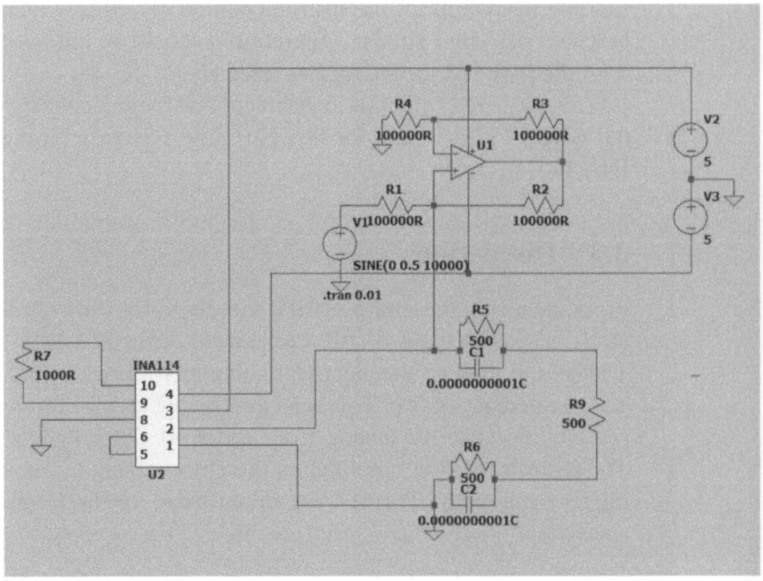

Figure 6: The simulated schematic of bioimpedance with two-pole. The injected voltage is 0.5 V and the resistors in VCCS are 100000 Ω, so the input current is 5 μA. The frequency is from 10 kHz to 40 kHz. The instrumentation amplifier has a magnification of 51.

system and the injected signal with 40 kHz is best for the two-pole system.

Table 1: Simulation of bioimpedance with 5 μA

Input-frequency(kHz)	10	20	30	40
Output-voltage(mV) for two-pole	315	234	180	141.6
Output-voltage(mV) for four-pole	110	79.36	120	48.1
Impedance for two-pole(Ω)	1235.29	917.65	705.88	555.3
Impedance for four-pole(Ω)	431.37	311.22	235.29	188.63

The actual measured values with four-pole are still different from the simulated values, as shown in Table 2. The error of simulated value is the error between measured impedance and simulated value and the error of test impedance is the error between measured impedance and test impedance. In the experiment, frequencies from 10 kHz to 40 kHz were tested with an amplitude of 0.5 V. The test impedance was 500 Ω.

Table 2: actual measured values with four-pole

Input-frequency(kHz)	10	20	30	40
Output-Voltage(mV)	129	111	94	80
Simulated value(mV)	109	79.36	60	48.1
Measured impedance(Ω)	505.88	435.29	368.63	313.73
Simulated value(Ω)	431.37	311.22	235.29	188.63
Error(%) of simulated value with respect to the simulated one	18.89	39.87	56	66.32
Error(%) of test impedance	1.18	12.94	26.27	37.25

Throught this experiment, it can be seen how much error of simulated value with respect to the simulated one is there in our system. From the table it can be concluded that the greater the frequency the greater the error. The reason is too low bandwidth of the instrumentation amplifier which reaches only up to 10 kHz. Therefore it should be replaced with the INA 128 for the further research.
It is also ensured from this experiment that the injected signal with 10 kHz is best for this four-pole system with the INA 114.

3.3 Discussion

From the result, the four-pole EIT with INA 114 works best at 10 kHz. But there is still a tolerance. Error is 1.18% . The reason may be the electrical components used, which have a tolerance of 5%. This is an important basis for future research because the analog front end works in principle. The instrumentation amplifier is thereby exchanged for a higher bandwidth. This is a important basic for the future research.

4 Conclusion

In this study an analog front end is designed for the usage in a low-cost EIT which will be the focus of the on going project. It may improve the control of prostheses. In addition, the EIT can also be combined with EMG in order to be adopted to prostheses and many other human-computer interfaces [4].

Acknowledgement

The work has been carried out and supervised at the Institute of Signal Processing. I would like to thank my tutor, Ole Thomsen.

Author's Statement

Conflict of interest: Authors state no conflict of interest
Informed consent: Informed consent has been told.

5 References

[1] Pease, Robert A, *AN-1515 A Comprehensive Study of the Howland Current Pump*.Texas Instruments, pp. 1–17, 2013

[2] S. Kaufmann, *Instrumentierung der Bioimpedanzmessung*. In: Optimierung mit Fokus auf die Elektroimpedanztomographie (EIT), Springer Publishing, Wiesbaden, pp. 15–16, 2015

[3] N. Leitgeb, *Sicherheit von Medizingeräten*, Springer Publishing, Berlin, Heidelberg, pp. 162–165, 2015.

[4] R. Kusche, M. Ryschka, *Combining Bioimpedance and EMG Measurements for Reliable Muscle Contraction Detection*. IEEE Sensors Journal. IEEE Publishing, pp. 11687–11696, 2019

[5] Y. Zhang, R. Xiao, C. Harrison, *Advancing Hand Gesture Recognition with High Resolution Electrical Impedance Tomography*. In Proceedings of the 29th Annual ACM Symposium on User interface Software and Technology. Association for Computing Machinery Publishing, New York, pp. 16–19, 2016

[6] Y. Zhang, C. Harrison, *Tomo: Wearable, Low-Cost, Electrical Impedance Tomography for Hand Gesture Recognition*. Proceedings of the 28th Annual ACM Symposium on User Interface Software & Technology. Association for Computing Machinery Publishing, New York, pp. 167–163, 2015

[7] S. Kaufmann, *Instrumentierung der Bioimpedanzmessung*. In: Optimierung mit Fokus auf die Elektroimpedanztomographie (EIT), Springer Publishing, Wiesbaden, pp. 1–2, 2015

[8] A. Krasoulis, I. Kyranou, M. Suphi Erden, K. Nazarpour, S. Vijayakumar, *Improved prosthetic hand control with concurrent use of myoelectric and inertial measurements*. Journal of Neuroengineering and Rehabilitation, Springer Publishing, pp. 1–14, 2017

2

Biomechanics

The Effect of Interference Fit and Loading Activity on Implant Fixation of a Titanium Press-fit Tibial Knee Implant

Carlos Javier Galdamez Calles [1], Robert Wendlandt [2], Corine Post [3]
[1] Biomedical Engineering, Universität zu Lübeck, carlos.galdamezcalles@student.uni-luebeck.de
[2] Clinic of Orthopedics, Universität zu Lübeck, robert.wendlandt@uk-sh.de
[3] Orthopaedic Research Laboratory, Radboud Institute for Health Sciences, Radboud University Medical Centre, Corine.Post@radboudumc.nl

Abstract

This investigation focused on exploring the effect of the interference fit and the loading activity on the resulting micromotions of a titanium tibial component. This was achieved by the generation of finite element simulations of the tibial bone and the implant. The results showed that the titanium implant generated higher resulting micromotions in a walking activity than in the knee bend activity. Then, by implementing an increase in the interference fit this showed that the micromotions increased too.

1 Introduction

Total Knee Arthroplasty (TKA) is one of the most common joint replacement procedures and has a primary goal of alleviating severe pain and inflammation caused by degenerative diseases such as osteoarthritis [1]. To restore the knee joint, the damaged joint is replaced by a tibial, femoral, and optionally a patellar component. Currently, the clinical default material of a tibial component is titanium due to its low elastic modulus compared to other metals and high biocompatibility [2]. During this investigation, the degree of response of utilizing a titanium implant was analyzed.

Understanding the potential of a certain material will help to provide a better prediction in the success of fixation of the tibial implant. A titanium implant has a particular material property; thus, it will act distinctively when it is exposed to a specific loading condition. Cemented implants are the usual practice for implant fixation but in this case, cementless press-fit implantation will be the studied scenario to properly evaluate its impact on the resulting micromotions. This type of implant obtains its stability through the interference fit between the tibia bone and the tibial component and this is surgically achieved by resecting the implant´s hole on the proximal part of the tibia slightly smaller compared the implant´s dimensions [3]. This parameter plays a key role in successful implant fixation as a balance needs to be met between a too small or a too large interference fit. If the interference fit is too large this can result in permanent damages in the bone and possible fractures. Then, if the value is too small this could result in a loose fixation and result in unwanted displacements from the implant [3].

The surface characteristics of cementless implants influences bone in-growth that would result in successful osseointegration [4]. The success of implantation is affected by the resulting micromotions. Micromotions can be defined as the relative shearing displacement of the implant with respect to the tibia [3]. The resulting micromotions should not surpass the permitted 50 μm boundary, as displacements larger than that will encourage the in-growth of fibrous tissue [5].

Loading in the knee can differ depending to the activity the implant is exposed to. Activities of such can include walking or squatting (Deep Knee Bend) and these will have a particular effect on the tibial implant due to the difference in their corresponding load distributions. Thus, the implant needs to be able to adapt to the exposure of multiple forces and stresses to avoid complications in the future.

The purpose of this investigation was to model relative micromotions of a titanium tibial implant using finite element simulations in a walking and knee bend activity. This would help to evaluate the response of the tibial implant by assessing the resulting micromotions on the base-plate whenever the implant was exposed to a particular loading activity or an increase in its interference fit.

2 Material and Methods

Finite Element models of both the tibial component and the tibial bone were generated to evaluate the resulting micromotions. The model for the bone was obtained by segmentation from a CT scan. The reliability of the titanium tibial implant was evaluated through different combination of parameters that were applied. This resulted in a specific value for the micromotions.

2.1 Meshing and Model Adjustment

The alignment of the tibial component and, the definition of the hole to fix the implant inside the bone were one of the first steps to consider. This alignment and hole resection were performed in the software Simlab 2018. After the mentioned steps were fulfilled the models were transferred to Hypermesh to create 3D meshes from the aligned surface meshes that were generated seen in Figure 1.

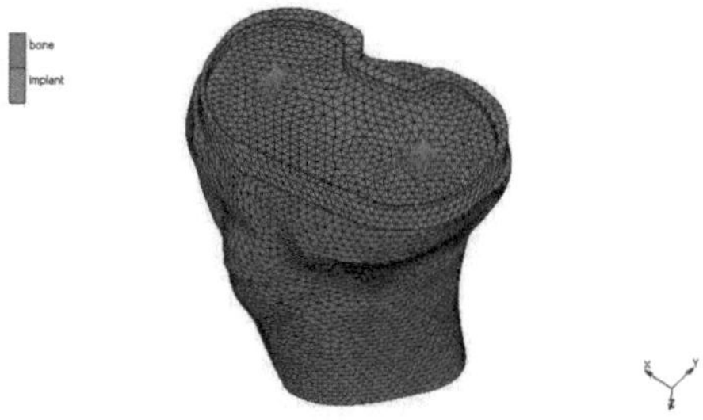

Figure 1: Aligned 3D meshes of tibia and implant models

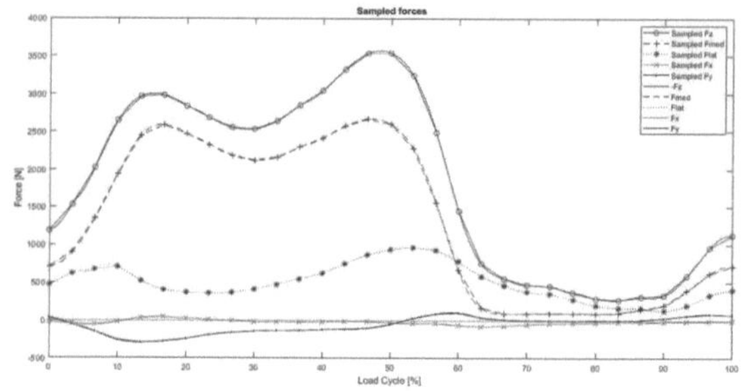

Figure 2: Sampled force distribution in a regular gait cycle

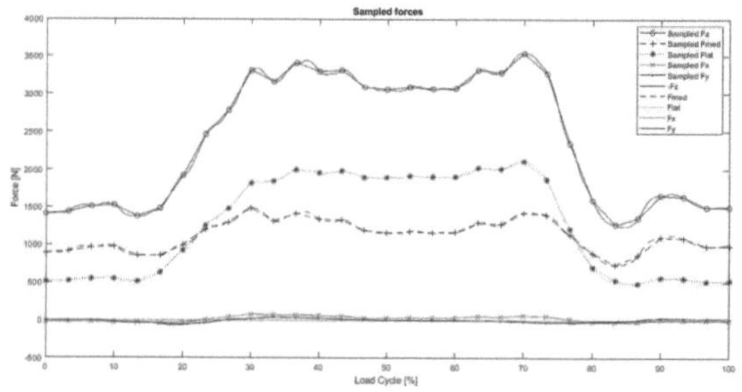

Figure 3: Sampled forces distribution in a deep knee bend scenario

2.2 Material Properties and Loading Conditions

For the titanium implant, the material property chosen was a Young´s Modulus of 109 GPa and a Poisson ratio of 0.33 as an elastic isotropic material. For the tibia bone, this was done with the use of a Matlab script that determined the material properties of the bone for each element of its finite element model, as the density in the bone changes depending in the location of the element. It consisted in matching the orientation of the created model including its resection to the complete CT scan of the tibia. Then with a calibration phantom the corresponding Hounsfield Units were converted to its calcium values and those calcium values were then used to calculate its Young´s modulus values [6]. The bone´s material was selected to be a elastic-plastic material.

The loading of the implant was divided into two types, for a regular gait cycle (Figure 2) and for a deep knee bend scenario (Figure 3) and the applied loads for these cases was obtained from the Orthoload database [7]. These forces in axial and shear direction were sampled using a Matlab script and from the 601 provided data points, a sampling rate of 20 was chosen that resulted in 31 sampled points. The mentioned forces were applied in two separate nodes where the forces were set accordingly to the medial and lateral side of the tibia as Figures 2 and Figure 3 can infer.

The medial forces (Fmed) and lateral forces (Flat) represent the distribution of the total axial force in the medial and lateral side of the tibia bone. The magnitude of these two forces differed depending on the activity that is taking place. The amount of force transferred to the medial side can be calculated using the moment that is generated in the varus-valgus direction (My), the total axial force (Fz) and the distance between the condyles [8] and this can be presented in the following formula (1):

$$F_{med} = \frac{|F_z|}{2} - \frac{M_y}{l}. \qquad (1)$$

Then the addition of Fmed and Flat must equal Fz, thus a simple subtraction can be done to calculate the values for Flat. Another important parameter to consider from this Fmed would be the medial force ratio (MFR) this helps to represent in what percentage is the total axial force distributed on the medial and the lateral side of the tibia plateau [8]. This can be expressed visually with the help of Figure 4 and Figure 5 as well as in a mathematical expression from equation (2):

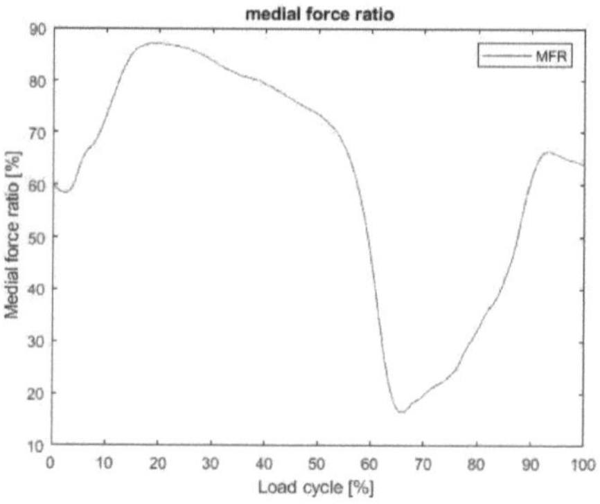

Figure 4: Medial force ratio for a walking activity

$$MFR[\%] = \frac{F_{med}}{|-F_z|} \times 100 \qquad (2)$$

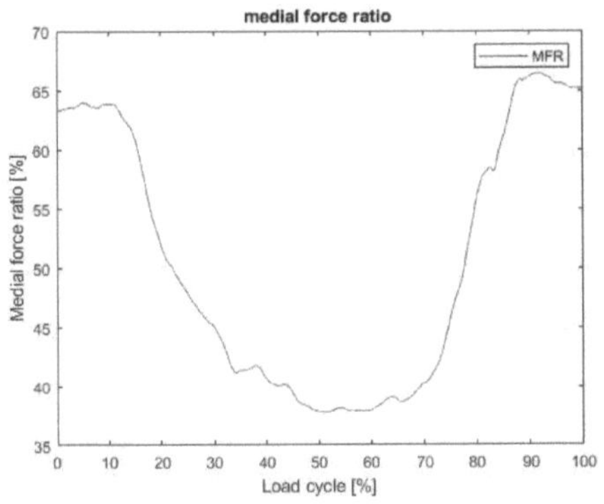

Figure 5: Medial force ratio for a knee bend activity

2.3 Boundary Conditions and Simulation Parameters

Two fixed displacements were set. One of them involved the fixation of the distal part of the tibia model, where an immobilization of these nodes was required. Secondly, the placement of the implant into the bone was also simulated, thus, the model of the implant was translated 50 μm away from the bone and linearly it was moved back to its wanted position once the simulation started in the initial phase. The two point loads were placed where the femoral component enters in contact with the polymer insert (Figure 6):

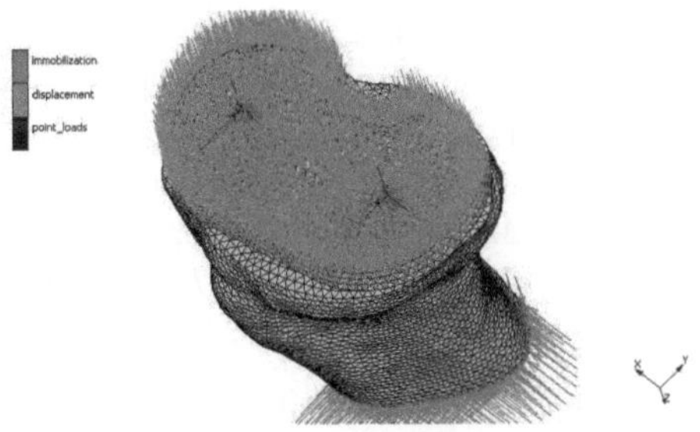

Figure 6: Chosen boundary conditions in the finite element model

Other important chosen parameters were the interference fit of the tibial component and the tibia bone that was set to 0.25 mm, 0.50 mm and 0.75 mm because this would cover a sensible range for this parameter and the friction coefficient between the contacts of the models that was set to 0.5. Additionally the total number of increments that were set was divided into the implantation phase where the interference fit would linearly increase up to one of the three values that were used. Followed by the loading phase that incorporated four full load cycles of the sampled forces that allowed the implant to settle in its position and where the interference fit remained constant.

The total number of simulated cases was six. This included the comparison between the walking and deep knee-bend scenario that used an interference fit of 0.25 mm, 0.50 mm and 0.75 mm for the titanium implant. The resulting micromotions helped to compare how the implant would react to various combinations of parameters that was present.

The resulting micromotions that were assessed was the 95th percentile of the simulated micromotions and this was done to avoid numerical errors that could generate sudden peaks in nodes and could also be interpreted as misleading when those type of results was considered.

3 Results and Discussion

The results of the micromotions were represented in one mayor table with the most significant data:

Table 1: Resulting micromotions of the titanium implant

Activity	Interference Fit [mm]	Micromotions [μm]
Walking	0.25	18.07
Walking	0.50	20.31
Walking	0.75	21.60
Knee Bend	0.25	10.72
Knee Bend	0.50	19.37
Knee Bend	0.75	20.11

The scenario that resulted in the highest micromotions was the walking activity with 21.60 μm with an interference fit of 0.75 mm. The resulting micromotions concentrated on the lateral side of the base-plate in this activity (Figure 7). In the knee bend scenario, the micromotions were in the posterior medial side of the base-plate (Figure 8) of the titanium implant and the highest value that was generated was 20.11 μm. Overall the resulting micromotions were lower in the knee bend activity than in the walking activity and this could be caused by the difference in MFR between the two activities. As medial forces are significantly higher than the lateral forces in the walking scenario the implant will be held very tight in that side making the lateral side looser generating a tilting motion towards the medial side seen in the titanium implant. In the knee bend activity, the MFR is not as large as in the walking activity and lateral forces are higher with less difference than the medial forces. That means that in this activity the implant will be held tighter on the lateral side and concentrate the micromotions in the medial side of the base-plate.

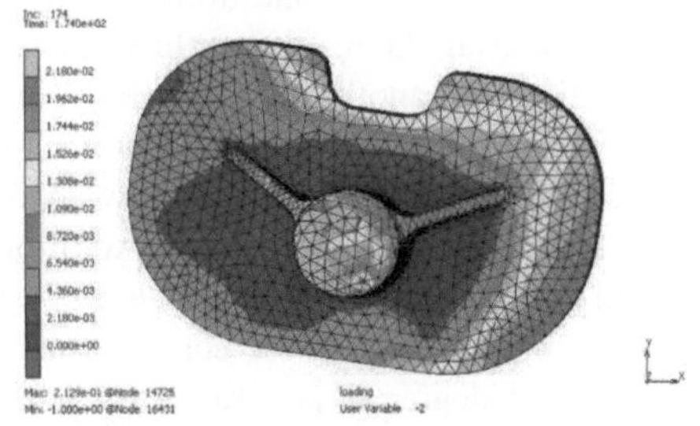

Figure 7: Resulting micromotions during walking activity with interference fit of 0.25 mm

As the results showed, increasing the interference fit resulted in higher resulting micromotions. This is the case because as the interference fit remains low, the easier it is to

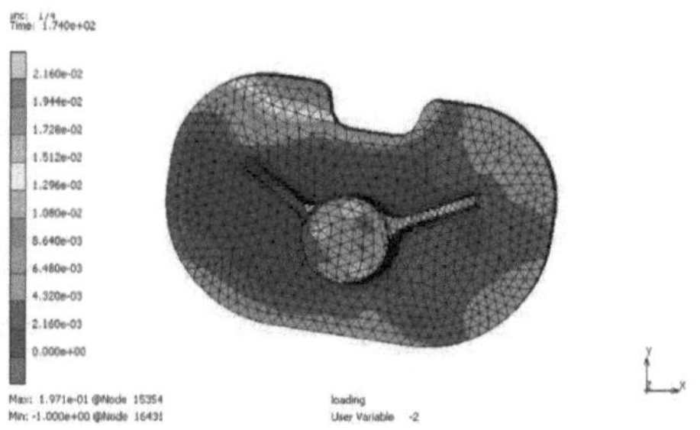

Figure 8: Resulting micromotions during knee bend activity with interference fit of 0.25 mm

introduce the implant to the bone. Then as less force is nec essary, the implant can successfully be fixed to its wanted position without permanently harming the bone. Nevertheless, too low interference fits could also generate high micromotions as the implantation would be too loose and the implant would not be able to fix properly. Then, when the interference fit is large, a higher force is necessary to introduce the implant to the bone and as this is performed, this could permanently damage the bone or create possible fractures that would compromise future stability. Thus, a clear compromise needs to be done in order to select an adequate value for this parameter. The values for the resulting micromotions when the interference fit was 0.25 mm were 18.07 μm for the walking activity and 10.72 μm for the knee bend activity.

4 Conclusion

A series of finite element simulations were carried out in order to evaluate the response of a titanium implant when it was exposed to walking and knee bend activity, as well as evaluating the effect a change in the interference fit would have in such response. The titanium implant showed resulting micromotions that were below the currently known limit of 50 μm. This reinforces the reliability of titanium as the default material for a tibia component. The resulting micromotions for the titanium implant were always higher in the walking activity than in the knee bend activity. An area of focus would be to compare the behavior of the titanium implant under the investigated conditions with the one from another type of material, the results could validate potential alternatives to utilize for another type of tibial component. Future research could include a higher number of different loading scenarios, this would cover a wider variety of activities that present themselves daily. Additionally, the cuts performed in the finite element models were generated completely straight. In reality these cuts are manually performed with a lower degree of accurateness. Trying to implement this change in the tibia model would be an area of interest because the response of the implant to this new surface could lead to a direct impact on micromotions. The depth of the research could be further developed by exploring a variation in set parameters like the coefficient of friction. This could give a larger foundation to evaluate how the implant would respond to other combinations because it influences the contact between the models thus, the resulting micromotions could also be affected by this.

Acknowledgement

The work has been carried out at the Orthopedic Research Laboratory in Radboudumc in Nijmegen, the Netherlands and supervised by the Clinic of Orthopedics at Universität zu Lübeck.

Author's Statement

Conflict of interest: Authors state no conflict of interest.

5 References

[1] J. ping Wang, D. Guo, S. hua Wang, Y. qiang Yang, and G. Li, 'Structural stability of a polyetheretherketone femoral component—A 3D finite element simulation', *Clin. Biomech.*, vol. 70, pp. 153–157, Dec. 2019, doi: 10.1016/j.clinbiomech.2019.09.001.

[2] M. Long and H. J. Rack, 'Titanium alloys in total joint replacement - A materials science perspective', Biomaterials, vol. 19, no. 18. Elsevier Sci Ltd, pp. 1621–1639, Sep. 1998, doi: 10.1016/S0142-9612(97)00146-4.

[3] Berahmani, M. Hendriks, D. Wolfson, A. Wright, D. Janssen, and N. Verdonschot, 'Experimental preclinical assessment of the primary stability of two cementless femoral knee components', *J. Mech. Behav. Biomed. Mater.*, vol. 75, pp. 322–329, Nov. 2017, doi: 10.1016/j.jmbbm.2017.07.043.Improbable Research, vol. 12, no. 5, pp. 16–21, 2006.

[4] P. V. Papas, D. Congiusta, and F. D. Cushner, 'Cementless versus Cemented Fixation in Total Knee Arthroplasty', *J. Knee Surg.*, vol. 32, no. 7, pp. 596–599, 2019, doi: 10.1055/s-0039-1678687.

[5] M. J. Cross and J. Spycher, 'Cementless fixation techniques in joint replacement', in *Joint Replacement Technology*, Elsevier Ltd., 2008, pp. 190–211.

[6] J. H. Keyak, T. S. Kaneko, J. Tehranzadeh, and H. B. Skinner, "Predicting proximal femoral strength using structural engineering models," *Clin. Orthop. Relat. Res.*, no. 437, pp. 219–228, 2005.

[7] 'Standard Loads Knee Joint OrthoLoad'. https://orthoload.com/test-loads/standard-loads-knee-joint/ (accessed Jan. 08, 2021).

[8] I. Kutzner, A. Trepczynski, M. O. Heller, and G. Bergmann, 'Knee Adduction Moment and Medial Contact Force – Facts about Their Correlation during Gait', *PLoS One*, vol. 8, no. 12, p. e81036, Dec. 2013, doi: 10.1371/journal.pone.0081036.

Design of a Biomechanical Test setup to analyze the Symphysis Pubic motion under physiological loads

Mouayad Boukai [1], Robert Wendlandt [2],
[1] Biomedical Engineering, Luebeck University of Applied Sciences, mouayad.boukai@stud.th-luebeck.de

[2] Biomechanics Laboratory, Clinic for Orthopedic and Trauma Surgery, University Medical Center, robert.wendlandt@th-luebeck.de

Abstract

The current state of the art in the orthopedic treatment of pubic symphysis rupture does not present an appropriate solution for the fixation technique. While in orthopedic surgery plate osteosynthesis is a routine practice to relink the two pelvic bones after fracture reduction, this method does not consider the special structure of the pubic symphysis, which often leads to detachment or failure of the implant. Due to the exceptional flexibility of the fibrocartilage connection between the two pelvic bones special mechanical requirements result for the used osteosynthesis method. In order to improve the current fixation techniques and develop new approaches, this work aims to establish a test-rig to determine the translational and rotational movability at the pubic symphysis using synthetic bone.

1 Introduction

A symphyseal pelvic rupture is known to have some serious consequences, because it could lead to instability of the entire pelvic ring. Any failure in the fracture treatment and the fracture fixation can lead to a permanent pain and a restricted movement. These kinds of symphysis ruptures might occur by severe accidents and sometimes it can be caused during childbirth to women [1]. Pelvic ring injuries without loss of stability are referred to as fracture type A, pelvic ring injuries with rotational loss of stability and retained vertical stability are classified as fracture type B and pelvic ring injuries with rotational and vertical instability, complete shift and displacement of half pelvis are fracture type C see figure 1 [2]. Stabilizing a pelvic ring after a fracture is not an easy work due to its physical and biomechanical behavior, which involves considerable physical stresses on the symphysis.
Several methods of bridging were previously established but different types of failures were a real challenge; dislocation of the implant, breakage of screws or complete material failure in the osteosynthesis plate could occur, that happens when the symphyseal bridge absorbs forces in different direction after treatment [5]. To avoid any failure or malfunction in the fixation of the symphyseal rupture and to increase the chance of healing outcome, mechanical tests should be done to measure the translation and the rotation at the symphysis without fixation. Afterwards, the best fixation method for different types of pelvic ruptures accompanying the symphyseal rupture could be determined.
For the purpose of determining the potential of the pelvic bone and the resulting force until mechanical failure of the test objects, different research groups developed some different techniques; cementing the femoral head into the acetabulum was one of the good approaches, where the symphysis joint has been fixed with a transducer and the load was applied from the other half of the pelvis [4]. Various approaches had been followed to described the simulation of muscle contraction; representing the transmitted forces at a hip using a loaded ball on the sacrum and the muscle pulls were implemented by nylon cords attached between the femur and the iliac [3]. Another work represented cyclic loads which were implemented as sinusoidal forces using a universal testing machine with a camera to measure the displacement, additionally, cable pulleys were attached to the iliac to stimulate hip abductor muscles contractions. [7].
In this work, a mechanical test setup is to be designed in which an unconstrained load is to be applied to the pelvis from its sacrum, in a simulated one-leg stance. A specimen is to undergo a testing procedure simulating consequences for the symphysis fracture and serves to determine the movements at the symphysis joint. The design has to take the actual orientation of the pelvic and its anatomical position into consideration. In addition to a simple model of the muscular forces applied in one hemiarthroplasty, these help to obtain almost realistic values which further analysis could rely on it later.

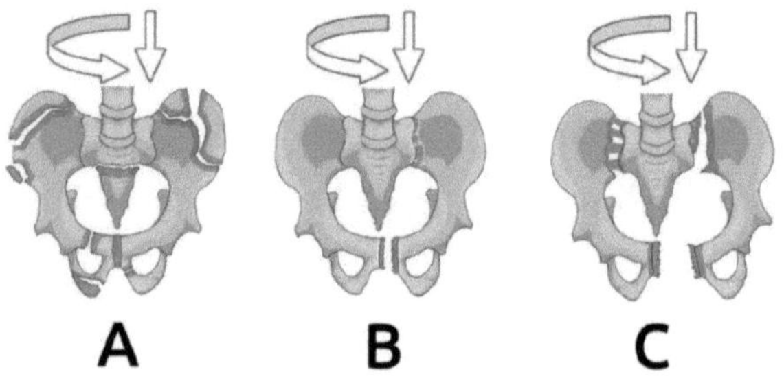

Figure 1: Classification of pelvic ring injuries (Amboss GmbH 2019).

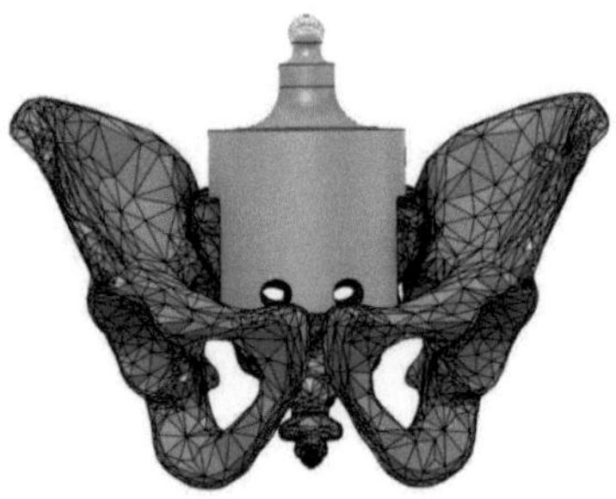

Figure 2: Load-hat fixed on the sacrum.

2 Material and Methods

The CAD program Autodesk Fusion 360 was used for design and modeling. The 3D-design comprises a setup which consists of a full pelvis (Data Base Center for Life Science, Source; BodyParts3D), fixed plastic hat located on the sacrum with a spherical top (to avoid constrained loading), femur and cables which are attached to the hemiarthroplasty to simulate the abductor pull and a third cable fixed in the ischium to prevent rotation of hemipelvis around the femoral head under loading. The cables tensioned to balance the system before loading from the sacrum [6]. These cables are made of high-performance PE-fiber which (Dyneema), which is more durable than nylon or steel cables of the same diameter. The remaining components were designed according to the requirements of the test setup and adapted to the dimensions of the testing machine.

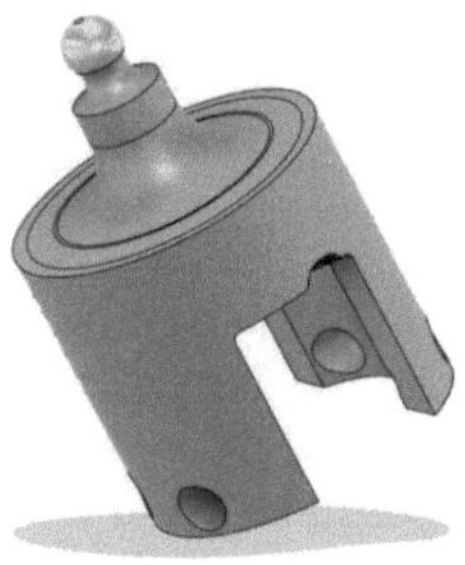

Figure 3: Load-hat detailed view

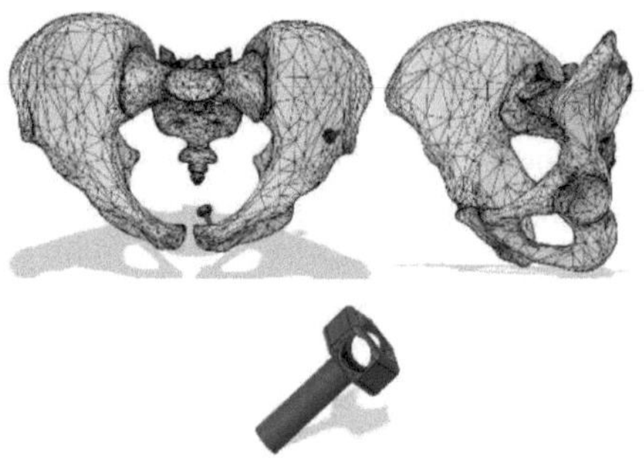

Figure 4: Hip control screws with its location on the pelvis.

3 Results and Discussion

The setup was specially designed for testing a full pelvis and aimed to determine the motions at the symphysis joint. The pelvis is positioned in such a way that the symphysis joint is visible from the front and the movement at this point can be determined that is shown in figure 2, 3. The load-hat is designed in a way that exactly fits the sacrum without any gap or space. The hat body is designed and set to be manufactured from plastic, which is assumed to be better for transferring the load, while the sphere is to be made from a femoral head component made out of CoCr-alloy with a diameter of 32 mm. The hat is fixed with two screws in the sacrum to avoid any motion which could lead to inconsistency of load transfer.

As shown in figure 4, three screws were designed to hold the tensioned cables which represent the muscle pulls. This is a simple method to simulate the muscle contractions which helps for easier control and less percentage of failure.
Figure 5 shows the femur and the femoral head, this special design consists of a metallic stick and a pulley. All components work as one system to help for more realistic functionality between the hip and the femur. The three cables which are to be rigidly attached to the iliac and the ischium have to be tightened by routing them through the metallic stick then wrapping them around the pulley to adjust their recommended tension.
The last version of the system shown in figure 6, illustrates the simple mechanism and the aim of this testing setup. The homogenous combination of the above components would easily interact to transfer the exerted load from the load-hat to the pubic symphysis, providing a simplified version of a complex body mechanics.
In comparison to existing test rigs, the developed test set-up differs from previous biomechanical tests through the high variability and adaptability to the test object. Monitoring of the pelvis has to be considered to take movement measurements at the pubic symphysis. The realized test setup in this work is characterized by its flexible application facilities and its simple and replicable composition.
For further optimization of the test setup, problems in prior studies were taken into consideration; nonuniform force distribution was one of the biggest challenges. However, in

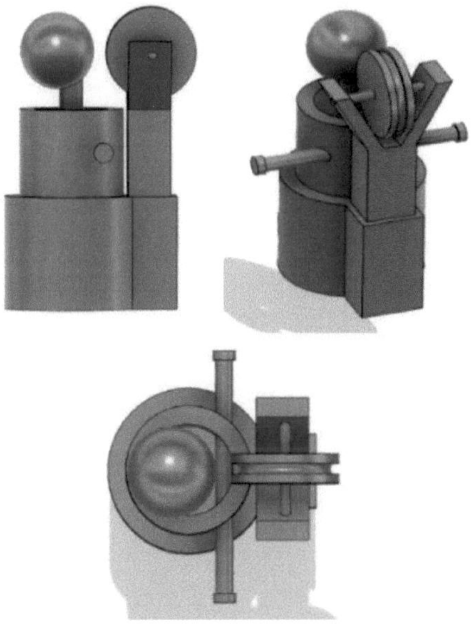

Figure 5: Femur and Abductor Pull Setup.

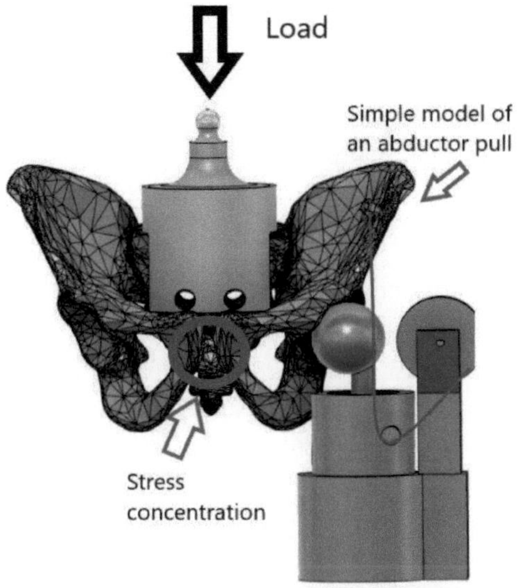

Figure 6: The full testing setup showing the load direction and stressing points.

this test setup, a whole pelvis model is used where the pressure is to be applied to the sacrum which in its turn would transfer the load towards the symphysis. The avoidance of the rotation in the whole system and creating a prior equilibrium to the pelvis model with three cables maintain a realistic functionality. Furthermore, a maximum load on pubic symphysis under specific adjustment and circumstances is achieved in this setup. One more challenge could make the procedure of establishing the setup harder than what is expected during the design phase, is the complex nature of the pelvis due to the presence of lots of curves and bends on its surface, which makes it difficult to manufacture the testing components and then fixing them accurately on the pelvis. Additionally, the unique orientation of the pelvis stands against the establishment of a simple setup, while positioning the pelvis during testing without affecting the load transfer from the sacrum to the symphysis is quite hard to manage.

Improvement in the design of the pelvis model with the screw would help to achieve more accurate movement. The number of screws can be increased to distribute the cables in a more complicated but realistic manner as in a real human muscle. Then the effect after applying pressure would allow more precise observation. A motor unit could also be installed in the whole system to simulate the actual physical muscle contraction. since the direction and strength of the muscle contractions cannot be exactly determined, the probability of obtaining a slight error in the testing outcome is present.

A determination of the load on symphysis is essential for force and moment measurements. For the movement measurement, an adjustment of the plastic hat and the modeled femur must be carefully selected. As the whole test setup is for determining the motion on the symphysis through the sacrum, it is planned to append additional elements and some existing components later, e.g. screws and a motor to properly include the muscle contraction. The determined final load would help to identify requirements for a setup of the real human pelvis. Furthermore, since the load is to be performed directly via a universal testing machine, there would be no need for osteosynthesis techniques to measure the loads.

4 Conclusion

The symphyseal pelvic rupture and the pelvic fracture can be determined from the modeled test setup in this work. The simulation of the real testing with this setup would ensure its efficiency and suitability, to analyze the symphysis pubic motion under different loading conditions. The overall tension value at which the femur setup will be simulated can be defined for a specific material type. Lastly, different loading situations can be stated and their effect can be examined to determine the maximum load before the clinical failure of the test objects by attaching the external elements to the pelvis.

Acknowledgement

The work has been carried out at Biomechanics Laboratory, Clinic for Orthopedic and Trauma Surgery, University Medical Center, University of Lübeck.

Author's Statement

Authors state no conflict of interest. Informed consent

5 References

[1] Hofmann, D. Vergleichende Untersuchung verschiedener stabilisierungsverfahren bei der Luxation der Beckenhalbgelenke. Unfallchirurgie 17, 247–252 (1991). https://doi.org/10.1007/BF02588402

[2] Baierlein, Sammy A., Frakturklassifikationen. Stuttgart: Georg Thieme Verlag, 2011.

[3] JANKU, D. Vergleichende biomechanische Untersuchungen zur internen Stabilisierung der Symphyse am Beckenring. Bringen winkelstabile Osteosynthesen Vorteile? (Doctoral dissertation, Saarland University, Saarbrücken , Germany), P.54-75, 2011.

[4] Hohlbaum,Harald, Vergleichende Stabilitätsmessung an der Symphyse zwischen einer herkömmlichen Doppelplattenosteosynthese und einem selbstentwickelten Fixateur interne am Knochenmodell (Doctoral dissertation, Ernst-Moritz-Arndt-University, Greifswald , Germany), P. 25–27, 2014.

[5] Kinzi, L. et al., Therapie der Symphysensprengung und Ilio- sacralgelenksluxationen. In: Hefte Unfallheilk. (140), P. 233–238, 1997.

[6] MacAvoy MC, McClellan RT, Goodman SB, Chien CR, Allen WA, van der Meulen MC., Stability of open-book pelvic fractures using a new biomechanical model of single-limb stance. J Orthop Trauma. 11:590–3, 1997.

[7] G. Osterhoff1 et al., Symphyseal internal rod fixation versus standard plate fixation for open book pelvic ring injuries: a biomechanical study. Eur J Trauma Emerg Surg, 42:197–202, 2016

Influence of high pressure balloon aortic valvuloplasty on the hydrodynamic result after valve-in-valve procedure

Denise Bruhn [1], Michael Scharfschwerdt [2], Stephan Ensminger [2] and Buntaro Fujita [3]
[1]Medical Engineering, Universität zu Lübeck, denise.bruhn@student.uni-luebeck.de
[2]Department of Cardiac and Thoracic Vascular Surgery, University Hospital of Schleswig-Holstein, Lübeck, Germany
[3]Department of Cardiac and Thoracic Vascular Surgery, University Hospital of Schleswig-Holstein, Lübeck Campus, Germany, buntaro.fujita@uksh.de

Abstract

Transcatheter valve-in-valve (ViV) procedures are performed to treat degenerated surgical bioprostheses in aortic position. In order to improve the functional result bioprosthetic valve fracture (BVF) using high pressure ballon aortic valvuloplasty (HP-BAV) has been introduced. The aim of this study was to evaluate the feasibility of BVF and its influence on the hydrodynamic result of a ViV procedure. The hydrodynamic properties of the Evolut R® 26 mm were evaluated after implantation as a ViV procedure in three surgical bioprostheses (Perimount Magna Ease®, Epic Supra® and Trifecta®) using a pulse duplicator. The Evolut R was evaluated before and after HP-BAV of the surgical valves using a non-compliant balloon with a diameter of 22 mm. The Evolut R® showed improved hydrodynamic function in all three surgical valves after HP-BAV compared to before HP-BAV. HP-BAV may be able to improve the functional result after a ViV procedure, even if BVF was not achieved.

1 Introduction

Within a person's life, over time, natural degeneration and changes in the physiological properties of the heart valves can occur. The aortic valve is particularly often affected by valve stenosis or insufficiency.
Surgical aortic valve replacement (SAVR) is used to treat aortic valve stenosis in young patients with a low risk of surgery. For this procedure, the chest is opened through sternotomy, cardiopulmonary bypass is established and the diseased valve is replaced with a prosthesis under direct vision.
In most cases, a biological prosthesis is used, which carries the risk of degeneration while still alive, which may require a redo SAVR. Transcatheter aortic valve implantation (TAVI) offers an alternative option, which allows to replace the valve without sternotomy and cardiopulmonary bypass. TAVI is a catheter-based procedure in which the insufficiently functioning heart valve is not removed. Instead, a biological valve prosthesis is crimped and delivered to the aortic valve using a catheter and expanded inside the old valve. This so called valve-in-valve (ViV) procedure is established as a safe and effective means of treating surgical bioprosthetic valve failure in patients at high risk for complications related to reoperation [1]. It has been shown that the hemodynamic result depends largely on the size of the previously implanted valve, as the maximum degree of valve expansion is limited by the inner diameter of the previously implanted surgical bioprosthesis [2], [3]. High pressure balloon aortic valvuloplasty (HP-BAV) is a novel technique to address this problem. Here, the stent frame of the old valve is fractured using a non-compliant balloon in order to enlarge the valve diameter.
In the past, few case reports have been published. However, there are no systematically collected data that quantify the improvement in the hemodynamic situation. The aim of this work was therefore to investigate this issue in a standardized *in vitro* setup.

2 Material and Methods

Small surgical bioprostheses with a labelled size of 21mm were used. Three different types of bioprostheses were chosen: the Trifecta (St. Jude Medical, Little Canada, Minnesota, USA), Perimount Magna Ease (Edwards Lifescience, Irvine, California, USA) and the Epic Supra (St. Jude Medical, Minnesota, USA), see Fig. 1.

2.1 Valve-in-valve procedure and high pressure balloon aortic valvuloplasty

The CoreValve Evolut-R 26 mm (Medtronic, Little Canada, Minnesota, USA) was used for ViV procedure (see Fig. 1D). The Evolut R was crimped according to the manufacturer's instruction for use and deployed inside the surgical valves under direct vision. The implantation position was chosen according to the "Valve in Valve Aortic app".

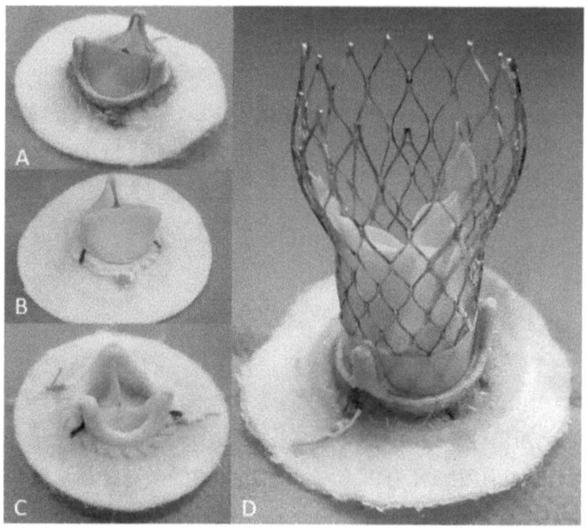

Figure 1: The picture shows three different biological valve prostheses which were used for the measurements in this project. **A** shows the Perimount (21mm), **B** is the Trifecta (21mm) and **C** the Epic (21mm). The TAVI prostheses CoreValve Evolut-R (26mm), which was used for the valve-in-valve procedure, is shown in D, in a valve-in-valve prostheses with the Perimount.

Fracture of the surgical bioprostheses was attempted by HP-BAV using a non-compliant balloon of the size 22 mm x 40 mm (ATLAS® PTA Dilatation Catheter, Bard Peripheral Vascular, Inc, Tempe, Arizona, USA, see Fig. 2). The balloon was placed within the surgical bioprostheses and inflated with saline. The pressure at which the valve fractured was recorded.

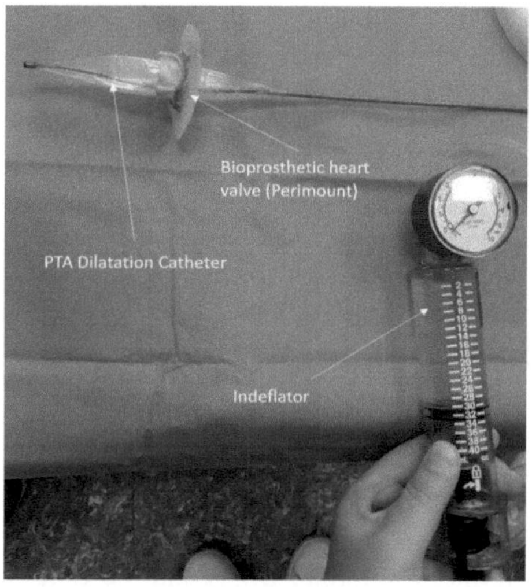

Figure 2: Detonation of the Perimount valve using a non-compliant balloon of the size 22 mm x 40 mm and indeflator.

2.2 Assessment of the functional performance of the Evolut R prosthesis

The hydrodynamic performance of the Evolut R prosthesis deployed inside the surgical valves was evaluated using a pulse duplicator, which was developed by Scharfschwerdt et al. [4]. The device mimics the essential functions of the left ventricle and enables to assess the hydrodynamic properties (e.g. transvalvular pressure gradient (TVP), effective opening area (EOA)) of the valve in accordance with ISO standards [4], [5], [6]. For the measurements, the pulse duplicator was perfused with isotonic saline at 37 °C. During the measurements, valve cusp kinematics were recorded using a high speed camera (Motionpro Y3-1000, Image Solutions GmbH, Eningen, Germany). The hydrodynamic performance of the Evolut R inside the surgical valves was investigated before and after HP-BAV.
Six measurements were made with each ViV combination. Subsequently the ViV was mounted in the aortic valve compartment of the pulse duplicator. One measurement cycle corresponds to 10 successive heartbeats. The measurements were made at a heart rate of 64 beats per minute and four different stroke volume settings for each ViV combination.

2.3 Statistical analysis

The hydrodynamic performance (EOA and TVP) of the Evolut R inside of each surgical valve was compared before and after HP-BAV. Numerical variables are expressed as mean ± standard deviation as they followed a normal distribution or graphically as box plots. EOA and TVP before and after HP-BAV were compared using Student's t-test. A two-sided p-value <0.05 was considered statistically significant. All statistical analyses were performed using SPSS Statistics for Windows, Version 26.0. (IBM Corp. Released 2019. IBM, Armonk, NY: IBM Corp) and R: A language and environment for statistical computing (R Foundation for Statistical Computing, Vienna, Austria).

3 Results and Discussion

HP-BAV led to BVF of the Perimount (PME) and Epic Supra (EP), while the Trifecta (TRF) could not be fractured. The PME and EP fractured at balloon pressures of 15 atm (**atm**ospheric pressure) and 8 atm, respectively. The TRF did not fracture until a pressure of 25 atm. Instead, at this pressure, the balloon ruptured. The Evolut R 26 mm showed significantly greater EOA after HP-BAV compared with before HP-BAV in all three bioprostheses as shown in Fig. 3. The following information of the two parameters (TVP and EOA) all correspond to the impact volume setting 5, because it becomes closest to the natural physiology of a heart valve. Table 1 below lists the measured values of all stroke volume settings. The values (before / after) for the Perimount were 1.64±0.06 / 1.99±0.02 cm^2, $p<0.001$, for the Trifecta 1.63±0.03 / 1.83±0.06 cm^2, $p<0.001$, and for the Epic 1.19±0.06 / 1.54±0.04, $p<0.001$. Similarly, TVP was significantly smaller after HP-BAV. The values for the Perimount were 7.73±0.68 / 5.69±0.18 cm^2, $p<0.001$, for the Trifecta 7.95±0.33 / 6.51±0.39 cm^2, $p<0.001$ and for the Epic 13.16±1.28 / 8.55±0.52, $p<0.001$ (see Fig. 4).
Still images of the Evolut R inside the EP in closed position before and after HP-BAV are shown in Fig. 5. After HP-BAV, the coaptation lines of the cusps of the Evolut R

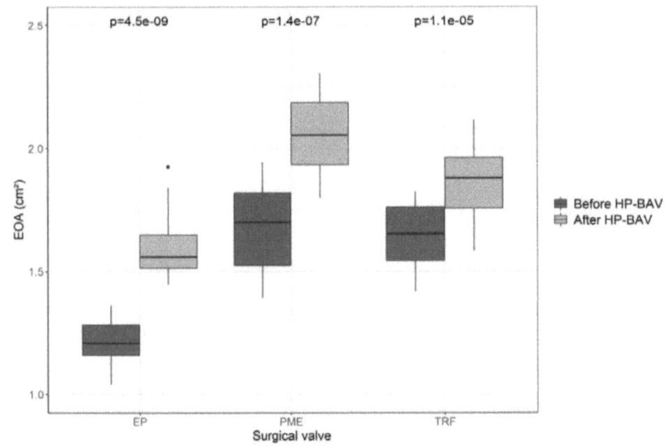

Figure 3: Effective orifice area (in cm²) of the Evolut R 26 mm prostheses before and after HP-BAV. EP= Epic, PME= Perimount and TRF= Trifecta.

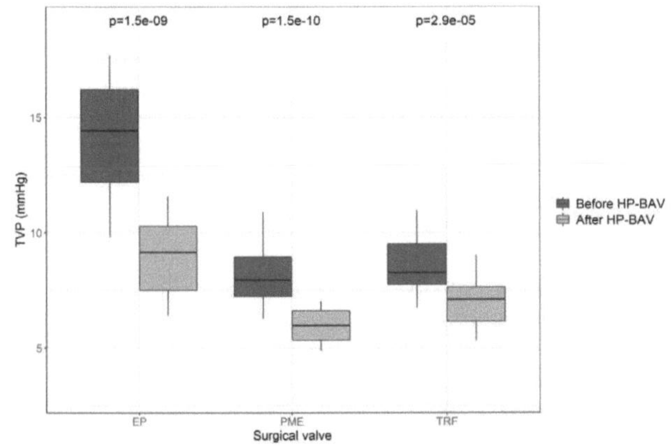

Figure 4: Mean transvalvular pressure gradient (in mmHg) of the Evolut R 26 mm prosthesis before and after HP-BAV. EP= Epic, PME= Perimount and TRF= Trifecta.

seemed more straight than before HP-BAV indicating a higher degree of expansion after HP-BAV.

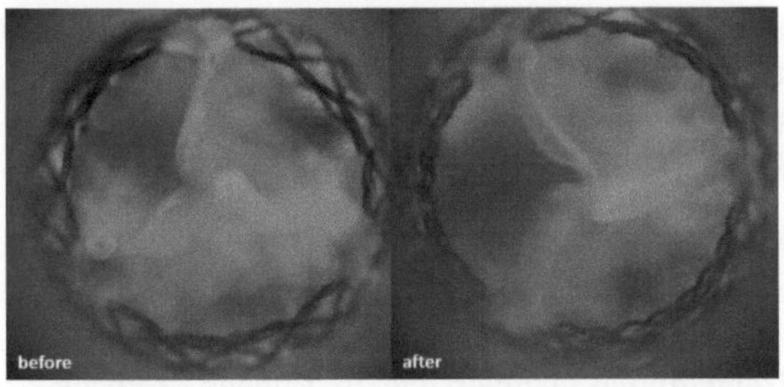

Figure 5: Closing behavior of the Epic valve before (left) and after (right) the valve fracture. In the closed position, the Evolut R appears expanded to a greater degree after HP-BAV compared to before HP-BAV.

3.1 Discussion

In this study the feasibility of BVF using HP-BAV of three surgical valves and its influence on the functional result after a ViV procedure was investigatet. The findings can be summarized as follows:

1) BVF using HP-BAV could be achieved with the PME and EP, while the TRF could not be fractured.

2) The diameter of all three valves incerased after HP-BAV, irrespective of BVF.

3) HP-BAV led to significantly improved hydrodynamic results of a ViV procedure using the Evolut R prosthesis.

Table 1: Values of the effective orifice area (in cm²) of the ViV prosthesis with the Evolut R before and after blasting. The stroke volume settings (SVS) correspond to different volumes (4= 57-59 ml, 5= 72-74 ml, 6= 88-90 ml and 7= 90-102 ml). EP= Epic, PME= Perimount Magna Ease, TRF= Trifecta.

Valve	SVS	Before	After	p value
PME	4	1,46 ± 0,04	1,83 ± 0,03	< 0,001
	5	1,64 ± 0,06	1,99 ± 0,02	< 0,001
	6	1,76 ± 0,09	2,13 ± 0,03	< 0,001
	7	1,86 ± 0,09	2,28 ± 0,02	0,001
TRF	4	1,46 ± 0,04	1,7 ± 0,06	< 0,001
	5	1,63 ± 0,03	1,83 ± 0,06	< 0,001
	6	1,73 ± 0,03	1,93 ± 0,06	< 0,001
	7	1,8 ± 0,03	2,03 ± 0,9	< 0,05
EP	4	1,13 ± 0,05	1,48 ± 0,33	< 0,001
	5	1,19 ± 0,06	1,54 ± 0,04	< 0,001
	6	1,23 ± 0,51	1,59 ±0,04	< 0,001
	7	1,33 ± 0,03	1,75 ± 0,08	0,001

HP-BAV has been suggested as a useful tool to improve the functional result after a ViV procedure. However, apart from the newest generation of prosthetic valves, surgical bioprostheses were not designed to be fractured later on in case of degeneration to facilitate treatment with a transcatheter heart valve. Therefore it seems very important to characterize the feasibility of BVF using HP-BAV as well as fracture pressures for individual prosthetic models. In this study, a 22 mm balloon for three commonly implanted surgical valves with a labelled size of 21 mm to investigate this issue was used. The *in vitro* study showed, the PME fractured at a pressure of 15 atm and the EP at 8 atm. This is an interesting finding as a previous study revealed exactly the same fracture pressures for these valves [3]. It seems that these valves do not show a significant batch-to-batch variability regarding their fracture pressure.

In general, bioprosthetic valves (BPV) with an alloy metal band ring (such as the Magna Ease) showed a higher breakage threshold (18–24 atm) than BPVs with a polymer ring (Biocor Epic, Mosaic, Mitroflow; 8–12 atm) [2]. Such clear characterization of the fracture behavior is important to plan a ViV procedure into these valves.

Similar to another study, we were not able to fracture the TRF. Bench tests (rupture tests) with various high-pressure balloons were performed on various biological valve prostheses, including Mitroflow, Magna, Magna Ease,

Mosaic and Biocor Epic and also the Trifecta. This was to investigate which valves could be broken and at what pressure a break occurred. The bench tests showed that the framework of most, but not all (including the Trifecta), bioprosthetic surgical aortic valves could be broken with high pressure balloons [2], [3]. Even at a pressure of 25 atm it was not able to provoke BVF of this valve. However, like the PME and EP, the TRF showed an increase of the inner valve diameter after HP-BAV suggesting that TRF can be dilated and may still be associated with an improved functional result.

This work confirmed this hypothesis with the pulse duplicator experiments as the Evolut R showed improved hydrodynamic function by means of significantly higher EOA and lower TVP in all three surgical bioprostheses after HP-BAV (Fig. 3 and 4). Fig. 5 shows that after HP-BAV and BVF of the EP, the Evolut R shows a greater degree of expansion due to the increased inner diameter of the valve. The degree of improvement was highest for the EP, followed by the PME and finally TRF.

These results suggest that HP-BAV with BVF is more effective than without BVF. However, the TRF also showed a significantly improved result by HP-BAV even without BVF through dilation of the valve stent frame. To investigate whether this effect is permanent, we determined EOA and TVP of the Evolut R inside the TRF 2 weeks after HP-BAV. Here, we could see that the results was still improved compared with before HP-BAV, but to a lesser extent compared with directly after HP-BAV. The dilation of the TRF is therefore probably not permanent and the functional result may decline again over time.

However, with a transcatheter heart valve in place, this results may become different. With the Evolut R, a continuous outward directed radial force could help to maintain the enlarged diameter. Similarly, implantation of a balloon-expandable valve may also help to keep the dilated diameter over time. These hypotheses need to be investigated in the future.

3.2 Limitations

This research work has some limitations. Tests were carried out *in vitro*, which does entirely not reflect human *in vivo* conditions in its whole complexity. Another limitation of the work is the experimental setup itself. Instead of blood, which has a different viscosity, saline was used. This means that there are different pressure losses and leakage values. Another factor would be the rigid fixation of the valve-in-valve prostheses. They do not represent a natural environment, as would be the case in the patient, because normally the surrounding tissue would move with the contraction.

4 Conclusion

This study showed that two of the three examined surgical valves can be fractured using a high pressure balloon, while one valve was not fractured but merely dilated. In all three valves, treatment with a high pressure balloon led to an improvement of the hydrodynamic result of the transcatheter heart valve when implanted in these valves as a valve-in-valve procedure. Therefore, this procedure may be an effective tool to improve results for a ViV procedure in selected patients.

This work represents a basis for *in vitro* experiments. However, a more detailed overview of the three biological valve prostheses must be examined, also with regard to the valve size in relation to the *Evolut-R*. The application and safety of this technique in (larger) patient populations, and also in relation to facilitating transcatheter ViV procedures with small surgical valves, must be carefully investigated in clinical trials to determine its safety and usefulness [2].

Acknowledgement

The work was carried out in the research laboratory of the Department of Cardiac and Thoracic Vascular Surgery of the University Hospital of Schleswig-Holstein, Lübeck Campus. The authors thank Tim Schaller and Najla Sadat for excellent support during the experiments.

Author's Statement

All authors declare no conflict of interest with respect to the contents of this manuscript.

5 References

[1] D. Dvir, *Transcatheter aortic valve implantation in failed bioprosthetic surgical valves*, JAMA, USA, 2014.

[2] J. T. Saxon, K. B Allen, D. J. Cohen and A. K. Chhatriwalla, *Bioprosthetic Valve Fracture During Valve-in-Valve TAVR: Bench to Bedside*. ICR Journal, Kansas City, 2017, p. 20.

[3] K. B. Allen and A. K. Chhatriwalla, *Bioprosthetic Valve Fracture to Facilitate Transcatheter Valve-in-Valve Implantation*, The Society of Thoracic Surgeons, Kansas City, 2017, pp.1501-1503.

[4] M. Scharfschwerdt and H. H. Sievers, *Entwicklung und Evaluation eines pulsatilen Linksherz- Simulators zur funktionellen Untersuchung nativer und artifizieller Herzklappen*, Universität zu Lübeck, Lübeck, 2009, pp.11-12.

[5] DIN EN ISO 5840-3, *Cardiovascular implants – Cardiac valve prostheses – Part 3: Heart valve substitutes implanted by transcatheter techniques*, Dezember 2015, Berlin.

[6] DIN EN ISO 5840-1, *Cardiovascular implants – Cardiac valve prostheses – Part 1: General Requirements*, Dezember 2015, Berlin.

Implementing a single-cell force spectroscopy set-up to investigate adhesion between *Plasmodium falciparum*-infected erythrocytes and various human endothelial receptors

Vincent M. Arriens[1], Jana Brehmer [2], Iris Bruchhaus [2], and Thomas Gutsmann [3]

[1] Biophysics, Universität zu Lübeck, vincent.arriens@student.uni-luebeck.de

[2] RG Protozoology, Bernhard Nocht Institute for Tropical Medizine, Hamburg, Germany

[3] Division of Biophysics, Research Center Borstel, Leibniz Lung Center, Germany

Abstract

Erythrocytes infected with *Plasmodium falciparum*, the most virulent parasite causing malaria, cytoadhere to endothelial cell receptors (ECR) to avoid splenic clearance for survival. Cytoadhesion can have serious consequences for the human host. It results from interactions between members of the *P. falciparum* erythrocyte membrane Protein 1 (*Pf*EMP1) family and various endothelial receptors. The aim of this project is to contribute to the picture of the various receptor-ligand partners by performing single-cell force spectroscopy (SCFS) on an atomic force microscope (AFM) and thus study their binding behavior. Two ECRs (receptor 1 (R1), receptor 2 (R2)) were chosen because of their known binding affinity to *Pf*EMP1. It could be shown that dwell times of 0.1 s and trigger forces below 1 nN are a good setup to perform biologically relevant measurements over a wide range of loading rates to distinguish between slip bond and catch bond mechanisms. The acquired data further emphasizes especially the binding affinity of R1 to *Pf*EMP1.

1 Introduction

The protozoic parasite *Plasmodium falciparum* is the most lethal species of *Plasmodium*, being responsible for the majority of malaria cases. In 2019, 409.000 malaria related deaths were registered [1]. Its complex life cycle includes infection of host red blood cells during which the parasite is growing and dividing. Those infected Erythrocytes (iE) undergo a change of shape from their characteristic donut-like shape towards a more rounded shape with a concurrent change in membrane rigidity and permeability. Due to their increased rigidity iEs are generally recognized by the spleen as deficient and therefore cleared from the blood. But at the same time iEs avoid their clearance by aggregating and binding to endothelial cells of the microvascular system. Thus leading to complete or partial blocking of the microvasculature contributing to the development of severe Malaria [2].

There are several surface proteins in iEs mediating the interaction with endothelial cells, with proteins of the variant surface antigen family *Plasmodium falciparum* erythrocyte membrane protein 1 (*Pf*EMP1) playing a predominant role. These antigens are exposed on the iE surface in electron-dense protrusions called 'knobs' [3]. There are about 60 different *var* genes per *P. falciparum* genome encoding *Pf*EMP1, but due to the mutually exclusive expression only one *Pf*EMP1 variant is expressed in the trophozoite and schizont state of the parasite. This variability in antigen expression allows for effective evasion of the host immune system. *Pf*EMP1 are large multi-domain proteins (250-350 kDa) with cysteine rich interdomain regions (CIDR) and Duffy binding-like (DBL) domains defining their adhesion characteristics [4].

On the endothelic side of the cytoadhesion interaction are various host receptors involved including receptor 1 (R1) and receptor 2 (R2). However, which receptor is taking part in the actual adhesion event depends on the present *Pf*EMP1 variant with its specific CIDR and DBL domains [5].

1.1 Single-Cell Force Spectroscopy

To analyze the binding behaviour between two types of surface proteins of living cells, single-cell force spectroscopy (SCFS) can be used. Based on atomic force microscopy (AFM) it provides force measurements with enough sensitivity to study single receptor-ligand interactions. In this method a single erythrocyte is attached to the cantilever of an AFM to function as a probe tip. The modified probe is then brought into contact with the receptor of interest. The receptor of interest can be recombinantly expressed and fused to a substrate via a binding tag or expressed on the surface of transgenic cells.

The measurement procedure in this study involves three phases: It begins with the approach phase, during which the probe is moved towards and gently pressed onto the adherent cell expressing the receptor of interest until a preset trigger force is reached. In the following short dwell time the probe remains at its current position and bonds can be formed. Finally, during the retraction phase the probe is removed with a constant speed until all binding interactions are fully separated. Throughout the entire experiment the deflection of the cantilever is monitored via the reflection of a laser on its rear side. From the known spring constant of the cantilever and its deflection it is directly calculated which forces are acting upon the probe. The captured forces are then plotted against the distance between probe and sample, which is extracted from the piezo element operating the cantilever movement. The majority of information can be derived from the retraction part of the force-distance curve [6]. As displayed in Fig 1, there are certain discrete steps in the curve, due to rupture events, that show a instantaneous change of force. In this study, the number and the height of these force steps, called jumps, have been analysed.

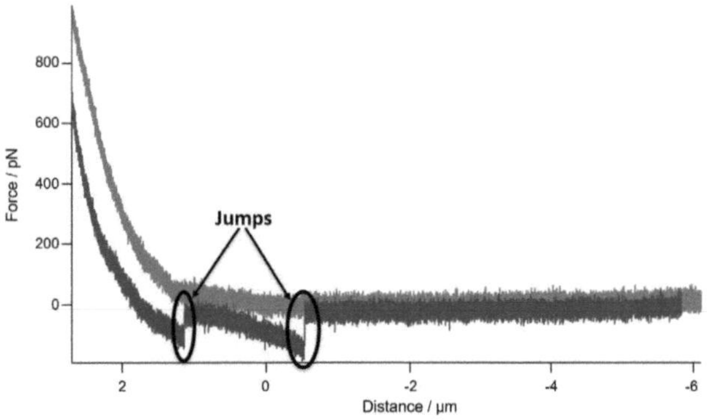

Figure 1: Characteristic force-distance curve obtained in an AFM-SCFS experiment. It displays the approach phase (red) and the retraction phase (blue) with two rupture events (Jumps).

1.2 Loading rate and bond characteristics

There are two distinct bond mechanisms (slip bond, catch bond) showing different lifetime behaviour, when the bonds are increasingly stressed. The rate at which a bond is stressed during cantilever retraction is called loading rate and is defined as the product of cantilever spring constant and retraction speed. Slip bonds show an exponential decrease in lifetime when they are loaded with an increased rate. Catch bonds, however, show an increasing lifetime over a distinct range of loading rates. Rupture forces can be used to distinguish between slip bonds and catch bonds due to the direct relation of bond lifetime and rupture force. Slip bonds exhibit a linear increase of rupture forces at increasing loading rates on a logarithmic scale, whereas catch bonds show a similar linearity only over a distinct range of loading rates. Especially below this range there are no ruptures observable [7].
The catch bond mechanism could explain how the iEs maintain adhesion to the endothelial cells under the continuous mechanical stress prevailing in the blood vessels. Furthermore, the identification of catch bond forming receptor-ligand pairs could indicate which proteins are contributing most to the adhesion.

2 Material and Methods

2.1 Parasite culture

The used *P. falciparum* isolate (*Pf*I) was cultivated with human O+ erythrocytes (5% haematocrit) in the presence of 10% human serum A+ (Interstate blood bank, Memphis, USA), according to standard procedures[8]. AFM measurements were performed with a parasite population only expressing the *Pf*EMP1-protein encoded by the *var*-gene of interest (VGI). This transfectant was generously provided by Tobias Spielmann (BNITM). It was measured with parasites in the trophozoite stage.
During measurement preparation the enrichment of knob-containing iEs was performed using gelatin (175g Bloom, Sigma-Aldrich, Germany) flotation [3]. The supernatant containing the iEs of interest was washed with binding medium (RPMI 1640 medium supplemented with 2% glucose, pH 7.2).

2.2 Substrate cell culture

Transfected CHO-745 cells (Chinese Hamster Ovary cells), with the receptor of interest (R1, R2) fused to cytosolic green fluorescent protein (GFP) and expressed on the surface, were cultivated at 37 °C and under 5% CO_2 in Ham's F-12 medium (PAN Biotech Aidenbach, Germany) supplemented with 10% foetal calf serum (Capricorn Ebsdorfergrund, Germany) and penicillin-streptomycin (PAN Biotech Aidenbach, Germany). Neomycin (G418 (Capricorn Ebsdorfergrund, Germany); stock concentration 50 mg/mL; with final concentration, 0.7 mg/mL) was used as a selective agent for the transfected cells. The CHO-cells were grown on petri dishes, which have been coated in advance with 0.1 mg/mL Poly-D-Lysine (PDL (Merck, Darmstadt, Germany)) solution. The PDL was used to mediate an adherence strong enough for the CHO-cells to stay attached to the petri dish during the experiment. CHO-cell concentration and growth time were adjusted to approximately 72 h, so that on the day of the experiment the petri dishes were covered with 'islands' of healthy CHO-cells and open spaces in between.

2.3 Force Spectroscopy

2.3.1 Cantilever

Tipless silicon nitride cantilever (MLCT-O10, Bruker) were used. To obtain an iE functioning as a probe tip it has to be attached tightly to the Cantilever. Therefore the Cantilever was functionalized with 1 mg/ml Concanavalin A (ConA (Merck, Darmstadt, Germany)) solution [5].

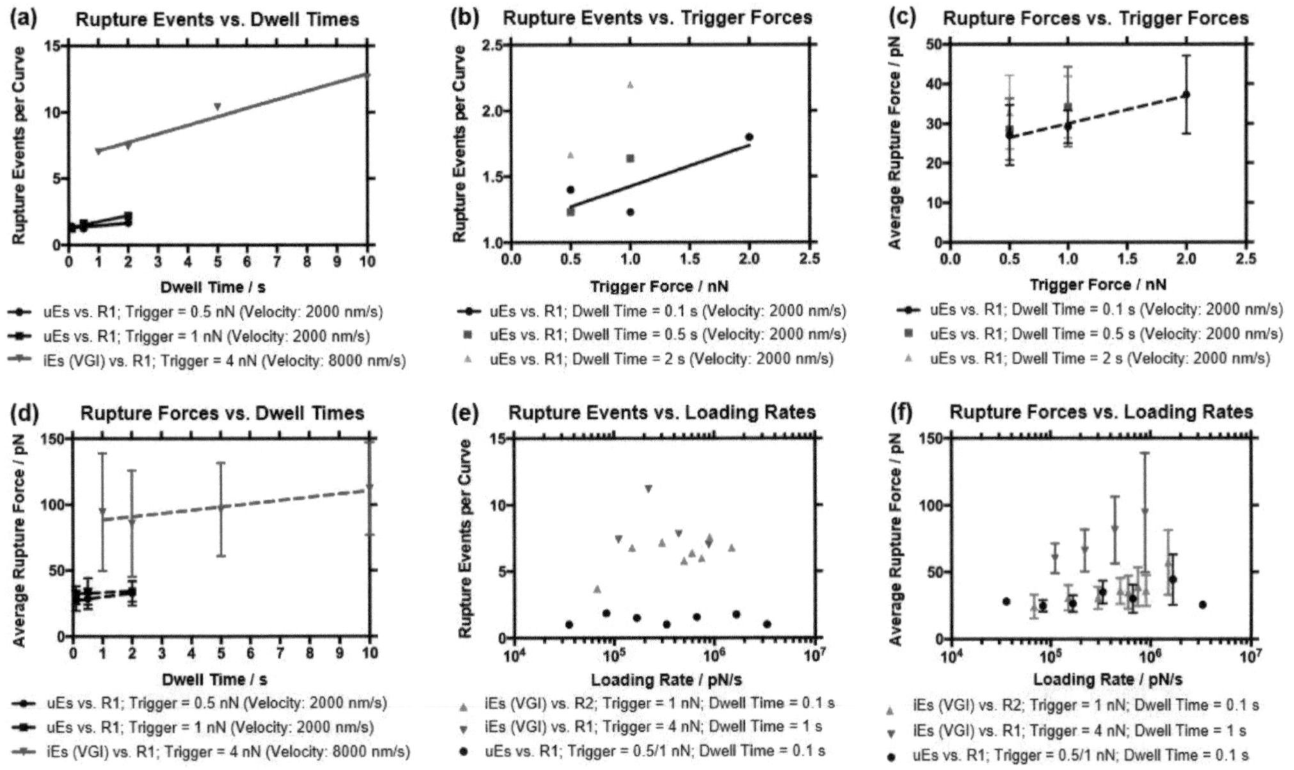

Figure 2: Data acquired by performing AFM-SCFS between erythrocytes (iEs and uEs) and CHO cells expressing either R1 or R2. Each data point corresponds to the mean of 5 to 20 analysed force-distance curves. **(a)** Number of rupture events per curve at different dwell times. **(b)** Number of rupture events per curve at different trigger forces. **(c)** Rupture forces at different trigger forces. **(d)** Rupture forces at different dwell times. **(e)** Number of rupture events per curve at different loading rates. **(f)** Rupture forces at different loading rates

2.3.2 Data Acquisition

The experiments were performed on an AFM (MFP3D, AsylumResearch) in combination with an optical microscope (Olympus IX70) and a heater stage. The spring constant of each Cantilever was calibrated in binding medium on a glass slide using the thermal method at measuring temperature (e.g. 37 °C).
At the beginning of the experiment the CHO cell culture medium was replaced by binding medium and afterwards erythrocytes in binding medium were added before placing the petri dish under the AFM. During temperature equilibration an erythrocyte was attached to the cantilever by pressing the cantilever onto the cell for 10-15 minutes, then withdrawing it from the substrate and subsequently waiting another 10-15 minutes to allow for further strengthening of the attachment.
With this modified probe, the force spectroscopy experiments were executed on one or few CHO cells with regard to various measurement parameters. Trigger forces were preset between 0.5 nN and 4 nN, retraction speeds ranged from 200 to 20000 $\mathrm{nm\,s^{-1}}$ under closed loop conditions to maintain a constant retraction speed and dwell times from 0 to 10 s were used. The sampling rate was adjusted at each retraction speed to 10 data points per second.
The reason for so much variation in the experimental parameters was to find a setup that generates reproducible and comparable results, and in addition, get a good overview on the adhesion properties of our samples.

3 Results and Discussion

For each set of parameters (trigger force, dwell time, retraction velocity) 5-20 force curves were acquired and analysed by hand with focus on rupture events, especially their mean number per force-distance curve and mean magnitude. The great variation of experimental parameters and so far small number of acquired data don't give detailed results yet, but already allow some initial interpretations.

3.1 Dwell Times and Trigger Forces

Different dwell times and trigger forces were tested to find the optimal values for these parameters. Analysing the number of rupture events per force-distance curve against different dwell times, as shown in Fig. 2 (a), gives an increase in the number of ruptures when using longer dwell times. This could be expected as it gives receptors and ligands which are spatially close to each other more time to form bonds. A similar effect can be seen in Fig. 2 (b) when plotting the number of rupture events against different trigger forces. Pushing the elastic surfaces of CHO cells and

erythrocytes with higher force onto each other leads to an increased contact area, thus bringing more receptor-ligand pairs in close contact to form bonds.
Fig. 2 (c) and Fig. 2 (d) both show a slight increase of rupture force when using longer dwell times and applying higher trigger forces. Regarding longer dwell times, an explanation might be that structural changes of the receptor-ligand complex take place or that additional nonspecific binding effects arise. But this could also be an artefact due to the lack of data. Nevertheless, all those effects must be considered when comparing rupture forces of different measurements.
Furthermore, the data allows for a first comparison of uninfected erythrocytes (uEs) to *Pf*I-VGI infected erythrocytes and their adhesion to CHO-R1. Fig. 2 (a) and Fig. 2 (d) show much more rupture events as well as higher rupture forces when probing iEs on R1 compared to uEs on R1. The differences are so distinct that they might still remain when taking into account the higher trigger forces and retraction velocities.

3.2 Loading Rates

Fig. 2 (f) shows the comparison of three different experimental setups (uE vs. R1, iE vs. R1, iE vs. R2) regarding their rupture force behaviour in dependence of the applied loading rates. It is already known that the VGI binds to both R1 and R2 [9] and the results in Fig. 2 (e) clearly emphasise this finding. In addition Fig. 2 (f) shows distinct differences, namely higher rupture forces, when comparing iE vs. R1 with iE vs. R2 as well as with uE vs. R1. But here again, the differences in trigger forces and dwell times have to be taken into account.
Furthermore, those plots can not yet meet their actual purpose. Additional measurements at even lower loading rates have to be performed to confidently determine the bond mechanisms.

4 Conclusion

The results obtained so far demonstrate that SCFS is a suitable tool to study binding forces and mechanisms between *P. falciparum*-infected erythrocytes and various human endothelial cell receptors. The strong dependence of rupture forces on measurement parameters requires a careful choice of the experimental setup. Furthermore, the biological relevance has to be taken into account. Due to blood flow in the vascular system erythrocytes don't dwell at the same spot for several seconds. We suggest to set dwell times at 0.1 seconds and to keep trigger forces below 1 nN, thus obtaining force-distance curves with a small number of rupture events. Otherwise ruptures can overlap and become less distinct.
After completing the aforementioned experiments, the subsequent goal will be to have measured at least three different biological replicates with different iEs and additionally perform control measurements on CHO cells, which are not expressing the receptor of interest. Furthermore, the same experiments could be carried out at higher temperatures to simulate febrile conditions.

Acknowledgement

The work has been carried out at Division of Biophysics, Research Center Borstel, Leibniz Lung Center, Germany and in cooperation with the Bernhard Nocht Institute for Tropical Medizine, Hamburg, RG Protozoology.

Author's Statement

Conflict of interest: Authors state no conflict of interest.

5 References

[1] W. H. Organization *et al.*, "World malaria report 2020: 20 years of global progress and challenges," 2020.

[2] L. H. Miller, D. I. Baruch, K. Marsh, and O. K. Doumbo, "The pathogenic basis of malaria," *Nature*, vol. 415, no. 6872, pp. 673–679, 2002.

[3] A. Tilly *et al.*, "Type of in vitro cultivation influences cytoadhesion, knob structure, protein localization and transcriptome profile of plasmodium falciparum. sci. rep. 5, 16766," 2015.

[4] J. Normark, *Surface antigens and virulence in Plasmodium falciparum malaria.* Department of Microbiology, Tumor and Cell Biology, Karolinska Institute, Stockholm, Sweden, 2008.

[5] P. Carvalho, M. Diez-Silva, H. Chen, M. Dao, and S. Suresh, "Cytoadherence of erythrocytes invaded by plasmodium falciparum: quantitative contact-probing of a human malaria receptor," *Acta biomaterialia*, vol. 9, no. 5, pp. 6349–6359, 2013.

[6] J. Helenius, C.-P. Heisenberg, H. E. Gaub, and D. J. Muller, "Single-cell force spectroscopy," *Journal of cell science*, vol. 121, no. 11, pp. 1785–1791, 2008.

[7] E. A. Evans and D. A. Calderwood, "Forces and bond dynamics in cell adhesion," *Science*, vol. 316, no. 5828, pp. 1148–1153, 2007.

[8] W. Trager and J. B. Jensen, "Human malaria parasites in continuous culture," *Science*, vol. 193, no. 4254, pp. 673–675, 1976.

[9] N. G. Metwally *et al.*, "Characterisation of plasmodium falciparum populations selected on the human endothelial receptors p-selectin, e-selectin, cd9 and cd151," *Scientific reports*, vol. 7, no. 1, pp. 1–14, 2017.

3

Biomedical Optics

Characterization of a diffractive phase mask for chromatic depth-scanning microscopy

Sabine Wünsche [1], Sebastian Karpf [2]
[1] Medical Engineering Science, Universität zu Lübeck, sabine.wuensche@student.uni-luebeck.de
[2] Institute of Biomedical Optics, Universität zu Lübeck, sebastian.karpf@uni-luebeck.de

Abstract

In this paper a diffractive phase mask is characterized for a potential application in chromatic z-axis scanning microscopy. The diffractive phase mask can lead to a large chromatic focal shift, which can be employed for depth-scanning microscopy employing wavelength-swept laser sources for illumination. To characterize the phase mask, two experimental setups were built and beam profiles and focal positions were measured. One setup employed two distinct wavelengths and the focus was recorded on a camera chip. The second experiment employed a rapidly wavelength-swept Fourier Domain Mode Locking (FDML) laser in a chromatic confocal microscopy setup. In contrast to the expected results, the analyzed beam profiles showed only a small influence of the phase mask. This deviation is analyzed and possible mitigation strategies discussed.

1 Introduction

For biological and medical imaging, it can be very useful to utilize three-dimensional images. These images can be used, for example, to better investigate structures and processes at the subcellular level. One technique that makes this possible is chromatic confocal microscopy [1]-[3]. Taking advantage of the chromatic aberration of a lens, it is possible to focus to different depths. By utilizing a wavelength-dependent reflection into the depth, this can be used to yield three-dimensional images.
An important imaging technique that allows excitation in only one plane is two-photon microscopy. It is applied in research at the Institute of Biomedical Optics at University of Lübeck. One focus is on the Spectro-temporal Lifetime Imaging by Diffracted Excitation (SLIDE) microscope, a two-photon microscope that can scan two-dimensional images at kHz speed. This is possible by utilizing a tunable laser light source, a Fourier Domain Mode Locking (FDML) laser, and a grating [4]. The ability to augment these ultrafast images with depth information could further enhance the microscope. High z-resolution in a short time over a larger area, e.g. 100 µm, is desirable.
This might be achieved by using a diffractive optical element (DOE) in the form of a phase mask [3]. The interference of different phases behind the phase mask is used here. This underlying phase shift is caused by different path lengths d within the material that makes up the phase mask. Since the light passes through the phase mask at a slower speed, depending on the refractive index n and the wavelength λ, the phase is delayed compared to the phase of the light in the surrounding air. The phase shift $\Delta\phi$ can be described by (1) [5].

$$\Delta\phi = \frac{2 \cdot \pi \cdot (n-1) \cdot d}{\lambda} \tag{1}$$

The given phase mask is designed for a wavelength of 635 nm and seems to be similar to a Fresnel zone plate as employed by Dobson [3]. Using (2) for the calculation of the focal length f_m of a diffractive optical zone plate, the influence of the wavelength becomes clear. With an increasing wavelength λ, constant zone plate radius r_1 and diffraction order m, the focal length decreases [3].

$$f_m(\lambda) = \frac{{r_1}^2}{m \cdot \lambda} \tag{2}$$

With a convex lens behind the phase mask, the beam is focused near the specified focal length of the lens (Fig. 1). This position on the z-axis is also wavelength dependent. For a good depth resolution, the distance between the foci caused by different wavelengths should be as clearly defined as possible and should be large enough for the application. This paper deals with the question whether z-axis scanning with an already existing phase mask is possible.

2 Material and Methods

To determine the effect of the phase mask, measurements are taken in two setups. They differ in the light sources and the kind of detection.

2.1 Experimental setup one

In the first experiment (Fig. 1), one of two laser diodes (517 nm or 655 nm wavelength) was used as a light source ⟨1⟩ in the form of a fiber checker in each case. By coupling into a single-mode fiber suitable for the wavelength, the light beam takes on approximately the shape of a Gaussian beam after out-coupling. Here, the radial expansions of the beam in x and y direction are approximately the same and become minimal at the beam waist ω_0.
During out-coupling, the beam was aligned as precisely as possible with the center of the phase mask ⟨3⟩, since this is where the circularly arranged structures of the used phase mask are located. Here, a cage system was useful. The beams diffracted by the phase mask were then focused using a convex lens ⟨4⟩. The three lenses used (L1, L2, L3) had different focal lengths (L1: f = 35 mm, L2: f = 50 mm, L3: f = 125 mm) and had no correction to suppress chromatic aberration. A camera chip on a manual stage ⟨5⟩ was utilized to record the spot. This made it possible to record the beam path at constant intervals of 50 µm around the focus in the z-direction. To prevent overexposure of the camera sensor, the light was attenuated with optical density filters ⟨2⟩ before the phase mask.

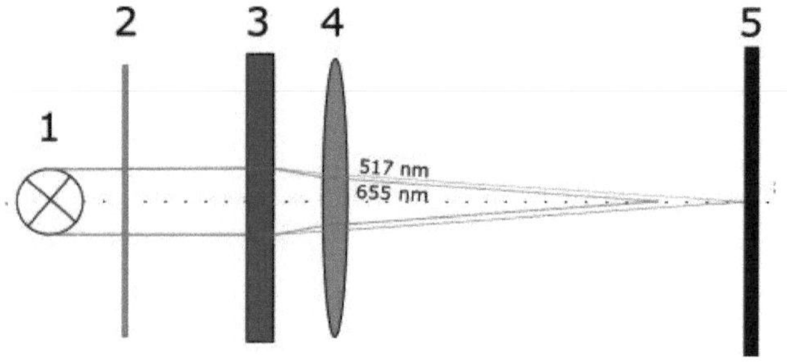

Figure 1: Setup containing of ⟨1⟩ laser light source, ⟨2⟩ optical density filter, ⟨3⟩ phase mask, ⟨4⟩ convex lens and ⟨5⟩ detector. The focus position depends on the wavelength.

The measurement of the width was done with the already existing LabVIEW program *mode field analyzer*. Using the LabVIEW function Gaussian Peak Fit (3), a Gaussian curve was estimated for each z-plane in x and y directions [6]. Here, a denotes the amplitude, μ the center, c the offset and σ the standard deviation. By transforming the formula, the width Δx is obtained (4).

$$f(x) = a \cdot \exp\left(-\frac{(x-\mu)^2}{2 \cdot \sigma^2}\right) + c \quad (3)$$

$$\Delta x = 2 \cdot \sqrt{2} \cdot \sigma \quad (4)$$

When measuring with the Gaussian peak fit function, two values for σ (standard deviation and estimated standard deviation) are passed for x and y respectively. A beam profile is now generated for all four values. Subsequently, the beam profiles were slightly smoothed with a mean filter taking into account the two surrounding measured values. From this, the position of the minimum for the four resulting beam profiles can now be determined. The average value of the minima was taken as the position of the focal point.
Using this method, beam profiles were measured several times with and without the phase mask. In order to be able to compare the results for the different measurement setups well, the beam profile measured with a wavelength of 517 nm and without the phase mask was then set as the reference value. Its minimum corresponds to the focal length indicated on the lens.

2.2 Experimental setup two

In the second experimental setup, a tunable FDML laser is used as light source. The FDML operates in a range ± 50 nm around 1300 nm. Wavelengths of 1275 nm, 1300 nm or 1325 nm were most commonly used for the measurements. After out-coupling from the fiber, the beam hits the phase mask and lens, as in the first experiment. It is then reflected back into the fiber by a movable mirror. A circulator (single mode fiber, best working around 1310 nm) separates the different directions of the light in the fiber.

With a power meter (PM100D) or an optical spectrum analyzer, the coupled power can be measured. How much light is returned to the fiber depends on the position of the mirror for the corresponding wavelength. By moving the mirror at equal intervals, this method can be used to create a beam profile. If the mirror is exactly in focus, then the measured power is maximum.

2.3 Analysis

The Rayleigh length (5) can be used to evaluate the beam quality. It is calculated from the beam waist ω_0 and wavelength λ [7]. Z_R calculates the point z on the optical axis where the cross section of the ideal Gaussian beam has doubled.

$$z_R = \frac{\pi \cdot {\omega_0}^2}{\lambda} \quad (5)$$

3 Results and Discussion

To evaluate the results, the beam profiles were compared. They result from the measurements with the different light sources with and without phase mask and different lenses. The beam profiles from the first experimental setup seem to be of good quality (Fig. 2). Especially the shift of the focus due to chromatic aberration is striking. It is much stronger than the shift due to the phase mask. The chromatic aberration increases with a larger focal length of the convex lens. The approximated focus shifts between the wavelengths 517 nm and 655 nm are listed in Table 1.
In contrast, the influence of the phase mask on the beam profiles and the position of the foci seems to be small. On

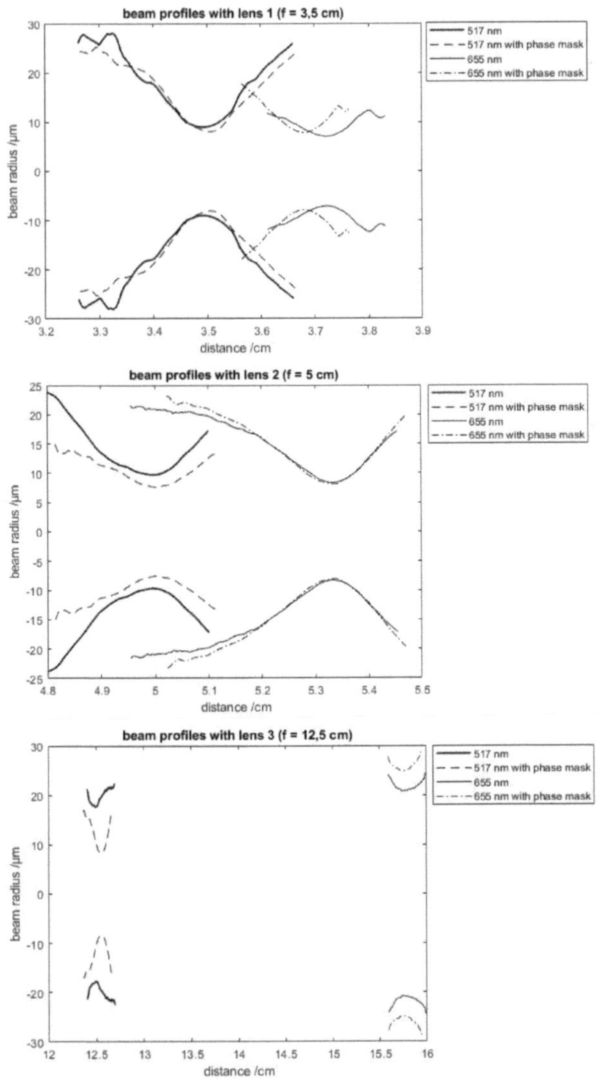

Figure 2: Beam profiles of 517 nm and 655 nm light with and without phase mask and different convex lenses. The chromatic shift is visible.

Table 1: Focus shifts of the beam profiles without phase mask

Lens	Focal shift
L1 (f = 3.5 cm)	≈ 0.226 cm
L2 (f = 5 cm)	≈ 0.339 cm
L3 (f = 12.5 cm)	≈ 3.240 cm

average, the absolute distance between the beam profiles for 517 nm and 655 nm decreases a little.

Table 2 shows the focal shift between the beam waist position without ($z(\omega_0 1)$) and with ($z(\omega_0 2)$) phase mask for each wavelength. On average the calculated mean of the focal shift was 95.9 µm/138 nm = 0.695 µm/nm.

Based on the data, the width of the beam waist ω_0 for most measurements is about 9 µm. For the measurement with lens L3 and phase mask the radius ω_0 is significantly wider

Table 2: Focal shift in µm between beam profiles without $z(\omega_0 1)$ and with phase mask $z(\omega_0 2)$ for respective single wavelengths

Wavelength λ [nm]	Lens L1	Lens L2	Lens L3
517	+ 72.7 µm	+ 48 µm	+ 500 µm
655	- 381.3 µm	- 68.5 µm	- 75 µm

with approximatly 18 µm. At this point it should be noted, that the diameter of the recorded spots is influenced by the optical density filters. They weaken the light and might reduce the measured radius. The comparison of the width of the beam profiles at the points of the calculated Rayleigh lengths z with the ideal values $\sqrt{2}\omega_0$ indicates that the beam quality is slightly below the ideal values.

Also the results from the second setup show the biggest effect due to chromatic aberration (Fig. 3). Although the beam profiles for 1275 nm, 1300 nm and 1325 nm show an increasing shift of the focus (Table 3), it is difficult to evaluate these results correctly. The main reason for this is the fluctuating values of the power, measured with the powermeter, by 1 %. This results on the one hand from the background noise. On the other hand, slight fluctuations in the power of the laser generally occurred over the period of the measurement. This should be considered as a possible source of error.

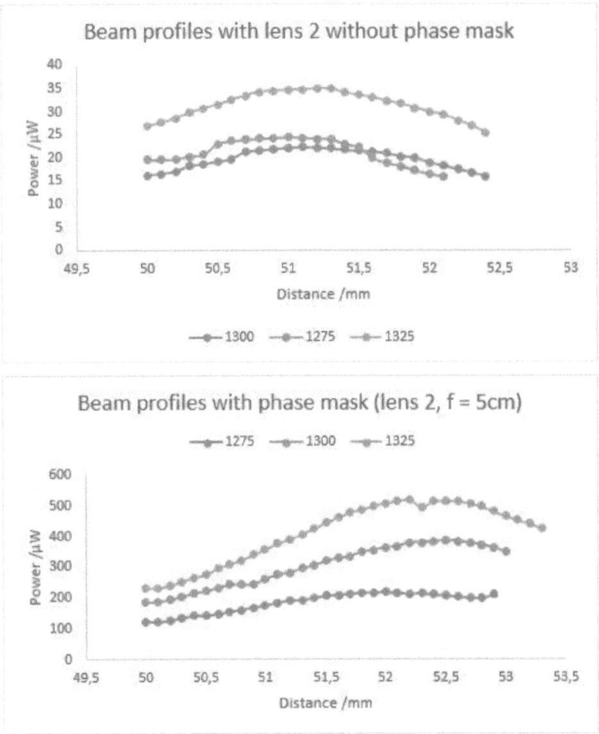

Figure 3: Excerpt of the measured beam profiles in the infrared spectrum.

Table 3: Chromatic focal shift measured with setup two

Lens	Focal shift without phase mask	Focal shift with phase mask
L1	4.6 μm/nm	3 μm/nm
L2	4 μm/nm	7.08 μm/nm
L3	32.2 μm/nm	53.6 μm/nm

A disadvantage in the second experiment could also be the higher loss of power due to the lens and the phase mask. To allow comparability of the results, the same lenses were used in both experiments. However, these are coated to transmit light particularly well only in the visible spectrum. At 1300 nm wavelength, for example, the phase mask reduces the measured power per pass by almost 45 %. Smaller fluctuations in the power due to background noise, for example, have a greater overall influence on the power measured at the end for this reason.
Furthermore, it was noticed that the positions of the intensity maximum were partly different in repeated measurements, with exactly the same experimental setup (same wavelength, same lens). A possible cause for this could be a change in the mirror angle, which follows from the movement of the manual stage.

Overall, it was therefore not always clear where the focus was exactly located for the corresponding measurement. For this reason, the results from the first experimental setup are to be preferred.

During the evaluation of setup one, it was found that the phase mask used behaves like a Fresnel zone plate. The shift in focal length of different wavelengths caused by the zone plate counteracts the shift caused by chromatic aberration. The effect of the phase mask on the focal length is largely determined by the radius of the first zone plate, which is constant but unknown. Nevertheless, the overall effect of chromatic aberration was much stronger. Therefore, it would probably be beneficial to consider using an achromatic lens for further measurements with the phase mask. Depth scanning based on the strongest possible chromatic aberration through specific lens selection might also be of interest for chromatic confocal microscopy.
It would also be possible that the orders would not be as well focused as required. This could be the case if the light beam is not exactly centered on the phase mask, but this has been attempted to be avoided. Additionally, defocusing of the diffraction orders could mean that the orders diffracted by the phase mask have been attenuated too much by the optical density filters and therefore have little effect on the focus shift.
Overall, however, the phase mask appears to be unsuitable for depth scanning microscopy for the SLIDE system.

4 Conclusion

In summary, the measurement results indicate little influence of the phase mask on the position of the focus. This is unexpected and leads to the fact that the phase mask probably does not have the desired effect. It was also noticed, that a lot of light is lost in the infrared spectrum due to the phase mask. Both are unfavorable for a later application in the SLIDE microscope. Reasons for the results could be that the design of the diffractive phase mask is unsuitable for a large focus shift or that the diffracted orders were not properly focused on the optical axis. Changing the convex lens or its position might improve this a little. Overall, however, it probably makes more sense to use a different diffractive phase mask for chromatic depth-scanning microscopy, ideally designed for wavelengths in the infrared spectrum. This could be an approach for further experiments.

Acknowledgement

The work has been carried out and supervised by the Institute of Biomedical Optics, Universität zu Lübeck.

Author's Statement

Conflict of interest: Authors state no conflict of interest.

5 References

[1] H. J. Tiziani and H.-M. Uhde, *Three-dimensional image sensing by chromatic confocal microscopy*, Applied Optics Vol. 33, Issue 10, pp. 1838-1843, 1994.

[2] F. Blateyron, *Optical Measurement of Surface Topography - Chromatic Confocal Microscopy*, Leach R, Springer, Berlin, Heidelberg, pp. 71-106, 2011.

[3] S. L. Dobson, P. Sun and Y. Fainman, *Diffractive lenses for chromatic confocal imaging*, Applied Optics Vol. 36, Issue 20, pp. 4744-4748, 1997.

[4] S. Karpf, C. T. Riche, D. D. Carlo, A. Goel, W. A. Zeiger, A. Suresh et al., *Spectro-temporal encoded multiphoton microscopy and fluorescence lifetime imaging at kilohertz frame-rates*, Nature Communications 11, 2062, 2020.

[5] C. A. Mack, *Field Guide to Optical Lithography*, SPIE Press, Bellingham, WA, 2006.

[6] LabVIEW 2018 Help, *Gaussian Peak Fit VI*, Available: https://zone.ni.com/reference/en-XX/help/371361R-01/gmath/gaussian_peak_fit, [last accessed on 2021-24-01].

[7] H. P. Huber, *Räumliche Charakterisierung von Laserstrahlung*, Hochschule München - Laserzentrum, München, pp. 16, 2012.

Design and construction of a motorized XYZ positioning stage for large field of view optical coherence tomography imaging

Sazgar Burhan [1], Madita Göb [2], Wolfgang Draxinger [2] and Robert Huber [2]
[1] Medical Engineering Science, Universität zu Lübeck, sazgar.burhan@student.uni-luebeck.de
[2] Institute of Biomedical Optics, Universität zu Lübeck, {m.goeb, wolfgang.draxinger, robert.huber}@uni-luebeck.de

Abstract

Optical coherence tomography (OCT) is a promising method to examine biological tissue non-invasively. With today's state-of-the-art technology, OCT volumes of high resolution are acquired in under a second. Therefore, it is a suited technique in dermatology for rapid, painless, and non-invasive diagnosis. At present, OCT systems are capable of capturing small field of views (FOV). However, with the Fourier Domain Mode Locking (FDML) laser developed in our research group, the OCT imaging speed can be increased, enabling the acquisition of large FOVs. However, the lateral FOV of the system remains limited to about 1 x 1 cm by the scan optics. Consequently, to scan large OCT volumes, a controllable XYZ stage with a long travel distance is required. In this study, a controllable and motorized XYZ positioning stage was designed, set up and evaluated for imaging large tissue samples with a scan area of 22,5 x 22,5 x 22,5 cm. A software, written in LabVIEW, was used to control the XYZ stage and first OCT images could be acquired.

1 Introduction

Optical coherence tomography (OCT) imaging technology is suitable for examining and visualizing scattering materials, such as biological tissue [1], [2]. Offering a high tissue penetration depth of several millimeters combined with a high resolution of a few micrometers, OCT enables cross-sectional imaging of the upper layers of the skin. In combination with FDML lasers, high repetition rates at large optical bandwidths are possible, enabling high-speed OCT imaging (MHz-OCT) [3], [4]. This allows us to achieve large-area and high-resolution OCT images rapidly. In the used setup, raster scanning is realized by fast galvanometer scanners and additional beam shaping optics. However, to precisely scan large tissue samples, it is necessary to have a freely movable scan head over a large area.
An additional beneficial application of the stage would be an automatic imaging of *in vitro* human skin models. In cooperation with the Lübeck Institute of Experimental Dermatology (LIED) an automated screening of wound healing processes has been established. For this study, the human skin of healthy plastic surgery patients is artificially injured with a punch followed by *in vitro* monitoring of the healing process. 3D OCT images from day zero and day six are used to quantify the wound volume and thus measure the wound closure process. This procedure has already been automated by using segmentation algorithms, but the manual imaging of each wound still consumes valuable time. Therefore, the use of a motorized XYZ stage could accelerate the entire screening process.
This work deals with the construction and design of a motorized and controllable XYZ positioning stage and its subsequent testing. The construction is based on an already created and self-built XYZ stage in our research group [5].

2 Material and Methods

The following section illustrates the design and structure of the positioning stage. An overview of the various components and their purpose is discussed in more detail. In addition, further information is given regarding the used stepper motors and their control via LabVIEW.

2.1 Mechanical Design

To keep the design simple, it is advisable to create many individual parts that can later be combined into an assembly. This has the decisive advantage that only some components have to be modified in case of a possible change later on. The modifications are then automatically transferred by the CAD software. Also, already created assemblies can be combined in this way.
The custom components (unlabeled parts in Fig. 1) were designed with the 3D CAD software SolidWorks 2018 (Dassault System SolidWorks Corporation, Waltham, MA, USA). Any other component is commercially available. All parts are provided with holes and milled holes that are needed to connect and place the different components. A 340 mm profile rail (HIWIN, EGR20R340H) is mounted centrally on each side surface, on which a carriage (HIWIN, QEH20CAZ0H) is attached in each case. These carriages can move along the profile rail and are

equipped with an aluminum plate that serves to hold the front slider. Each linear slider is provided with a mechanical aluminum stopper on the upper and lower side of the profile rail to prevent the carriages from falling off. Two limit switches (Marquardt, 01050.5202-00) are also mounted on each stopper to make sure that the carriages cannot collide with components behind them. When a moving object hits a limit switch, a signal is sent to the driver, which stops the stepper motor immediately.
In this setup, right-hand thread 500 mm trapezoidal threaded spindles with a pitch of 2 mm are applied (drylin, PTGSG-10X2-01-R), which convert rotary into linear motion.
To accommodate large axial forces, also trapezoidal threaded spindle nuts with flange and anti-backlash were used (drylin, JFRM-AB-2525-TR10X2). As a result, the frictional resistance increases slightly, which prevents the axis from sagging when the stepper motor is released and leads to higher stability of the axis. Hence, this allows exact positioning of the screw nut with no potential backlash in both directions of the trapezoidal lead screw.
Furthermore, for each axis, two pulleys and a timing belt are used. In belt drives, one pulley rotates the belt, which in turn drives the other pulley. The advantage of belt drivers is that the stepper motor and the lead screw can be easily connected and disconnected mechanically, which solves design-related problems. Also, with pulleys systems, resolution and speed can be changed. If a smaller pulley drives a larger one, the larger pulley rotates slower, but with a higher torque and a finer resolution. In the opposite case, a lower torque and lower resolution is obtained. Belts and pulleys are available in various shapes and sizes. In this setup HTD-3M pulleys with a belt width of 9 mm and teeth numbers of 30 or 44 (maedler, 17023000 and 17024400) were used. Accordingly, on the Z and Y axis, the timing belts have an effective length of 318 mm with 106 teeths (maedler, 17113500). The timing belt on the X axis has a length of 255 mm at a teeth number of 85 (maedler, 17112800).
Moreover, a locating/non-locating bearing arrangement is used. In this case, the accommodation of the axial and radial forces in both directions is taken over by pillow block bearing units for the fixed side (maedler, 64200310), the locating bearing. The function of the locating bearing is to act as an axial guide for the shaft and can in principle be realized by a single bearing. However, for very high axial or radial loads, two bearings are commonly used to ensure the locating bearing function. Therefore, pillow block bearing units for the support side (maedler, 64200412), also called non-locating bearing arrangement, absorbs axial displacements that may occur during operation.
To reduce the lateral forces acting on the shaft and to prevent it from escaping from the guide, right-handed thread clamping rings (igus, CRR-01-TR10X2) were used and mounted on top and underneath each locating bearing.
The completely assembled XYZ positioning stage is shown in Fig. 1.

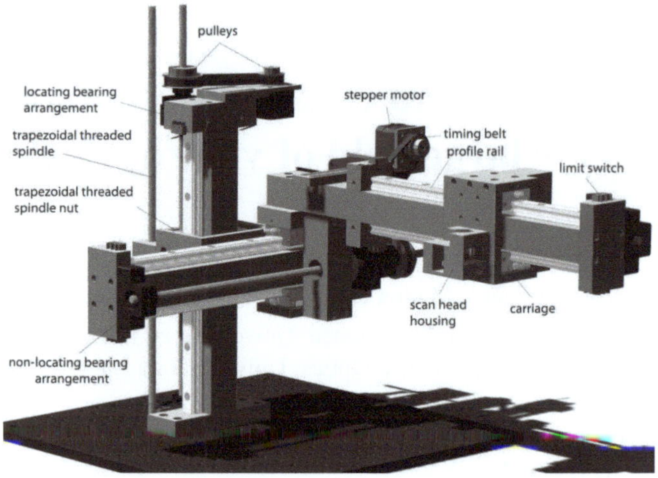

Figure 1: Final version of the XYZ positioning stage with custom-designed (not labeled) and commercially available components. The scan head housing will include scanners and scanning optics of the OCT system.

2.2 Stepper Motors and Driver Board

The used stepper motors are linear motors (Trinamic, QSH4218-51-10-049-AT) designed with a step angle of 1.8 ° (200 steps per rotation). For precise positioning and monitoring of the stage, an incremental encoder (TMCS-28-5-10000-AT-01, TRINAMIC Motion Control GmbH & Co. KG, Hamburg, Germany) is mounted on the motor with a resolution of 10.000 lines (40.000 counts). By counting the number of pulses per revolution, encoders can determine position, angle and revolution of the stepper motors. Whenever the shaft rotates through a certain angle, two square pulses, A and B, are generated with a 90 ° phase shift. With the output values of these signals, the direction of rotation can be easily determined. Equal values point to a counterclockwise rotating encoder, whereas varying output signals indicate clockwise turning. To drive the motors and read out the encoders and limit switches, a triple axis stepper motor driver (TMCM-3110-TMCL, TRINAMIC Motion Control GmbH & Co. KG, Hamburg, Germany) is used. It has a self-developed software for operating the stepper motor via computer. For example, the TMCL-IDE (Trinamic Motion Control Language - Integrated Development Environment, TRINAMIC Motion Control GmbH & Co. KG, Hamburg, Germany) graphical user interface offers a fast setup through commands in direct mode.

2.3 Motion Control Software

For controlling the motorized stage with a self-developed software, all programming is done in LabVIEW 2017 (National Instruments Austin, Texas, USA), a graphical programming language commonly used as a control software. LabVIEW's ability to easily communicate between commercial software and third-party hardware has made it become a standard in the industry, education, and research. The most practical and convenient advantage of

LabVIEW is the easy implementation of typical real-time system functions, e.g., process synchronization and events handling.
Individual function elements are available as building blocks, so-called VIs (Virtual Instruments) in extensive function libraries. The Virtual Instrument Software Architecture (VISA) supplies an interface to test and measurement equipment. Since the connection between the driver and the computer is established via USB, the implementation of VISA commands is required. In the following LabVIEW program, the stepper motor is controlled by binary commands, although a control via ASCII-commands is also available.
To control each motor manually, but also generate a matrix scan, two interacting LabVIEW programs were developed. In the Main VI, the user controls the motors by setting relevant operating axis parameters, while the the Scan VI enables a stepwise movement of each axis. To communicate data between the two VIs, notifier operations functions are used. In principle, notifiers can send messages and temporarily halting the execution of loops. The distinct advantage is the ability to send notifications to numerous VIs.
Before starting the program, the operator can configure general stepper motor control settings, e.g., adjust the maximum acceleration, positioning speed and steps per mm. Parameters to calculate the number of steps per millimeters are thread pitch, number of teeth on the pulleys, and number of motor steps per revolution. Considering the parameters described in section 2, we obtain a step size of 68,1 steps per millimeters.
When the positioning stage is turned on, the current stage position is unknown. It only knows the maximum travel distances of the axis. Thus, after starting the main program it is necessary to execute a reference search and to hit at least one of the two limit switches to move to a specific position. The zero position is then the point where the limit switch is being last activated. The program also shows the user the current motor and encoder position of each axis. Flashing LEDs indicate the current TMCL application status and warn the user immediately if a zero or position error occurs. A slide for each axis enables the manual movement of the stage to any desired position.
However, to scan a large area, an automatic positioning is advantageous. Therefore, with the Scan VI, the user can move to the desired positions after configuring the parameters scan starting position, scan ending position, and step size. To monitor the stage, the current position of each axis is visualized in graphs. LEDs indicate when a position change occurs and are used as triggers to communicate with other programs.
All three stepper motors could be controlled and configured by the Main VI. Besides, each axis could be moved manually to the desired position. The Scan VI also showed promising results and an automatic scanning was possible. Nevertheless, the program still needs to be implemented appropriately in the existing OCT imaging system to ensure full validation of the matrix scanning function.

3 Results and Discussion

In the following section, the results of the different OCT measurements are presented and discussed. In addition, potential improvement strategies and a corresponding outlook on future optimizations are given.

3.1 Stage Design

We have developed and successfully assembled a motorized XYZ positioning stage with a scan area of about 22,5 x 22,5 x 22,5 cm. Still, it became apparent that the stage was heavy with a strong lever arm loading on the X-axis, which resulted in a slight skewing. Since the Z-axis has a high load on it, a weight reduction of the other two axes is advantageous. One possibility is to make some parts narrower or to mill out specific areas. Another possibility is the use of two Z-axes, which would significantly stabilize the entire stage. Alternatively, the use of lighter material instead of aluminum could also achieve the desired result. It would be beneficial to print some components of the X- and Y-axis with the help of 3D printers, as these can be produced quickly at low cost and would lead to a significant reduction in weight. However, the stage showed promising results and could already be moved propitiously by the stepper motors.

3.2 OCT Imaging

To preliminary study the functionality of the stage for OCT imaging and at the same time obtain important knowledge about the tilt angle in X- and Y-direction, nine 1.65 mm thick polyamide PA washers (plastic washers), placed in a 24-well plate, were acquired with the OCT imaging system and evaluated by the image processing program ImageJ (version 1.52q, Wayne Rasband, NIH, USA). The test setup is shown in Fig. 2A. Using the existing OCT imaging system, 1000 B-Scans from each well were acquired, while the 500th one was evaluated. The evaluation showed that the washer had a thickness of 273.05 pixels, which could be used to calculate the inclination of the X- and Y-stage in millimeters. The deviations of the plane bottom surface position of the wells were determined in relation to the buttom surface position of well A1. Deviations of A2: 0.22 mm, A3: 0,44 mm, A4: 0,68 mm, A5: 0,89 mm, A6: 1,11 mm, B1: 0,19 mm, C1: 0,39 mm and D1: 0,56 mm were observed. The obtained results are shown in the diagrams in Fig. 2A. The measurements indicate a tilting in x- and y-direction.
Since the future intention is to use this setup to scan biological tissue, we also acquired OCT data of human skin to study the consequences of the axes inclination under real conditions. For this purpose, on day six of the wound healing screening study described above, a 24-well plate was examined containing the human skin organ cultures. 24 OCT images of each wound at constant Z-axis height were acquired, as exemplarily shown in Fig. 2B. The results showed that the tilt of the stage in x-direction leads to significant artifacts in the OCT images. In contrast to D1, well

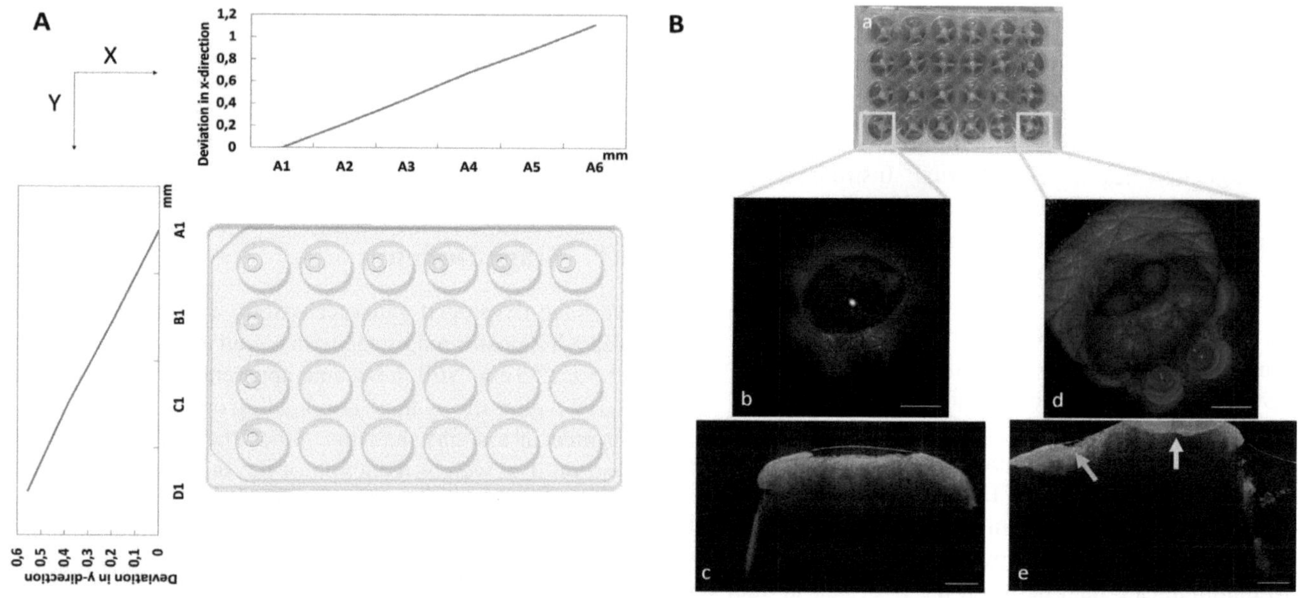

Figure 2: A) In the first row and column of the 24-well plate, a plastic washer is placed in the same position. Two graphs show the deviation of the surface position in X- and Y-direction in millimeters. B) A 24-well plate (a) contains human skin with lesions. Subsequently, en face OCT (b, d) and B-Scans (c, e) of the skin samples in the wells D1 (left) and D6 (right) were acquired. The green arrow points to the wound, while the yellow one shows the significant flipping-artifact. Scale bar in the OCT images (b – e) corresponds to 1000 µm.

D6 showed distinct flipping-artifacts that made the quantification of wound volume impossible.
Accordingly, possibilities to make the stage significantly more stable and accurate would have to be considered in the future since even small fluctuations in OCT images lead to considerable artifacts. One option would be to apply the improvement options discussed in section 3.1.

4 Conclusion

This paper presents the design and construction of a motorized and controllable XYZ positioning stage. The complete setup of the stage as well as the motor control software could be demonstrated. However, a slight tilt of the X- and Y-axis were observed, which can be corrected by reducing the weight of the components and slightly modifying the assembly. The results of the LabVIEW program were promising. The entire stage is now controllable with the interactive motion control software. The preliminary imaging results demonstrate that OCT measurements are feasible with the stage, but further testing is required. Besides, complete integration into the imaging system is needed. In long term, the implementation of an automatic stitching of the processed OCT volumes is planned to obtain large area OCT volumes.

Acknowledgement

The work has been carried out at the Institute of Biomedical Optics, Universität zu Lübeck.

Author's Statement

Conflict of interest: Authors state no conflict of interest.

5 References

[1] J. Welzel. *Optical coherence tomography in dermatology: a review*. Skin Research and Technology, vol. 7, pp. 1 - 9, 2010.

[2] D. Huang, E. A. Swanson, C. P. Lin, J. S. Schuman, W. G. Stinson, W. Chang, M. R. Hee, T. Flotte, K. Gregory, C. A. Puliafito, and J. G. Fujimoto, *Optical Coherence Tomography*. Science, vol. 254(5035), pp. 1178–1181, 1991.

[3] R. Huber, M. Wojtkowski and J. G. Fujimoto, *Fourier Domain Mode Locking (FDML): A new laser operating regime and applications for optical coherence tomography*. Optics Express, vol. 14, pp. 3225 - 3237, 2006.

[4] T. Pfeiffer, M. Petermann, W. Draxinger, C. Jirauschek, and R. Huber, *Ultra low noise Fourierdomain mode lockedlaserfor high quality megahertz optical coherence tomography*. Biomed. Opt.Express, vol. 9, pp. 4130-4148, 2018.

[5] J. P. Kolb, D. Weng, H. Hakert, M. Eibl, W. Draxinger, T. Meyer, T. Gottschall, R. Brinkmann, R. Birngruber, J. Popp, J. Limpert, S. Karpf and R. Huber, *Virtual HE histology by fiber-based picosecond two-photon microscopy* . Proc. SPIE 10882, Multiphoton Microscopy in the Biomedical Sciences XIX, pp. 108822F, 2019.

Comparison of light sources with different spatial and temporal characteristics for full-field swept-source OCT

Svea Höhl[1], Salim Melikov[1], Clara Pfäffle[2], Gereon Hüttmann[2], and Dierck Hillmann[2,3]

[1] Medical Engineering, Universität zu Lübeck, {svea.hoehl,salim.melikov}@student.uni-luebeck.de
[2] Institute of Biomedical Optics, Universität zu Lübeck, {cl.pfaeffle,gereon.huettmann,d.hillmann}@uni-luebeck.de
[3] Thorlabs GmbH, dhillmann@thorlabs.com

Abstract

Full-field swept-source optical coherence tomography provides high-resolution depth-resolved images. With its tunable laser source and fast CMOS camera, volumetric images can be generated in 8.5 ms. However, acquired datasets suffer from crosstalk due to multiply scattered light, which corrupts the images with white shadows beneath strongly scattering tissue. Additionally, the used light source may limit the axial resolution and, when applied to functional retinal imaging, may cause undesired background stimulation of the acquired retinal area. In this work, it is shown that a deformable membrane to modulate the light source can effectively reduce the crosstalk. Furthermore, two laser sources covering different spectral ranges are compared in terms of achieved signal-to-noise ratio, axial resolution, and background stimulation of the retina.

1 Introduction

Optical coherence tomography (OCT) is an imaging modality that acquires volumetric images with a resolution in the μm range and is particularly important in ophthalmological diagnostics. One possible variant is full-field swept-source OCT (FF-SS-OCT), which uses a tunable laser source combined with an area illumination and detection. Its Fourier-domain signal detection and parallel data acquisition enable very high imaging rates and sensitivity.

Due to the high speed and resulting phase stability, path-length changes in the sub-wavelength range can be observed, which provide new applications of FF-SS-OCT such as the imaging of retinal function [5]. However, the activation potentials of the neurons yield only small optical changes and are therefore hard to detect, especially as the signal gets overlayed by inevitable eye motion [6]. Additionally, the laser, with wavelengths around 841 nm, leads to unwanted stimulation of the retina. Finally, the spatial coherence of the laser and the associated interference of multiple scattered photons leads to a degradation of the image quality by so-called crosstalk, which hides important sample features of deeper retinal layers [2]. In scanning systems, a confocal pinhole in front of the detector prevents the laterally travelling light from being detected. As a pinhole cannot be implemented in a full-field system, an alternative option was suggested by [1] and will be presented by using a deformable membrane (DM).

In this paper, two possible improvements will be investigated by altering the spatial and temporal characteristics of the light source used. First, we investigate the suppression of multiple scattered photons by a DM, and, second, we compare two light sources with different spectral ranges concerning the axial resolution, signal-to-noise ratio, and wavelength used for imaging retinal functions to reduce unwanted retinal stimulation.

2 Material and Methods

2.1 Deformable Membrane

OCT measures light run-time interferometrically to obtain depth information about the imaged tissue. FF-SS-OCT offers great advantages in image speed over scanning OCT systems due to parallel detection of the backscattered light instead of lateral and axial scanning.

However, the area illumination of the sample also has disadvantages. For example, if a sample scatteres light multiple times, it can travel laterally and may be mapped incorrectly in the volume [3]. Consequently, this multiply scattered light overlays the deeper layers of the sample and limits the imaging depth. This effect is called crosstalk and manifests itself as bright shadows below strongly scattering tissue. To supress the multiply scattered photons, a DM can be implemented in the optical setup, which works analogous to the confocal filtering in scanning OCT systems. The corresponding setup is shown in Fig. 1.

To acquire a volume, the laser is tuned from 816 to 867 nm. The laser beam enters the setup via a single-mode fibre, is collimated and then reflected by the DM, which consists of a membrane that can be excited by an actuator into chaotic oscillations at a frequency of up to $500,000$ Hz. With the

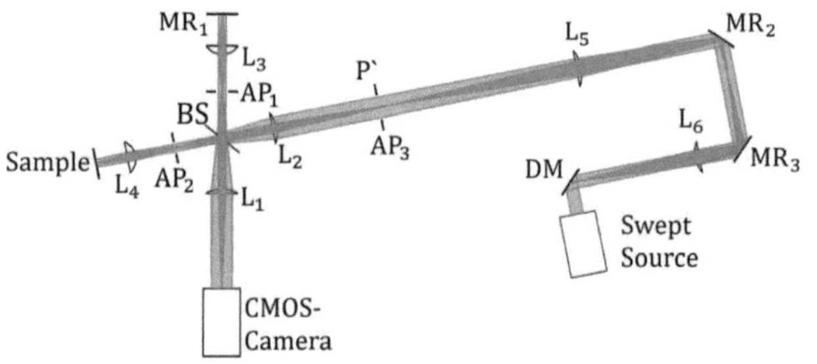

Figure 1: Optical setup to reduce crosstalk. The path of the collimated laser beam, as well as the mapping of the DM plane are shown. The DM is imaged onto the P'-plane, sample, reference mirror and camera. L_1 - L_6 – lenses; MR_1 - MR_3 – mirrors; BS - beam splitter; DM – deformable membrane; P' – plane conjugate to the DM.

subsequent lenses L_5 (focal length $f = 200$ mm) and L_6 ($f = 75$ mm), the beam diameter is enlarged to about 2.5 times its previous size. Together with the two mirrors MR_2 and MR_3, this part serves to map the DM onto a plane conjugated to the sample plane (P'-plane). The following Michelson interferometer is designed to keep the plane of the DM conjugated to the sample, the reference mirror, and the camera. In the reference arm, the plane P' is imaged onto a mirror MR_1. The sample arm is identical, with the exception of a scattering sample instead of the mirror.

In case the DM is off, it effectively acts as a mirror. Backscattered and reflective light from the sample and reference arm, respectively, are recombined by the beam splitter and imaged onto the camera through the lens L_1 ($f =$ 100mm).

When the DM is turned on, it applies a phase error to the incident beam, creating small areas of spatial coherence. The resulting beam does no longer have a flat wavefront and can be seen as incoherent over the exposure time of the camera. To ensure that identical phase patterns are imaged onto the sample and the reference mirror, the DM is placed in front of the interferometer. Thus, light from the reference- and the sample arm can only interfere with each other if they originate from the same coherence volume – that is, if the same phase error has been applied to both beams. Otherwise, the interference pattern is washed out, suppressing the crosstalk.

Similarly, the phase patterns of reference and sample arm decorrelate when one arm is moved out-of-focus. Therefore, it is essential that both arms of the interferometer are carefully aligned. In addition, sacrifices must be made in the usable depth of field with an active DM.

The interference image is detected by a CMOS camera, which records a sample volume of $640 \times 368 \times 256$ pixels in 8.5 ms. The rate of the chaotic oscillations of the DM is far higher than the inverse exposure time of the camera of about $60,000$ Hz, which is necessary to average the incoming light to a uniform distribution. For the reconstruction, the time series is then converted to OCT volumes by Fourier transformation.

2.2 Retinal Measurement

Three-dimensional tomograms of the retina with a resolution in the μm range can be acquired by FF-SS-OCT. The optical setup shown in Fig. 2 can be used to detect retinal function in the living human eye. It is based on a Michelson interferometer and uses a tuneable light source for the acquisition of an OCT volume.

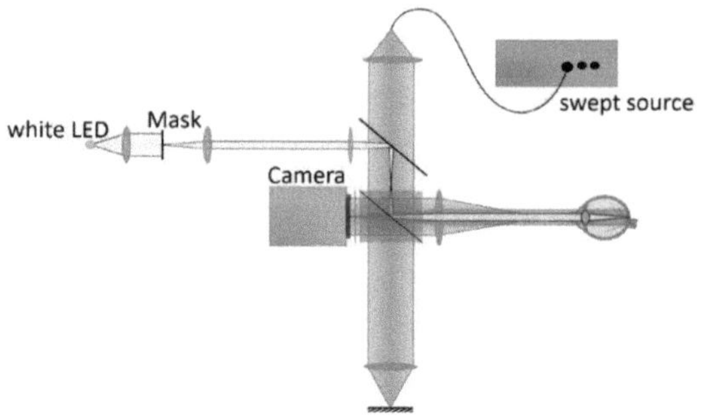

Figure 2: Optical setup to obtain a tomogram of the human retina. A Michelson interferometer is used to split the beam from the tuneable light source into a reference beam and a sample beam. The backscattered light from the eye in the sample beam is then imaged onto the CMOS-camera where it is superimposed with the reference light. A projector with a white LED source is used to stimulate the retina.

A collimated laser beam, operating in the infrared range, is split into the reference beam and the sample beam by a beam splitter. While the reference beam focusses on a single spot on a mirror, the sample beam illuminates a rectangular area of the retina of 3.6×1.5 mm through an aperture and a system of lenses with a radiation power of 5.2 mW. To ensure that the sample- and the reference arm have the same length, the reference arm can be adjusted individually. A CMOS camera captures the interfering light of reference- and the sample beam and acquires a volume of the retina in 8.5 ms, containg 512 images. Such high acquisition speeds and parallel imaging are important properties to obtain a stable phase across the whole field of view and permits computational aberration compensation that can significantly enhance image quality [1].

The phase stability allows detection of small photoreceptor changes in the optical path length $l = n \cdot d$ of the imaged tissue, which depends on the refractive index n and the distance d that the light has passed through. In this case it is used to visualize the physiological response of the retina to the stimulation by an X-shaped white light pulse, which is included in the optical setup by an LED-based projection system and irradiates a 0.6 mm^2 area of the retina. The optical stimulation activates the photoreceptors of individual cones and thereby leads to a change in optical path length, which can be detected by FF-SS-OCT, as shown in [4].

These small changes in optical path length are hard to detect and make an accurate measurement of the retina essential and can be further optimised by choosing a suitable laser. The first laser is tuned in the wavelength range of $816 - 867$ nm. Thus, it has a bandwidth of $\Delta\lambda = 51$ nm and a central wavelength of $\lambda_0 = 841$ nm. The second laser can be tuned in a higher wavelength range from $875 - 961$ nm, has a wider bandwidth of $\Delta\lambda = 86$ nm and its central wavelength is $\lambda_0 = 918$ nm.

3 Results and Discussion

3.1 Deformable Membrane

Images of an aloe vera plant with and without the DM being activated are shown in Fig. 3. It can be seen that the activated DM significantly suppresses crosstalk and leads to an improved contrast in the images.
The areas circled in light and dark blue demonstrate how the active DM improves the image quality. While the structure within the dark blue ellipse is imaged clearly with an active DM, it is barely visible when the crosstalk is not suppressed. Also, at deeper layers, a bright shadow appears in the images when the DM is off, as the scattering light is mapped incorrectly to these layers. The average pixel intensity within the light blue ellipse is 43.87 dB for DM off and 41.87 dB for DM on, which proves an increase in intensity for the inactive DM.
The reduction of crosstalk can also be estimated by the variance of the intensities σ^2 from self-selected regions in the reconstructed OCT image as shown in [1]. These regions are highlighted in Fig. 3 by the red squares and do not include any specific object structures. Thus, a low variance is desirable, as the selected region shall only include pixels of similar low intensity. If, however, light is mapped wrongly to this region due to crosstalk, the intensity of some pixels and therefor the variance increases. In this case we obtain a variance of $\sigma^2_{\text{off}} = 0,158$ and $\sigma^2_{\text{on}} = 0,126$ for DM off and on, proving that with an active DM, the variance and hence crosstalk is reduced.

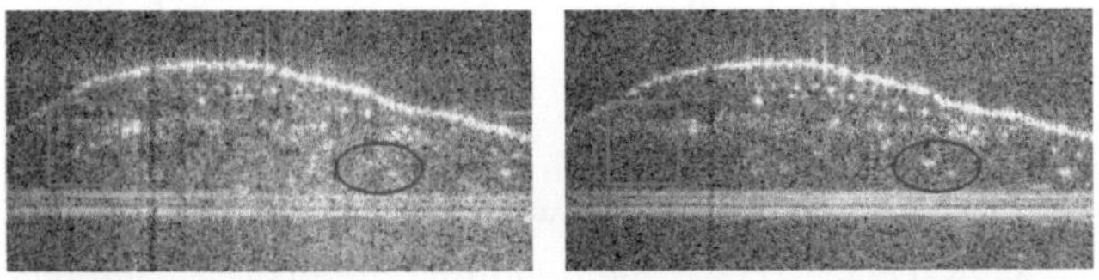

Figure 3: B-scans of an aloe vera plant. On the left side, the DM was off. Thus, the crosstalk was not suppressed. The right side shows the image with an active DM. Hence, a reduction of crosstalk can be seen. The red squares in the B-scans mark the areas which have been used for a quantitative analysis of the crosstalk. The blue ellipses highlight areas where the difference of crosstalk is clearly visible.

3.2 Retinal Measurement

For retinal measurements, two different lasers were implemented in the setup and compared to each other. Fig. 4 shows two B-scans of the retina taken with both lasers. The B-scans illustrates the different layers of the retina very well. However, some layers seem to be more sharply imaged in the B-scan with the 918 nm laser, which could be

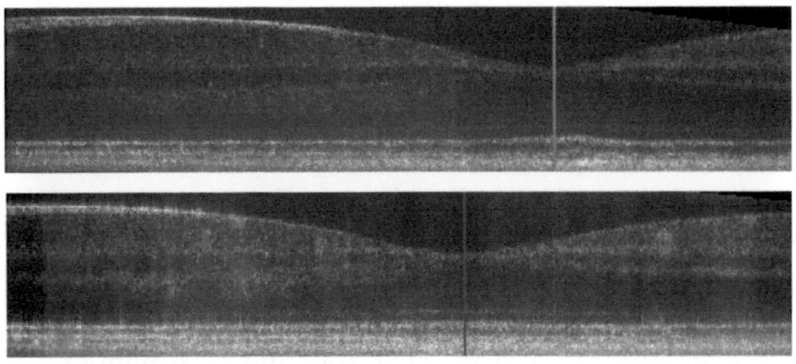

Figure 4: B-scans taken with the 918 nm laser (top) and the 841 nm laser (bottom). The red and blue lines correspond to the A-scans in Fig. 5.

explained by an improved axial resolution.
The axial resolution can be determined by the full width at half maximum (FWHM) and the assumption of a rectangular spectrum. In theory, the axial resolution is calculated via the formula $\frac{1{,}21 \cdot \pi}{\Delta k}$, and therefore depends on the bandwidth Δk of the laser, given in wave numbers. With $\Delta k = 452.94 \cdot 10^3 \frac{1}{\text{m}}$ for the 841 nm laser, a resolution of 8.39 μm in air can be calculated. This value is slightly better than the actual resolution of 8.5 μm in [4]. The same applies to the axial resolution of the 918 nm laser. Theoretically it lies at 5.92 μm, given that $\Delta k = 642.61 \cdot 10^3 \frac{1}{\text{m}}$. Although its actual resolution is slightly worse. This can be determined by measuring a single reflecting surface, such as a glass plate which has been used in this case. In order to determine the FWHM of the reflection accurately, the camera image is first enlarged to five times its original size using zero padding of the spectra. Next, the enlarged camera image is Fourier transformed to obtain a B-scan of the glass plate. To determine the FWHM of the intensity peak, all pixels whose value is above half of the maximum intensity value are added up. With an axial pixel spacing $\frac{\pi}{\Delta k}$ and the $5\times$ oversample, this yields the actual width of the intensity peak of 6.11 μm, which in turn corresponds to the axial resolution of the 918 nm laser in air.

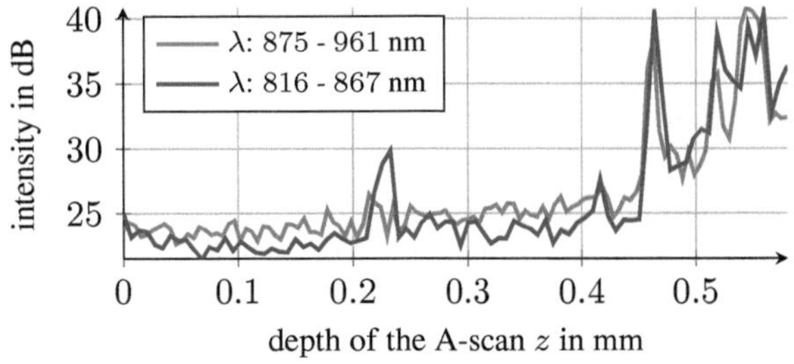

Figure 5: Intensity values of the A-scans of both lasers from the area of the fovea plotted against its depth. The A-scans correspond to the vertical red and blue lines in Fig. 4.

Due to the different bandwidths of the lasers, the axial pixel spacing in the OCT images also changes as it is inversely proportional to the scanning in frequency space. Thus, the z-distance between the pixels in the Fourier transformed image also changes. Here, we obtain an axial pixel spac-

ing of 9.23 μm for the 841 nm laser and 6.50 μm for the 918 nm laser. However, the B-scans and A-scans for Fig. 4 and 5 have been scaled to the same size.
The peaks in Fig. 5, corresponding to different layers of the retina, have very similar shapes. However, the peak at the center of this A-Scan is more pronounced with the 841 nm laser (blue line) and is therefore easier to recognise. In addition, the signal-to-noise ratio (SNR) can be determined very well from the A-scan. Therefore, the maximum ($x_{\max}$) and minimum ($x_{\min}$) intensity values are determined, and afterwards the SNR in dB is calculated by [5]

$$\mathrm{SNR} = 20 \cdot (\log_{10}(x_{\max}) - \log_{10}(x_{\min})). \qquad (1)$$

We thus get an SNR of 17.2 dB for the 918 nm laser and a slightly better SNR of 18.9 dB for the 841 nm laser.

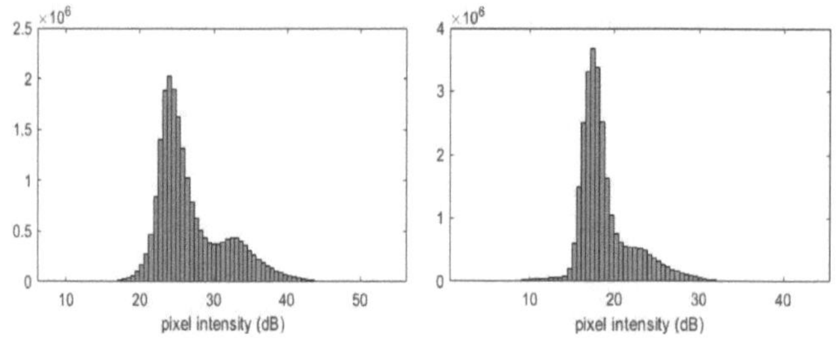

Figure 6: Histograms of OCT volumes of the 841 nm laser (left) and the 918 nm laser (right). The volumes contain different numbers of pixels, thus the height of the bars differ accordingly. A maximum intensity of 43 dB can be observed for the 918 nm laser, while most of its intensity values lie around 17 dB. The 841 nm laser has its maximum intensity at 54 dB and most pixels at 24 dB.

In Fig. 6 two histograms can be seen, which were created over all pixels of the respective volumes. Even though the two histograms have a similar shape, there are some differences. Firstly, the volumes consist of a different number of pixels, due to the different pixel spacing. As a result, the height of the bars is greater in the histogram of the 841 nm laser. Also, the dB values themselves differ. The intensity in the image with the 918 nm laser reaches values of 43 dB, while the maximum value of the 841 nm laser is at 54 dB and thereby much higher. The difference can be explained by the fact that the camera is less sensitive to the photons at a higher wavelength range. Also, the absorption by the water of the eye becomes more dominant at higher wavelengths. Thus, fewer photons are detected, decreasing the intensity of the OCT images. To counter this phenomenon, a higher irradiation power could be used. However, care must be taken to permissible irradiation power for the human eye.

4 Conclusion

It was described how two different approaches may help to further improve the illumination of FF-SS-OCT.
The first part demonstrated an efficient way to suppress interference of multiple scattered photons in FF-SS-OCT by extension with a DM. This results in a reduced crosstalk in the images, which makes previously invisible structures visible again. Additionally, it is a low-cost and robust add-on to any existing FF-SS-OCT system, requiring only simple modifications [3], that would make this technique also attractive for clinical applications. After further image enhancement with computational aberration correction and optical system improvements it might even become an alternative to scanning OCT systems.
The second part dealt with the comparison of two lasers for FF-SS-OCT, that is used for visualisation of optical path length differences in the retina after stimulation with white light. It could be shown that the 841 nm laser has a higher SNR, while the 918 nm laser provides a better axial resolution. As both are important image features, it cannot yet be said which laser fulfils this task best. As the radiant flux directed into the eye was not yet limited by safety standards, a further increase in sensitivity is possible [5].

Acknowledgement

The work has been carried out and supervised by the Institute of Biomedical Optics, Universität zu Lübeck.

Author's Statement

Conflict of interest: Authors state no conflict of interest.

5 References

[1] E. Auksorius, D. Borycki and M. Wojtkowski, *Crosstalk-free volumetric in vivo imaging of a human retina with Fourier-domain full-field optical coherence tomography*. In: Biomedical Optic Express, vol. 10, pp. 6390–6407, 2019.

[2] D. Borycki, M. Hamkalo, M. Nowakowski, M. Szkulmowski and M. Wojtkowski, *Spatiotemporal optical coherence (STOC) manipulation suppresses coherent cross-talk in full-field swept-source optical coherence tomography*. In: Biomedical Optic Express, vol. 10, pp. 2032–2054, 2019.

[3] P. Stremplewski, et al. *In vivo volumetric imaging by crosstalk-free full-field OCT*. In: Optica, vol. 113, pp. 608–617, 2019.

[4] D. Hillmann, et al. *In vivo optical imaging of physiological responses to photostimulation in human photoreceptors*. In: PNAS, vol. 113, pp. 13138–13143, 2016.

[5] D. Hillmann, et al. *Off-axis reference beam for full-field swept-source OCT and holoscopy*. In: Optics Express, vol. 25, pp. 27770–27784, 2017.

[6] C. Pfäffle, et al. *Simultaneous functional imaging of neuronal and photoreceptor layers in living human retina*. In: Optics Letters, vol. 44, pp. 5671–5674, 2019.

Investigation of intracellular Localization of the Photosensitizer Amphinex and the Antibody TuBB-9 for their potential Use in photochemical Internalization

I. Knor [1], P. Enzian [2], A. Link [2], and R. Rahmanzadeh [2]

[1] Medical Engineering Science, Universität zu Lübeck, igor.knor@student.uni-luebeck.de

[2] Institute of Biomedical Optics, Universität zu Lübeck, {p.enzian, astrid.link, ramtin.rahmanzadeh}@uni-luebeck.de

Abstract

Photochemical internalization (PCI) is a drug delivery technology, developed for cancer therapy. PCI is based on the use of photosensitizers (PS), which are incubated with the cells, accumulate in the membranes of endocytosed vesicles and induce the membrane to rupture after light irradiation. Thus, the desired macromolecules can be delivered to their targets before they are degraded in lysosomes. Accurate localization of the photosensitizer and drugs in the cell is very essential for efficient triggered release. For this reason, the focus of this work is to analyze the localization of photosensitizer Amphinex and the antibody TuBB-9 in HeLa cells prior to light exposure for subsequent applicability intended for PCI. The results show a localization of the photosensitizer at the cell- and endosomal membrane at various time points between 5 minutes and 24 hours of incubation. In addition, it was shown that the antibodies reached their target in the cell nucleoli, providing a good basis for subsequent light irradiation.

1 Introduction

Photochemical internalization is a novel technology based on the principle of photodynamic therapy (PDT), but in addition to the biological effects of reactive oxygen species after PDT, it allows photochemical release of drugs trapped in endocytic vesicles into the cytosol. PCI, like PDT, is based on light activation of photosensitizers, which have a high affinity to accumulate in tumor tissues. Moreover, photosensitizers have no strong side effects in the absence of light irradiation [1].

These above properties of photosensitizers are the basis of both PDT and PCI methods. However, PCI can be called a more detailed-focused continuation of photodynamic therapy [3]. Not all molecules are able to penetrate the cell membrane, particularly therapeutic drugs that are intended to treat cancer. Those drugs that penetrate the cells by endocytosis finally end up in lysosomes, where they are degraded and thus lose their therapeutic effect. The innovativeness of PCI is based on the approach that the therapeutic drugs are released from endocytic vesicles and lysosomes and enter the cytoplasm, avoiding the degradation stage in lysosomes [2]. The photosensitizer will rupture the endosomal membrane and enable the endocytosed drug to enter the cytosol [1]. In this way, the potential of drugs that have to reach the nucleolus of the cell directly, for example, can be exploited much better. A scheme of this process can be seen in Fig. 1.

Each of the above PCI stages is very important. The first part of this work is focused on analyses of the photosensitizer Amphinex. The amphiphilic photosensitizers used in PCI are strongly bound to the membranes of endocytic vesicles [4]. However, for PCI it is necessary to know exactly where the PS is localized in the cell, otherwise the drug cannot be released into the cytosol under light irradiation. Thus, the first aim was to characterize the photosensitizer Amphinex in terms of its intracellular binding characteristics. An equally important preliminary stage of PCI is the preparation of the drug or antibody, which requires prior demonstration that it will recognize its target in the cell. Therefore, the second part of the work is focused on the TuBB-9 antibody. This antibody recognizes the antigen Ki-67 in proliferating cells, which is located in the cell's nucleoli. Accordingly, light irradiation would destroy the cancer cell originating from the nucleus. Thus, the second aim of this study was to investigate whether the TuBB-9 antibody is useful for targeting the nucleus.

2 Material and Methods

2.1 Cell Culture and Cell Number

HeLa is cervical cancer cell line used in scientific research and was purchased from American type tissue culture (ATCC, No. ACC 57, headquarters in Manassas, Virginia). It is the oldest and most commonly used human cell line [5]. These cells were taken from a 31-year-old patient, Henrietta Lacks, at a cancer clinic at Johns Hopkins

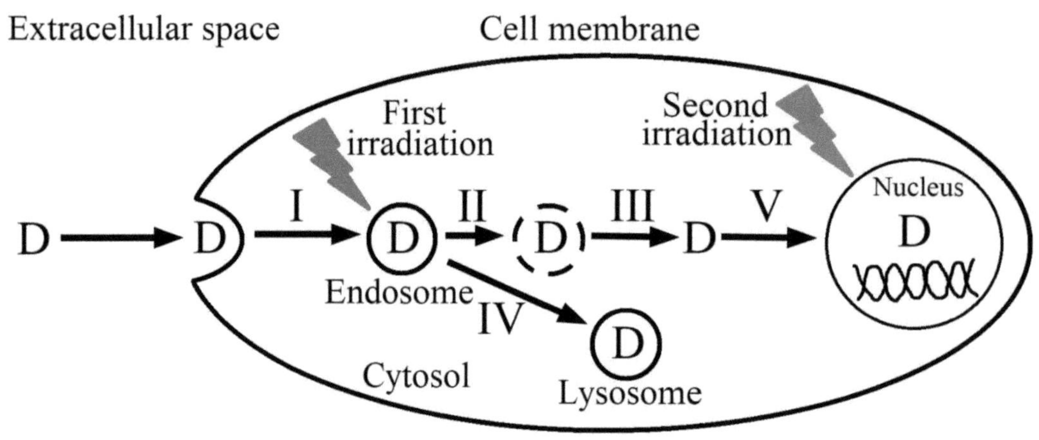

Figure 1: Schematic illustration of the PCI process.The drug (D) is endocytosed (I). The photosensitizer is localized in the membrane of endosomal vesicles. Under light exposure, the photosensitizer generates reactive oxygen species that degrade the endosomal membrane (III), leading to release into the cell cytosol (IV). Even in the cytosol, the drug can reach the cell nucleolus (V), where, if fluorescent dye is used, the drug can be exposed to light of a second wavelength (e.g., green), which can be used to affect the cell nucleolus directly, thus increasing the efficiency of the therapy. Alternatively, the drug enters the lysosome and is degraded (II), for example, due to the missing irradiation of the photosensitizer.

in Baltimore in 1951. This adherent cell line is cultivated in Dulbecco's Modified Eagle's Medium (DMEM) containing 4500 mg/l glucose (Sigma-Aldrich, USA) supplemented with 10% fetal bovine serum (FBS, Sigma-Aldrich, USA) and 1% penicillin-streptomycin (10 000 units/mL penicillin and 10 mg/mL streptomycin, Sigma-Aldrich, USA).

Cells were cultured in T-75 cell culture flasks in an incubator at 37°C and a 5% CO_2 concentration. At confluence of about 80%, the cells were split.

Cell number was determined microscopically using a Neubauer counting chamber. To separate living and dead cells, the cell suspension was mixed in a ratio of 1 : 1 with 0.5% trypan blue solution. The hemocytometer was filled with 10 µl from the resulting solution and counted under a light microscope. The dead cells take up the dye and appear blue and are not counted.

2.2 Photosensitizer Amphinex

In this study, the photosensitizer Amphinex (disulfonated tetraphenyl chlorine with the sulfonate groups on adjacent phenyl rings (4, 4'-(15, 20-diphenyl-7, 8(or 12, 13 or 17, 18)-dihydro-21 H, 23 H - porphine-5, 10-diyl) bisbenzenesulfonic acid, $TPCS_{2a}$) was evaluated [4].

To determine a wavelength for future PCI irradiation at which the reactive oxygen species can be generated, the absorption spectrum of Amphinex was measured. A HITACHI U-2900 UV-VIS Double Beam Spectrometer was used for this purpose. Therefore, Amphinex (stocksolution 30 mg/ml) was diluted 1:20 000 in dimethyl sulfoxide (DMSO, Sigma-Aldrich, USA). The fluorescence spectrum was measured by using the spectrometer SpectraMAX M4 (Molecular Devices, USA) after excitation at 420 nm.

2.3 Antibody TuBB-9-700DX

The antibody TuBB-9 was described in 2006 by Bullwinkel et al. at the Borstel Research Center. The antibody binds to the antigen Ki-67 and is produced from hybridoma cells. The labeling of TuBB-9 with IRdye700DX was performed according to a protocol of the company LI-COR Biosciences at the Institute of Biomedical Optics.

2.4 Immunofluorescence Microscopy

The cellular localization of Amphinex was analyzed by fluorescence microscopy. The images were captured using the Nikon Eclipse Ti inverse fluorescence microscope with NIS-Elements software. All fluorescence images were taken with a 60x oil immersion objective.

2.4.1 Microscopy on fixed HeLa Cells

The localization of the antibody was observed on fixed HeLa cells. HeLa cells were seeded with a cell density of 80 000 cells/ml in cell culture dishes with a glass bottom (CELLView™ Cell Culture Dish with four compartments, Ø 35 mm, Greiner Bio-One). Before staining, cells were fixed and permeabilized. For this purpose, the medium was removed and cells were washed three times with 500 µl Dulbeccos's Phosphate Buffered Saline (PBS, Sigma-Aldrich, USA) without calcium chloride ($CaCl_2$) and magnesium chloride ($MgCl_2$). Afterwards, the cells were incubated in 4% formaldehyde ROTI®Histofix (pH 7, Carl Roth, Germany) for 15 min. For permeabilization of the cells, they were treated with 0.25% Triton X-100 for 3 min. Subsequently, HeLa cells were washed three times with PBS. TuBB-9-700DX (TuBB-9 concentration: 1mg/ml) was used for detection of the Ki-67 protein. 1:100 and 1:50 dilutions were prepared in PBS with 10% FBS and incubated at room

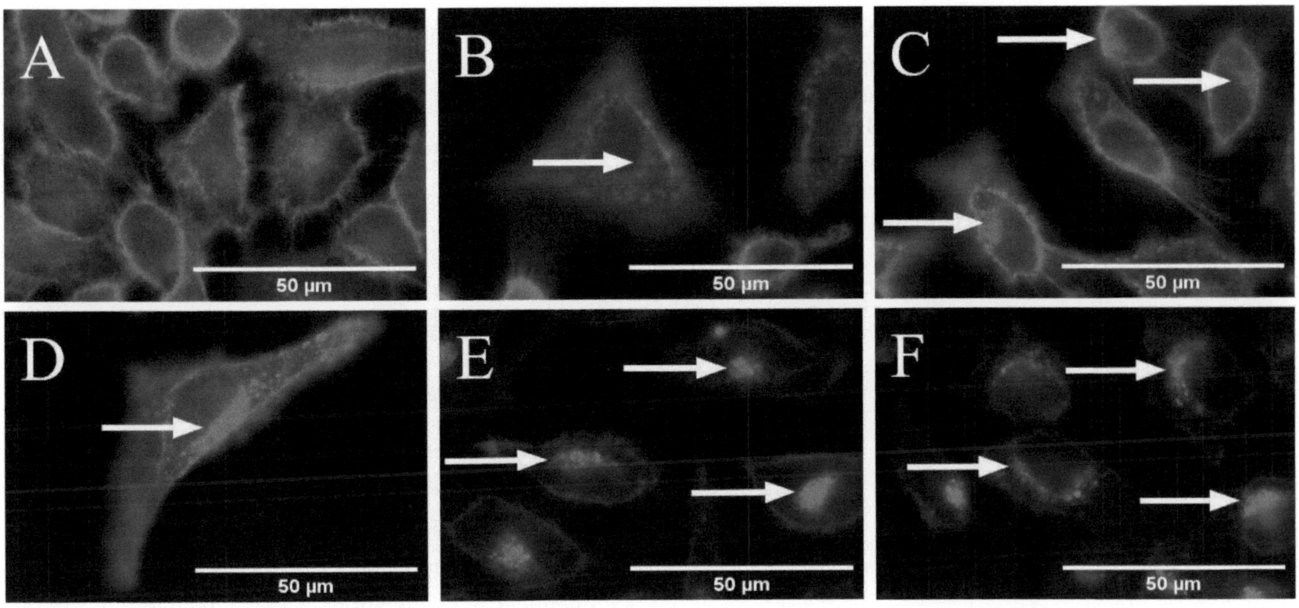

Figure 2: Localization of Amphinex in HeLa cells after different incubation times. (A) 5-Minute sample, (B) 30-Minute sample, (C) 2-Hour sample, (D) 4-Hour sample, (E) 18-Hour sample, (F) 24-Hour sample. The photosensitizer is localized in the cell membrane even in the 30-minute sample, but the localization is much more obvious in later samples, with a visible localisation in the cell cytoplasm. (indicated by white arrows).

temperature for 1h. Before capturing images under the fluorescence microscope, cells were washed three times with PBS and examined in 500 µl PBS.

2.4.2 Microscopy on living HeLa Cells

The localization of Amphinex was examined on living HeLa cells. One day before incubation with Amphinex, cells were seeded with a cell density of 80 000 cells/ml. After 24h the medium was removed and Amphinex (0.2 µg/ml in DMEM) was added to the cells. The incubation times (5min, 30min, 2h, 4h, 18h, 24h) were varied to observe the uptake of the photosensitizer. Amphinex was removed after these incubation times. Cells were washed with Dulbecco's Phosphate Buffered Saline (PBS^+, Sigma-Aldrich, USA) with calcium chloride ($CaCl_2$) and magnesium chloride ($MgCl_2$) and were examined under the microscope in PBS^+.

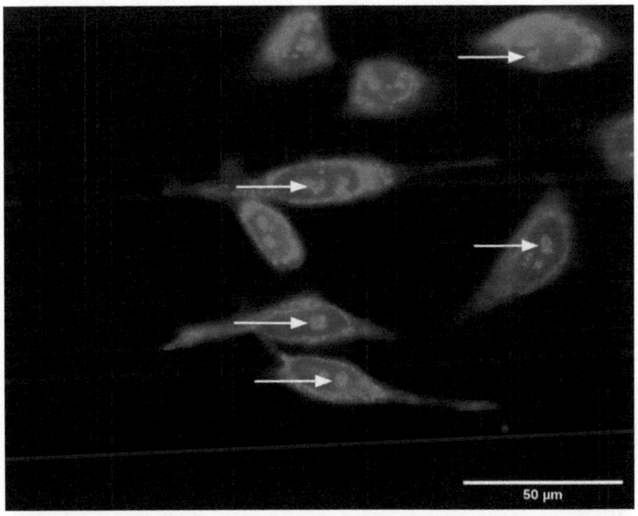

Figure 3: After incubation of antibodies TuBB-9-700DX on fixed and permeabilized HeLa cells, they are localized in the nucleoli of cells (indicated by white arrows). The characteristic dotted pattern of the antibody can also be seen in the image.

3 Results and Discussion

In this study, two important pre-stages of PCI were evaluated. Specifically, the localization of TuBB-9 antibodies and the photosensitizer Amphinex in HeLa cells was observed. The use of PCI to treat cancer enables the delivery of drugs either into the cytosol or directly into the nucleoli of the cells. The endosomal membrane must contain a photosensitizer to release the drug after passing through the cell membrane. By irradiation, the membrane is supposed to be disassembled and the drug can enter the cytosol [6]. Therefore, it is important to determine which incubation time ensures the optimal localization of Amphinex in the cells.

The localization of Amphinex in HeLa cells is shown in Fig. 2. All samples showed a localization of the photosensitizer at the cell membrane. As the incubation period of Amphinex increased, localization also occurred in the cytoplasm and mitochondria. Since the drugs are taken up into the cells via endocytosis, they are trapped in endosomes. The detected localization of Amphinex possibly allows a release of the drugs after irradiation, since it would then also accumulate in the endosomal membrane. This could allow

drug release into the cytosol in later experiments.
The second important pre-stage of PCI represents the drugs that have to be delivered through the cell membrane. In this study, IRdye700DX-labelled TuBB-9 antibodies were used that are directed against the antigen Ki-67 [7]. On fixed HeLa cells TuBB-9-700DX was located in the nucleoli. These results indicate that the labelled antibodies bind to Ki-67. This antibody might provide a good target for PCI irradiation. The characteristic dotted pattern of the TuBB-9 monoclonal antibody can be seen on the Fig. 3.

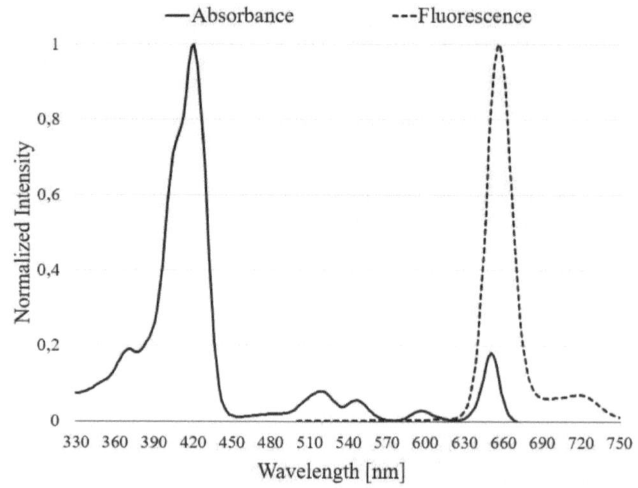

Figure 4: Normilized absorption spectrum and normilized fluorescence spectrum of Amphinex. The main peak of Amphinex absorption is at 420 nm.

To perform irradiation, it is necessary to determine the absorption and fluorescence spectra of Amphinex in advance. Depending on the wavelength, light can penetrate the tissue to diffrent depths, so it is important and preferable that the absorption maximum is in the range of 600-800 nm [4], where the depth of penetration is the deepest. The measurement showed that although Amphinex has an absorption maximum at 420 nm, it also has a peak at 650 nm, where PCI irradiation would be possible. Fig. 4 shows also the fluorescence peak of fluorescence at 656 nm.

4 Conclusion

Despite the fact that the main absorption peak of Amphinex lies at 420 nm, the localization of this photosensitizer in cells allows an optimistic prognosis about the future application of this photosensitizer in PCI. The next part of the study should be to determine more precisely the time point in which the photosensizier accumulates in the cells in sufficient amounts for further drug delivery (e.g. antibodies) into the cell cytosol. In addition, it should be investigated which amphinex concentration achieves the best results for this purpose. Also, important properties about the localization of TuBB-9 were provided. Specifically, the localization of TuBB-9 in the nucleoli could be a promising approach for subsequent research. To expand the understanding of the proliferation-associated antigen Ki-67, the next step is to investigate the viability of the cells after light irradiation.

Acknowledgement

The work has been carried out at the Institute of Biomedical Optics, Universität of Lübeck.

Author's Statement

Conflict of interest: Authors state no conflict of interest.

5 References

[1] Berg, Kristian; Weyergang, Anette; Vikdal, Marie; Norum, Ole-Jacob Selbo, Pål Kristian (2014). Photochemical Internalization: A novel Technology for Targeted Macromolecule Therapy, In Mahmoud H. Abdel-Kader (ed.), *Photodynamic Therapy - From Theory to Application.* Springer. ISBN 978-3-642-39629-8. III. s 119 - 130

[2] Høgset, Anders; Prasmickaite, Lina; Selbo, Pål Kristian; Hellum, Marit; Engesæter, Birgit Øvstebø; Bonsted, Anette Berg, Kristian (2004) Photochemical internalisation in drug and gene delivery. *Advanced Drug Delivery Reviews.* ISSN 0169-409X. 56(1), s 95- 115 . doi:10.1016/j.addr.2003.08.016

[3] O-J. Norum, 1.K. Selbo, A. Weyergang, K-E. Giercksky, K. Berg, (2009) Photochemicalinternalization (PCI) in cancer therapy; from bench towards bedside medicine, *Journal of Photochemistry and Photobiology B: Biology*, doi:10.1016/j.jphotobiol.2009.04.012

[4] Jerjes W, Theodossiou TA, Hirschberg H, Høgset A, Weyergang A, Selbo PK, Hamdoon Z, Hopper C, Berg K (2020) Photochemical Internalization for Intracellular Drug Delivery. From Basic Mechanisms to Clinical Research, J Clin Med, 9 (2), doi:10.3390/jcm9020528

[5] Rahbari R, Sheahan T, Modes V, Collier P, Macfarlane C, Badge RM (2009) A novel L1 retrotransposon marker for HeLa cell line identification, *BioTechniques.*, 46 (4): 277–284. doi:10.2144/000113089

[6] Bayona, A. M. D. P., Moore, C. M., Loizidou, M., MacRobert, A. J., Woodhams, J. H. (2016) Enhancing the efficacy of cytotoxic agents for cancer therapy using photochemical internalisation. *International Journal of Cancer, 138 (5),* 1049-1057. doi:10.1002/ijc.29510

[7] Wang S, Hüttmann G, Scholzen T, Zhang Z, Vogel A, Hasan T, Rahmanzadeh R. (2016) A light-controlled switch after dual targeting of proliferating tumor cells via the membrane receptor EGFR and the nuclear protein Ki-67. *Sci Rep.* Jun 1;6:27032. doi: 10.1038/srep27032.

4

Biophysics

-Development of a more sensitive and more reliable LC-QqQ MS method for detecting endocannabinoids and related structures-

Tuomas Mikael Lindeman [1]
[1] Biomedical Engineering, Luebeck University of Applied Sciences, tuomas.mikael.lindeman@stud.th-luebeck.de

Abstract

Liquid chromatography tandem mass spectrometry (LC-MS) techniques are essential to quantifying metabolites such as endocannabinoids(ECs) from organic samples. This this paper demonstrates the development and implementation of an LC-MS method with simultaneous online solid-phase extraction (SPE) capability. The SPE is needed to concentrate and purify low levels of these lipids in serum to make them detectable using MS. The finished result of the work for this paper is a functional system setup and a unique method providing improved capability for EC detection, identification and quantification. This method platform is then available to researchers and enables further studies.

1 Introduction

Endocannabinoids (ECs) are a key signalling lipid in both the central nervous system and the periphery. The interplay of cannabinoid receptor types 1 and 2, ECs and enzymes forms the endocannabinoid system (ECS).[1] The ECS is involved in regulating physiological and cognitive processes, including fertility, various activity of immune system, appetite and memory.[2] As these molecules play a key role in a wide range of biological systems and their changes in human disease they present a key focus of research.

Such analyses require quantitative analysis of ECs from human serum samples and there are already existing methods utilizing cartridge-based sample prepaparation. In example for a study showing that during first episode psychosis there is a clear dysregulation of the central nervous system and peripheral EC systems.[3] The existing method already provides valuable data. However, this method required improvement regarding a large sample volume required (200 μL of blood serum), limited number of metabolites and high background noise in blank samples. It was therefore the aim of this study to improve upon the existing method. It is important to mitigate the volume of blood as there is a limited amount of blood available for all the desired assays. This can be affected by removing a currently used large dilution step for the SPE. The existing assay covers 8 ECs and for control purposes it also quantifies the primary metabolite of tetrahydrocannabinol which is the active ingredient in cannabis. The new method seeks to expand this assay to cover other endo- and exocannabinoids primarily cannabidiol(CBD) and its metabolites. The aforementioned background noise is largely caused by plasticiser leaching from the plastic materials used in sample preparation. The leached plasticizers have similar structures with the ECs, which can make quantification challenging. The online SPE method would allow this step to be performed in a metal high-performance liquid chromatography (HPLC) setup thus reducing the chances of leaching.

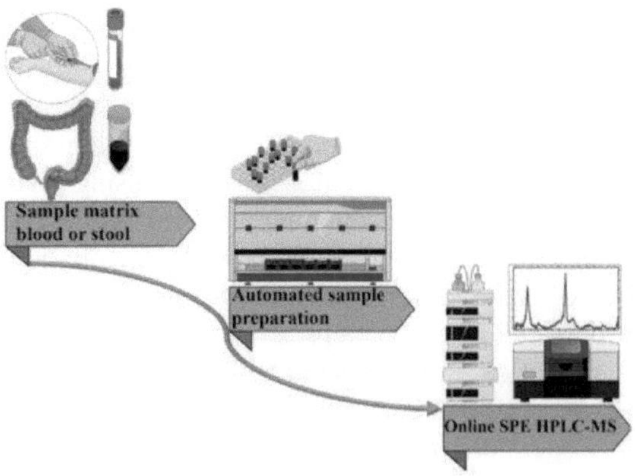

Figure 1: Illustration flowsheet of the entire process from sample to data acquisition

The improved workflow overview can be seen in Fig 1. The overview illustrates the steps that are the main focus of development for this method. The method is expanded to be compatible with fecal samples and automated sample preparation is streamlined as preparation requirements change due to the developed simultaneous online SPE in the third step. Changes in the SPE approach could improve or disadvantage the individual step, but there may be trade-offs in other aspects. Therefore, the entire workflow must be taken into account when evaluating the success of the developed method.

2 Material and Methods

Online solid-phase extraction system design

Oasis HLB (Hydrophilic-Lipophilic Balance) was selected as sorbent material after a successful cartridge-based trial. The material is capable of hydrophilic retention of polar compounds and lipophilic reverse-phase retention. These properties are suitable for selectively binding the target ECs while letting other debris pass to waste.[5] The system model for SPE was chosen to be catch and release with backflush. This approach is ideal for small sample volumes for concentration of the captured analytes. The approach for combining the sample streams of the analytical solvent gradient and the elution flow was done using a flow mixer. The mixer was chosen for reliability and the possibility to run the different flows also in parallel independently of each other. During the design phase, the SPE solvents were chosen based on the pre-existing cartridge method. Initially, the system was set to mimic the loading, washing and elution phases of the cartridge method. The pre-existing method only required an injection volume of 10 µL pre-treated extract while when injecting raw supernatant into to the online SPE system 100 µL was required to have the same amount of serum content. This was an issue as the system has a maximum injection volume of 50 µL. A new pre-treatment method was programmed for the injector which performed the desired amount of injections as several injections for a single run are not supported directly by the software.

Automated sample preparation method

Without protein precipitation or with poorly performed separation the organic solvents used in liquid chromatography would result in precipitation in the system and cause clogging.[4] The precipitation was done using a Hamilton Microlab STAR liquid handling platform. In the old workflow this platform handled the protein precipitation, filtration and cartridge-based SPE. For the new online SPE system only the first two steps are required. Also, the drying done after cartridge-based SPE to concentrate samples could be omitted. By using an automated method, the required operator knowledge and manual work could be minimized. To use the robot the operator only needs to turn on the system, load tips, samples, and solutions into the system based on a standard operation protocol, and then run a pre-built method. The sample preparation method run takes approximately 40 minutes to complete and samples are outputted in a 96-well plate format.

Online solid-phase extraction liquid chromatography mass spectrometry method

The auto-sampler was set to maintain the samples at 15 °C. At the loading-phase the flow was set to 500 µL/min the flow path A for the SPE column seen in Fig 2 schematic was used with valves A(1) and A(2) open while the valves B(1) and B(2) were closed. In other words the flow direction on the column was the primary one and after the column the flow was directed to waste. From the start of the loading-phase the acetone concentration was linearly increased to 20% over 10 minutes preforming a mild organic wash on

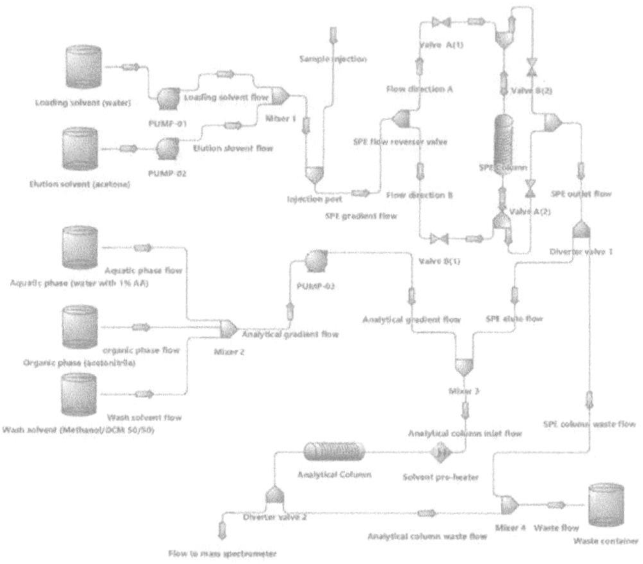

Figure 2: Schematic presentation of the online SPE system..

the SPE column and removing unwanted material. After 10 minutes the elution-phase is started by reversing the flow direction on the column by switching to flow path B for the SPE column. The reversed flow direction is achieved by switching valves B(1) and B(2) open while the valves A(1) and A(2) are closed. In other words, the analytes that were caught at the start of the column were now at the end of the column ready to be mixed to the analytical gradient that the diverter valve 1 had switched the flow path to. During the first 0.5 min of the elution-phase the flow speed is decreased from 500 µL/min to 350 µL/min and the acetone concentration is linearly increased to 50%. Then between 10.5 min and 11.75 min the acetone concentration is increased to 100% and kept stable until 14 min. After 14 minutes the B flow path is maintained while the diverter valve directs the flow into waste and the 100% acetone flow is directly increased to 1000 µL/min to clean any remaining material from the SPE column. Shortly after the acetone wash the gradient is switched to 100% water while maintaining the 1000 µL/min flow rate to push out acetone from the tubing in preparation for loading the next sample. At the start of the new sample the valves switch to the flow path A and the system is ready for injecting the next sample. In this manner the SPE system works in parallel with the LC-MS by preparing the next sample while the previous one is in the data acquisition-phase.

Liquid chromatography method conditions

Thermo Accela pump is used for creating the analytical gradient flow by mixing the two phases from separate reservoirs. The solvents used were 100% acetonitrile (ACN) for the organic phase and water with 1% acetic acid for the aqueous phase. The analytical gradient starts from 500 µL/min 40% ACN and the solvent ratio is linearly changed 10% per minute to 70% ACN over 3 minutes. The increase is slowed down and only increases from 70% to 80% over 1.5 minutes. This is done to achieve better separation for the analytes overlapping around this retention point specifically

2-AG and 2-AGe, but it is good for the separation of retention times of other analytes with similar RT as well. At 4.5 minutes, when 80% ACN has been reached, the concentration is quickly shifted to 100% to elute the compounds with greater retention on the column. The 100% ACN with 500 µL/min flow is maintained until 8 minutes at which point all of the analytes will have passed through the column. After 8 minutes the ACN concentration is kept at 100%, but the flow rate is increased to 800 µL/min for cleaning the column. The cleaning settings are maintained for 2.75 minutes after which the pressure caused by the increased cleaning flow needs to be quickly decreased for the next loading phase. This is done by directly decreasing the flow rate to 100 µL/min while switching from 100% ACN to 90% water 10% ACN over 0.25 min. Now at 11 minutes into the method the loading flow for the next sample starts where a flow of 90% water at 400 µL/min is maintained until 15 min. The 10% ACN is maintained in the mixture to prevent analytes from crashing out of the solution when the elution flow from the SPE system is mixed into the analytical gradient loading flow.

Mass spectrometry method conditions

The mass spectrometer used for this method is Sciex QTRAP 5500, which can run a scheduled multiple reaction monitoring mode. In this mode, the detection is based on parent and product ion pairs where the analyte molecule is first ionized in either negative or positive mode and this resulting parent ion is detected. Then the parent ion is fragmented using nitrogen as a collision gas and product ions are produced. The most intense or characteristic product ions are then selected to optimise the detection of the analyte. Each analyte was set up with a main parent and product ion pair, which is used for quantifying the analyte-, but also had a second pair with the same parent ion and a different product ion. This second pair was used as an additional qualifier to confirm the detection of an analyte only when both pairs are detected at the same retention timepoint. Each analyte also had an internal standard(IS) appointed to it which was a deuterated form of the same molecule which does not occur in the organic sample matrix. The internal standard was set up with two parent and product ion pairs in the same manner as the analytes.

Data analysis method

The data produced from the experiments was analysed and quantified using MultiQuant software. The quantification method is relying on comparing the measured analyte peak area or height to the internal standard peak area or height. The internal standards are analytical standards that were injected in set concentration and present the known factor which can be used to quantify the unknown concentration the sample peak area or height corresponds to. To take this a step further standard curves are implemented. The standard curve consists of several sample solutions where the internal standard concentration is kept constant while the analyte standard concentration is increased on each step. Since the analyte concentration is known at each point a curve can be plotted to represent the relative increase in analyte concentration. Based on this information and the known IS any sample peak that is within the range of the standard curve and has an IS injected with it can be quantified.

3 Results and Discussion

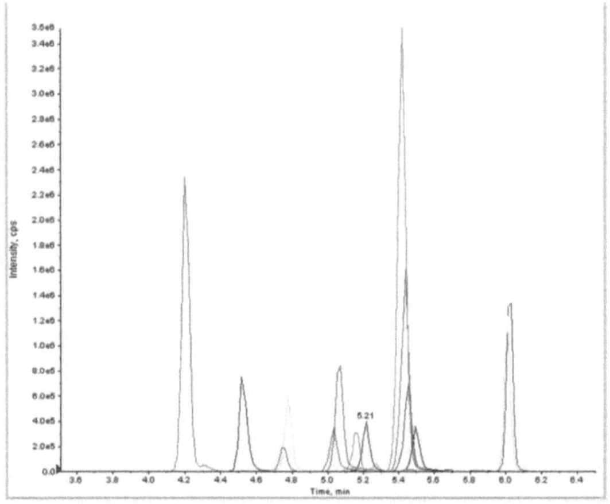

Figure 3: Analyte standard peaks detected in scheduled multiple reaction monitoring positive mode.

In Fig 3 it can be seen that many of the pure analyte standards can be successfully extracted and detected with the system. The results shown in Fig 3 are acquired from the standard curve with 7.5 parts per billion concentration for most of the analytes. Overall the scheduled multiple reaction monitoring method was sensitive enough to detect all the target analytes even from the lower concentrated samples and the signal to noise ratio was good enough to distinguish the actual peaks.

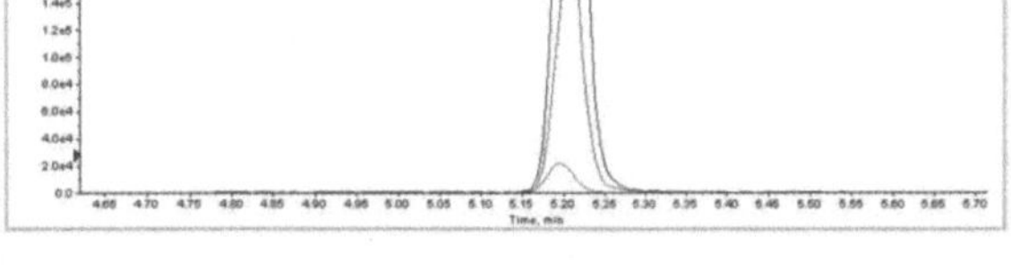

Figure 4: MRM detection of CBD and CBD-d3 from human serum using the online SPE system. Showing CBD is present in blood after administration in a clinical study.

The number of analytes and internal standards was increased by adding Stearoyl ethanolamide -d3, Alpha-linolenoyl ethanolamide -d4, Oleoyl ethanolamide -d4, N-arachidonoyl-L-serine, N-Arachidonylglycine, CBD and CBD-d3. A key analyte for this method was CBD which was not included in the pre-existing method. The blue and red peaks in Fig 4 present the quantifying and qualifying ion pairs for CBD. The green peak is for the quantifying ion pair for CBD-d3 used as an internal standard for CBD. When the serum samples of the same individual at different time points of the clinical study were analysed it was possible to pinpoint the time when CBD administration had started as some of the serum samples only presented the internal standard peak. This is crucial in determining the resulting CBD concentration in blood for different administration systems and times.

4 Conclusion

The end result of the development is a 15-minute method capable of simultaneously extracting new sample matrix while acquiring MS data of the previous sample.

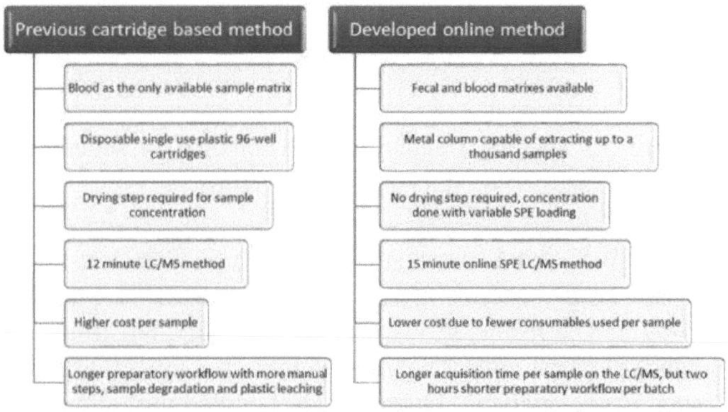

Figure 5: Direct comparison between the old and new methods in key areas with significant differences

This new method and the whole workflow rely heavily on the previous cartridge-based method and were developed as an imitation of it in a different form. In the end the new method can exceed the capabilities of its predecessor in key areas. Direct comparisons between several main features can be seen above in Fig 5. Most importantly the developed method is cheaper as fewer consumables are used per sample. For approximately the same cost the SPE column is able to run ten times more samples than a single use 96-well SPE cartridge. Also, as the online method can completely omit the drying step which means that the nitrogen gas and the one hour spent on drying each plate separately is saved. In terms of time the online method takes 3 minutes longer per sample on the LC-MS, but time is saved in the shorter preprocessing of the samples as the drying step is omitted and the automated liquid handling method previously lasting more than an hour is cut to 40 minutes. This time saved in the sample preprocessing is especially important as during the drying procedure the samples need to be heated which increases sample degradation speed. With the online method, the preprocessing can be done using a 4°C cooling rack and only the short filtration step is performed in room temperature. This is a major improvement from heating the samples up to 45 °C for an hour. The previous method was only tested with blood serum while the new method has been set up with the capability to also handle lower concentrated faecal samples.

The online method has comparable sample extraction efficiency to the previous cartridge-based SPE method. Individual sample extraction with minimized degradation time and plastic leaching alleviate the issues related to the previous method.The system was used for sets of 30-40 samples without issues or need to preform extra cleaning in between sets. Still the robustness of the system needs to be further tested by running sets of several hundreds of samples. A prestudy consisting of a few hundred samples will be conducted prior to implementing the method on a larger scale clinical trial. Contact with plastic could be completely avoided by replacing the filtration step in the workflow. This is possible to for small sample sets using manual glass tools and centrifugation, but utilizing a leaching resitant filter would be a better scaling future development.

Acknowledgement

This work has been carried out at Turku Bioscience. The work has been supervised by Prof. Ralf Moll from Technische Hochschule Lübeck and Adj. Prof. Alex Dickens from University of Turku.

Author's Statement

Conflict of interest: The author states no conflict of interest.

5 References

[1] Iannotti FA, Di Marzo V, Petrosino S. Endocannabinoids and endocannabinoid-related mediators: Targets, metabolism and role in neurological disorders. Prog Lipid Res. 2016 Apr;62:107-28. doi: 10.1016/j.plipres.2016.02.002.

[2] Pertwee, R. G. (Ed.). (2015). Endocannabinoids. Handbook of Experimental Pharmacology. doi:10.1007/978-3-319-20825-1

[3] Dickens, A.M., Borgan, F., Laurikainen, H. et al. Links between central CB1-receptor availability and peripheral endocannabinoids in patients with first episode psychosis. npj Schizophr 6, 21 (2020). https://doi.org/10.1038/s41537-020-00110-7

[4] Kong, R. (2005). 17 LC/MS application in high-throughput adme screen. Handbook of Pharmaceutical Analysis by HPLC, 413–446. doi:10.1016/s0149-6395(05)80061-3

[5] Poole, C. F. (2020). Core concepts and milestones in the development of solid-phase extraction. Solid-Phase Extraction, 1–36. doi:10.1016/b978-0-12-816906-3.00001-7

Detection of Helminths eggs in stool samples using Hyperspectral Imaging

Manikwadura Dilini Tharindika [1]

[1] Biomedical Engineering, Lübeck University of Applied Sciences, dilini.tharindika.manikwadura@stud.th-luebeck.de

Abstract

Billions of people get infected by Gastrointestinal (GI) helminths globally. The standard procedure to diagnose these parasitic infections is to examine stool samples of patients under a light microscope and search for GI helminths eggs, which is often a time consuming and a laborious task. Hyperspectral imaging could provide a non-invasive approach for much faster detection of GI helminths in stool samples. A simple optical setup was custom built to obtain images using narrow bands of visible and near-infrared (VIS-NIR) spectrum of four types of helminths egg samples. After examining the data collected during the experiment, limitations of the current setup were recognized and possible modifications are suggested for future improvements.

1 Introduction

Global helminths infection rate is very high in underdeveloped and developing regions of the world. It is estimated that global prevalence is 1221 million for *Ascaris lumbricoides*, 795 million for *Trichuris trichiura* and 740 million for hookworm species *Ancylostoma duodenale* and *Necator americanus* in the regions of Latin America and the Caribbean, Middle East and North Africa, South and East Asia and the Pacific Islands, China and India [1]. *Enterobius vermicularis* and *Strongyloides stercoralis* has infected respectively 209 million and 30 million people world wide, especially in tropical regions [2].

Here in Germany, soil-transmitted helminths (STH) infections and gastro intestinal (GI) helminths infections are very rare. However when patients are diagnosed with high blood eosinophil levels, it could be an indication of a parasitic infection, a chronic inflammatory disease or even cancer. Physicians often prescribe a stool test for suspected patients in order to rule out the possibility of STH or GI nematode infection. Most common method for this investigation is a microscopic examination which requires many man hours in laboratories.

Studies have used different spectral methods for the successful identification of helminths eggs. One such study discuses the possibility to use auto-fluorescence of the eggs for the identification of five different types of helminths eggs from waste water and sludge samples. This experiment further makes use of Raman microscopy and confocal microscopy for the investigation [3].

Another study had been able to assess the viability of eggs from different nematode species by staining the sewage sludge sediments with LIVE/DEAD kits and then by investigating them under a fluorescent microscope [4]. Reference [5] discuses the use of chemiluminescence for successful identification of *Schistosoma mansoni* eggs in human fecal samples, with the help of luminol-H_2O_2, Helmintex method and spectrophotometry.

To the extend literature research was conducted for this work, previous studies were not found where hyperspectral or multispectral imaging was used for the detection of helminths eggs. But hyperspectral imaging allows optical sensors to obtain specific chemical and spatial information by correlating a narrow wavelength band with a chemical compound of a system [6]. Hyperspectral imaging has been used in many fields of applications; such as satellite investigation to estimate the conditions of farming lands in agricultural industry and also medical hyperspectral imaging (MHSI) was used in a study to determine the healthiness or diseases in animal and human tissue [7].

Hyperspectral imaging also has the advantages of non-invasive, non-contact based investigation, potential to avoid the usage of dyes or tags for further processing of samples and the ability to automate the detection process. Hence this experiment is designed to find out the possibility to use hyperspetral imaging for the detection of helminths eggs. This work is set to investigate four different types of GI helminths egg samples namely, *Enterobius vermicularis*, *Ascaris lumbricoides*, *Trichuris trichiura* and *Taenia s.* using hyperspectral imaging in order to detect the eggs by obtaining their respective spectral signatures.

2 Material and Methods

2.1 Optical setup and Sample slides

A simple custom built microscopic setup was used for the experiment as shown in Fig.1. The optical arrangement comprises with a halogen optic lamp (L) of 12V/50W, with a color temperature of 3350K as the light source, which emits VIS-NIR radiations. A mirror (M) to redirect light to the illumination path. An aspheric condenser lens (C) of 25mm in diameter and focal length of 16mm, along with an iris diaphragm (I) was used to gain more concentrated and controlled light beam throughout the setup. Two polarisers (P) were used to get rid of the direct reflected light from the cover slip of the sample slide.

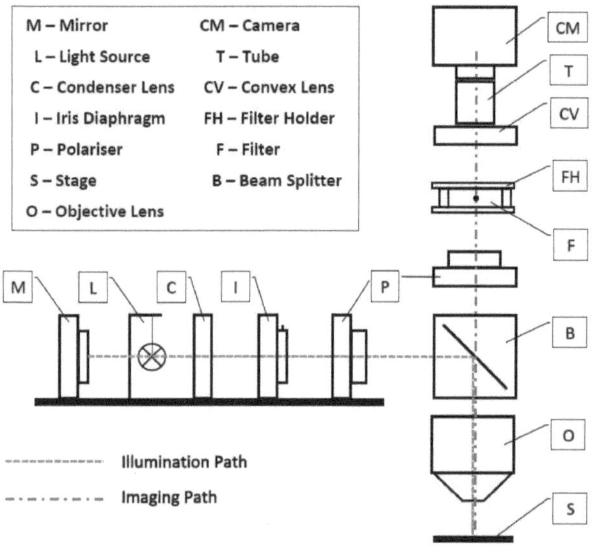

Figure 1: *Schematic of the Optical setup*

A non-polarized beam-splitter (B) was used to direct the light through the objective lens on to the specimen and back on to the camera sensor. An objective lens (O) of 20x magnification, 0.40 numerical aperture and 9mm focal length was integrated to the system. Different filters (F) were inserted into the light path for the sample investigation with the help of a fixed filter holder (FH). Narrow band filters which are of 450nm, 500nm, 550nm, 600nm, 650nm, 700nm, 750nm, 800nm, 850nm and 900nm with a bandwidth of 10nm were used to gain the remission spectra of specimens. An achromatic convex (CV) lens of 31mm of diameter and focal length of 200mm was included in the optical system along with a tube (T) 150mm in length. The microscopic setup has a total of 50x nominal optical magnification.

AVT Manta G-283 monochromatic camera (CM) was used as the optical sensor which had the resolution of 1936 × 1458 - 2.8 MP, interline CCD sensor 4.54 µm × 4.54 µm cell size. The camera was connected to a computer system with the driver software in order to observe the live samples.

Sample slides of the three different types of nematodes namely *Enterobius vermicularis*, *Ascaris lumbricoides*, *Trichuris trichiura* and one type of cestode namely *Taenia s.* which are already prepared, were borrowed from the laboratory of Microbiology and immunology for the investigation.

2.2 Image acquisition

A microscopic slide was placed on the stage and objective lens was focused on an egg, then filters were integrated to the setup one by one to obtain images using different wavelengths.

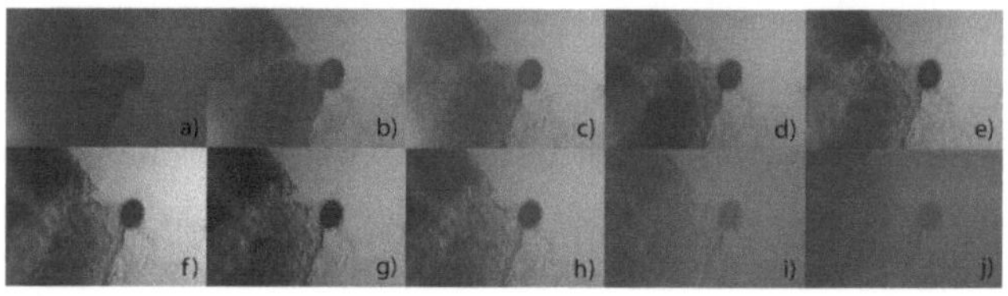

Figure 2: *Ascaris lumbricoides* helminths egg captured using a) 450nm, b) 500nm, c) 550nm, d) 600nm, e) 650nm, f) 700nm, g) 750nm, h) 800nm, i) 850nm and j) 900nm wavelength filters

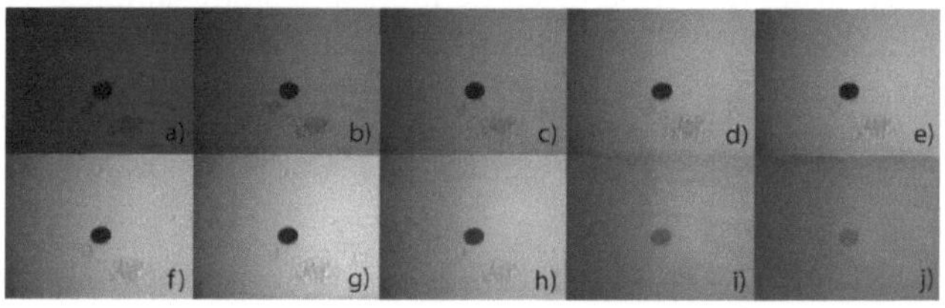

Figure 3: *Taenia s.* helminths egg captured using a) 450nm, b) 500nm, c) 550nm, d) 600nm, e) 650nm, f) 700nm, g) 750nm, h) 800nm, i) 850nm and j) 900nm wavelength filters

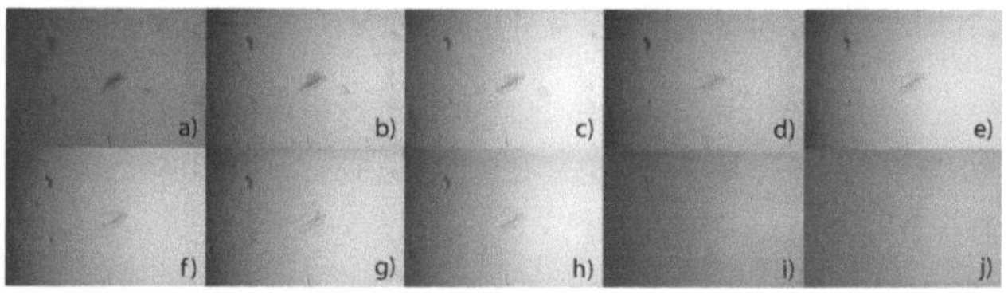

Figure 4: *Enterobius vermicularis* helminths egg captured using a) 450nm, b) 500nm, c) 550nm, d) 600nm, e) 650nm, f) 700nm, g) 750nm, h) 800nm, i) 850nm and j) 900nm wavelength filters

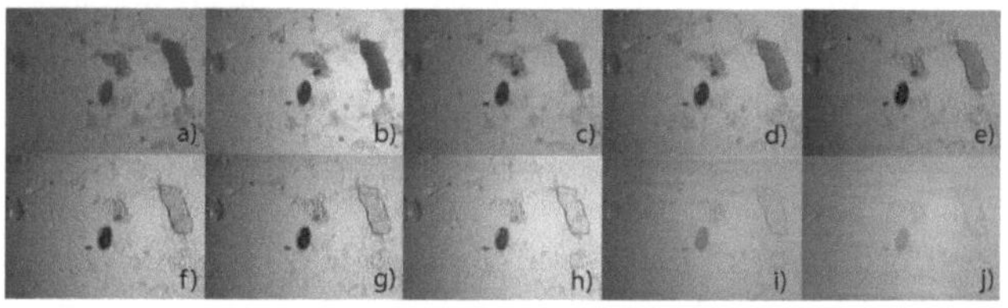

Figure 5: *Trichuris trichiura* helminths egg captured using a) 450nm, b) 500nm, c) 550nm, d) 600nm, e) 650nm, f) 700nm, g) 750nm, h) 800nm, i) 850nm and j) 900nm wavelength filters

The images of *Ascaris lumbricoides*-Fig.2 and *Taenia s.*-Fig.3 samples were taken by keeping the sensitivity of the camera constant while changing brightness of the light source. As for *Enterobius vermicularis*-Fig.4 and *Trichuris trichiura*-Fig.5 samples, images were captured by changing both camera sensitivity and brightness of the light source.

2.3 Obtaining spectral information

As shown in Fig.2 through Fig.5, images were taken for all four types of specimen samples and they were aligned on top of each other using an image processing software tool to create a stack of hyperspectral images/hyper-cuboid per specimen.

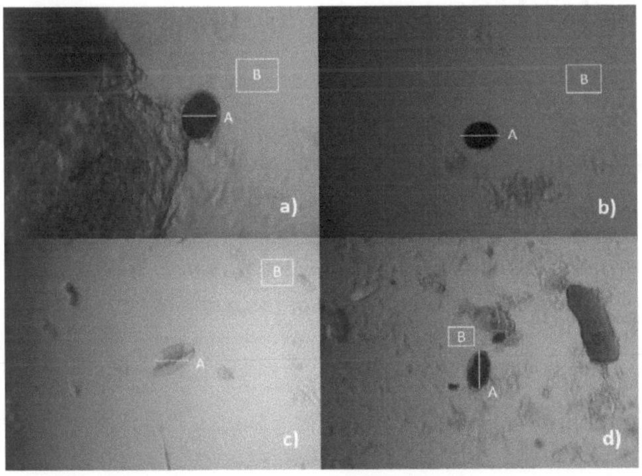

Figure 6: Selected planes and areas for evaluation from a) *Ascaris lumbricoides*, b) *Taenia s.* c) *Enterobius vermicularis*, d) *Trichuris trichiura* . A - a line through the egg, B - area selected as white reference

First, the dark image was subtracted from each respective layer of the hyper-cuboid to remove any camera generated noise in the images. Then in the orthogonal view of the egg through line A-Fig.6, a pixel column was chosen and the grey values are obtained which represents the same pixel position for each wavelength. This step is repeated for a couple more pixel columns to calculate mean grey values of the egg. Then mean value of B-Fig.6 as white reference was calculated for each wavelength channel. This background signal of the sample (B) is generated from the *white* color stage where the sample slides were kept during image acquisition.

3 Results and Discussion

3.1 Remission spectra of specimens

Mean grey values from A (calculated as described in section 2.3) was normalized using the respective white reference from B for each image in the image stack Fig.6. These normalized grey values from Egg was plotted against wavelength to investigate spectral details of helminths samples. The obtained remission spectra are shown below in Fig.7 through Fig.10.

In a normal scenario, light absorption by objects in the 450nm - 500nm wavelength range should be greater than

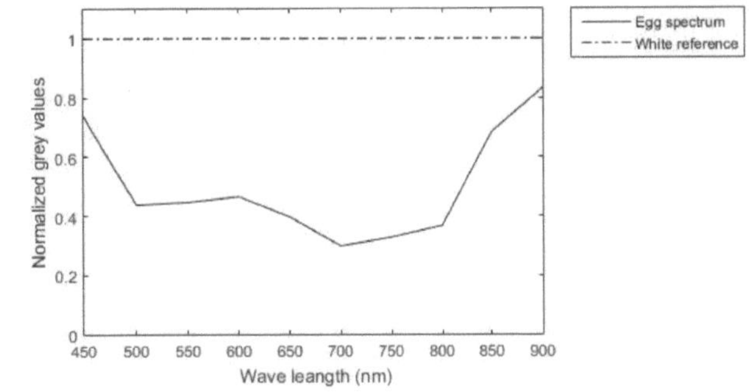

Figure 7: Remission spectrum of *Ascaris lumbricoides*

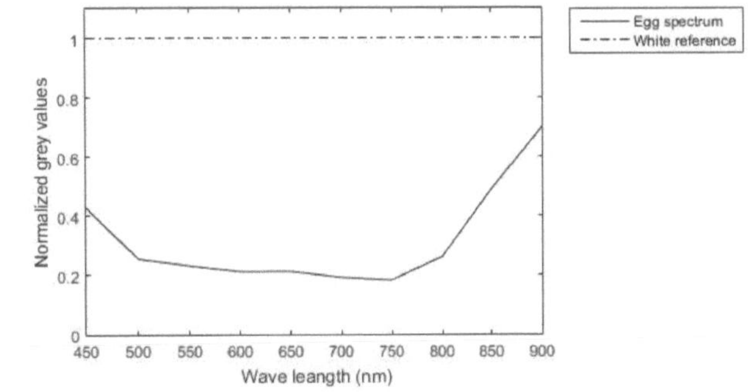

Figure 8: Remission spectrum of *Taenia s.*

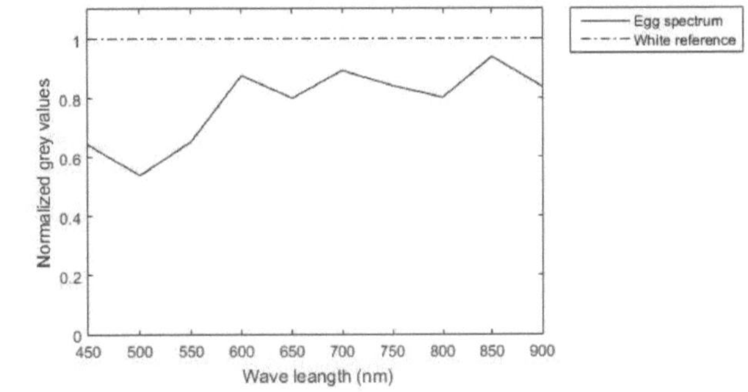

Figure 9: Remission spectrum of *Enterobius vermicularis*

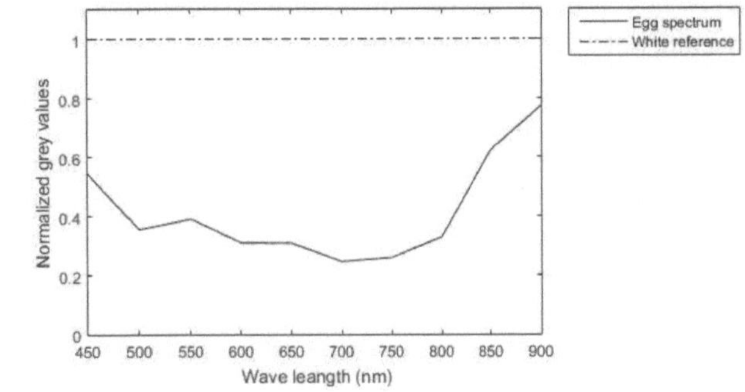

Figure 10: Remission spectrum of *Trichuris trichiura*

the 550nm - 650nm wavelength range. But from the Fig.7, Fig.8 and Fig.10, we can see that light absorption is comparatively lower in 450nm - 500nm range for egg spectra. It was found out that this was due to low light efficiency of the light source.

All three helminths eggs except *Enterobius vermicularis*-Fig.9 seem to be more black and do not contain bright enough spectral signature. This problem can be corrected by using some other illumination method like *dark field illumination* for the optical setup. The reason for *Enterobius vermicularis*-Fig.9 being different from other egg spectra could be due to the fact that they have a different morphological structure (translucent build) compared to other eggs. However more experiments should be carried out to support this statement.

When images were taken with the 450nm and 500nm wavelengths, highest possible intensity of the halogen lamp was used in order to obtain a decent image of the specimen, still the spectral details collected in those regions of the spectra are not sufficient. Images captured using wavelengths from 800nm - 900nm appears to be darker/unclear due to the low transmission and reflection rate of the beam-splitter after 800nm Fig.2 - Fig.5.

A white stage was used for easy observation of the eggs via the optical setup Fig.1. Due to this, Fig.7, Fig.8 and Fig.10 shows similar spectra as the obtained remission spectra contains spectral details from both egg and the background and the exposure time/maximum brightness of the images are determined by this background as well. To avoid this, a dark background should be used where only the scattered light from the sample could be collected.

3.2 Future improvements

This setup needs to be improved by integrating a high efficiency light source, a highly sensitive optical detector and a beam-splitter which supports transmission and reflection of the whole VIS-NIR wavelength range. Changing the illumination from direct illumination to dark field illumination method could also improve the result significantly. In the experiment only one filter was used in the light path to gain a bit brighter image. But in principle an illumination filter and an emission filter should be used to obtain more wavelength specific results. A hyper-cuboid with many layers of images has to be created by imaging with continuous narrow bands of VIS-NIR spectrum.

Once the optical setup is improved by overcoming its current limitations, a characteristic spectral signature could be created for each of the sample specimen. Then an automated system could be built to search for the spectral signature of the eggs instead of manually observing samples under a light microscope.

4 Conclusion

The optical setup built for this experiment uses very basic optical elements which are easily available in an optical laboratory. A more sophisticated and modified optical arrangement is in need to explore the full capacity of hyperspectral imaging. Once the characteristic spectral signature for all the helminths eggs are recorded, it could make way for easy detection of helmiths eggs.

Acknowledgement

The work has been carried out at Laboratory for optical metrology, Lübeck University of Applied Sciences, under the supervision of Malte Gienow-Broers who also helped with the optical setup. Project idea, proposal and laboratory by Prof. Mathias Beyerlein - Laboratory of Optical metrology. Technical support in the laboratory from Mario Wiegleb. Microscopic slides provided by Prof. Dagmar Willkomm - Department of Applied Natural sciences.

Author's Statement

Conflict of interest: Authors state no conflict of interest.

5 References

[1] Nilanthi R de Silva, Simon Brooker, Peter J Hotez, Antonio Montresor, Dirk Engels, Lorenzo Savioli, *Soil-transmitted helminth infections: updating the global picture.* In: Research focus| Volume 19, issue 12, P547-551, December 01, 2003

[2] Gillian Stepek, David J. Buttle, Ian R. Duce, Jerzy M. Behnke, *Human gastrointestinal nematode infections: are new control methods required?.* Available: https://doi.org/10.1111/j.1365-2613.2006.00495.x,29 August 2006

[3] Farah Qazi, Asma Khalid, Arpita Poddar, Jean-Philippe Tetienne, Athavan Nadarajah, Steven Prawer et al. *Real-time detection and identification of nematode eggs genus and species through optical imaging.* Published online 2020 Apr 29. doi: 10.1038/s41598-020-63747-5

[4] Joanna Dąbrowska, Jolanta Zdybel, Jacek Karamon, Maciej Kochanowski¸ Krzysztof Stojecki et al. *Assessment of viability of the nematode eggs (Ascaris, Toxocara, Trichuris) in sewage sludge with the use of LIVE/DEAD Bacterial Viability Kit.* Ann Agric Environ Med. 2014; 21(1): 35–41.

[5] Vivian Favero, Carolina De Marco Veríssimo, Angela R. Piovesan, Alessandra L. Morassutti et al. *A new diagnostic strategy which uses a luminol-H2O2 system to detect helminth eggs in fecal sediments processed by the Helmintex method.* Published: July 30, 2020 https://doi.org/10.1371/journal.pntd.0008500

[6] Pina Colarusso, Linda H. Kidder, Ira W. Levin, James C. Fraser, John F. Arens, E. Neil Lewis, *Infrared Spectroscopic Imaging: From Planetary to Cellular Systems.* Appl Spectrosc Rev 1998; 52:106A-20A

[7] Svetlana V. Panasyuk, Shi Yang, Douglas V. Faller, Duyen Ngo, Robert A. Lew, Jenny E. Freeman, *Medical Hyperspectral Imaging to Facilitate Residual Tumor Identification During Surgery.* Cancer Biology Therapy 6:3, 439-446; March 2007 40407248

Immunological Analyses of Tumor Samples and Cultured Tumor Stem cells with the Aim of Approaching the Role of the Blood-Brain Barrier in Pathologic Microenvironments

Faryal Soomro[1] and Christina Zechel[2]

[1] Biomedical Engineering, Lübeck University of Applied Sciences, faryal.soomro@stud.th-luebeck.de

[2] Experimental Neuro-oncology, CBBM, Department of Neurosurgery, University Clinic Lübeck, christina.zechel@uni-luebeck.de

Abstract

Endothelial cells (ECs) and neighboring specialized astrocytes form the blood-brain barrier (BBB), which functions as barrier for cells (e.g. microglia) and macromolecules (e.g. chemotherapeutic drugs). During this study, I focused on the proteins characteristically expressed by astroglia, microglia and endothelial cells. I used different staining protocols (H&E staining, immunofluorescence) and worked with specimens from human malignant glioma and orthotopic tumors from a mouse model. Furthermore, I assessed the effect of treatments, the chemotherapeutic drug Temozolomide on stem-like glioma cells (SLGCs) in the presence and absence of chloroquine. Overall, I was able, (i) to specifically detect blood vessels and microglia in the tumor specimens and, (ii) to monitor the responsiveness of SLGCs and the survival of cells with a high degree of stemness.

1 Introduction

The Blood-Brain Barrier (BBB) is an essential structure present in the Central Nervous System. It is largely made up of endothelial cells (ECs) [1]. The principal function of the BBB is to control the exchange of the brain to the neurons [1]. The supplementary extensions of the BBB are astrocytic projections, i.e. specialized astrocytes, which are recognized as important regulators of the BBB. It has been shown that mature astrocytes might act as the initiation spark for the development of malignant gliomas, such as the glioblastoma (GBM). GBMs might grow continuously, invade healthy brain tissue and might spread over to spinal cord [2]. GBM have a very heterogeneous cell morphology. The population of GBM cells is constituted by differentiated and un-differentiated cells, in which the undifferentiated GBM cells express markers, such as Sox2, CD133 and Nestin [3][4][5]. Both, the survival of GBM cells as well as tumor progression depend on the availability of oxygen, nutrients and diffusible factors, which are transported by the blood cells or the blood plasma [6]. Analytically, the cross-talk between the GBM cells and the BBB is exceedingly diagnostic for the decision whether the tumor growth is fast or slow. Notably, the BBB is quite a challenge in perceiving, investigating and evaluating the brain tumors, in particular when conducting clinical trials to treat the brain tumor. The cornerstone would be to observe and analyze the treatment responses in relation to the characteristics of the BBB. This includes studies on the growth of blood vessels (vascularization, angiogenesis) and the molecular changes in nearby healthy tissues. In order to recognize how substances would migrate over the BBB or how molecules (e.g. chemotherapeutic drugs) are taken up by the ECs that contribute to the BBB suitable models need to be applied. For this purpose, orthotopic mouse models or in vitro cultures of tissue slices or cells might be used. Such models have been set up in the host laboratory during the last years [4][5]. The aim of the present study was to analyze the differences in the tissue architecture between healthy brain tissues and various types of brain tumor tissues in tissue from orthotopic mouse models and human tumors. Moreover, the responsiveness of GBM cells to various treatments were evaluated.

2 Material and Methods

Tumor tissue and tumor cells: Paraffin embedded human tumors or mouse orthotopic tumors were provided by the host laboratory. Glioma Stem Cells were grown in serum-free medium and treated with Temozolomide (TMZ, Temodal®; Essex Pharma GmbH, Munic, Germany) and/or the autophagy inhibitor Chloroquine (CQ; Sigma-Aldrich, Munic, Germany)

2.1 Microtome Cleavage

For slicing, the Leica RM2245 (Leica Mikrosysteme Vertrieb GmbH, Germany) was used. The block was trimmed with 4.5 μm and 3-4 slices were placed into a container with warm water to flatten the slices.

2.2 Staining of tissue slices

To study the tissue structure (connective tissues) and cellular components (DNA) H&E (Hematoxylin and Eosin) staining was performed using standard H&E protocol [4][5]. Firstly, the deparaffinization of slices by Ethanol bathing. Afterwards, the slides were placed in Hematoxylin solution (Roth Industries GmbH Co. KG, Germany) for 10 minutes. Then, the slides were placed in 1% Eosin solution (Roth Industries GmbH Co. KG, Germany) for 2 minutes. Lastly, the slides were mounted and dried overnight. To analyze the expression of proteins specifically associated with endothelial cells (CD31), astroglia (GFAP), or microglia Immunohistochemistry was performed using standard IHC protocol [4][5]. Firstly, the deparaffinization, same as in H&E protocol. After that, in order to demask the epitopes, the slides were cooked in the pressure cooker containing citrate buffer. Then, a mixture containing the primary antibody as well as 10% FCS (fetal calf serum) and 0.02% sodium-acid was pipetted onto the tissue pieces and incubated overnight in 4°C. Next day, the slides were incubated for with the mixture containing the secondary antibodies and otherwise identical to the previous mixture. After that, the slides were incubated with DAPI(4',6-diamidino-2-phenylindole; Thermo Fischer Scientific; Loughborough, UK) dilution (1:200) in 1xPBS(Phosphate Buffer Saline) for 10 minutes. Orthotopic mouse tumors in Table 1 and human brain tumor pieces in Table 2 were analyzed by the methods indicated in the respective Tables.

Table 1: Orthotopic Samples obtained for H&E and IHC

Cell Line	Tumor Origin	Primary anti-bodies
T436,T430, T447,T150	Orthotopic	Iba/GFAP
T571,T570, T563,T561	Orthotopic	Iba/GFAP &Iba/CD31

Table 2: Human Tumor Samples obtained for H&E and IHC (Primary antibodies: Iba/GFAP & Iba/CD31)

Cell Line	Human Tumors
T1593-1,T1593-2, T1681,T1661	GBM
T1594,T1620	recurrent GBM
T1653,T1637	Malignant glioma
T1659	Astrocytoma III
T1662	Ependymoma

2.3 Staining of Glioma stem cells (GSC, SLGCs)

In order to analyze the expression of stem cells markers and proteins induced by cytotoxic stress, two distinct SLGC lines were plated on chamber slides. After five days of treatment, the cells were fixed for exactly 7 minutes at -20° C using ethanol/acetic acid (95%:5%). Until staining, the chamber slides were stored at 4°C. However, the following staining procedure and the preparation of staining mixtures were identical to above. The only variance was, the different combinations of primary antibody mixtures were used shown in Table 3.

Table 3: Cell cultured tumor samples obtained for ICC

Chamber Slides	Treatment	Antibodies
T1371-16/1464	Untreated SLGC lines	SOX2/CD133
T1464 sub-clone A3,T1442 subclone E1	DMSO;TMZ 100μM; CQ5mg/ml& mixture of TMZ/CQ	SOX2/CD133& γH2AX/Nestin

2.4 Antibody mixtures

Primary antibodies: αCD31 (mouse; Cell Signaling; 1:100); αCD133/Prominin-1(mouse; W6B3C1; Miltenyi Biotec, Bergisch Gladbach, Germany; 1:200); γH2Ax (rabbit, Cell Signaling; 1:200); αGFAP (mouse, MAB360; Merck; 1:100); αIba (rabbit, Wako Chemicals GmbH, Germany; 1:500); αNestin (mouse, Chemicon; 1:100); αSox2 (rabbit; temlite pluripotency kit; clone D6D9; Cell Signaling; 1:100). Secondary antibodies: Goat anti-mouse DyLight® (Thermo Fischer Scientific; Loughborough, UK; 1:400); Goat anti-rabbit Cy3(Jackson Immuno-Research, Newmarket, Suffolk, UK; 1:300).

2.5 Microscopy

The microscope Keyence Fluorescence Biozero BZ 8100E used with Lens Plan Apo 2x0.10 or 20x0.75. The exposure times had been empirically determined by the colleagues in the laboratory also using Multilayer&Z-stack. Identical exposure times were used for a given primary antibody.

3 Results and Discussion

This present research, encompasses the first steps to the analysis of the function of the BBB in the normal and diseased brain. The first aim of the study was the characterization of tumor specimens from different human brain tumors. Secondly, I analyzed orthotopic tumors from SCID mice. Lastly, treatment responsiveness of cultures of SLGCs.

3.1 Human tumor specimen

In order to scrutinize the presence of connective tissue structures (pink), tumor cells (revealed by staining of the DNA content in the nucleus of cells; blue-violet) and blood vessels, H&E staining was used for human tumors. It turned out that all specimens contained regions with few nuclei and regions with many nuclei, organized in irregular patterns; shown in Fig.1. The regions with few nuclei corresponded to healthy tissue, the presence of increased numbers of nuclei in irregular patterns to tumor tissue. In addition, smaller and larger spaces without any connective tissue were observed. In some cases, the spaces were lines with cobble-stone like cellular structures, resembling the epithelial lining blood-vessels. In many cases, the spaces contained single (sometimes many) small, oval structures with a dark pink color, which are erythrocytes shown in Fig.1. In order to confirm the above assumptions, stains with two antibody pairs were performed: (a) αCD31/αIBA-1 and (b) αGFAP/αIBA-1 shown in Fig.2: T1593, GBM; T1659, astrocytoma III; T1661, GBM; compare Table.2. The presence of IBA-1 positive immune cells was observed in all cases. They had the typical star-like phenotype and showed variable densities in the stained tumor specimen. Also, their density varied between distinct regions of the same tumor specimen and was highest in the proximity of blood vessels. Blood vessels became best visible by the presence of dark spaces in the otherwise dense and structured tissue. Typically erythrocytes were present in these spaces (oval-shaped green-orange small structures without any blue [DAPI+] nucleus). A very large dark gap was observed in T1659, which did not resemble a blood vessel but a ventricle. Ventricles are hollow structures in brain filled with cerebral fluid[8]. The endothelial cells lining the blood vessel could be detected, but only at higher magnifications. The specialized astrocytes typically present at the BBB, did not become apparent in the GFAP stain exerted here. Additional antibodies will be included in the study to solve this problem in future experiments.

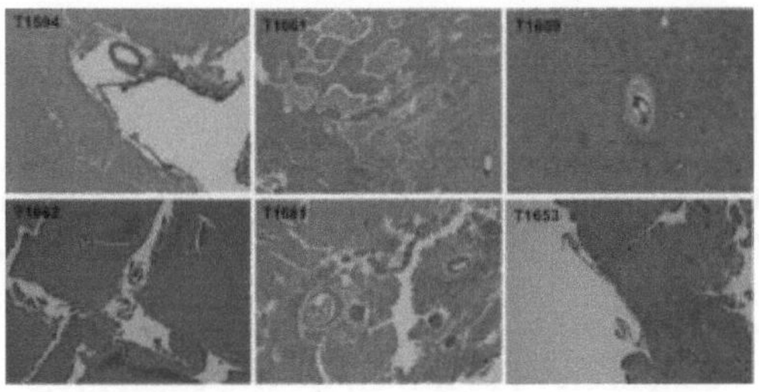

Figure 1: H&E stain of Human Tumor Cells. Eiosin stained cytoplasmic structures (pink). Hematoxylin stained nuclei of cell (light bluish). –Bar, 50 μm.

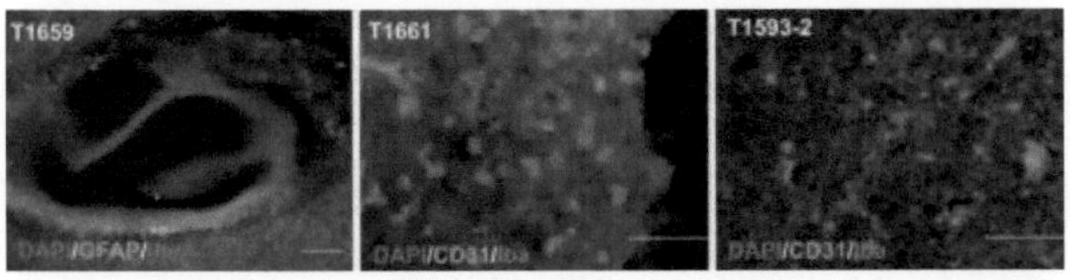

Figure 2: IHC analysis of Human Tumors. Antibody combinations used: (i) Iba/Cy3 (red) with CD31/Dylight (green); Magnification x40; (ii) Iba/Cy3 (red) with GFAP/Dylight (green); Magnification x20. Nuclear counterstain with DAPI (blue). –Bar, 50 μm.

3.2 Orthotopic mouse tumors

Human tumor specimen are not available in unlimited amounts. Moreover, when used up for any type of analyses, biological replicates with the same tumor specimen can no longer be investigated. Therefore, the SLGCs were isolated from the tumor specimens, cultivated in vitro and inoculated in the brain of immunosuppressed mice (SCID mouse model)[4]. Notably, not all inoculated SLGC samples generated huge tumors in short time [4]. Mouse brain from two of these previously generated series of orthotopic tumors were subjected to analysis. The mouse brains were analyzed by H&E stain and IHC. The H&E stains in Fig.3 reveal healthy mouse brain parenchyma with equally distributed nuclei. Though some tumors were observed (identifiable by high numbers of nuclei), most mouse brains did not reveal large tumors. What is apparent in Fig.3 are regions with blood vessels, filled with erythrocytes (see e.g. lower panels). The erythrocytes were also apparent in the immunohistochemical stains shown in Fig.4(green-orange clusters of small oval structures). Moreover, the antibody IBA-1 detected clusters of microglia in the mouse brains in Fig.4. Whereas the IBA-1 antibody could detect mouse and human cells, the CD31 antibody used in the study, would only detect human cells, i.e. endothelial cells derived from the human SLGCs. As only a few orthotopic tumors were observed, the analysis of the CD31+ cells could not be completed. Additional tumor samples, preferable with huge orthotopic tumors, will be analyzed in future experiments.

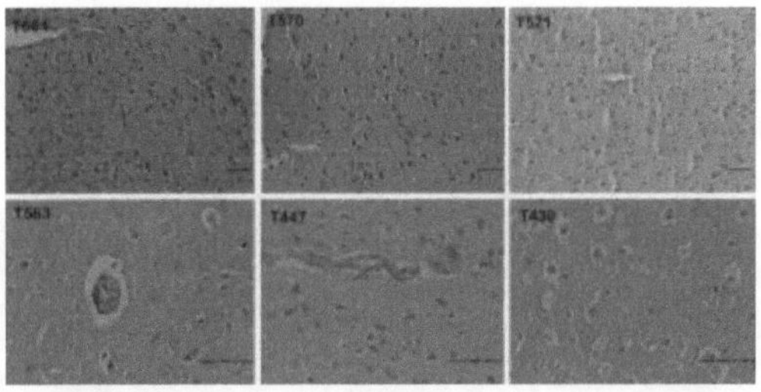

Figure 3: H&E stain of Human Tumor Cells. Eiosin stained cytoplasmic structures (pink). Hematoxylin stained nuclei of cell (light bluish). -Bar, 50 μm.

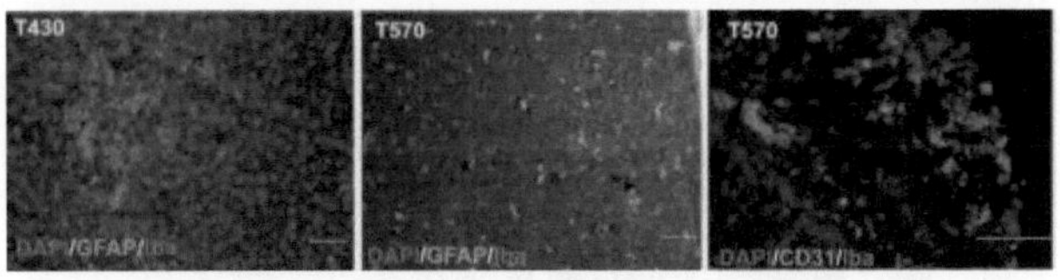

Figure 4: IHC analysis of Orthotopic Tumors. Antibody combinations used: (i) Iba/Cy3 (red) with CD31/Dylight (green); Magnification x40; (ii) Iba/Cy3 (red) with GFAP/Dylight (green); Magnification x20. Nuclear counterstain with DAPI (blue). -Bar, 50 μm.

3.3 Treatment responsiveness of cultures of SLGCs

In order to judge the degree of stemness, the SLGC cells were stained with an antibody against the transcription factor Sox2 [5]. It became obvious, that most cells in the T1371 control expressed very high Sox2 levels shown in

Fig.5. In contrast, the intensity of the Sox2 signal varied between weak and very strong in the cases of T1442 and T1464, indicating that the cells had established a cellular hierarchy in the culture. This is a typical phenomenon observed for SLGC cultures[7], which was present in all three SLGC cultures, but more prominent in T1442 and T1464. The expression of the marker CD133 was at best very low in all three cultures, indicating that the cultures did not significantly differentiate. The intermediate filament Nestin is a protein expressed in all neural cells and in SLGCs [4][5][7] which was confirmed by the present ICC stain. Cytotoxic stress or treatment with chemotherapeutic drugs leads to the phosphorylation of the histone γH2AX. Hence, cells staining positive for the γH2AX show a responsiveness to treatment or underwent cytotoxic stressing. Fig.6 shows a strong responsiveness of T1442 to treatment with chloroquine(i.e. no or faint γH2AX signals in the control and strong signals in most cells after treatment). On the contrary, T1464 cells were already showing a strong γH2AX signal in the controls, which was not increased by chloroquine. This indicated that the T1464 culture underwent cytotoxic stress, which was not due to the treatment. Note, that the images resemble only part of the analysis. They indicate, however, the usefulness of the in vitro cultures as a measure for the outcome of treament and could constitute a helpful control for future experiments with chemotherapeutic drugs.In addition, I was able to identify GFAP+ cells in a parallel assay (data not shown).

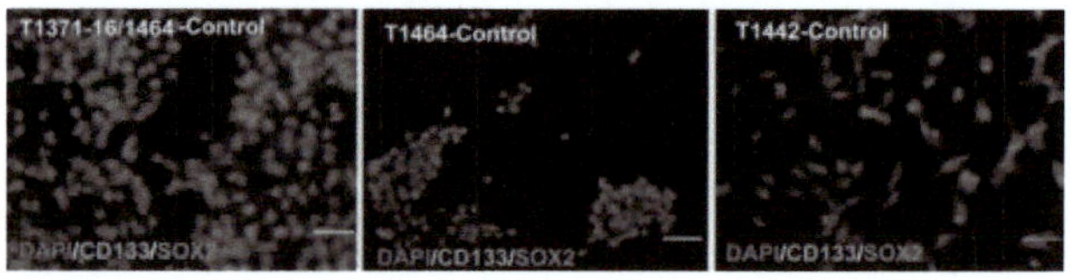

Figure 5: IHC analysis of SLGC plated in chamber slides. Antibodies used: CD133 (green)/DyLight with SOX2 (red)/Cy3. Nuclear counterstain with DAPI (blue). Magnification x20; -Bar, 50 µm

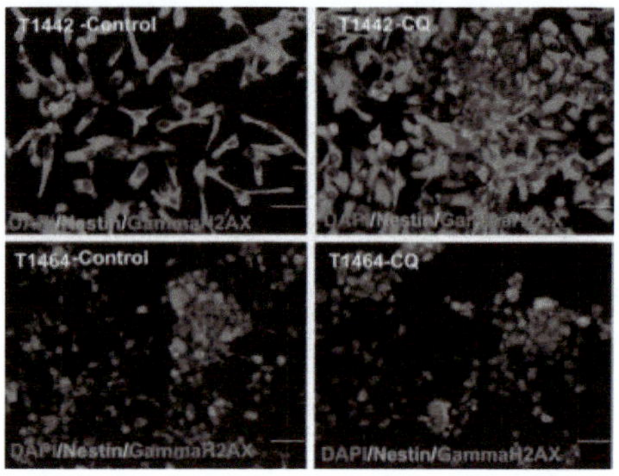

Figure 6: IHC analysis of SLGC plated in chamber slides. Antibodies used: Nestin (green)/Dylight with γH2Ax (red)/Cy3. Nuclear counterstain with DAPI (blue). Magnification x20; -Bar, 50 µm

4 Conclusion

In order to approach the future analysis of the BBB, I was able to carry out the histo-(patho-)logoical analyses of human tumor specimens and orthotopic tumors as well as the treatment of stem-like glioma cells in culture. I confirmed the usefulness of the antibodies directed against Nestin, CD133, Sox2, CD31, GFAP and IBA-1. I acquired knowledge in the interpretation of stains (H&E, IHC, ICC) and histological structures. This will open me the option to test further antibodies helpful for the analysis of the BBB and to investigate aberrant forms of BBB in human tissue in future experiments.

Acknowledgement

The work has been carried out at Experimental Neurooncology, CBBM, Department of Neurosurgery, University Clinic Lübeck .

Author's Statement

Conflict of interest: Authors state no conflict of interest.

5 References

[1] R. Daneman and A. Prat, *The Blood Brain Barrier.* ColdSpring Harb Perspect Biol;Jan;2015.

[2] E.G. Van Meir, C.G. Hadjipanayis, et. al, *Exciting new advances in neuro-oncology: the Avenue to a cure for malignant glioma.* CA Cancer J Clin;60:166-193;2010.

[3] DL. Schonberg, TE. Miller, Q. Wu, et. al, *Preferential-Iron Trafficking Characterizes Glioblastoma Stem-like Cells.* Cancer Cell;28(4), 441–455;Oct 12;2015.

[4] E.N.S. Raju, C. Zechel, S. Sridhar, et. al, *Maintenance of Stemlike Glioma Cells and Microglia in an Organotypic Glioma Slice Model.* Neurosurgery;77:629-643;2015.

[5] I. Choschzick, C. Zechel, et. at, *Responsiveness of stem-like human glioma cells to all-trans retinoic acid and requirement of retinoic acid receptor isotypes α, β and γ.* Neuroscience;279:44-64;2014.

[6] F. Galeffi and D.A. Turner, *Exploiting metabolic differences in glioma therapy.*Current drug discovery technologies;9(4);280–293;2012.

[7] R. Chen, M.C. Nishimura, et. al, *A Hierarchy of Self-Renewing Tumor-Initiating Cell Types in Glioblastoma.* Cancer Cell;17, 362–375;2010.

[8] E. Crisan, 2016, *Ventricles of the Brain.* Available: https://emedicine.medscape.com/article/1923254-overview [last accessed: 2021-01-25]

Investigation of surface-active therapeutics on lipid monolayers

Priscillia Y. Masalle [1], Thomas Gutsmann [2], Christian Nehls [2]

[1] Medical Engineering Science, Universität zu Lübeck, priscillia.masalle@student.uni-luebeck.de
[2] Division of Biophysics, Priority Area Infections, Research Center Borstel, {tgutsmann, cnehls}@fz-borstel.de

Abstract

The behavior of all biologically active substances including drugs on living cells in the body begins with their interactions with the membrane. Therefore, the aim of this study is to investigate the interaction between the pulmonary surfactant monolayers and the inhalable drugs. The behavior between active surfactant and drugs was studied by evaluating the change in lateral pressure of lipid monolayers due to drug injection using a computer-controlled Langmuir-Blodgett (LB) film balance. 1,2-Dipalmitoyl-sn-glycero-3-phosphocholine (DPPC) was applied as the lipid membrane agent to be evaluated. The lipid monolayers were compressed to a lateral pressure of $20\,\mathrm{mN/m}$. After compression, Tyloxapol was injected at various concentrations into water as the subphase. The stability of the monolayers was dependent on the monolayer composition as well as the lateral pressures. In this work, the maximum lateral pressure could be determined. Comparison of phase separation in presence of Tyloxapol was investigated using Atomic Force Microscopy (AFM).

1 Introduction

Active pharmaceutical compounds which are inhaled into the lungs after nebulization interact initially with the surfactant layer coating of lungs alveoli. This surfactant layer consists of a lipid-protein monolayer [1]. An established method to characterize lipid monolayers is the Langmuir film balance. In this method, a lipid monolayer can be spread at the water-air interface and its area can be varied by means of one or two movable barriers. The lateral pressure is measured with a Wilhelmy plate. Generally, the interaction between drugs and lipid monolayers is measured by injecting the drugs into the subphase. This, however, does not depict the real situation in a treatment with such pharmaceutical, where the active compounds of the pharmaceutical have to be transferred from the gaseous phase into the lipid monolayer. The aim of this practical project is to compare the interaction of the pharmaceutical compound Tyloxapol with lipid monolayers applied through the water phase (injection) and the air (nebulization). The latter will be done in the future in a separate work. 1,2–dipalmitoyl–sn–glycero–3–phosphocholine (DPPC) is one of the main components that constructs pulmonary monolayers. Tyloxapol is a non-ionic liquid polymer of the alkyl aryl polyether alcohol, which is widely used as pharmaceutical due to its surface-active and approved for human use properties [2]. To investigate the stability of the lipid monolayer on the subphase, the lateral pressure vs time isotherms (π-t) were determined [3]. The interaction between the change in lipid interaction in the lipid monolayers and drug injection method was performed with different concentrations in the trough during compression-decompression of isotherm measurement. This interaction of the DPPC and Tyloxapol after injection can be further investigated through imaging with Atomic Force Microscopy (AFM). Atomic Force Microscopy is widely used to study the morphology and phase behavior of large domains in monolayer films (Langmuir) [4, 3].

2 Material and Methods

2.1 Material

DPPC was obtained from Avanti Polar Lipids, Alabama, USA; Tyloxapol was purchased from Sigma-Aldrich, Darmstadt, Germany. The Wilhelmy plate was made of a rectangular filter paper with a dimension of 10 mm x 25 mm. Water was used as subphase in these experiments. The application of $40\,\mu l$ Tyloxapol solution in the subphase was carried out by using a Hamilton syringe. Atomic Force Microscopy (AFM) was used to study the interaction between Tyloxapol and the monolayer after injection of Tyloxapol. For AFM imaging, the monolayers must be transferred to a solid substrate (LB film). The LB support itself is a mica plate ($20\,\mathrm{mm} \times 16\,\mathrm{mm}$).

2.2 Methods

In order to determine the applicability of different drug delivery methods on the lipid monolayer, the KSV Nima KN2001 Langmuir Blodgett trough (Biolin Scientific, Gothenburg, Sweden) was utilized. KSV NIMA Langmuir Troughs was used to study floating lipid monolayer. Figure 1 describes the setup of a Langmuir trough. The lipid monolayer consists of $9.5\,\mu l$ DPPC ($1\,\mathrm{mg/ml}$) dissolved in chloroform. $40\,\mu l$ Tyloxapol diluted in water will be injected into the subphase using a Hamilton syringe with various concentrations leading to final concentration of 125 μg/ml, 100 μg/ml, 70 μg/ml, 50 μg/ml, 20 μg/ml, 10 μg/ml, 5 μg/ml and 0.5 μg/ml. But before this experiment with injection method was performed, the optimal lipid amount had to be determined by a series of DPPC isotherms [6]. The amount of DPPC in chloroform that was used for injection method is 9.5 μl, as detailed in the following section. The surface pressure of subphase can be determined with the help of Wilhelmy plate. The plate itself is in the upper (less dense/lighter) phase (3) in Fig.1, where it has a certain lifting force.

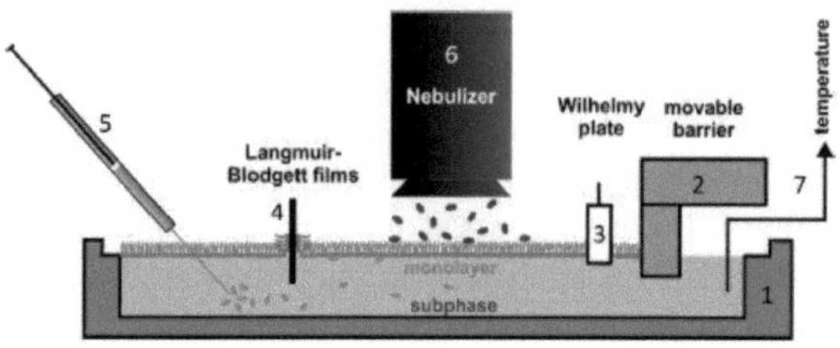

Figure 1: Schematic setup of a Langmuir trough. (1) Telfon trough; (2) Moveable barriere; (3) Wilhelmy plate, lipid monolayers are in surface subphase; (4) Langmuir Blodgett films; (5) Hamilton syringe, the red substances are Tyloxapol solution; (6) Nebulizer, the blue substances are nebulized Tyloxapol solution; (7) Temperatur controller. The part of the Langmuir Blodgett film is further used for AFM imaging.

2.2.1 Measurement of Isotherms

The lateral pressure between the movable barrier were obtained in a computer-controlled KSV Nima. The apparatus consisted of a teflon trough, two movable barriers (compared to nebulization method, which only required one moveable barrier) and a Wilhelmy plate, which served as a pressure sensor. The temperature during the experiments was $21 \pm 1°C$, maintained by a thermostated circulating water system. Prior to each experiment, the trough was cleaned using ethanol and rinsed twice with distilled water. Following this, the trough was filled with distilled water as subphase and DPPC solution in chloroform was applied dropwise onto water surface. After evaporating the solvent for 5 min the compression of the phospholipid monolayer was performed by closing the barriers at a pre-set speed of 10 mm/min. This method provide a way to obtain information on compressibility of lipids and confidently reproduced the surface pressure/area per lipid isotherms of monolayers in different states and can also explain the area expansion and compression generated in particles/substances. So after performing a few isotherm measurements, 9.5 μl DPPC was chosen as the optimal lipid amount.

2.2.2 Injection Method

In the injection delivery method, the substance was injected directly into the subphase below the lipid monolayer. For this purpose, the compression of the monolayer was performed until the lateral pressure reached the given value of 20 mN/m, which was shown in the operating programme. 40 μl of the Tyloxapol solution was injected with a Hamilton syringe after 20 min equilibration. In addition, injection of water into the subphase serves as a control experiment.

3 Results and Discussion

3.1 Injection Method

Figure 2 presents the relative change of area between the movable barriers as a function of time under constant lateral pressure of 20 mN/m and at various Tyloxapol solution concentrations in the trough, and also injection of water as control experiment. The injection of Tyloxapol solution with various concentrations, as described in section 2.2.2, leads to an increase in lateral pressure of the lipid monolayer. To maintain the lateral pressure of 20 mN/m, which represents the natural pressure in cell membrans, the area of the monolayer is adjusted by moving the barriers. The time dependence of the tyloxapol intercalation into the monolayer is measured. In Figure 2 it can be seen, that the area increases after Tyloxapol injection are greater than 100 %.

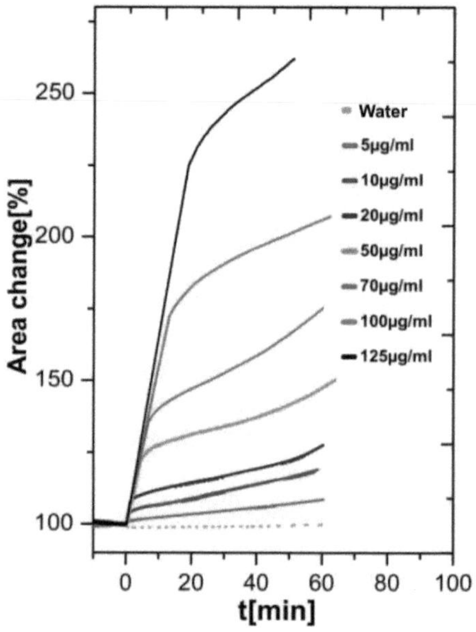

Figure 2: Change of monolayer area as function of time in regards to various Tyloxapol concentrations. From bottom to top, the Tyloxapol concentration is increased.

The change of the area at a given concentration increased with increasing concentration of Tyloxapol. The injection of water as control measurement results in no area change and the highest area change was achieved with a Tyloxapol concentration of 125 μg/ml, which also required least time to acquire the maximum area. In the beginning, the increase of area is rapid and linear, which corresponds to the maximum barrier movement speed to maintain the 20 mN/m lateral pressure. This is caused by a technical problem, that directly after Tyloxapol injection the circuit loop in the computer programme could not move the barrier fast enough to maintain the 20 mN/m lateral pressure. After reaching certain time, the area change increased gradually and after 60 min a saturation was not reached, which should be indicated by flat curves. This indicates, the circuit loop can adjust the barrier movement to adequately follow the increase in lateral pressure. It is also remarkable that from 50 μg/ml the curve bends upwards at 40 min after injection, which does not occur on all curves. To investigate the area expansion more closely, measurements were conducted with Tyloxapol concentrations of 50 μg/ml; $PM041$, $PM055$, $PM055_1$ and 70 μg/ml; $PM062$, $PM066$, $PM070$, whose results are presented in Fig. 3. In Figure 3 it can be observed, that the measurement with Tyloxapol concentration of 70 μg/ml results in greater data deviation from their mean value, which is indicated by larger error bars.

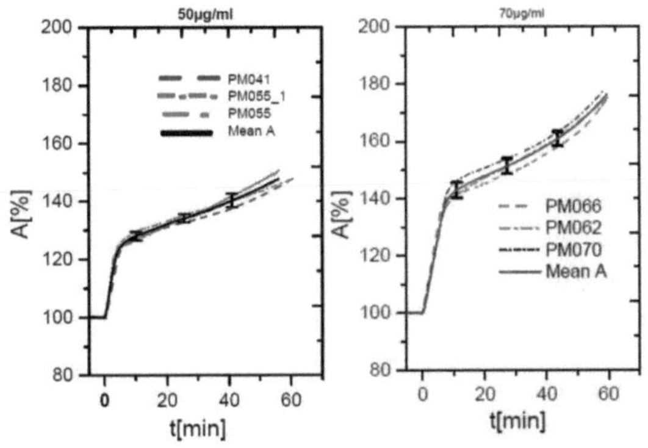

Figure 3: Comparison between injection of 40 μl 50 μg/ml (left) and 70 μg/ml (right) Tyloxapol at 20 mN/m lateral pressure. The dotted lines show the result of three independent measurements. The mean of plotted data is depicted as solid line respectively, the error bars give the standard deviation for 3 timepoints.

3.1.1 Schwarz plot

To better understand the relation between the Tyloxapol concentration and the increase of the monolayer area, can be estimated with the help of Schwarz plot [5]. In Figure 4 the area change at time = 40 min for all Tyloxapol concentrations is plotted against the respective Tyloxapol concentration. A linear regression of the plotted data was done, whose slope indicates the Tyloxapol molecule's density per area 0.385 03 μg Tyloxapol/cm^2.

3.1.2 Expansion at constant lateral pressure of 40 mN/m

In this part of the experiment, the lateral pressure of the lipid layer was held constant at 40 mN/m. Thereafter, 40 μl of 50 μg/ml Tyloxapol was injected into the subphase. After 40 min equilibration, decompression was started until the maximum distance between moveable barrier and Wilhelmy plate was achieved, which corresponds to the minimum lateral pressure of the monolipid layer. As the pressure increased during compression, DPPC molecules rearrange themselves, resulting in bending and partial penetration into the subphase. Figure 5 shows the decompression curves after 40 μl 50 μg/ml Tyloxapol injection and water as control measurement.

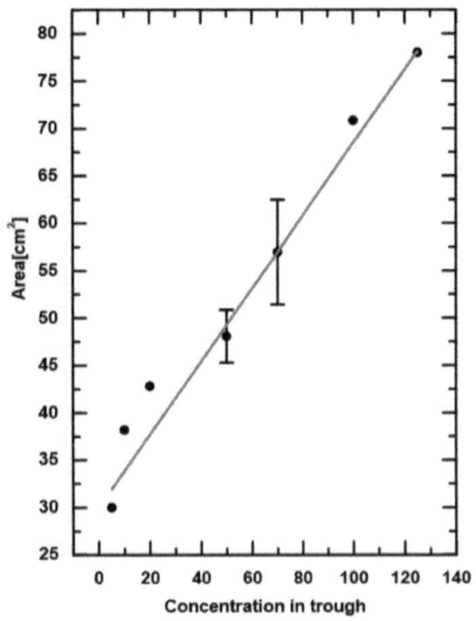

Figure 4: Schwarz plot of area change at t = 40 min of all Tyloxapol concentrations. Linear regression is shown in red.

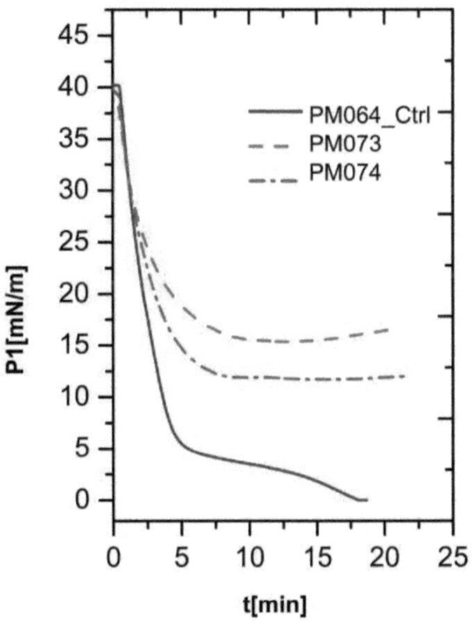

Figure 5: Lateral pressure as function of time after injection of 50 μg/ml Tyloxapol. The red and green lines show the result of two separate measurements. Control measurement using water is depicted in blue.

Compared to injection of 50 μg/ml Tyloxapol (PM073 and PM074), which resulted in 16 mN/m and 12.5 mN/m pressure, injection of water resulted in 0 mN/m lateral pressure after decompression. In Figure 5, PM073 and PM074 created an exponential curve at 30 mN/m right after decompression began. The PM073 curve shows constant lateral pressure of 16 mN/m for 10 minutes, which is then followed by slight lateral pressure increase. This indicates that 20 mN/m lateral pressure is not the optimum lateral pressure for the Tyloxapol and DPPC integration into DPPC monolayers.

3.2 AFM Imaging of Lipid domains in monolayer

AFM studies of LB films of biological interest have typically been performed using mica, which provides a very flat hydrophilic surface support. When the lipid monolayer is transferred onto the mica surface, the polar head groups of the lipids will face the mica surface, while the hydrophobic tails are exposed to air (Fig.6). On this part, DPPC and Tyloxapol in the subphase at 20 mN/m after 40 min equilibration was transferred onto the mica as LB film. AFM images are presented in Fig. 7, where AFM scans of LB films containing different substances, thus resulting in different surface of LB films, can be observed. The phase domains appear in lighter color at >0.5 nm (higher domain) surrounded by a darker zone.

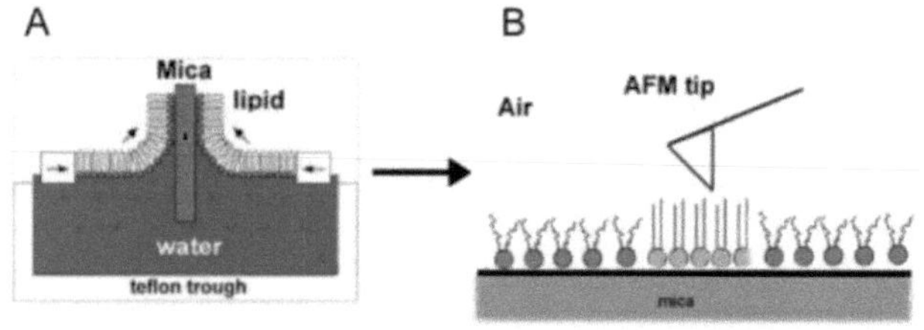

Figure 6: Schematic Figure of LB film on mica surface. (A) After spreading of lipids at the air/water interface of a Langmuir trough, the film is compressed up to the chosen surface pressure by two Teflon barriers and transferred onto mica film; (B) the sample is placed under the AFM tip and examined using the non-contact method.[4]

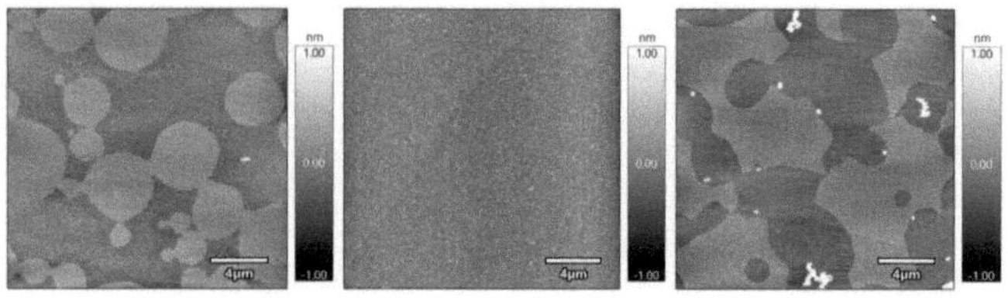

Figure 7: AFM imaged of DPPC and Tyloxapol solution in subphase at 20 mN/m. (Left) DPPC film with injected water; (Middle) Only Tyloxapol; (Right) DPPC film with injected Tyloxapol

As can be seen in Fig. 7 (left), lipids form round-shaped domains, whereas Fig. 7 (middle) shows that Tyloxapol itself does not form any domain. However in Fig. 7 (right) of DPPC with injected Tylpxapol, there is an obvious change of the domain structure, which indicates interaction between the lipid monolayer and Tyloxapol.

4 Conclusion

In this study, the Langmuir technique was used to investigate the interaction between Tyloxapol, an active pharmaceutical compound, and DPPC on the water interface. Based on injection experiment, Tyloxapol solution increases the average distance between DPPC and Tyloxapol molecules and thus also the average area per molecule, especially for higher Tyloxapol solution concentration in the trough. Based on expansion at 40 mN/m (3.1.2), the most optimal intercalation into monolayers were found at surface pressure of 16 mN/m. AFM delivers direct information of the shape and the size of formed domains on top of the LB film. This experiment is helpful in gaining better insight into the interaction between pharmaceutical drug compound and lipid monolayer.
In further studies, the nebulization method will be performed and then compared with the injection method, whose result is presented in this work.

Acknowledgement

The work has been carried out at the division of biophysics, Research Center Borstel, supervised by Thomas Gutsmann, head of the division of biophysics and Christian Nehls, postdoc at the division of biophysic

Author's Statement

Conflict of interest: Authors state no conflict of interest.

5 References

[1] H. Halliday *Surfactants: past, present and future*. In: Journal of Perinatology 28, Nature Publishing, 2008.

[2] Drugbank, *Tyloxapol*. Available: https://go.drugbank.com/drugs/DB06439 [last accessed on 20.01.2021].

[3] C. Nehls, *Charakterisierung der Wechselwirkung zwischen dem bakteriellen Protein VapA und der Phagosomenmembran an Modellmembransystemen*. Forschungszentrum Borstel, 2016.

[4] P.E. Mielhiet, M.C. Giocondi, and C. Le Grimellec, *AFM Imaging of Lipid Domains in Model Membranes*. Mini-Review The Scientific World Journal (2003), 59–74 ISSN 1537-744X; DOI 10.1100/tsw.2003.12.

[5] T. Gutsmann, *A short introduction into biology*. In: Vorlesung Instrumentierung der Biophysik, 2020.

[6] B. Alfred, *A comparative study of the phase transitions of phospholipid bilayers and monolayers*. In: Biochimica et Biophysica Acta (BBA)-Biomembranes 557 (1979), Nr. 1, S. 32–44.

Characterisation of the interaction between mast cells, α-synuclein and the enteric nervous system in Parkinson's disease

Catrin Przibylla [1] and Francois Cossais [2]

[1] Biophysics, Universität zu Lübeck, catrin.przibylla@student.uni-luebeck.de

[2] Institute of Anatomy, Christian-Albrechts-Universität zu Kiel, f.cossais@anat.uni-kiel.de

Abstract

Currently, there are no diagnostic tools available to identify early phases of Parkinson's disease (PD). At the time when first symptoms of the disease become apparent and where treatments start, already more than half of dopaminergic neurons are lost. Glial-mediated neuroinflammation has been proposed to be involved in the pathological aggregation of α-synuclein in the central nervous system. Gastro-intestinal disorders represent a common non-motor symptom in PD. However, the interplay between α-synuclein and the intestinal neuroimmune system is still not clearly characterised. In this study, we provide first data on the potential alteration of mast cell numbers in PD as well as on α-synuclein expression in the enteric neuroimmune microenvironment. This approach may help to find specific diagnostic markers to predict the onset of PD symptoms in the early course of PD or to find new innovative treatments against this disease.

1 Introduction

Parkinson's Disease (PD) is a neurodegenerative disorder which is characterized by a loss of dopaminergic neurons in the substantia nigra in the brain stem, thus leading to symptoms like bradykinesia, rigidity, resting tremor or postural instability. A second pathological hallmark of the disease is the presence of aggregates, containing misfolded alpha-Synuclein (α-Syn), called Lewy bodies. These pathological aggregates are not only affecting the central nervous system (CNS). Indeed, several clinical reports indicated the presence of Lewy bodies and neurites in the enteric nervous system (ENS) of almost every investigated PD patient [1] but also in healthy control individuals [3]. Functions of α-Syn are still not clearly identified. Since the protein preferentially enriches in presynaptic terminals, one can assume that the protein is involved in the regulation of synaptic transmission, synaptic plasticity and neurotransmitter synthesis. It is also still unknown if the aggregation of pathological α-Syn is the cause or a consequence of PD [2]. The ENS is an integrative, complex network within the gut wall, organized in two ganglionated plexuses, the submucosal plexus, as the name implies located in submucosa, and the myenteric plexus which lies between circular and longitudinal muscle layers. Because of its similarities to the CNS, the ENS is often described as "the-brain-in-the-gut". The ENS regulates several functions like gastrointestinal (GI) motility, mucosal blood flow, ion and water transport and resorption [3]. It contains a large population of enteric glial cells (EGCs) which can be considered as the digestive equivalent of brain astrocytes [1]. EGCs may take an important part in neuroinflammatory events and in the regulation of α-Syn life-cycle in the GI tract [1], [4]. In addition to typical motor symptoms, 60-90% of the PD patients suffer from GI dysfunctions and develop some degree of gastrointestinal inflammation which may contribute to the initiation and progression of PD [5]. Increased expression levels of various pro-inflammatory markers like cytokines have been observed in the gut of PD patients in previous studies [5], [6]. Therefore, several authors suggest a bidirectional link between PD and GI inflammation [6]. In this study, we aimed to provide first evidence in support of the involvement of the enteric neuroimmune system in the regulation of α-Syn life-cycle and intestinal neuroinflammation in PD. Colocalization of α-Syn with EGCs, enteric neurons and mast cells was characterized in the colon of control individuals. In addition, we made a quantitative analysis of colonic mast cells, which are part of the neuroimmune system, in PD patients and controls.

2 Material and Methods

2.1 Immunohistochemistry

2.1.1 Tissue Source

For each PD patient or control, deep mucosal biopsies were obtained from the upper dorsal rectal wall. Control patients (n = 12) were recruited from the Department of Internal Medicine I at the University Hospital Schleswig-Holstein, Campus Kiel, undergoing colonoscopy for colorectal cancer screening or GI symptoms without clinical evidence of neurological diseases. Patients (n = 10) were recruited from the Department of Neurology at the University Hospital Schleswig-Holstein, Campus Kiel. Diagnosis of PD was based on clinical examination by neurologists according to UK Parkinson's Disease Society Brain Bank Clinical Criteria. The study protocol received approval from the Local Ethics Committee of the Faculty of Medicine, Christian Albrecht's University of Kiel, Germany (D455/10; B299/07).

2.1.2 Tissue Processing

After surgical removal, all specimens were transferred into phosphate-buffered saline (pH 7.2) to allow adaption and further dissection. Full-thickness rectangular tissue blocks (30x10 mm) were pinned out flat on a cork plate by fine needles without artificial stretching or shortening, thereby preserving the original size. After fixation (4% paraformaldehyde in phosphate-buffered saline) for 24 hours and dehydration, tissue blocks were transferred into paraffin wax and cut into orthogonal sections (5 µm) along the longitudinal gut axis for immunohistochemistry. Paraffin-embedded tissue sections of controls (n = 5) or PD (n = 3) were pretreated with citrate buffer (pH 6.0, 95°C, water bath) for 25 minutes, followed by overnight incubation with rabbit-anti-MJFR (abcam, Cambridge, UK), mouse-anti-PGP (OriGene, Rockville, US), mouse-anti-S100β (Millipore, Darmstadt, Germany), goat-anti-c-Kit (Santa Cruz, California, US), diluted in antibody diluent (Life Technologies, Karlsruhe, Germany). Secondary antibodies, including anti-rabbit AlexaFluor488, anti-goat Alexafluor555, anti-mouse AlexaFluor555 (all from Invitrogen, California, US) and anti-rabbit star red, anti-mouse abberior 580 (both from Abberior, Göttingen, Germany) were diluted in antibody diluent (Life Technologies) and incubated for 2 hours at room temperature. Nuclei were stained with Bisbenzimid (Sigma-Aldrich, Darmstadt, Germany). To correct for unspecific signals, blank controls were performed by processing adjacent sections for each individual omitting primary antibodies.

2.2 Detection and Analysis

For quantification of mast cells, immunohistochemical findings were acquired with a 10x (Plan Apo 10x NA 0.45) and 40x (Plan Apo 40x NA 0.95) objective magnification using a Keyence BZ-X810 microscope and BZ Analyzer software (Keyence, Neu-Ilsenburg, Germany). Mast cells were quantified manually using the cell-counting plug-in of the software QuPath and Fiji to determine the number of cells per area. For confocal and Stimulated Emission Depletion (STED) microscopy, tissue was imaged with a 100x, NA 1.4 (UPLan SApo) objective on a Aberrior Instruments facility line STED microscope and Imspector software (version 16.3.13030) (Abberior, Göttingen, Germany). Confocally acquired images were prepared using the software Fiji and Adobe Photoshop Elements 9. For STED imaging, Abberior star red labelled proteins were excited with a wavelength of 635 nm and depleted with a 775 nm STED laser while Abberior STAR 580 labelled proteins were excited with a wavelength of 580 nm and depleted with a STED laser of 775 nm. STED images were acquired with a pixel size of 25 nm and a pixel dwell time of 10 µs. Deconvolution of STED data was carried out using the STED module in Huygens Professional software (version 20.10).

2.3 Statistical Analysis

Statistical analysis was performed using the GraphPad Prism 8.4.2 software (PrismTM, San Diego, CA). Results are expressed as mean ± SEM.

3 Results and Discussion

3.1 Immunoreactivity of MJFR, CD117, S100β and PGP in colon of controls

Parkinson's disease is one of the most common neurodegenerative diseases with a rising incidence in the elderly. Because of the increasing life expectancy, the number of individuals suffering from PD will grow in the coming decades [1]. Braak suggested in 2006 that the hallmark of PD, pathology of α-Syn, develops in the ENS in the early course of PD prior to the pathology in central dopaminergic neurons and thus prior to the occurrence of motor symptoms. Therefore, Braak assumed that the ENS may be critically involved in pathophysiology of PD [6]. In order to gain further insight on α-Syn expression in the enteric neuroimmune system of control individuals, double labeling immunohistochemistry for α-Syn (MJFR) and markers of enteric neurons (PGP, Fig. 1i), EGCs (S100β, Fig. 1f) and mast cells (CD117, Fig. 1c) was performed and analysed using confocal microscopy. Expression of α-Syn was observed in close proximity to all analysed cell types. Generally, α-Syn immunoreactivity was detected in ganglia of both the myenteric and submucosal plexus but never in the nucleus of cells. Furthermore, STED microscopy was used to enhance resolution and to investigate presence of α-Syn in EGCs more precisely. As shown in Fig. 2, α-Syn was detectable in the immediate surroundings of EGCs, but no positive staining was found within the glia cells in control individuals. Whereas astrocytes which are glial cells of the central nervous system, are involved in α-Syn life-cycle in the brain, further work is required to determine whether EGCs play similar functions in the ENS [10]. Presence of pathological α-Syn aggregates in the ENS is still a subject of intense debate in the literature. In this regard, development of isoform-specific α-Syn antibodies has been an important research focus in the recent years. The MJFR-14 antibody used in this study was shown to bind not only α-Syn oligomers and fibrils but also α-Syn monomers [8]. The broad immunoreactive signals detected in tissue samples of control individuals suggest that MJFR-14 also binds to the non-pathological form of α-Syn aggregates which can be found in healthy ENS. A recent study reports a monoclonal antibody against α-Syn (5G4) which distinguishes pathological α-Syn from healthy ones [11].

It may be of high interest to retry dual-labeling immunohistochemistry using this antibody to differentiate between pathological and non-pathological forms and compare the

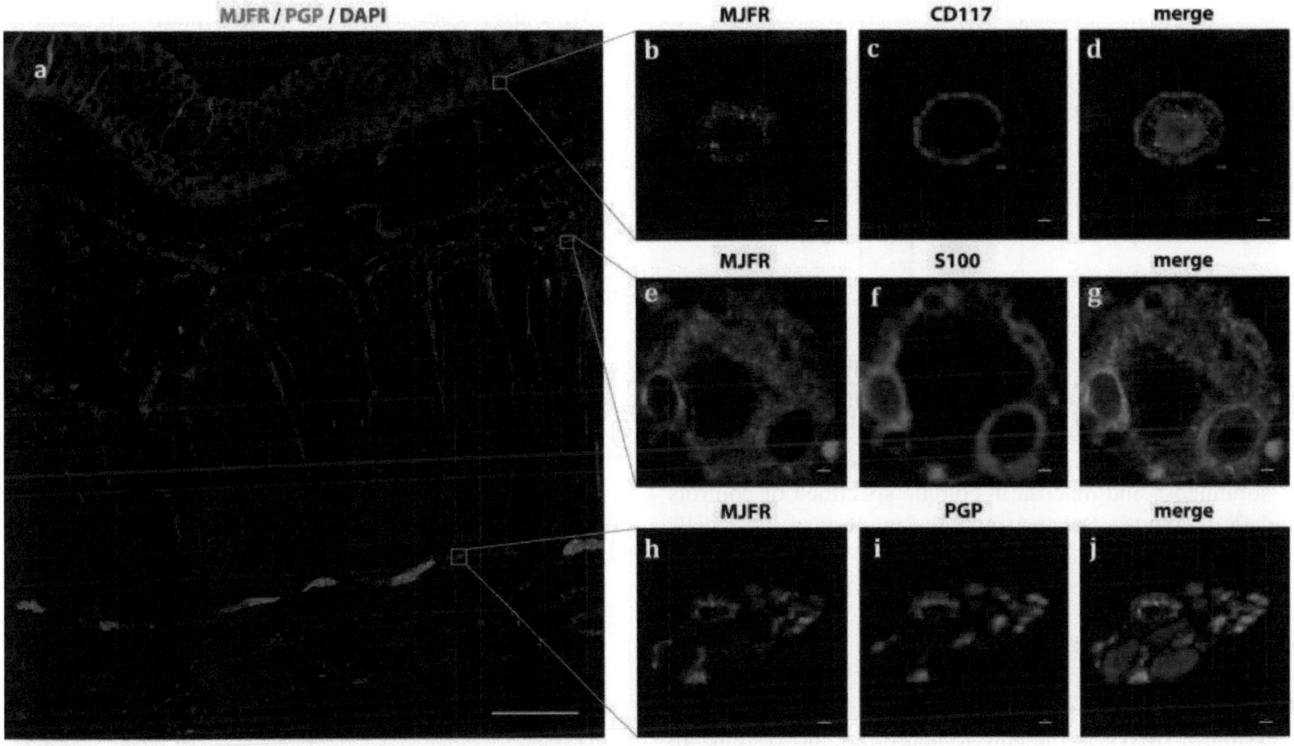

Figure 1: Dual-label fluorescence immunohistochemistry of MJFR, CD117, S100β and PGP in colonic specimen of controls. MJFR (marker for α-Syn; green) was detected in mast cells, visualized in b-d, EGCs (e-g) and neurons (h-j) using confocal microscopy. Red signals show the specific markers for mast cells (CD117 in c), EGCs (S100 in f) and enteric neurons (PGP in i), respectively. Nuclear counterstain with Bisbendzimid (blue; a, d, g, j), scalebar in a = 500 µm; scalebar in b-j = 2 µm.

amount and localization of pathological aggregates in enteric neurons, EGCs and mast cells in colon of PD patients and controls. It is worth noting that processed tissues were used which may also have an impact on posttranslational modifications of α-Syn aggregates.

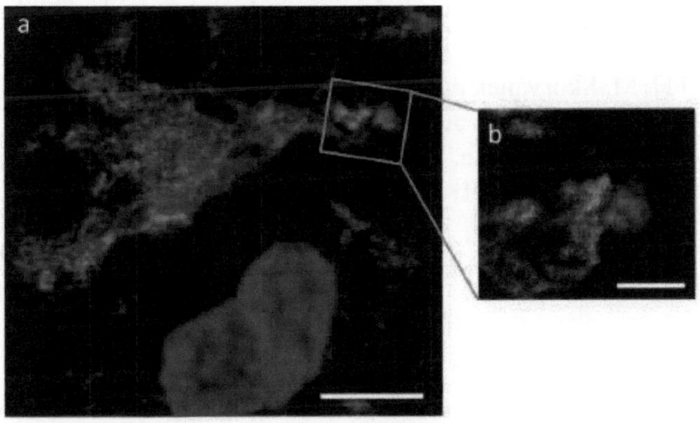

Figure 2: Localization of α-Syn and EGCs in colonic wall of control individuals. Double labeled immunohistochemistry was performed and detected by STED microscopy to investigate colocalization of EGCs (S100β, green) and α-Syn (MJFR, red). Findings revealed no colocalization of α-Syn and EGCs. Nuclear coutnerstain with Bisbendzimid (blue). Scalebar in a = 5 µm; scalebar in b = 2 µm.

3.2 Quantification of mast cells in PD patients and controls

Neuroinflammation has been associated with several neurodegenerative diseases, e.g. PD. Since mast cells release mediators such as TNF-α, histamine and proteases, they have the ability to potentiate neuroinflammation, neurodegeneration and blood-brain-barrier permeability. Therefore, Jones et al. suggest that mast cell interactions with neurons and EGCs may play a role in PD pathogenesis [9]. Because of these assumptions, we compared the number of mast cells in mucosa and submucosa of PD patients and control individuals. Therefor, CD117, a marker of mast cells, was stained and quantified using fluorescence microscopy in 10 controls and PD patients, respectively. As depicted in Fig. 3, the mean mast cell number was slightly increased in PD patients (mean: 101.7 $\pm$ 11.15 mast cells/mm²) in comparison with controls (mean: 90.67 $\pm$ 13.66 mast cells/mm²). We assume that there is a correlation between the amount of colonic mast cells and PD. Further experiments to increase the number of observed samples for quantification analysis of mast cells in controls and PD patients will be carried out to confirm our assumption and the present results. Additionally, immunohistochemical experiments with the use of a marker for activated mast cells would be of interest to compare neuroinflammatory events in colonic specimen of PD patients and controls.

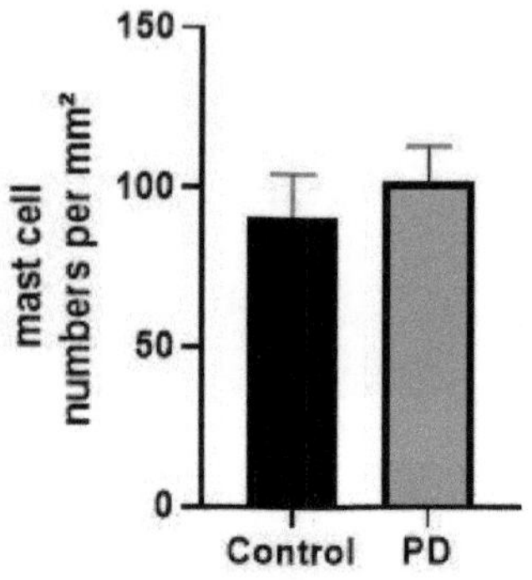

Figure 3: Quantification of mast cells in colon of PD patients and controls. Immunohistochemistry and expression of CD117 were used to quantify the number of mast cells in submucosa and mucosa in colonic specimen of controls and PD patients. Subsequently the number of mast cells was normalized to the area of interest (n= 10).

4 Conclusion

There is still a lack of research regarding the cellular expression of α-Syn in the enteric neuroimmune system. In further experiments, potential alterations of α-Syn expression patterns within enteric neurons, EGCs and mast cells will be investigated in colonic specimen of PD patients and compared to controls. Additionally, STED microscopy will be used to obtain further insight on the subcellular expression of α-Syn in enteric neurons and mast cells. Characterization of the interplay between α-Syn and the enteric neuroimmune system should bring important knowledge on PD pathogenesis along the gut-brain-axis.

Acknowledgement

The work has been carried out at Institute of Anatomy, Christian-Albrechts-Universität zu Kiel and supervised by Dr. Young-Hwa Song, Institute of Physics, Universität zu Lübeck.

Author's Statement

The authors declare no conflict of interest.

5 References

[1] L. Benvenuti *et al.*, "Enteric glia at the crossroads between intestinal immune system and epithelial barrier: Implications for Parkinson disease," *Int. J. Mol. Sci.*, vol. 21, no. 23, pp. 1–16, 2020.

[2] M. Böttner *et al.*, "Expression pattern and localization of alpha-synuclein in the human enteric nervous system," *Neurobiol. Dis.*, vol. 48, no. 3, pp. 474–480, 2012.

[3] M. Barrenschee *et al.*, "Distinct pattern of enteric phospho-alpha-synuclein aggregates and gene expression profiles in patients with Parkinson's disease," *Cerebellum and Ataxias*, vol. 4, no. 1, pp. 1–14, 2017.

[4] D. Devos *et al.*, "Colonic inflammation in Parkinson's disease," *Neurobiol. Dis.*, vol. 50, no. 1, pp. 42–48, 2013.

[5] F. Cossais *et al.*, "Expression profiling of rectal biopsies suggests altered enteric neuropathological T´traits in Parkinson's disease patients," *J. Parkinsons. Dis.*, pp. 1–6, 2020.

[6] M. Rolli-Derkinderen *et al.*, "Is Parkinson's disease a chronic low-gradc inflammatory bowel disease?," *J. Neurol.*, vol. 267, no. 8, pp. 2207–2213, 2020.

[7] H. Braak, R. A. I. De Vos, J. Bohl, and K. Del Tredici, "Gastric α-synuclein immunoreactive inclusions in Meissner's and Auerbach's plexuses in cases staged for Parkinson's disease-related brain pathology," *Neurosci. Lett.*, 2006.

[8] S. T. Kumar, *et al.*, "How specific are the conformation-specific α-synuclein antibodies? Characterization and validation of 16 α-synuclein conformation-specific antibodies using well-characterized preparations of α-synuclein monomers, fibrils and oligomers with distinct structures and morphology," *Neurobiol. Dis.*, vol. 146, no. August, p. 105086, 2020.

[9] M. K. Jones, A. Nair, and M. Gupta, "Mast cells in neurodegenerative disease," *Front. Cell. Neurosci.*, vol. 13, no. April, pp. 1–9, 2019.

[10] A. Filippini, M. Gennarelli, and I. Russo, "α-Synuclein and Glia in Parkinson's Disease: A Beneficial or a Detrimental Duet for the Endo-Lysosomal System?," *Cell. Mol. Neurobiol.*, vol. 39, no. 2, pp. 161–168, 2019.

[11] M. Skorvanek *et al.*, "α-Synuclein antibody 5G4 identifies manifest and prodromal Parkinson's disease in colonic mucosa," *Mov. Disord.*, vol. 33, no. 8, pp. 1366–1368, 2018.

On the theoretical determination of protein volumes using solvent accessible surface areas and crystallographic data

Finja Rike Klare [1], Niclas Ludolph [2], and Hauke Paulsen [3]
[1] Medical Engineering Science, Universität zu Lübeck, finja.klare@student.uni-luebeck.de
[2] Institut für Physik, Universität zu Lübeck, niclas.ludolph@student.uni-luebeck.de
[3] Institut für Physik, Universität zu Lübeck, paulsen@physik.uni-luebeck.de

Abstract

The volume is a very important property of proteins and its accurate determination is of great importance for a deeper understanding of the folding process of proteins. Experimental determination of protein volume is difficult and for some purposes does not have sufficient accuracy, so precise computational determination of protein volumes is highly desirable. As a starting point for the theoretical calculation of protein volumes, this work uses protein structural data provided in the Protein Data Bank. Initially all protein files are downloaded and subsequently filtered in order to obtain a limited number of proteins for further investigations. Shell scripts were designed to examine the large number of structures automatically. The first filtering consists in defining a certain number of residues the protein should have. Subsequently proteins with disulfide bridges were filtered out. Due to the immense abundance of proteins, this procedure was supplemented by searching for proteins with specific volumes.

1 Introduction

The study of proteins and their structural behavior has been an important area of research for many years. These versatile macromolecules possess a wide range of functions depending on the special sequences of amino acids. They are essential for many different reactions in the body. For instance actin and myosin as contractile proteins for the muscle activity or immunoglobulins for the formation of defence mechanisms. Protein folding is an important process which is essential for the entire human organism and all other living organisms. Disturbances in protein formation especially in the folding process can cause devastating consequences in the human body [10]. Many diseases arise due to misfolded proteins such as Alzheimer or sickle cell anemia. That is why research into the behavioral properties of proteins has become very important. The primary structures of an organism's proteome, i.e. the sequences of amino acids in the protein chains, are encoded in the genome and thus known for many organisms. From the primary structure of a protein, good predictions of the secondary and tertiary structure, i.e. the three-dimensional arrangement of the residues, can now be made using bioinformatics methods. However, for an exact determination of the tertiary structure, very elaborate experimental methods such as X-ray crystallography, NMR spectroscopy or cryo-transmission electron microscopy are still required. The basic interactions responsible for the specific tertiary structure of a protein are known, but no simple model exists that describes the process of protein folding and allows it to be predicted. Protein folding is therefore an active field of research that is being investigated using both experimental and theoretical methods. The most important macroscopic parameters that can be used to influence the folding state of a protein include temperature, the concentration of denaturants (such as urea or guanidinium hydrochloride), and hydrostatic pressure. For the interpretation of the folding process, pressure-driven protein folding and unfolding offers several advantages [9]. The natural variables of Gibbs energy, the thermodynamic potential of the isothermal-isobaric ensemble, are temperature and pressure, and the variables conjugate to them are entropy and volume, respectively. The latter is much more accessible to the imagination than the entropy. An example of a protein whose folding state can be altered by applying hydrostatic pressure, as has been shown by single molecule spectroscopy and theoretical simulations [1], is cold shock protein A (CspA) [2], whose structure is shown in Fig. 1. While the mass of a protein can be determined exactly experimentally, the protein volume can only be determined approximately, with the aid of the average density of proteins of about 1.35 g/cm^3. Accuracy of volume determination, as necessary to explain pressure-induced conformational changes of proteins, can only be achieved by theoretical methods. The two most important methods for this are the determination of the Archimedean displacement volume [3] and the calculation of the solvent accessible surface area (SASA) [4], a method first described by Lee and Richards 1971 [5]. The volume determined with the first method comes closest to the volume as a variable of the

Gibbs energy. However, this method is much more complicated than the calculation of the volume with the help of the SASA. Therefore, only the second method will be considered in this paper.

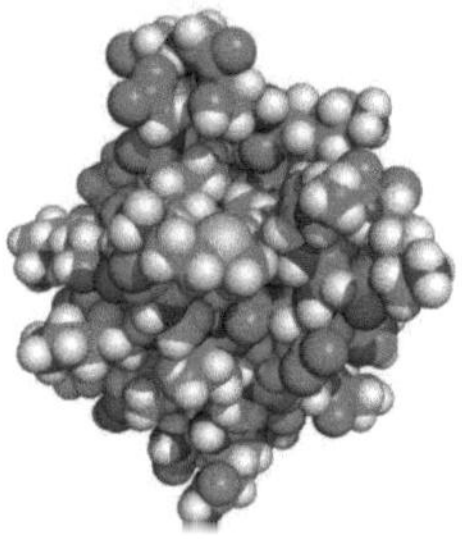

Figure 1: Coldshock protein CspA. Colored spheres with van der Waals radius represent the atoms of the molecule.

1.1 Protein structure

As already indicated, the sequence is not directly responsible for the function of the proteins. The folding of the amino-acid-chain and the resulting three-dimensional structure largely determine the function. There are several methods to determine these structures, x-ray crystallography being the one most frequently used, next to nuclear magnetic resonance (NMR), which allows to study proteins in aqueous solutions and thus in almost physiological conditions. Especially suitable for very large proteins is the method of cryoelectron transmission spectroscopy. As a result of investigations using these techniques more than 160 000 protein structures are currently stored in the Protein Data Bank (PDB) [6]. The entries in the Protein Data Bank contain the type and the position of all atoms constituting the protein as well as the covalent bonds between the atoms. A particular case of these bonds is the so called disulfide bridge between two sulfur atoms, that can occur between two cysteines in the same or in two separate amino acid chains, thus forming disulfide cystines. Disulfide bridges are particularly important for the stability of the protein structure, but are problematic for the biotechnological production of proteins [10].

1.2 Molecular surface

The protein structures of the protein data bank as well as structures obtained from molecular dynamics calculations can be used to calculate the volume of the proteins in order to better understand the influence of cavities and voids in the native protein structure. The above mentioned SASA method is the most prominent approach for such calculations. As shown in Fig. 2 the protein volume calculated with SASA is composed of the intrinsic volume of the protein atoms (van der Waals volume) and of the intramolecular cavity volume (void volume). The latter has a special importance in understanding the folding process since voids in the protein structure do, for instance, affect the pressure unfolding. Starting from the atomic coordinates as provided by the protein data bank the SASA method generates the surface area of the protein by using the so-called rolling ball approach [8], that is illustrated in Fig. 2. There are different ways to implement this approach into an efficient algorithm.

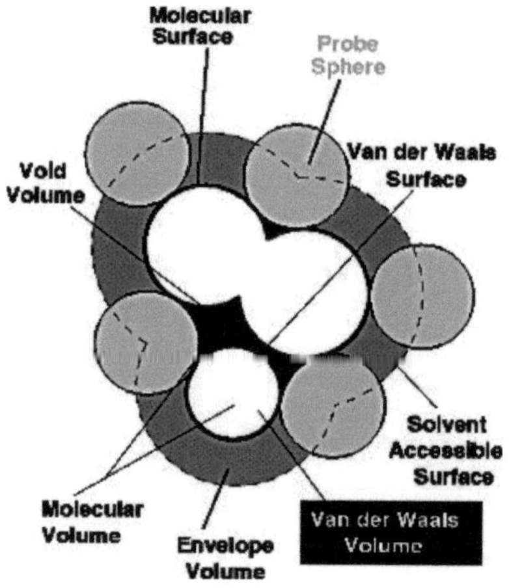

Figure 2: Volumes and surfaces of a molecule [8].

A specific way to calculate the solvent accessible surface SAS within the framework of the SASA method is provided by the algorithm developed by Eisenhaber and coworkers, which uses the double cubic lattice method [8], which describes SAS as

$$SAS = \sum_{i=1}^{N} 4\pi r_i^2 \frac{n_{\mathrm{surf},i}}{n_{\mathrm{tot},i}} , \tag{1}$$

were N describes the number of atoms of which the protein consists, r_i is the radius of atom i, $n_{\mathrm{surf},i}$ is the number of points on the solvent accessible surface of atom i and $n_{\mathrm{tot},i}$ is the total number of points placed on atom i.

2 Material and Methods

2.1 Protein Data Bank

The Protein Data Bank (PDB) has an archive that provides experimentally obtained three-dimensional structural data of macromolecules. It is freely accessible and can easily be used for research work. The data provides information concerning atomic coordinates, crystallographic structure factors, primary and secondary structures, and details on data collection.

The entire directory containing the protein files was downloaded via the PDB FTP pages (ftp.wwpdb.org), which are updated every week with regard to new and revised data entries. The pool of proteins is further sorted in the following process of this research.

2.2 Protein files

Coordinate files of biological macromolecules list all atoms of the molecule and their position in space. These coordinate files exist among others in the pdb format. There is a certain order how such files should be constructed. A row generally consists of 80 columns as can be seen in Fig. 3. The first six columns provide the name of the record type, which specifies what information is listed in these associated rows. The record type EXPDTA can be used to find out which experimental technique was used for the structure determination. The REMARK record type contains general information that can often be freely described. There are mandatory entries and optional entries, which makes comparability and standardization difficult but provides an extraordinary wealth of information. Information regarding the understanding of a pdb file can be found out via the website wwpdb.org.

```
         1         2         3         4         5         6         7         8
12345678901234567890123456789012345678901234567890123456789012345678901234567890
SEQRES   1 A   21  GLY ILE VAL GLU GLN CYS CYS THR SER ILE CYS SER LEU
SEQRES   2 A   21  TYR GLN LEU GLU ASN TYR CYS ASN
SEQRES   1 B   30  PHE VAL ASN GLN HIS LEU CYS GLY SER HIS LEU VAL GLU
SEQRES   2 B   30  ALA LEU TYR LEU VAL CYS GLY GLU ARG GLY PHE PHE TYR
SEQRES   3 B   30  THR PRO LYS ALA
SEQRES   1 C   21  GLY ILE VAL GLU GLN CYS CYS THR SER ILE CYS SER LEU
SEQRES   2 C   21  TYR GLN LEU GLU ASN TYR CYS ASN
SEQRES   1 D   30  PHE VAL ASN GLN HIS LEU CYS GLY SER HIS LEU VAL GLU
SEQRES   2 D   30  ALA LEU TYR LEU VAL CYS GLY GLU ARG GLY PHE PHE TYR
SEQRES   3 D   30  THR PRO LYS ALA

SEQRES   1 A    8   DA  DA  DC  DC  DG  DG  DT  DT
SEQRES   1 B    8   DA  DA  DC  DC  DG  DG  DT  DT

SEQRES   1 X   39    U   C   C   C   C   C   G   U   G   C   C   C   A
SEQRES   2 X   39    U   A   G   C   G   G   C   G   U   G   G   A   A
SEQRES   3 X   39    C   C   A   C   C   C   G   U   U   C   C   C   A
```

Figure 3: Example for the record type SEQRES
Chain A contains 21 residues, whereas Chain B contains 30 residues.

In order to be able to sort the downloaded proteins according to their size, it is necessary to determine the number of residues of each protein. For this purpose, the data set type SEQRES is used, which is mandatory if atom sets are available. SEQRES contains a listing of the chemical components such as standard amino acid residues or nucleic acid residues that are covalently bonded to a polymer. Not listed are chemical components attached to side chains or sugars and bases. The number of residues in a chain is given in columns 14 to 17. Another record type that is useful in filtering the available protein data is SSBOND, which must always be listed if a disulfide bridge exists. This entry allows omitting proteins that contain disulfide bridges.

2.3 GROMACS

An important and powerful program in the field of molecular simulations is GROMACS. It is a free software package, which is primarily used in the field of simulation and evaluation of molecular dynamic processes. It was developed at the University of Groningen and is now used at research institutes and universities worldwide [7]. In order to be able to investigate the selection of proteins, the GROMACS version 2019.4 was installed.

3 Results and Discussion

First, 158.647 protein files were downloaded in pdb format. A script was written, which determines the number of residues. For this purpose the record types SEQRES and CHAIN were used. The script runs through all files automatically and extracts the number of residues of each chain. If the number is within a set interval the protein is copied to the appropriate folder containing only proteins within this interval. After this initial sorting, it could be seen that most proteins have chain lengths with a number of 0 to 600 residues. One problem arose after closer examination of all the folders created in the process. If a protein contains more than one polypeptide chain, it can be assigned to different folders. That means that it can appear several times after filtering and is not only assigned to a single range with a certain residue number. Thus, after sorting, the total number of proteins in all folders was higher than the initial number of downloaded proteins. What remains to be clarified is how to proceed with proteins that have several chains of different lengths and how the script can be modified accordingly.

Table 1: Example for the categorization of proteins based on the number of residues. The proteins were assigned to the appropriate intervals with respect to the residue number of their chains. Subsequently, all proteins showing disulfide bridges (SSBOND) were sorted out.

Residue Range	protein number incl. SSBOND	protein number without SSBOND
30 - 60	6	1
60 - 90	19	9
90 - 120	41	32
120 - 150	37	31
150 - 180	23	11
180 -210	38	25
210 - 240	25	15
240 - 270	20	17
270 - 300	30	22

The next step was to filter with respect to disulfide bridges present. Each protein that has disulfide bridges in its structure receives an entry via the record type SSBOND in the pdb file. Based on this, a new script was written. Before applying this to all protein files, a test run was performed with three randomly selected folders containing 207 proteins. The results are shown in Table 1. Here it can also be seen that after the first sorting with respect to the residue number, some proteins must appear multiple times due to different chain lengths, because the initial number of 207 proteins is exceeded after adding the protein numbers located in the folders.

It is planned to use SASA method in order to calculate the volume of the filtered pdb files. To calibrate the SASA method, the volume of a sodium chloride nanocrystal was calculated using the GROMACS command gmx sasa. An important parameter of this method is the radius of the spheres with which the molecule is scanned.

Fig. 4 shows the calculated volume of the nanocrystal versus the probe radius. In the limit of an infinitesimal small probe radius the calculated volume approaches the volume of union van der Waals spheres. Instead for infinitely large probe radii the convex envelope of the molecule is obtained.

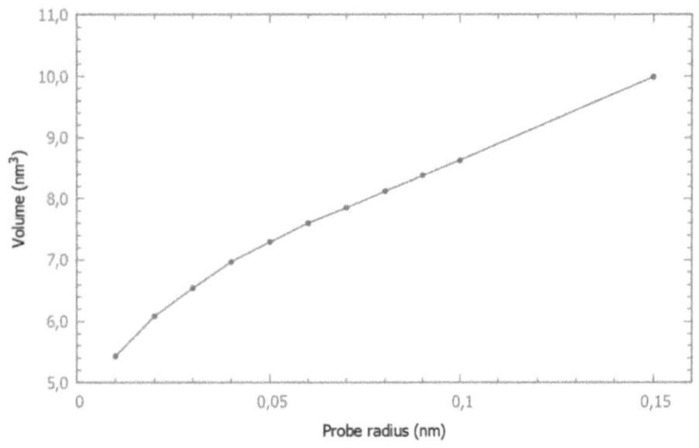

Figure 4: Calculated volumes of a sodium crystal versus probe radius.

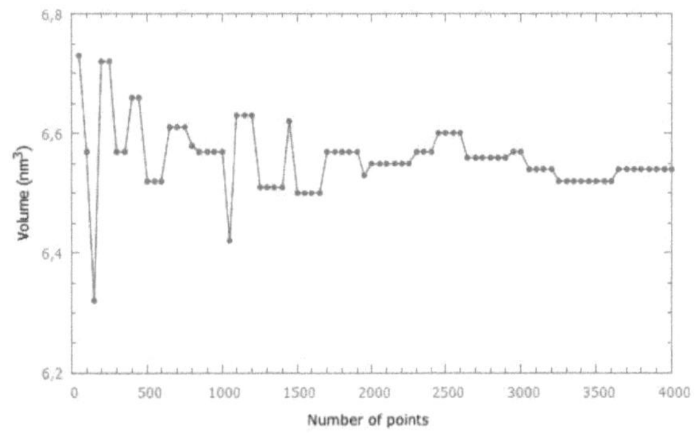

Figure 5: Calculated volumes of a sodium crystal versus number of points.

A second important parameter of the SASA method is the number of points on the van der Waals sphere, which indicates how fine the grid of the scanning is. Fig. 5 shows the calculated volume plotted against this parameter. Using the sodium chloride nanocrystal as an example, it is shown that a number of 4000 points is necessary to obtain stable results for the volume.

4 Conclusion

In the course of this project, it became apparent that the initial approach of extracting all proteins from the PDB archive and only examining certain proteins with special filtering could not be implemented due to the amount of existing proteins. The pdb files provide numerous possibilities and information regarding the protein but the creation of a script to automatically run through all files is very extensive, which is why this approach was initially abandoned. However, this approach could be further elaborated in a more comprehensive framework such as the problem of multiple sorting of some proteins. Future projects could also focus on volume determination of particularly interesting proteins whose structure has already been experimentally determined for different states. Another approach could be the volume calculation using the SASA method of protein structures calculated with GROMACS.

Acknowledgement

The work has been carried out at the Institute of Physics, Universität zu Lübeck.

Author's Statement

Authors state no conflict of interest.

5 References

[1] S. Schneider, H. Paulsen, K.C. Reiter, E. Hinze, C. Schiene-Fischer and C.G. Hübner, *Single molecule FRET investigation of pressure-driven unfolding of cold shock protein A*. In: The Journal of Chemical Physics, vol. 148, no.12, 2018.

[2] Y. Tang et al., *Fully automated high-quality NMR structure determination of small 2H-enriched proteins*. In: Journal of Structural and Functional Genomics, vol. 11, no. 4, pp. 223–232, 2010.

[3] R. DeVane et al., *A Molecular Dynamics Method for Calculating Molecular Volume Changes Appropriate for Biomolecular Simulation*. In: Biophysical Journal, vol. 85, no. 5, pp. 2801–2807, 2003.

[4] F. Eisenhaber, P. Lijnzaad, P. Argos, C. Sander and M. Scharf, *The double cubic lattice method: Efficient approaches to numerical integration of surface area and volume, and to dot surface contouring of molecular assemblies*. In: Journal of Computational Chemistry, vol. 16, pp. 273–284, 1995.

[5] B. Lee B and F.M. Richards, *The interpretation of protein structures: Estimation of static accessibility*. In: Journal of Molecular Biology, vol. 55, no. 3, pp. 379–380, 1971.

[6] wwPDB consortium, *Protein Data Bank: the single global archive for 3D macromolecular structure data*. In: Nucleic Acids Research, vol. 47, no. D1, pp. D520–D528, 2019.

[7] M. J. Abraham, D. van der Spoel, E. Lindahl, B. Hess and the GROMACS development team, *GROMACS User Manual version 2019*. Available: https://www.gromacs.org.

[8] M. S. Till, G. M. Ullmann, *McVol- A program for calculating protein volumes and identifying cavities by a Monte Carlo algorithm*. In: Journal of Molecular Modeling, vol. 16, pp. 419–429, 2009.

[9] J. Roche and C. A. Royer, *Lessons from pressure denaturation of proteins*. In: Journal of the Royal Society Interface, vol. 15, 2018.

[10] J. M. Berg, J. L. Tymoczko and L. Stryer, *Stryer Biochemie*. Springer Spektrum, 2014.

5

Medical Electronics

High Power LED Driver for Multispectral Flash Illumination

Roshanak Talebi [1], Caitlin Toogood [2], and Malte Gienow-Broers [2]
[1] Biomedical Engineering, Luebeck University of Applied Sciences, roshanak.talebi@stud.th-luebeck.de
[2] Laboratory for Medical Optics, Luebeck University of Applied Sciences, {caitlin.toogood, malte.gienow-broers}@th-luebeck.de

Abstract

To overcome the disadvantages of spectral scanning such as wavelength filtering, light efficiency, and scanning time in multispectral imaging, an alternative light source for image acquisition was developed and investigated. As a light source apparatus, an appropriate high-power Light Emitting Diode (LED) driver controlled by a high clock speed microcontroller was developed. The light source consists of 24 LEDs, which use 12 wavelength pairs to produce fast sequential flash illumination in the visible and near-infrared range. An LM317 was used to control the current and ensure a stable flash sequence of each wavelength. It was found that adjustable resistors for each LED are useful for adjusting the light brightness to achieve uniform illumination and avoid overexposure.

1 Introduction

In various applications, spectral imaging is used to identify the composition and structures of organic and inorganic samples or (bio)chemical processes based on the wavelength-dependent light-matter interaction. Such applications include agriculture and food industry, cultural heritage research, remote sensing, biomedical and biological analysis [1]. Depending on the resolution, band quantity, width, and band contiguity, spectral imaging could be called multispectral imaging, hyperspectral imaging or ultraspectral imaging [2]. Multispectral imaging (MSI) is a noninvasive and comprehensive method that has been used recently for clinical outcomes in various medical applications for instance ophthalmology, tissue-wound management, and dermatology [3]. For example, using MSI to facilitate the internal examination of the eye provides information not only about eye-specific diseases but also about general health conditions such as diabetes [4]. Based on spatially resolved spectral data, MSI plays an essential role in obtaining certain anatomical characteristics of the target and has the ability to potentially identify several physiological conditions. MSI techniques make it possible to measure a defined spectrum of each pixel in the image, accordingly, an image cube is acquired which provides not only the spatial but also the spectral information from the observed scene. This is remarkable compared to other methods such as conventional monochrome or RGB color imaging which are unable to differentiate a biological specimen of the target from the background [3]-[4]. Nowadays, a major focus is on mobile diagnostics and telemedicine. For this reason, smartphones in particular have become the center of attention as mobile diagnostic devices. The capability of data transfer, high resolution, cost-effectiveness, and portability, smartphones are considerable advantages in order to use their camera for acquiring the images in medical imaging [5]. One way to generate MSI is to spectrally scan the light source with, for example, narrow band Light Emitting Diodes (LEDs). Over the last few decades, due to considerable advances in LEDs, they are widely utilized as light sources. The availability of many different LEDs, narrow spectral band, durability and cost efficiency as well as low radiant heat are advantages of using them in spectral imaging [6]. In this paper, a spectral light source is presented which enables a fast flash sequence using high power LEDs of different wavelengths. To resolve the spectral images of this sequence, the frame rate of the camera and the light source must be matched. In this project, a smartphone camera is used for spectral reflectance capture. This snapshot-like approach of a fast spectral scanning light source thus combines the advantages of both methods - fast image acquisition with full spatial resolution. Due to the high current of the LEDs, a custom LED driver needed to be developed. The wavelengths are chosen in this project cover the visible and near-infrared light spectrum through 12 wavelengths from 400 nm to 750 nm, which are in the sensitivity range of the smartphone's RGB sensor.

2 Material and Methods

2.1 Selection of LEDs

In the visible light range, many different LEDs are commercially available. Aside from size, availability, brightness, and freedom of design, being the first considerations in selecting LEDs, there were also some clinical considerations in selecting wavelengths. Reference [7] shows all wavelengths from 400 to 500 nm were selected to capture the spectral information of the exterior layers of the retina, especially the inner limiting membrane and nerve fiber layer (NFL) and also the fluorescent retinal components. Wavelengths in the range of 500 and 680 nm were chosen to distinguish between oxygenated and deoxygenated arteries or veins. Reference [8] describes the retinal arterioles become optically less dense compared to the retinal venules at wavelengths greater than 590 nm. Notably, other dominant ocular components such as hemoglobin, lutein, and rhodopsin are also visible when the fundus is illuminated at wavelengths of 450 to 600 nm [7]. Therefore, a series of new high-power LEDs with related wavelengths were chosen to achieve the illumination, offering high design flexibility. The new LUXEON Z Color Line LEDs in micro-footprint were the best choice due to their size for the prototype. Since the LEDs were only offered with dominant wavelengths per data-sheet, careful measurement with a spectrometer was done to measure the peak wavelengths. The miniature spectrometer (RGB Photonics) with a sensitivity of wavelength range from 220 nm up to 1100 nm was used and the observations resulted in the wavelengths listed in table 1. The Two wavelengths 700 nm and 750 nm (SMB1N series from Roithner LASER Technik) were also added, but no micro sizes were available. The printed circuit board (PCB) was designed to fit the optical setup performed in an earlier experiment in the lab. The surface-mounted device (SMD) LEDs with micro footprints were soldered to the PCB in a ring shape. Two different LEDs types and sizes were also mounted in the center of this ring. The fabricated LED ring is shown in Fig. 1 and contains 24 LEDs. Aside from measuring peak wavelengths, all the

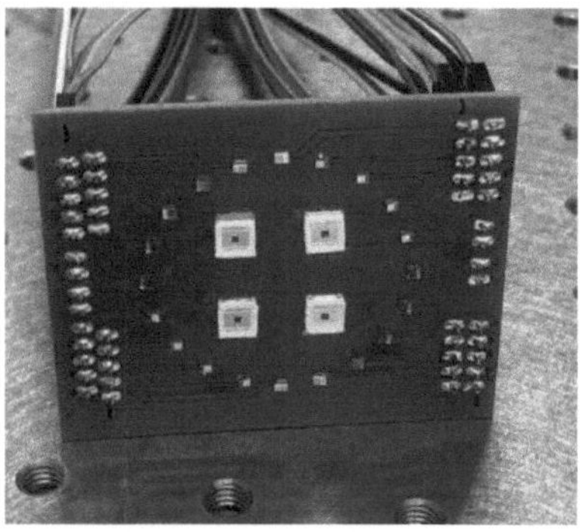

Figure 1: The manufactured PCB with soldered LEDs.

LEDs were tested at maximum current to investigate the predicted wavelength shift at different exposure times. Although the exposure time for this experiment was in the millisecond range, the LEDs were tested at an exposure time of approximately three seconds and also at longer exposure times. The goal in this step was to measure all specifications of the LEDs to compare them with the data-sheet and provide information for the next step. For example, the measured values for forward voltages of LEDs are shown also in Table 1.

Table 1: Comparing the data-sheet and measured wavelengths, also forward voltage values for the LEDs at 600 mA at room temperature (circa 21°C).

Data-sheet Wavelength (nm)	Measured Wavelength (nm)	Forward Voltage (v)
750-770	754.70	3.3
700-740	701.27	3.3
650-670	660.54	2.7
620-645	640.63	2.8
610-620	622.77	2.8
585-590	593.23	2.8
588-592	588.57	2.7
566-569	547.66	3.1
520-540	533.34	3.3
490-510	500.69	3.3
460-484	473.12	3.3
440-460	452.32	3.3

2.2 LED Driver

The electronic circuit of the short pulse illumination control was also designed and developed. The circuit needed to be capable of driving the LEDs at maximum power in short flash sequences. There were many design considerations such as space limitations, cost, performance, type of microcontroller, efficiency, forward voltage, and current of the LEDs. The schematic of the circuit is shown in Fig. 2. A DC-DC converter was used to provide the desired constant voltage for each pair of LEDs in a channel using a 9 v battery. The LM2596 step-down power module which is commercially available was utilized as a DC-DC converter. It was cost-effective and flexible to provide the desired voltage from 1.25 to 37 volts. The DC-DC step-down converter module LM2596 with voltmeter provides the ability to change the voltage during the design to get the maximum power and brightness of the LEDs. The maximum output current is 3 A, which meets the requirement of the LEDs. The output voltage of the DC-DC converter was tested to check the consistency of the voltage. To obtain the expected wavelengths, it is necessary to have a constant and stable current through the LEDs. This is because the current and temperature affect the efficiency of the LEDs. Therefore, the output current of the DC-DC step-down converter module LM2596 was examined with a multi-meter, and it was considered to be stabilized by a precision current limiting circuit with a LM317 working as current regulator. According to the LM317 chip data-sheet, there is a special circuit that works as a current limiter, and the current was adjusted for the load with a resistor calculated with regards to (1).

$$I = 1.25/R. \quad (1)$$

The two LEDs were chosen in parallel to consume an efficient voltage. The N-channel metal-oxide-semiconductor field-effect transistor (MOSFET-IRL2203NPbF) was used as a switch for each channel due to the suitable gain to source voltage for connection to the microcontroller pin, and also the drain current was sufficient for the high current LEDs. The DC-DC converter (LM2596) and current limiting circuit (LM317) were used only once for the whole design as the flash design allows only one channel to be considered during lighting. To control the flash illumination, a microcontroller part is used, which will be explained in more detail in the next section. The microcontroller with 3.6 V input voltage also was supplied by the 9 V battery. The designed schematic was transferred to the breadboard and was connected to the DC-DC board to be power supplied.

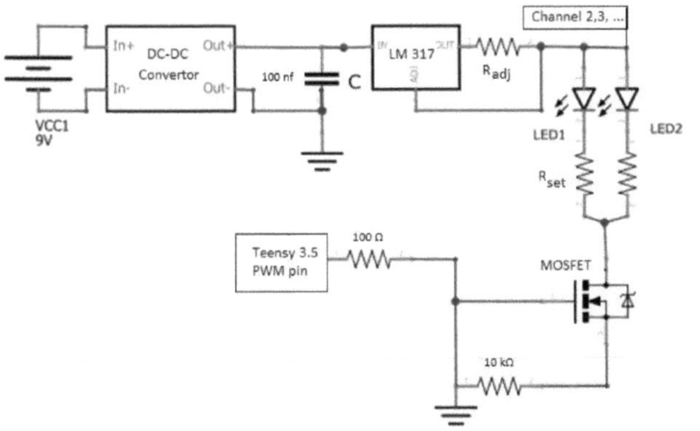

Figure 2: The schematic of the circuit.

2.3 Flash matching with defined frame rate

Fast imaging or fast flash illumination is used to reduce image shift caused by motion artifacts when observing dynamic specimens [4]. Timing the rapid flash succession with the capture rate is critical because it prevents two different colors or wavelengths from being captured in one single shot. For a correct acquisition of the sequential spectral images, the flash sequence has to be timed to basically match the frame rate of the camera. The smartphone camera used in this work is the iPhone11 with a frame rate of 120 fps. Therefore, the frame capture period is around 8.333 ms. To avoid aliasing, the flash time interval for one single wavelength should be larger than one frame duration. This approach allows the camera to capture at least one single shot with one color. To prevent the image from shifting, the LED is switched ON for 12.500 ms and switched OFF for half of a frame or 4.200 ms refers to Fig. 3.

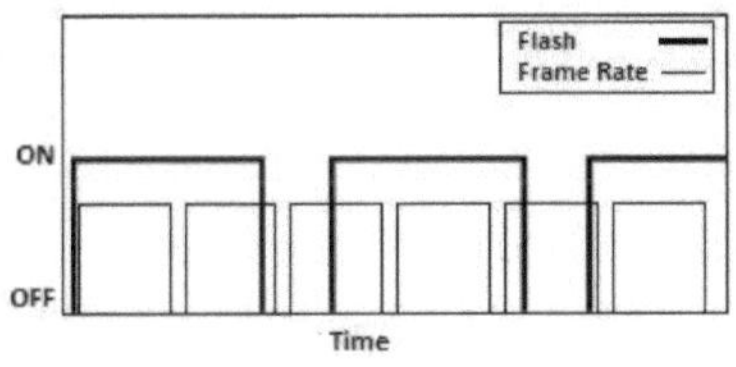

Figure 3: The illustration for matched frame rate with flash illumination.

The Teensy 3.5 microcontroller board (120 MHz ARM Cortex-M4) with 20 pulse width modulation (PWM) pins was programmed to perform the flash illumination of the LEDs. The reason for choosing the Teensy was the sufficient number of PWM pins, the internal clock speed and also the sufficient voltage. The whole flash sequences of all colors were repeated three times.

3 Results and Discussion

The measured normalized intensity of each peak wavelength is shown in Fig. 4. The graph shows the bandwidth of each wavelength and it is obvious that the 547 nm the 588 nm wavelength have a wider bandwidth.

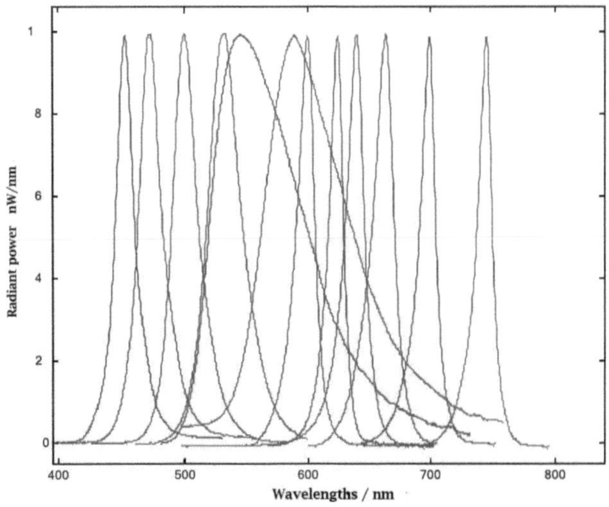

Figure 4: Normalised spectra of the LED wavelengths.

The measured LED spectra at different exposure times in Section 2.1 shows that the peak wavelength of some LEDs hardly changed after four minutes of illumination. For short exposure times such as one second, no shift was observed even at maximum current. In regards to the circuit design, the function of LEDs depends mainly on the current through them. To get the same lighting result from two identical LEDs, one could connect the LEDs in series, due to the magnitude of the voltage, considering the advantages of parallel LEDs, two LEDs in parallel with two separate load resistors can give the same result.

Multispectral imaging of the artificial eye, had been performed at the lab using an optical setup with a different light source in an earlier study. As an initial test to evaluate the function of the light source and the frame rate adjustment, the prototype was tested on the artificial eye. The artificial eye, HEINE Retinoscope Trainer, with a focal distance of 32 mm and pupil sizes of 2, 3, 4, 5, 6, 8 mm, was available in the laboratory. The iPhone11 was used to record a short slow-motion video (1080 pixels at 120 fps) of the artificial eye illuminated by the light source. The pupil size of the artificial eye was set to 8 mm during the test. The best images extracted from the slow-motion video without post-processing are shown in Fig. 5. Notably, the images at the 701 nm and 754 nm wavelengths are dark and of poor quality. According to the data-sheet, nitrogen reflow soldering should be used to fixate these LEDs but this technology was not available in the laboratory. Instead, these LEDs were soldered by hand and it was noted that these solders were smoked. One other possible assumption could be that the sensitivity of the RGB sensor is too low for this wavelength. These wavelengths may have clinical relevance so future work on this project should include research into improving images captured in this spectral range. Testing the light source on the artificial eye will allow for further improvements such as designing the circuit board for the final circuit to optimize the prototype against movement and reduce noise. Moreover, the whole prototype will be handheld and therefore a reduced size and weight of the device is necessary to make the device convenient for the end-user. Additionally, the light hazard protection which is described in ISO 15004-2:2007 for ophthalmic instruments should be considered in the next steps.

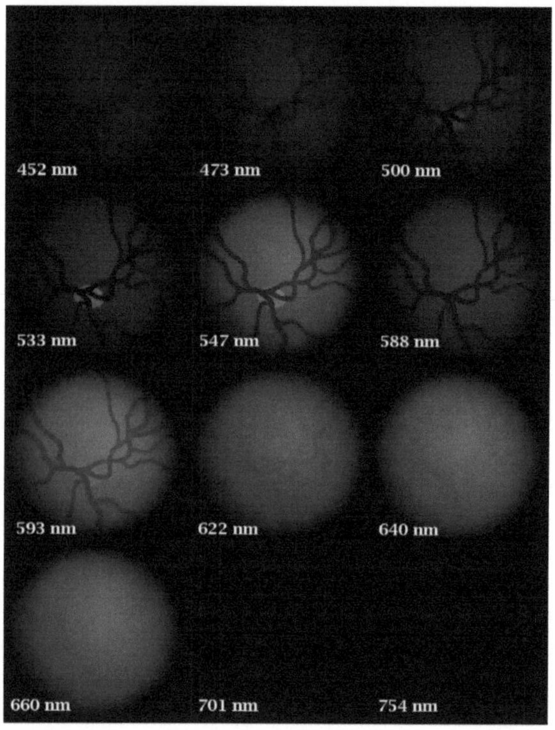

Figure 5: Images of different wavelengths captured by the iPhone using the developed light source.

4 Conclusion

In this paper, a high-power LED-based multispectral flash illumination source with 12 wavelengths was presented. The use of a smartphone to capture spectral data could have many beneficial aspects, such as telemedicine application, data transmission, high-resolution camera, convenience, and availability. A spectrally tunable light source based on high-power LEDs is a promising approach, especially when fast acquisition rates with short integration times are used. The light source could improve the brightness and quality of the images to facilitate post-processing. In further investigations sequencing and timing of image capture could improve the image quality. Images of some wavelengths (622, 640, 660 nm) are overexposed due to the high reflectivity of the artificial eye for these wavelengths. This problem can be solved by decreasing the brightness of LEDs and controlling them separately with a combination of resistor and potentiometer. In that case, the DC-DC convertor could be deleted. Due to the type of spectral imaging the wavelength range could be extended easily and inexpensive.

Acknowledgement

The work has been carried out at Laboratory of Medical Optics and supervised by Professor Dr. rer. nat. Mathias Beyerlein, Technical University of Applied Sciences Luebeck.

Author's Statement

Conflict of interest: Authors state no conflict of interest.

5 References

[1] J. Herrera-Ramírez, M. Vilaseca, and J. Pujol, *Portable multispectral imaging system based on light-emitting diodes for spectral recovery from 370 to 1630 nm*.Appl. Opt., vol. 53, no. 14, p. 3131, 2014.

[2] Q. Li, X. He, Y. Wang, H. Liu, D. Xu, and F. Guo, *Review of spectral imaging technology in biomedical engineering: achievements and challenges,*J. Biomed. Opt., vol. 18, no. 10, p. 100901, 2013.

[3] S. Kim et al, *Smartphone-based multispectral imaging: system development and potential for mobile skin diagnosis*. Biomed. Opt. Express, vol. 7, no. 12, p. 5294, 2016.

[4] N. L. Everdell, I. B. Styles, A. Calcagni, J. Gibson, J. Hebden, and E. Claridge, *Multispectral imaging of the ocular fundus using light emitting diode illumination*. Rev. Sci. Instrum., 2010.

[5] T. N. Kim et al., *A smartphone-based tool for rapid, portable, and automated wide-field retinal imaging*. Transl. Vis. Sci. Technol., 2018.

[6] P. Bartczak, A. Gebejes, P. Falt, J. Parkkinen, and P. Silfstein, *Led-based spectrally tunable light source for camera characterization*. 2015 Colour Vis. Comput. Symp. CVCS 2015, no. August, 2015.

[7] T. Alterini et al, *Fast visible and extended near-infrared multispectral fundus camera*.J. Biomed. Opt., 2019. , doi: 10.1117/1.jbo.24.9.096007.

[8] D. J. Mordant et al., *Spectral imaging of the retina*. Eye, vol. 25, no. 3, pp. 309–320, 2011.

Control of an electrosurgical generator

Niklas Schmid [1], Jelle Dijkstra [2], Hossam Abbas [3] and Philipp Rostalski [3]

[1] Medical Engineering Science, Universität zu Lübeck, niklas.schmid@student.uni-luebeck.de

[2] Olympus Surgical Technologies Europe, jelle.dijkstra@olympus-oste.eu

[3] Institute for Electrical Engineering in Medicine, Universität zu Lübeck, {h.abbas, philipp.rostalski}@uni-luebeck.de

Abstract

Goal of this work is to control the output-voltage of an electrosurgical generator (ESG) such that it follows a predetermined signal-waveform with maximum amplitude without violating power-, voltage- or current-constraints. This is a challenging task since the output-impedance is varying greatly during operation. The underlying ESG-architecture can be approximated by a linear model but suffers from actuators with a bandwidth only one order of magnitude higher than the applied signal frequencies. The performance of the proposed controller was evaluated in simulation and limitations of the design are discussed. The results confirm that the proposed control structure is applicable for the control problem.

1 Introduction

Electrosurgical generators (ESG) are used for cutting and coagulation of tissue by transmitting heat inducing, high-frequency current through the tissue. In some cases the surrounding air and vapor will be ionized by the applied high voltage which leads to sparks between the electrodes and tissue. This mainly happens during monopolar applications and is exploited for contactless surface coagulation but also occurs during cutting modes. The intensity of the sparks correlates with a so called spark-voltage U_{Spark} within the system. The dominating effect on the tissue is determined by the output voltage and spark-intensity as well as the waveform of the applied voltage, which is either a continuous sinewave or pulses of truncated sinewaves down to a single sinewave-period [1].
While the majority of the literature focusses on the control of ESGs based on inverters and purely resistive loads [2], [3], this paper models the output by a more realistic output-impedance in section 2 and deals with the control of another ESG-architecture which allows to derive a linear model. To control the output-voltage of the system a cascaded controller is designed in section 3 and evaluated in a simulation whose results are discussed in section 4.

2 Model of the output-impedance

In order to analyse the system and to evaluate the proposed control structure in simulation, an adequate model for the output needs to be found. While the impedance of many tissue types has been measured and tabulated [4] and good tissue-models using a combination of resistors and constant phase elements exist [5], the tissue impedance may vary greatly depending on the measurement setup [6]. It may be sufficient for this control task to model the tissue as a time-varying resistor R since the reactance of the impedance of the tissue is expected to be low compared its resistance and the reactance of the cables and electrodes at the output of the generator. Thus a simple RLC-circuit as depicted in fig. 1 is used to model the output-load of the generator where the inductance and capacitance are used to model the impedance of the cable and electrodes.

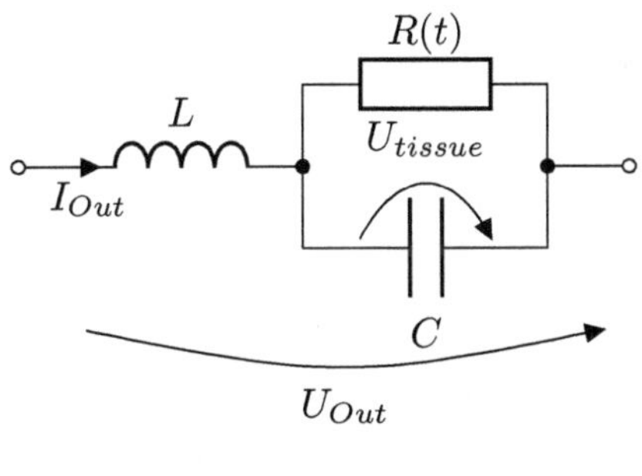

Figure 1: Model of the output load.

The voltage U_{tissue} across the tissue is not easily measurable and the tissue's resistance is unknown and time-varying. While one could use an observer to estimate U_{tissue} it is easier and generally sufficient for the application to control the output-voltage U_{Out} of the generator.
While [7] and [8] describe the electrical characteristics of arcs in arc furnaces, similar measurements have been made by the authors of this work for spark-discharges at the output of an ESG-unit. In order to simulate a load which has the electrical characteristics of spark-discharges, a parametrization for a dead-zone type hysteresis has been designed. The spark-discharge is assumed to be purely resistive and nonlinear. A simple illustration of the model can be found in fig. 2. Once a certain breakthrough-voltage is reached, current starts to flow. The current scales linearly with a further increase of the voltage with a fixed rate of

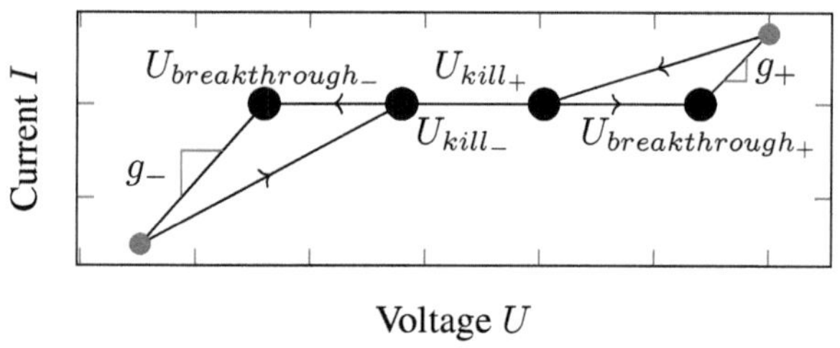

Figure 2: Spark-Model. Only the slopes and the black dots are required to describe the spark-behaviour. To describe a specific measurement also the grey dots are necessary.

$g = \frac{dI}{dU}$ and decreases linearly with the absolute value of the voltage such that it crosses a specific kill-voltage at the current-axis. The overall resistive value R may be calculated as the resistive value of the tissue plus the resistive value of the spark-discharge using Ohm's law.

3 Controller-architecture

Goal of the controller design is to generate a voltage at the output of the ESG-unit which has a predetermined waveform with the highest possible amplitude without violating constraints for the power-, voltage- or current at the output. The controller design is thus splitted into two tasks: First it is ensured that the desired waveform for the output-voltage is generated. In a next step the amplitude of the output-voltage is maximised such that non of the given constraints are violated.

An obvious challenge for controlling the output-voltage of ESG-units arises from the fact that the output-impedance may rapidly change between high and low. For the case of the ESG-unit which is subject of this work the system can be manipulated by an input-voltage which is applied to the ESG-circuit via actuators. These actuators suffer from restrictive saturation-limits and a bandwidth only one order of magnitude higher than the applied signal-frequency. The described actuator and dead-times limit the maximum controllable frequency which complicates the controller-design. Due to critical dead-times, more elaborate nonlinear and thus computationally demanding control methods are not easily applicable.

The proposed control architecture is depicted in fig. 3 and consists of four different control elements. The system is denoted as G, its input- and output-voltages are denoted as u and y respectively. The signal e_{sat} is the difference between the desired and applied input due to actuator-saturation. The variable y_A is calculated as product of the reference-waveform times $\hat{A}$, which is the input-amplitude and adjusted such that $\hat{y}$ converges to $\hat{y}_{ref}$. The actually desired output would be calculated as $\hat{y}_{ref}$ times the reference-waveform. The state-feedback-controller K_{fb} and an adaptive low-pass-filter C_{lp} are used to ensure the generation of a correct waveform with low distortions such that the output y follows the waveform y_A, while their amplitudes may differ. The value of $\hat{y}_{ref}$ is determined by $C_{High-level}$ in such a way that the output voltage amplitude is maximised and no constraints for the spark-voltage, the peak- and rms-voltage and current at the output as well as for the applied power are violated, which can be formulated as the following problem that will be referred to as high-level problem

$$\begin{aligned} \underset{\hat{y}_{ref}}{\text{maximize}} \quad & \hat{y} \\ \text{subject to} \quad & \frac{\gamma_{meas}}{\gamma_{constr}} \leq 1. \end{aligned} \tag{1}$$

where $\gamma \in \{|U_{Spark}|, I_{rms}, U_{rms}, U_{peak}, I_{peak}, P\}$, γ_{meas} is the measured value for variable γ and γ_{constr} is the constraint for variable γ. The input voltage amplitude $\hat{A}$ is determined by $C_{Amplitude}$ such that the output voltage amplitude $\hat{y}$ tracks the reference amplitude $\hat{y}_{ref}$ while taking input saturation into account.

3.1 Control of the waveform

As a first step it is ensured that the output-voltage follows a predetermined waveform using a state-feedback-controller K_{fb} and an adaptive low-pass-filter C_{lp}.

3.1.1 State-feedback-controller

While a state-feedback-controller K_{fb} could not ensure robust reference-tracking due to the actuator's bandwidth, it was possible to use it in order to increase the damping of the system-poles. The high system damping combined with the fact that for ESGs only pulsed or continuous sinewaves need to be generated at the output will be exploited to design a heuristic for an adaptive phase-correction that reduces signal distortions introduced by the system.

3.1.2 Adaptive phase-correction

Depending on the value of the output-resistor R the output-impedance may be dominated by the inductance and capacitance of the cables such that the system's transfer function varies depending on R.

Recall that the desired waveform of the output-voltage either represents a continuous sinusoidal signal or repeated pulses of several sinewave-periods down to a single period. The system's transfer-function may introduce signal-distortions when directly applying the desired waveform as input. Furthermore, this effect may vary depending on R. This may be compensated by a heuristic approach via an adaptive phase-correction. Therefore a second-order low-pass filter $H_{2nd}(s, \omega_p)$ has been used which consists of a critically damped complex pole-pair with a natural frequency ω_p. Depending on the direction of the phase-mismatch, ω_p will be increased or decreased such that the phase of the desired sinewave will be corrected. Fig. 4 is an example for the correction effect where ω_p is decreased to further decrease the phase of the sinewave thus correcting the waveform. Note that C_{lp} will not be used for continuous sinewave signals since, assuming a critically damped, linear and stable system and a continuous sinewave as input, the system output will, in certain cases, oscillate with

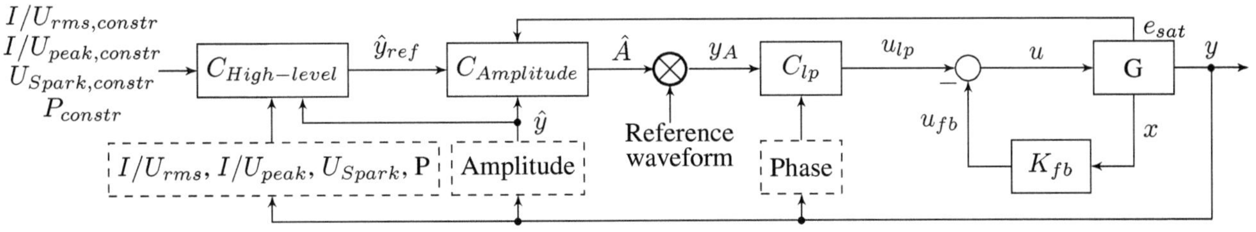

Figure 3: Proposed control structure. The system G is controlled by the controllers $C_{High-level}$, $C_{Amplitude}$, C_{lp} and K_{fb}. The dashed boxes calculate the phase-shift, rms- and peak values of the output-voltage y as well as the rms- and peak-current, the spark-voltage and the output-power for the respective controllers.

the input-frequency and the applied phase of the system will only result in a time-shift which is irrelevant for the given control problem.
To compensate changes in the signal-amplitude at the underlying frequency of the sinewave of the waveform-reference $\omega_{carrier}$ when changing ω_p the output is normalized to $|H_{2nd}(j\omega_{carrier}, \omega_p)|$. The frequency $\omega_p = \omega_p(t)$ is used to adapt the amount of the introduced phase.
Whether the phase needs to be increased or decreased may be determined by comparing the peak-heights of the first and second peak A_1 and A_2 of the sinewave that is seen at the output. The phase is assumed to be correct if A_1 equals A_2. The algorithm 1 presents a heuristic for an adaptive phase-correction along with a calculation of an error signal that is not dependent on the signal-amplitude including. The gain k_{lp} may be used as tuning-variable.

Algorithm 1: Adaptive phase-correction

$x_{\omega_p} = 0$;
while *true* **do**
  if *pulse over* **then**

$$e_{lp}(A_1, A_2) = \begin{cases} \frac{A_1}{A_2} - 1 & \text{if } A_1 \geq A_2 \\ 1 - \frac{A_2}{A_1} & \text{if } A_1 < A_2 \end{cases};$$

$x_{\omega_p} = x_{\omega_p} + k_{lp} e_{lp}$;
$\omega_p = exp(x_{\omega_p})$;
$C_{lp}(s, \omega_p, \omega_{carrier}) = \frac{H_{2nd}(s,\omega_p)}{|H_{2nd}(j\omega_{carrier},\omega_p)|}$;
  else
    detect the first two peaks A_1, A_2 of y
  end
end

3.2 Control of high-level constraints

So far, only the generation of a correct waveform has been considered while neglecting the signal amplitude. In order to solve the proposed high-level problem given in 1 two additional feedback-controllers are used.

3.2.1 Amplitude controller

In order to track a specific reference signal-amplitude $\hat{y}_{ref}$ an additional amplitude-controller in the form of an integral-controller is added. In case the actuator saturates the absolute difference between the desired and applied output e_{sat} is used in an antiwindup manner for the controller's integrator leading to

$$\Delta\hat{A} = k_{amp}(\hat{y}_{ref} - \hat{y}) - k_{sat} e_{sat} \tag{2}$$

where $k_{amp} \in \mathbb{R}$ and $k_{sat} \in \mathbb{R}$ are tuning-gains and $\hat{y}$ is the measured signal-amplitude. All i calculated values for $\Delta\hat{A}$ are accumulated leading to the input-signal amplitude $\hat{A} = \sum_i \Delta\hat{A}_i$. The reference-signal y_A is generated by scaling the signal of the waveform-generator with $\hat{A}$. An additional low pass filter suppresses undesired, high frequencies introduced by truncated sinewave-signals.

3.2.2 High-level controller

Let $i \in \{U_{Spark}, I_{rms}, U_{rms}, U_{peak}, I_{peak}, P\}$, $y_{meas,i}$ be the measured value for variable i and $y_{constr,i}$ be the constraint-value for variable i.
The reference amplitude $\hat{y}_{ref}$ is determined by a final control loop in order to solve the proposed high-level problem. One may calculate individual error-signals for each constraint as

$$e_i = \frac{y_{constr,i} - y_{meas,i}}{y_{constr,i}} \tag{3}$$

while the overall error-signal is calculated as

$$e_{hl} = min(e_{U_{Spark}}, e_{I_{rms}}, e_{U_{rms}}, e_{U_{peak}},, e_{I_{peak}}, e_P). \tag{4}$$

The minimal value of all normalized error signals will then be used for an integral controller. In case the reference amplitude is larger then the measured signal amplitude $\hat{y}$ times some predetermined factor α the reference amplitude is only allowed to decrease leading to

$$\Delta\hat{y}_{ref}(\alpha) = \begin{cases} k_{hl} e_{hl} & \text{if } \hat{y}_{ref} \leq \alpha\hat{y} \text{ or } e_{hl} \leq 0 \\ 0 & \text{otherwise.} \end{cases} \tag{5}$$

where $k_{hl} \in \mathbb{R}$ is a tuning-gain. The second case is useful to prevent the reference amplitude from increasing when the system's actuator saturates and the signal amplitude can not further be increased. All i calculated values for $\Delta\hat{y}_{ref}(\alpha)$ are accumulated leading to $\hat{y}_{ref}(\alpha) = \sum_i \Delta\hat{y}_{ref,i}(\alpha)$.

4 Results and Discussion

The proposed control structure was evaluated in simulation. It was possible to ensure reference-tracking of commonly used waveforms and solve the proposed high-level problem for arbitrary output-loads and such with spark-like dynamics. As an example, a load with spark-like characteristics and a waveform with repeated pulses of single sinewave-periods has been chosen. The waveform-correction due to a phase-correction can be seen within a few periods in fig. 4. Fig. 5 shows the convergence of the error values of $C_{high-level}$.

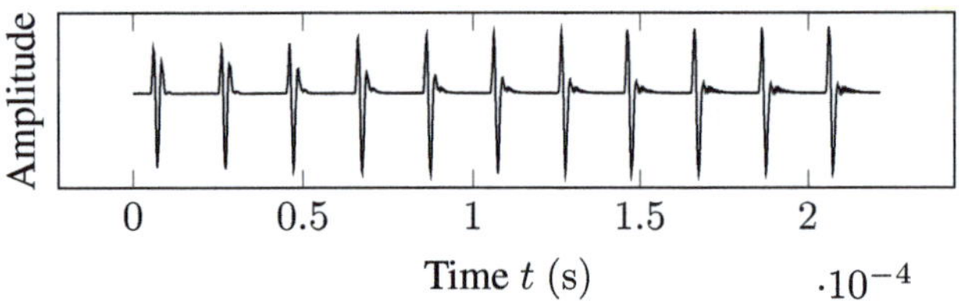

Figure 4: Correction of the waveform by the phase-correction method. An output-impedance with spark-like characteristics and pulses of single sinewave-periods have been chosen.

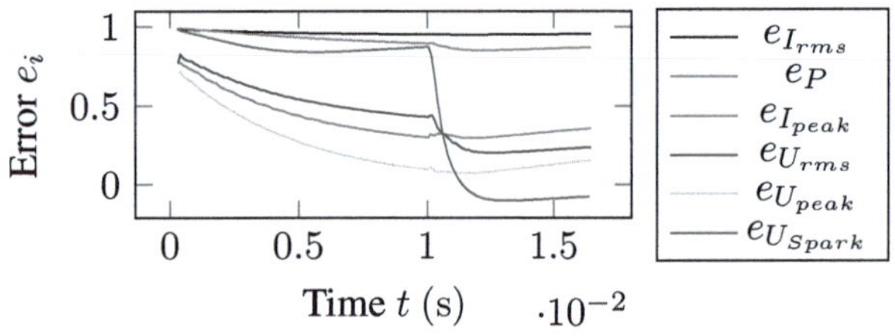

Figure 5: Convergence of high-level control variables. The output impedance changes at $t = 0.01$ s. The second output-impedance enforces a higher spark-voltage. In this case, first $e_{U_{peak}}$, then $e_{U_{Spark}}$ yields the lowest error value.

The topology to be controlled does not exist in practice, yet. Therefore, no experimental data exists and comparisons with classical designs still have to been done.

Special care has to be taken for C_{lp}. The amplitude of u_{lp} tends to increase with low values for ω_p and for low frequencies and may exceed the saturation limits of the system's actuator. Furthermore, this control architecture can only be used to control sinusoidal signals comparable to such used for ESGs and an adequate transfer-function for C_{lp} has to be found. Ensuring reference-tracking via feedback-control may be superior whenever applicable. However, using a heuristic for an adaptive phase-correction helped to circumvent feedback-control limitations due to a band limited and saturating actuator.

Continued research on nonlinear and adaptive controller-designs may lead to an applicable solution with a control law which is simple and robust enough to ensure faster reference-tracking of the waveform.

5 Conclusion

A method has been proposed to control an ESG while tracking high-level constraints as well as generating a predefined waveform. It consists of a cascaded controller with several feedback-loops and a heuristic for an adaptive phase-correction. The performance of the proposed control-architecture has been evaluated in simulation and its applicability has been verified.

Acknowledgement

The work has been carried out at Olympus Surgical Technologies Europe and supervised by the Institute for Electrical Engineering in Medicine, Universität zu Lübeck.

Author's Statement

Conflict of interest: Authors state no conflict of interest.

6 References

[1] B. Hug, R. Haag „Hochfrequenzchirurgie“ in *Medizintechnik - Verfahren - Systeme - Informationsverarbeitung*, vol. 3, R. Kramme, ch. 28, pp. 518-541, 2007.

[2] S. Fahad, N. Ullah, A.J. Mahdi, *A new robust closed-loop control system for electrosurgical generators*. Research on Biomedical Engineering, vol 36, pp. 213-224, 2020.

[3] M.M. Rafiq, M. Ishfaq, M. Ali, A. Ibeas, J. Herrera, N. Ullah (2019). *A closed loop robust control system for electrosurgical generators*. Control Applications for Biomedical Engineering Systems, pp. 466, 2019.

[4] C. Gabriel, S. Gabriel, E. Corthout *Compilation of the Dielectric Properties of Body Tissues at RF and Microwave Frequencies*, 1996.

[5] T. K. Bera, J.Nagaraju. *Electrical Impedance Spectroscopic Studies on Broiler Chicken Tissue Suitable for the Development of Practical Phantoms in Multifrequency EIT*, Journal of Electrical Bioimpedance, vol. 2(1), 48-63, 2011.

[6] D. Miklavcic, N. Pavselj, F.X. Hart. *Electric Properties of Tissues*. In Wiley Encyclopedia of Biomedical Engineering, M. Akay (Ed.), 2006.

[7] H. Schnack, *Schnelle Stromregelung von Drehstrom-Lichtbogenöfen mit Halbleiter-Stufenschaltern*, Ph.D. dissertation, Department of Mechanical Engineering, Helmut-Schmidt-Universität / Universität der Bundeswehr Hamburg, Hamburg, 2016.

[8] A. Novitskiy. *Elektromagnetische Verträglichkeit und Blindleistungskompensation in Elektrostahlwerksnetzen*, 2007.

LTE Measurements Using a Cellular-Connected Drone

Ann-Catrin Schurig [1], and Jonas Gruner [2]

[1] Medical Engineering Science, Universität zu Lübeck, anncatrin.schurig@student.uni-luebeck.de
[2] Institute for Electrical Engineering in Medicine, Universität zu Lübeck, j.gruner@uni-luebeck.de

Abstract

Drones can be used to provide a reliable data link over the cellular network during rescue operations. For this purpose, mobile radio parameters and influences on them have to be investigated. In this work, the spatial dependence of the cellular link's measured signal strength is investigated. For the analysis, several measurement flights were conducted using a drone and a smartphone to collect telemetry and cellular data. For this purpose, the drone flew identical routes in different locations at different altitudes. These data sets were revised, synchronized and analyzed. The study shows that altitude is a relevant factor for the strength of the received signal.

1 Introduction

When it comes to a rescue operation, rescue workers at the scene are cut off from the flow of information when caring for patients and cannot claim assistance. On the hospital side, preparatory measures are taken without specific knowledge about the patient. MOMENTUM stands for "Mobile Medizintechnik für integrierte Notfallversorgung und Unfallmedizin" [1] and is a national research project. The project deals with the problem of optimal communication along the rescue chain with the aim of improving it. One subtask of this project is to find a suitable concept for drones to extend the radio range of ambulances via the mobile network, thus securing communication channels. The use of drones has the advantage of being able to fly over obstacles or fly around them when ground reception is poor, allowing them to reach an area with better connectivity. For reliable data transmission to be possible, the drone must autonomously find the location with the optimal signal when the signal strength on the ground is not sufficient for a good connection. In order for the drone to automatically find the area with the best reception, an analysis of the spatial properties of performance indicators in cellular networks is essential. There already works that use drones to measure cellular network performance [2]. However, most of the works consider the challenges of cellular connected drones at altitudes above 50 m. For the use of drones in rescue operations values of the mobile radio parameters in the immediate vicinity of the rescue vehicle are of interest. Therefore, it is necessary to study the location- and altitude-dependent relationship to exclude areas with poor connectivity and identify those with good reception. Knowing how signal strength changes with relation to altitude and location is important, and new data is also needed to have a basis for training models for autonomous positioning of the drone as the project progresses. From this aspect, measurement flights were carried out with a drone at different heights and locations, during which mobile radio parameters were measured by a cell phone to identify changes in signal strength. Basic knowledge about the mobile radio parameters and the measurement setup is explained in section 2. In section 3 the measurement results are presented, interpreted and discussed. The paper concludes with section 4.

2 Material and Methods

2.1 LTE performance parameters

LTE is a cellular technology and stands for Long Term Evolution. There are several LTE performance parameters like the reference signal received power (RSRP), the received signal strength indicator (RSSI), the reference signal received quality (RSRQ) and the signal-to-interference plus noise ratio (SINR). The RSRP value indicates for the signal strength and is measured directly by the user equipment. With the help of the RSRP parameter, different transmission cells can be compared and decisions about the data transmission can be made based on the result [3]. RSSI is an indicator of the total reception performance of all sources, including signals from neighboring cells, background noises and interference [3]. RSRQ is calculated from the ratio of RSRP and RSSI [4]. The SINR is defined as the ratio of the received average signal to the sum of the interference and the noise [4]. The RSRP and RSRQ values are mainly used to determine the ranking between different neighboring cells according to their signal strength and signal quality. If the values of the parameters of the serving source fall below the values of the neighboring cell over a certain period of time, a handover occurs. The RSRP parameter alone is not sufficient to determine the signal quality, but the RSRP allows for a rough, performance assessment of whether LTE reception is possible in principle [3]. E. Eyceyurt et al. studied the uplink throughput prediction in cellular mobile networks with the result that the RSRP value is the most influential factor for predicting algorithms [5]. For these reasons, the focus of this work is on the study and evaluation of the measured RSRP values.

2.2 Measurement procedure

The German Drone Regulation contains instructions and rules for the use of unmanned area vehicles. The regulations in force at the time of the measurements state that there is a general ban on flying over sensitive places such as residential properties, hospitals, crowds and natural reserves. Similarly, drones may generally only be flown within sight and below an altitude of 100 meters. An exception exists for model airfields, where they are allowed to fly higher [6]. Therefore, the selection of suitable airfields is limited. The flight missions were carried out in two different locations. One place is a sports field closer to the city, and the other is more than six kilometers from the city center on the edge of an industrial area, a ground of a model flying club. For data acquisition, measurement flights were carried out with the Mavic Air drone from DJI, a small and stable flying drone. The commercially available drones do not match the requirements for measuring mobile network parameters. Therefore, the Unihertz Jelly Pro, a small LTE smartphone, was attached to the underside of the drone. NetMonitor Pro is an app installed on the Jelly Pro that can measure LTE performance parameters and save them to a file. Litchi is an alternative app to control the Mavic Air drone. With the Litchi app it is possible to plan the flight routes via a browser on the computer with a graphical interface and import the missions to the smartphone app for execution. A completed mission results in two data sets: one with the LTE performance parameters and one with the telemetry data of the drone. In order to continue working with this data, data processing must be carried out to delete incorrect and irrelevant data sets. After the data has been filtered and processed, the two data sets are synchronized via a timestamp.

2.3 Flight routes

The drone must not unnecessarily hinder the rescue operation by its flight and should be connected to the ambulance via a cable in the future final model. Therefore, it is important to investigate the changes in the mobilfunk parameters in the immediate vicinity of the ambulance. Various flight routes were planned to determine the differences in signal strength as a function of altitude and location. The drone flew identical routes with the same latitude and longitude, but at different altitudes. On the grounds outside the city, the drone flew at heights of 2 m and 15 m, and on the sports field at heights of 2 m and 12 m. To investigate the altitude dependency in more detail, flights were done where the drone flew 50 m up and down at a fixed local point at the model airfield. The LTE antenna was pointed in the direction of the next waypoint.

3 Results and Discussion

3.1 Results

In order to decide whether the height-dependent and not the location-dependent differences should be investigated more closely, both results were first examined. Fig. 1 shows the location-dependent linear interpolation of the RSRP values of a 2 m high measurement on the model airfield.

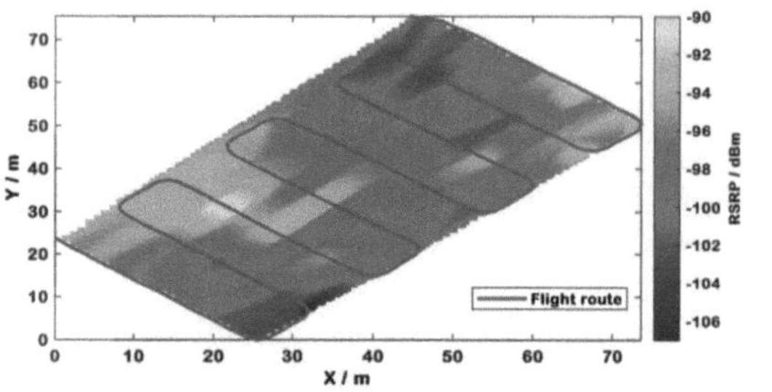

Figure 1: Location-dependent linear interpolation of the RSRP values of a measurement at 2 m height on the model airfield. The origin is the point of the minimum.

Table 1 shows mean values and standard deviation of the missions at the model airfield where the drone flew the same routes at different altitudes. The RSRP values of the flight missions at a height of 2 m are on average -102.71 dBm with a standard deviation of 3.2 dBm. According to [7], this area has a weak signal in terms of reception strength. The values of the measurements at a height of 15 m are in a range with good connection with an average of -83.75 dBm with a standard deviation of 2.5 dBm. The standard deviation values of the 2 m measurements are more widely scattered than those of the 15 m measurements. The mean values and the standard deviation of the measurements from the sports field where the drone flew the same routes at different altitudes are also shown in Table 1. The RSRP values of the 2 m measurements are -88.63 dBm on average with a standard deviation of 3.3 dBm, while those of the 12 m measurements are -84.53 dBm with 3.5 dBm. According to the definition in [7], the mean values of the individual measurements are all within the range of good signal strength. Thus, based on this height difference, only a small difference in signal strength can be determined. The standard deviation values are more spread around the mean and vary in both measured heights if compared to those from the model airfield. Fig. 2 shows the distribution of the RSRP measurement points from missions at 2 m and 15 m at the model airfield and at 2 m and 12 m at the sports field. For both measurements, a difference in signal strength as a function of altitude can be seen. The difference in altitude for measurements at the model airfield has more influence. There is also a recognizable difference when comparing the 2 m measurements at the two different locations. Likewise, it shows the distribution around the mean values. The stan-

Table 1: RSRP mean values (MV) in dBm and standard deviation (STD) in dBm for the flights at the model airfield (Route 1 to 5) and at the sports field (Route 6 to 9)

Route	MV 2 m	STD 2 m	MV 15 m	STD 15 m
1	-97.76	3.5	-80.64	1.4
2	-106.96	1.8	-84.66	1.8
3	-99.55	3.9	-83.39	2.9
4	-106.16	2.5	-85.85	2.8
5	-103.11	4.3	-84.20	3.2
	MV 2 m	STD 2 m	MV 12 m	STD 12 m
6	-91.60	2.9	-84.47	3.8
7	-80.03	4.6	-84.87	2.5
8	-90.67	3.1	-83.97	3.1
9	-92.21	2.5	-84.82	4.8

dard deviation of the measuring points at 15 m height is less scattered than in the other three measurements.

Fig. 3 shows the RSRP values in relation to altitude for flights up to 50 m height. It is obvious that the change in altitude affects the strength of the received signal. The results of the flights at 50 m show that the RSRP value increases to its maximum of -85 dBm for measurement 1 and -83 dBm for measurement 2 at a height of about 14.5 m, and decreases again further up to 50 m. Between 10 m and 50 m, all ranges are within the boundary between good and sufficient signal strength for a stable connection to the core network. For measurement 1 the mean value is -89.34 dBm and the standard deviation is 2.4 dBm and for measurement 2 it is -86.82 dBm and 2.1 dBm.

The average distance to the active cellular tower is 1358 m at the model airfield and 2500 m at the sports field.

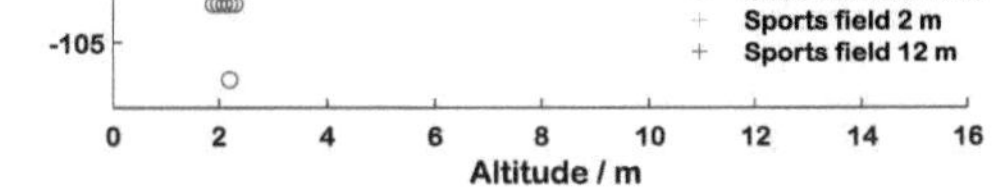

Figure 2: RSRP values in relation to altitude from measurements at the model airfield with the same route at 2 m and 15 m altitude and at the sports field with the same route at 2 m and 12 m.

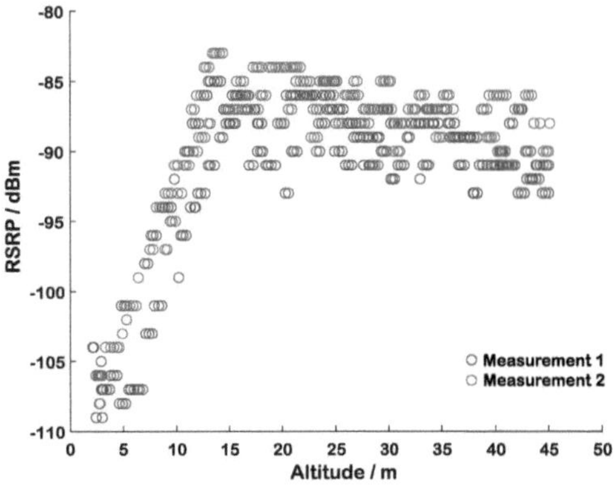

Figure 3: RSRP values in relation to altitude from measurements at the model airfield where the drone flew up and down 50 m with fixed local coordinates.

3.2 Discussion

The measurements indicate that the received signal strength is more dependent on height than on location. Fig. 1 shows a rather negligible difference in the dependence of the signal strength. The measurements at higher altitudes achieved higher values at both measurement locations. A probable reason for this could be the line of sight between the end device and the base station. The closer the device gets to the ground, the more obstacles tend to prevent a direct line-of-sight [8]. The distance and the alignment of the LTE antenna to the cellular tower can also influence the strength of the connection. Just a few meters after transmission, the field strength of the radiated wave decreases drastically due to signal attenuation [8]. However, a cellular tower covers an area of several kilometers, so the fluctuations in the values seem to be location-dependent and cannot be justified by the linear decrease in the strength of the signal with greater distance from the tower. Similarly, it is possible that the location of the measurement might affect the signal strength. The signal strength at the measurement location in the city center is in an acceptable range for all measurements, while the value at the model airfield is only in a good range at a height of 15 m. The reflection and absorption by buildings and other obstacles or simply signal attenuation, could explain the different results. The standard deviations of the measurements on the sports field are equally wide scattered. A denser and more developed network in the urban area also causes more interference from neighboring cells and the user equipment has more cellular towers available for switching when the mobile radio parameters are poor. The course of the RSRP values in the flights high to 50 m can also be explained by the attenuation of the signal and that in this case the strongest signal is present at an altitude of about 14 m, since the path of the waves seems to be the most direct there. Possibly this is a threshold from which the RSRP decreases steadily due to signal attenuation since the distance to the cell tower is increased with the altitude. To prove this, further measurements have to be performed, where the drone would fly much higher. Other possible causes could be that radio signals from other stations on the same frequency influence the signal as an interferer, and the orientation of the antenna or the number of subscribers at the same time can weaken it. Weather conditions as e.g. rain, heavy snowfall or fog can significantly affect the propagation of waves [8]. The influences of time and day of the week should be investigated to examine variations due to the number of users. In the case of the model airfield, it can be assumed that there is poorer connectivity due to company employees on weekdays and that better values could be measured on weekends. This assumption could be investigated and confirmed by performing the same flights at different times on each day of the week. Measurements of the 50 m altitude flights at many different locations could give further perspective in terms of changes in the value. In addition, further measurements should be made with revised equipment, as a more sensitive antenna may provide more accurate results. To enable exclusion of elevation areas that have a high probability of poor connectivity, the sample needs to be increased with constant test sizes. When analyzing the new data, influences of the confounding factors could be considered and investigated. By increasing the size of the sample, the result could be repeatable and therefore reproducible.

4 Conclusion

This work shows that there are tendencies in signal strength that depend on the height of the user equipment and the location of the measurement. In particular, the altitude difference shows a relevant influence on the strength of the RSRP value. For the use of drones for signal propagation, other parameters need to be investigated and facts need to be obtained from the conjectures. To investigate the influence of the orientation of the antenna to the cellular tower on the changes in signal strength, further flights with a grid route at different heights are already planned. When analyzing the data, it is possible to define the boundary between areas with good and insufficient and, on this basis, to declare an area between two heights where there could be a permanently good, stable signal for the cellular connection. For MOMENTUM, in addition to the influence of the altitude on the signal strength, the differences of the location-dependent measurements in comparison of the urban to rural area are also important. The drone is to be used in an emergency service operation to establish a secure and uninterrupted connection. This is especially necessary if the reception in the area of the ambulance would not be sufficient for a stable connection. In well-connected areas such as city centers, the drone may not need to be used. In rural areas, where a poorer connection is to be expected in comparison, the drone can reach areas with good and stable connection by ascending. With a good reliable connection, emergency workers can request telemedicine support. 5G is the latest development in mobile technology and is expected to provide increased speed and real-time communication, which is very important for the use of telemedicine. Measurements of parameters in the 5G network could therefore provide interesting results. Since the frequencies used for 5G waves are higher, stronger signal attenuation is to be expected, as radio waves are also more attenuated with increasing frequency.

Acknowledgement

The work has been carried out at Institut for Medical Electrical Engineering, Universität zu Lübeck.

Author's Statement

Research funding: The work was funded by the German Federal Ministry of Education and Research under grant no. 16KIS1027.
Conflict of interest: Authors state no conflict of interest.

5 References

[1] Bundesministerium für Bildung und Forschung, (2019), *Mobile Medizintechnik für die integrierte Notfallversorgung und Unfallmedizin.* Available: https://www.forschung-it-sicherheit-kommunikationssysteme.de/projekte/momentum [last accessed on 2021-01-21].

[2] A. A. Khuwaja, Y. Chen, N. Zhao, M.-S. Alouini and P. Dobbins, *A survey of channel modeling for UAV communications.* In: IEEE Communications Surveys and Tutorials, 2018.

[3] F. Afroz, R. Subramanian, R. Heidary, K. Sandrasegaran and S. Ahmed, *SINR, RSRP, RSSI and RSRQ measurements in long term evolution networks.* In: International Journal of Wireless & Mobile Networks , Vol. 7, No. 4 , pp. 113–123, 2015.

[4] A. R. Mishra, *Fundamentals of network planning and optimisation.* John Wiley & Sons, Ltd, pp. 255, 2018.

[5] E. Eyceyurt, and J. Zec, *Uplink throughput prediction in cellular mobile networks.* In: International Journal of Electronics and Communication Engineering, Vol. 14, No. 6, pp. 149–153, 2020.

[6] Bundesministerium für Verkehr und digitale Infrastruktur (BMVI), (2020), *Drohnen - die wichtigsten Regeln im Überblick.* Available: https://www.bmvi.de/SharedDocs/DE/Publikationen/LF/flyer-die-neue-drohnen-verordnung.pdf?__blob=publicationFile [last accessed on 2021-01-25].

[7] D. Rosigkeit, S. V. Baumgartner and A. Nottensteiner, *Usabilty of long term evolution (LTE) in DLR's research aircraft DO 228-212.* In: 2015 German Microwave Conference, 2015.

[8] LTE Anbieter Info, *Einflussfaktoren auf den LTE-Empfang.* Available: https://www.lte-anbieter.info/ratgeber/faktoren-fuer-empfang.php [last accessed on 2021-01-21].

MSP430: Realization of an interface converter from SPI to 1-wire – Integration of an EEPROM on a medical sensor's PCB –

Joshua Kirsch [1],
[1] Medical Engineering Science, Universität zu Lübeck, joshua.kirsch@student.uni-luebeck.de

Abstract

This paper deals with the implementation of an interface converter from SPI to 1-Wire on the PCB of a medical sensor. It is introduced as part of the planned integration of an EEPROM DS2431 on the PCB of the sensor. While the DS2431 communicates via 1-wire, the remaining electronics of PCB communicate via SPI. The interface converter was realized with a microcontroller of the MSP430FR2xx family, which receives data as a SPI signal and forwards the 1-wire translation of the data to the EEPROM and vice versa. A STM32-Nucleo-F103RB microcontroller board is used to simulate the signals of the sensor's device and to generate the SPI signal. The implementation of the interface converter was successful.

1 Introduction

During the development of the PCB of a medical sensor, a new EEPROM module is to be integrated. The selected chip DS2431 communicates with the master via a 1-Wire interface [1]. However, the bus system of the PCB of the medical sensor communicates via a SPI protocol. For the integration of the EEPROM it is therefore necessary to realize an interface converter from SPI to 1-Wire. For this function, a microcontroller of the MSP430FR2xx [2] family was selected and integrated into the PCB together with the EEPROM. It serves the task of translating the SPI data into 1-Wire data packages. For testing purposes, a simulation of the signals of the medical devices, where the sensor is used, must be ensured. This is implemented by a STM32-Nucleo-F103RB, which enables communication with the MSP430 via SPI and with a GUI on a PC via UART [3].

2 Material and Methods

2.1 Setup

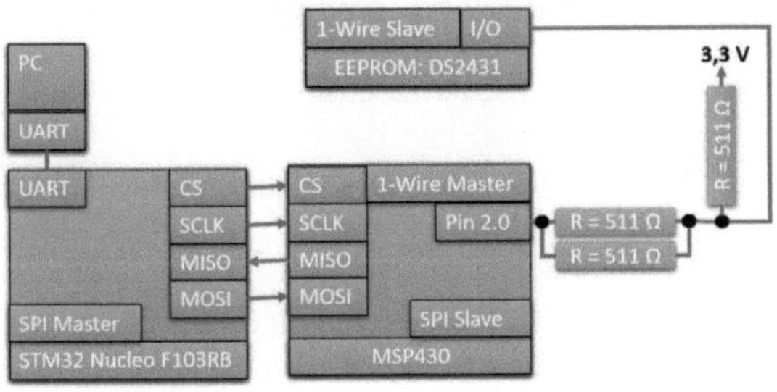

Figure 1: Wiring of the devices.

As it is shown in Fig. 1 the PC sends data via UART to the STM32 Nucelo F103RB, which serves as the SPI master. It sends commands to access the memory of the DS2431 with associated data to be written via SPI to the MSP430, which acts as a SPI slave and translates the SPI data as a 1-Wire master and forwards it to the 1-Wire slave DS2431.

2.2 MSP430

2.2.1 SPI

SPI is a bus system that has four lines. The data transfer between master and slave is synchronized by a clock signal. The three common lines to which each participant is connected are: SCLK (Serial Clock), which is generated by the master for synchronization, MOSI (Master Output, Slave Input) and MISO (Master Input, Slave Output) [4].

Table 1: MSP430: Relevant Registers for the 1-Wire interface. *if Pin x is Output, **if Pin x is Input [2].

Name	Access	Bit = 1	Bit = 0
P2DIR	R/W	Pin is Output	Pin is Input
P2IN	R	Input is HIGH	Input is LOW
P2REN	R/W	Internal R enabled	Internal R disabled
P2OUT*	R/W	Output HIGH	Output LOW
P2OUT**	R/W	Pullup selected	Pulldown selected

Table 2: MSP430: Relevant Registers for the SPI interface. *Flag is set if ... [2].

Name	Description
UCB0TXBUF	Holds data waiting to be sent.
UCB0RXBUF	Contains the last received character.
UCB0IFG	Contains UCRXIFG and UCTXIFG.
UCRXIFG	*UCB0RXBUF has received a complete character.
UCTXIFG	*UCB0TXBUF is empty.
UCB0STAT	Contains the flag UCBUSY.
UCBUSY	*there is an ongoing transmit or receive operation.

2.3 STM32 Nucleo F103RB

The STM32 Nucelo F103RB microcontroller board acts as the SPI master. It sends an array to the MSP430, which is structured like it is shown in Table 3. Index 0 shows whether data should be written to or being read out from the target address on index 1. The size of the data can be found at index 2, followed by an error-flag and the data to be written to the DS2431. 128 is the maximum of number of bytes per page in the EEPROM [1], which is why the array can include a maximum of 132 bytes.

Table 3: Structure of the data array sent by the F103RB.

Index	0	1	2	3	4:131
Description	R/W?	Address	Size	Success?	Data

2.4 EEPROM - DS2431

The DS2431 is a 1024-bit, 1-Wire EEPROM organized as four memory pages of 256/bits each. The communication follows the 1-Wire protocol. In addition to the main memory, an 8-byte volatile scratchpad is included [1].

2.4.1 1-Wire

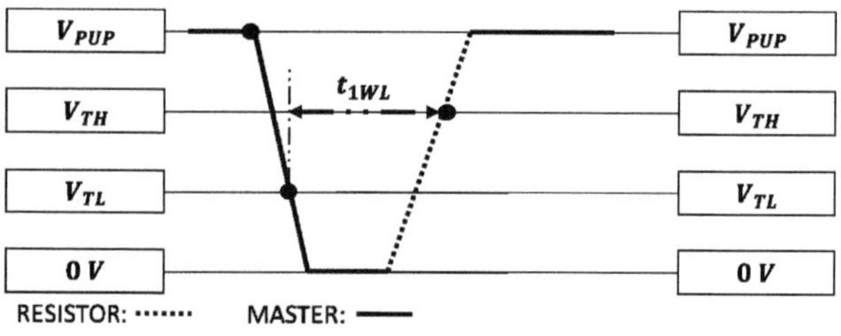

Figure 2: Example: 1-Wire write "1" operation [1]. For values of timings and voltages see Table 4.

Unlike most bus systems, the 1-Wire interface has only one data line and must therefore synchronize the transfer of the data without a clock signal [5]. This is realized with defined time slots, in which the voltage of the data line can be pulled down by the master or the slave for fixed time slots. Hence the timing and sequence of the signals are important. The voltage in Fig. 2 is pulled down from the stable state V_{PUP} (see Table 4) by the MSP430 to 0 V. It crosses the high-to-low-switching threshold voltage V_{TL} (see Table 4) and the time measurement of the slave begins. After e.g., 5 µs the master releases the line, and the voltage rises to pullup voltage V_{PUP}. It crosses the low-to-high-switching threshold voltage V_{TH} (see Table 4) and the time measurement of the slave ends. If the time measurement result is between 1 and 15 µs, the slave knows that a "1" should be written [1] (see Table 4).

Table 4: DS2431: Voltages and Relevant Timings [1].

Name	Sym.	Min	Max	Unit
1-Wire Pullup Voltage	V_{PUP}	3,0	5,25	V
High-To-Low-Switching Thres.	V_{TL}	Typ.:	$V_{0,65*V_{PUP}}$	V
Low-To-High-Switching Thres.	V_{TH}	Typ.:	$V_{0,75*V_{PUP}}$	V
1-Wire Pullup Resistance	R_{PUP}	300	2200	Ω
Reset Low Time	t_{RSTL}	480	640	µs
Presence Detect High Time	t_{PDH}	15	60	µs
Presence Detect Low Time	t_{PDL}	60	240	µs
Presence Detect Sample Time	t_{MSP}	60	75	µs
Write-Zero Low Time	t_{W0L}	60	120	µs
Write-One Low Time	t_{W1L}	1	15	µs
Read Low Time	t_{RL}	5	15- δ	µs
Read Sample Time	t_{MSR}-δ	5	15	µs
Programming Time	t_{PROG}		12	ms
Recovery Time	t_{REC}	5		µs
Time Slot Duration	t_{SLOT}	65		µs

3 Results and Discussion

3.1 Software on the MSP430

3.1.1 SPI interface: MSP430 to F103RB

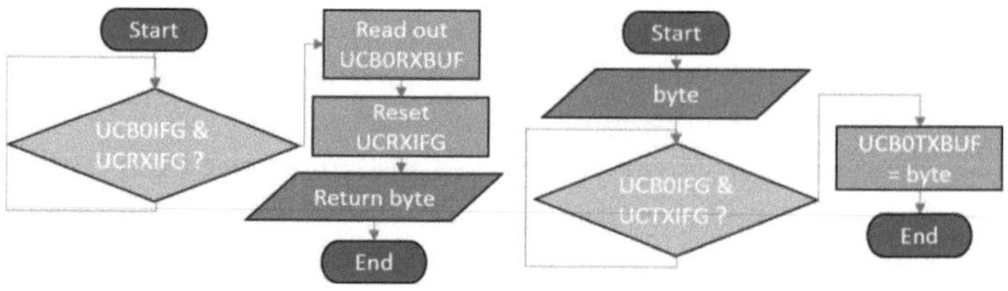

Figure 3: Functions to write (right) and read (left) a byte of data via SPI.

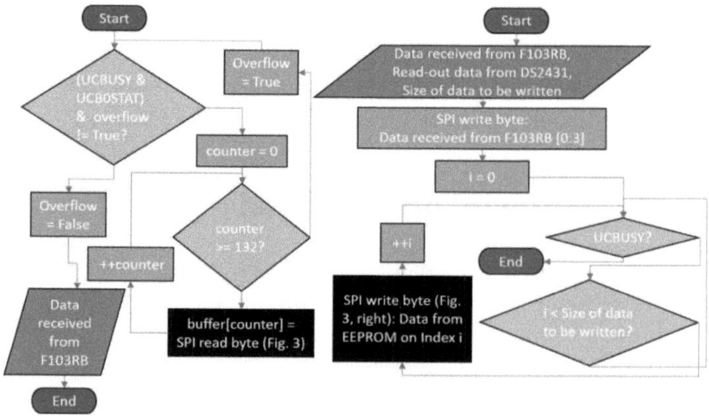

Figure 4: Functions to write (right) and read (left) data via SPI.

The MSP430 and F103RB send each other data arrays like the one shown in Table 3 via SPI. Two basic functions have been developed for this communication. The purpose of the left function in Fig. 3 is to enable the MSP430 to read a byte via SPI. Therefore its UCB0IFG register is checked repeatedly until the UCRXIFG flag is set (see Table 2). Then the receive buffer UCB0RXBUF (see Table 2) is read out and assigned to a buffer variable. The receive interrupt flag UCRXIFG must then be reset manually to be able to act as a trigger again. The return value of the function is the byte of data, which was received via SPI. To send the read-out data of the DS2431 back to the F103RB, the function on the right side in Fig. 3 was developed. As input, it receives a variable named byte, which contains the data to be sent to the F103RB. First, the interrupt flag register UCB0IFG is checked repeatedly again until the transmit interrupt flag UCTXIFG is set (see Table 2). In this case the input variable is assigned to the UCB0TXBUF, which then transfers the byte of data to the F103RB (see Table 2). The function on the left side of Fig. 4 was developed to receive data from the F103RB via SPI. First it checks the status register UCB0STAT, to see whether the UCBUSY flag is set (see Table 2). If the flag is set, a maximum of 132 bytes are read out from the F103RB iteratively and stored in an array, which is the output value of the function. To send back the read-out data of the DS2431 to the F103RB, the function on the right side in Fig. 4 is passed the read-out data of the DS2431 in an array and the received data of the F103RB in a second array as input values. The first four bytes of this array are sent back to the F103RB for verification of the read-out data and the detection of errors (see Table 3). After that, the array containing the read-out data of the DS2431 is sent iteratively back to the F103RB.

3.1.2 1-Wire interface: MSP430 to DS2431

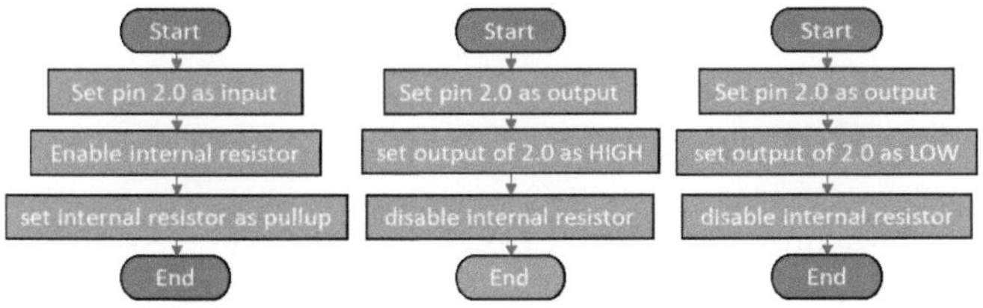

Figure 5: Functions for the MSP430 to release the 1-Wire line (left), push the line up to high (middle) or pull the line to low (right).

To enable the MSP430 to communicate with the DS2431, three basic functions of 1-Wire communication have been developed to manipulate the voltage on pin 2.0 of the MSP430, which is connected to the I/O port of the DS2431, like it can be seen in Fig. 1. The function in the middle of Fig. 5 was developed to pull the 1-Wire line to logical high. Therefore the first bit of the direction register P2DIR (see Table 1) is set. Then the first bit of the output register P2OUT (see Table 1) is set. Pin 2.0 is now an output and its output value is high. The voltage exceeds the high threshold voltage V_{TH}, like it can be seen in Fig. 2 and ends in the stable state of the pullup voltage V_{PUP} (see Table 4). The function on the right side of Fig. 5 was developed to pull the voltage of the 1-Wire line to logical low. Therefore the first bit of the direction register P2DIR (see Table 1) is set and the first bit of the P2OUT register (see Table 1) is reset. Pin 2.0 is now an output and its output value is low. The voltage drops from the idle state V_{PUP} to 0 V and crosses the low threshold voltage V_{TL}, like it can be seen in Fig. 2. To end the influence of the MSP430 on the line, the function on the left side of Fig. 5 was developed, in which the first bit of the direction register P2DIR is reset (see Table 1). After that, the first bit of the pullup or pulldown resistor enable register P2REN as well as of the output register P2OUT are set. As one can see in Table 1, pin 2.0 is now an input and the voltage on the 1-wire line increases due to the pullup resistor to pullup voltage V_{PUP}. The DS2431 now has the possibility to pull the 1-Wire line to low and to answer the MSP430.

The 1-Wire protocol of the DS2431 consists of four types of signaling on the 1-Wire line: reset sequence with reset pulse and presence pulse, write-zero, write-one, and read-data [1], which are implemented with the basic functions of Fig. 5 and delays of strictly defined time slots, which can be found in Table 4. Except for a presence pulse, which is the answer of the DS2431 to a reset pulse, the MSP430 initiates all operations with falling edges of the voltage of the 1-Wire line [1], which is why all functions in Fig. 6 start with the MSP430 pulling the line to low. As a result of different sequences of the MSP430 and DS2431 pulling the 1-Wire line for defined time intervals to low and releasing the line through the functions in Fig. 5, the functions in Fig. 6 implement the four types of signaling on the 1-Wire line. The function on the left side of Fig. 6 implements the reset sequence with reset and presence pulse, while the one in the middle of Fig. 6 implements the write-one or wirte-zero sequence. The function on the right side of Fig. 6 implements reading one bit via 1-Wire.

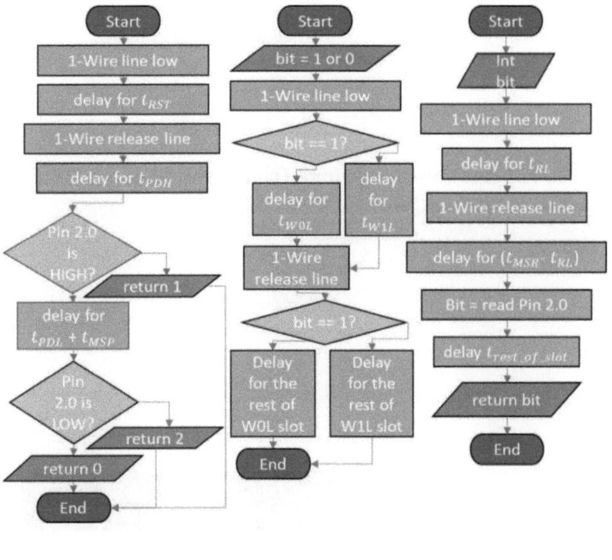

Figure 6: Functions to reset (left), to write one bit (middle) of and read one bit from the DS2431 (right).

3.1.3 Read/Write DS2431

The functions of Fig. 6 enabled the development of functions to write to and read from the memory of the DS2431, which are shown in Fig. 7. The write operation, which is shown on the left side of Fig. 7, is a four-step process. First, data is written to the scratchpad in a Write Scratchpad operation (see [1]), as shown in Fig. 7. To verify the data written to the scratchpad, its content as well as the E/S control register (see [1]) of the DS2431 is read out. If it is proofed, that the transaction of the data was successful, a Copy Scratchpad operation (see [1]) is executed and the data is copied from the scratchpad to the main memory of the DS2431. The function on the right side of Fig. 7 was developed to read data of a certain target address, e.g. the address of one of the four pages of the main memory, from the main memory of the DS2431. After sending a SKIP ROM and READ MEMORY command (see [1]), the low and high byte of the target address are transmitted, to which the DS2431 answers with the data located at the certain target address, which is then read out iteratively.

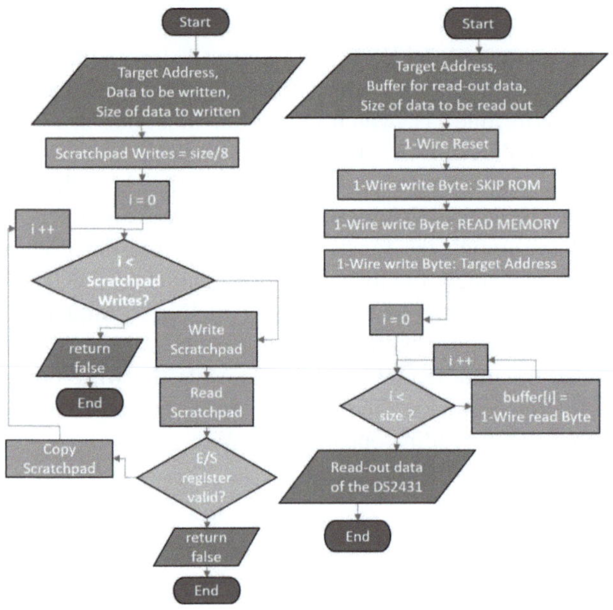

Figure 7: Functions to write to (right) and read out (left) the memory of the DS2431.

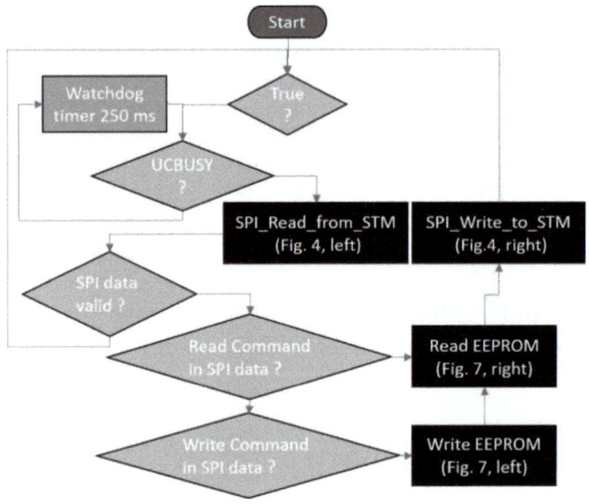

Figure 8: Main loop of the MSP430.

3.1.4 Main Loop of the MSP430

The main loop in Fig. 8 combines all developed functions and realizes the function of an interface converter from SPI to 1-Wire through software. It listens continuously for data form the F103RB via SPI, analyses the received data, writes to or reads from the DS2431 via 1-Wire and sends the data of the memory of the EEPROM back to the F103RB via SPI. After that, it listens for a new command from the F103RB via SPI.

4 Conclusion

The function of the interface converter was implemented successfully with the MSP430. Communication between the DS2431 and the SPI master has been realized and the EEPROM can thus be integrated into the PCB of the medical sensor.

Acknowledgement

The work has been carried out at Drägerwerk AG & Co. KGaA, Lübeck and supervised by Prof. Dr.-Ing. Mladen Berekovic, Institute of Computer Engineering, Universität zu Lübeck.

Author's Statement

Conflict of interest: Authors state no conflict of interest.

5 References

[1] Maxim Integrated, *DS2431 Datasheet*. Available: https://datasheets.maximintegrated.com/en/ds/DS2431.pdf [last accessed on 2021-01-20].

[2] Texas Instruments, *MSP430FR4xx and MSP430FR2xx family User's Guide*. Available: https://www.ti.com/lit/ug/slau445i/slau445i.pdf?ts=1611484595735&ref_url=https%253A%252F%252Fwww.ti.com%252Fproduct%252FMSP430FR2000 [last accessed on 2021-01-20].

[3] STMicroelectronics, *STM32F103xB Datasheet*. Available: https://www.st.com/resource/en/datasheet/stm32f103rb.pdf [last accessed on 2021-01-20].

[4] li, li and He, Jing and Zhao, Yong and Yang, Jianhong, *Design of Microcontroller Standard SPI Interface*. Applied Mechanics and Materials, 2014.

[5] M. Cina, *Das 1-Wire-Praxisbuch*. Elektor Verlag GmbH, Aachen, 2020.

6

Safety and Quality

Establishment of a Digitized Final and Cross Product Inspection in the Medical Industry

Marc Freitag [1], Jinghua Groppe [2]

[1] Medical Engineering Science, Universität zu Lübeck, marc.freitag@student.uni-luebeck.de

[2] Institute for information systems, Universität zu Lübeck, groppej@ifis.uni-luebeck.de

Abstract

As medical devices become more complex in order to improve accuracy in diagnosis and potency in therapy, the inspection of the devices becomes more complex as well. This leads to the need of smart inspection systems in order to assure high quality standards in the industry of medical devices. Next to software, quality and device failure, mislabelling is one of the most common defects. Deep learning-based object detection has shown promising prospects in order to minimise defects such as mislabelling. A potential solution to implement such an advanced inspection technique is to develop a system, which is based on an inspection garage, object detection algorithm and a digital interface, containing the checklist parameters. The scope of the system transcends the medical industry since it can be adapted to any visual product inspection by configuring of the parameters of the checklist.

1 Introduction

When medical devices are distributed on a market many regulations defined by various institutions such as the International Electrotechnical Commission (IEC)[1], the United States Food and Drug Administration (FDA)[2] or the International Organization for Standardization (ISO)[3] assure the safety and quality for customers in the market sector. The product compliance to these standards are visualised by labels and safety signs placed on specific regions of the device. The labels hold crucial information about:

- name and address of the company, country of origin
- model or type reference, batch identifier, individual identification
- components of equipment, detachable components
- voltage or ampere range and time frame for safe usage
- responsibility for the disposal
- warning symbols

Warning symbols contain high voltage, ionising radiation, hazardous chemicals etc. An example of a medical device label can be seen in Fig. 1. Mislabelling or labels placed in the wrong position lead to possible misuse by the customer, thus can be potentially dangerous and can therefore end in product types being banned from a market. A way of minimising quality defects is to split the final inspection into two parts. The final check, being the general final inspection with all important features and as second part the cross check, which purpose is to double check frequent sources of mistakes being made throughout the manufacturing process. The parameters used in the cross check vary between companies and are chosen on the basis of the companies' product recall statistics. The beneficial effect of the cross check is the advantage of the *four eyes principle*, meaning that two operators can detect defects better than one. That is why the cross check is performed by a different operator. Even though various operators checked and double checked the device for quality defects, errors in the way of mislabelling or even false production still occur due to the complexity of labeling. During the last decade 1491 medical devices were recalled due to errors concerning *labelling* from the the United States Food and Drug Administration alone [2]. Moreover *mislabelling* has been identified as one of the top five reasons for recalls in the first quarter of 2020 within the United States of America [2].

Considering the rise of technology and digitisation, imple-

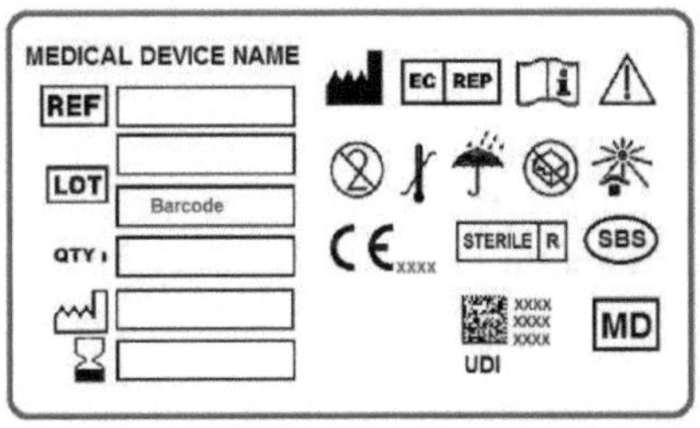

Figure 1: Example of labels used on a medical device [6].

[1] https://www.iec.ch/homepage

[2] https://www.fda.gov/

[3] https://www.iso.org/home.html

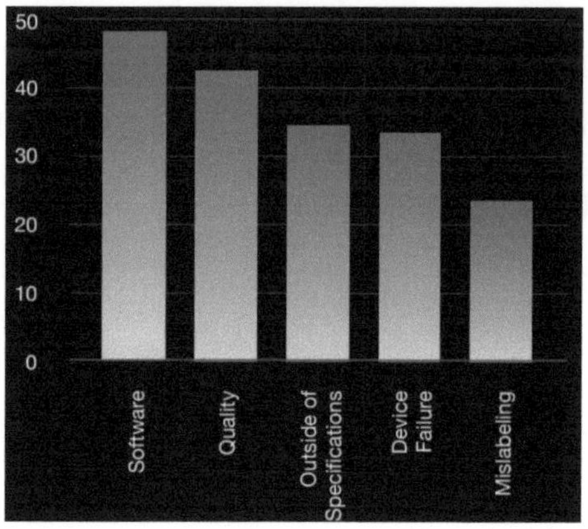

Figure 2: Absolute number of recalls for medical devices by reason for the first quarter of 2020 in the united states.

mentation of smart object detection systems is going to play a key role to minimise the occurrence of such errors. It has been shown that a real-time object detection model on an edge artificial intelligence (AI) optimized device can be used for detection of labels with a precision of 91,3 % [3]. In order to include the output of such an artificial neural network, in this work a digital checklist was developed containing all the specific parameters of each inspection in reference to the individual product type. In addition the data needs to be connected with a comprehensive manufacturing execution system (MES) such as SAP ME[4] , where the result from the inspection can be automatically transferred to and stored for further analysis. Moreover an inspection garage as a frame for the tools necessary for the automation of the final and cross product inspection was developed and constructed. Such an interface and inspection garage will be described in later sections.

2 Material and Methods

In this work we develope a digital checklist and an inspection garage to detect mislabelling of products and reduce waste of resources.

2.1 Process optimization with a digital checklist and an inspection garage

In order to reduce resource waste and mislabelling a process analysis was first performed applying the *Toyota production system* (TPS). It is a framework consisting of 14 principles for conserving resources by eliminating *waste* (muda) of all kinds. The seven different types of waste are: Overproduction, waiting (time on hand), unnecessary transport or conveyance, over-processing or incorrect processing, excess inventory, motion and defects [4]. The current system uses a paper based checklist, which the operator has to fill out firstly on paper before transferring the analogue parameters individually into the MES. This type of muda is considered *waiting* and *motion*, since the operator has to wait on the response of the MES during each transfer and has to walk to the printer and back in order to use the checklist. As written in the *Corrective and Preventive Actions* (CAPA) paragraph, "unfavorable trends" such as the occurrence of mislabelled devices have been identified [5]. Therefore *defects* in the way of mislabelled devices have been classified. The root cause for the mislabelled devices is insufficient accuracy in the final product inspection. A more accurate way of inspection is the use of an edge AI optimized device using deep learning-based object detection [3]. In order to use such a smart detection system, general tools have to be developed. A digitized checklist needs to be programmed as well as an inspection garage. The digital checklist software needs to have a user friendly interface that contains all the parameters of the paper based checklist, as well as an automatic data transfer to an MES. The digitization of the checklist would eliminate the *waiting* and *motion* wastes consequently, since the transfer will be automatically and no paper needs to be printed out anymore. The requirements for the inspection garage are the ability to mount the single board computer (SBC), where the AI will be installed and operated on and a movable camera bracket needed for the AI, a monitor, the power supply and the capability to include further upgrades of the system. The general concept and connection between the different tools for automation of the final and cross product inspection can be seen in Fig. 3.

[4]https://www.sap.com/products/execution-mes.html

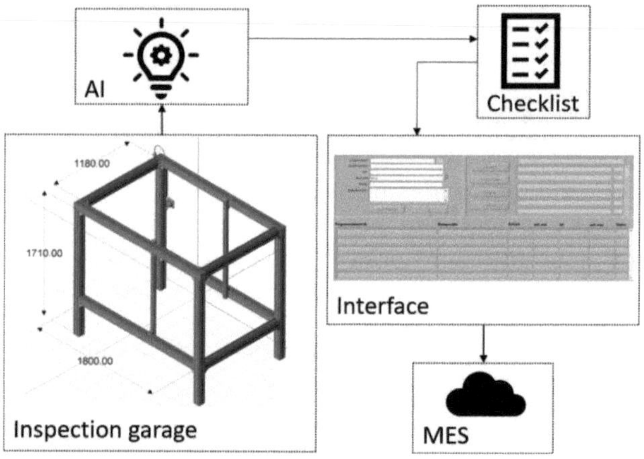

Figure 3: General structure of information flow. The dimensions of the inspection garage are in [mm].

2.2 Design of the digital Checklist

The digitized checklist should have a user friendly interface, where the operator can perform the inspection on. The parameters of the checklist should be *Boolean*, meaning that the value can be either *true* or *false*. In order to minimise future maintenance of the software, a system based on configuration files should be used. Configuration files (config. files) are used to set initial parameters for programs. Since any change to a software used in the medical industry has to be validated, the usage of config. files minimises the maintenance of such a program. Any change of parameters leads to a validation of the configuration file which contains those settings instead of the entire program. Two different sets of config. files should be used. The first set being the ones containing all the parameters and commands needed to perform the final and cross product check. The second set is a single config. file which holds the address to the MES and the different types of devices that are included in the inspection as well as the information whether those parameters will be transferred to the MES. The program should run on two types of settings: automatic and single step setting. The automatic setting continuously goes through the checklist point by point without stopping. The single step setting will let the operator choose one single step of the checklist and will set the result only for that parameter. In addition, the checklist should only transfer the data if all parameters are marked as *true* and the inspection was successful. The general structure of the checklist interface can be seen in Fig. 4.

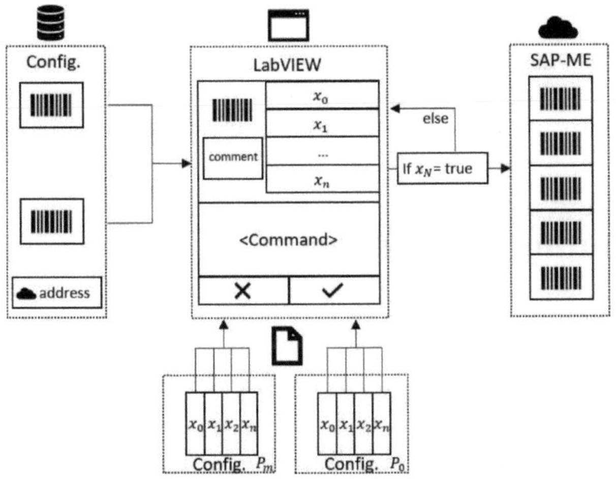

Figure 4: Structure of the checklist. Different checkpoints are marked as $[x_{0,...,n}]$. N being the closed set of [0,1,...,n]. The $[P_{0,m}]$ symbolises the m different medical device products.

3 Results and Discussion

3.1 Digitized Checklist

The digital checklist is programmed using the system-design platform and development environment *Laboratory Virtual Instrument Engineering Workbench* [5] (LabVIEW) by national instruments in the 2016 Version. A scanner reads a string into the program which can be compared to a specific product code. This code is used to connect the medical device to its specific checklist and all its components. Afterwards the system works as described in the previous section 2.2. Moreover a *comment* function was implemented into the program, where the operator can write a comment in the end of the inspection, that is being stored in the MES as well. An example of the syntax of the config. file code can be seen in following:

```
Title = Aufkleber focal spot
SingleStepName = Aufkleber focal spot
ShortName = Aufkleber_focal_spot
MeasurePoint = Operator
Command = Pruefe: Aufkleber focal spot angebracht
SAP_ME = 1
```

The first line represents the title, which defines what the operator sees as name for the step. The second line is the single step name and can be seen in the drop down list of parameters when choosing the single step setting. The *shortname* stands for the corresponding parameter within the MES and has to match exactly to the one used in the code. The *MeasurePoint* will always be equal to Operator as long as the inspection is not embedded with the AI yet, thus is performed by the operator. The command section defines the specific work instruction in order to perform the check. The last line refers to the Boolean question, whether the parameter shall be transferred to the MES. If it is set to *=1*, the transfer of data will be done. The interface can be seen in Fig 5.

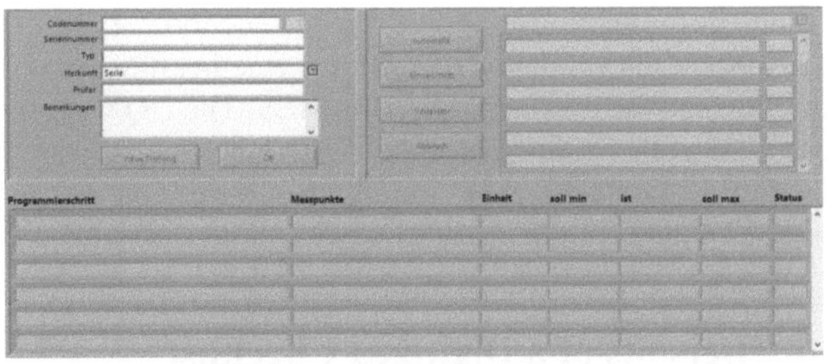

Figure 5: LabVIEW interface for the digitized checklist.

Further improvement of the program can be done by including numerical values next to the Boolean. That way other type of checklist parameters such as measuring of lengths could be included as well. This would increase the range of use for the tool. Moreover next to the command function, which gives the instructions to perform the inspection, the implementation of visual aid through pictures could benefit the operator.

3.2 Inspection Garage

The garage was designed using the *iCAD Assembler 3.3.4 CAD* tool by *MiniTec GmbH & Co. KG*. It is made of 90 x 90 mm aluminum profiles on the outside and two 45 x 45 mm aluminum profiles, where the cameras will be mounted. The height was set to 1710 mm in order to have the best angle for detection. The length (1800 mm) and width (1180 mm) were adapted to the medical device that is being inspected. Forty 90° mounting angles were used to give the construction stability. A monitor support with ball joint and a seven way multiple socket outlet was added in order to be able to add a monitor and electrical supply for the electronic components of the construction. A scheme of the garage can be seen in Fig. 3. Future modifications could be the use

[5] https://www.ni.com/da-dk/shop/labview.html

of a motorized camera racket as well as the addition of further cameras. In order to give the detecting cameras a better contrast, walls made of coated glass could be implemented. Another possibility for improvement would be the use of an assembly line. In that case the back of the garage needs to be removed and the garage would have the assembly line going through the center section.

3.3 Validation of the Checklist

As tool for the validation, the operational qualification (OQ) was used. It is a functional test of the different features of the software. The OQ was performed using the program configuration files, a LabVIEW run-time engine in the 2016 version, a bar-code scanner and the bar codes to every product type. The first test is the review of the scanning. Every scan lead to a correct connection of medical device product type. The second test is the comparison of the parameters of the paper based checklist to the digitized as well as the review of the commands displayed for every parameter, both for the final and cross inspection. The parameters and commands matched to the requirements as well. Afterwards the OQ included the evaluation of the automatic and single step setting. Both functioned as described in section 2.2. The final aspect of the validation was the test whether the data was correctly and fully transferred to the MES. The OQ was successful, thus the validation of the digitized checklist was. It has shown that the software functions as described and can be used in the manufacturing process.

3.4 Benefits of a Digitized Checklist

The biggest benefit is estimated to be the increase in quality of the products due to minimisation of mislabelled medical devices. The change from paper based to digitized checklist will show various benefits for manufacturing processes. Using paperless methods is good for the environment and leads to a green and positive customer image of the company. The annual costs for printing out the paper based checklists are estimated to 700 € on average for one product group. On top of that comes the time that is considered *waste* according to the TPS as described in section 2.1. The data necessary for calculating the costs were gathered through interviewing of operators and supervisors about the mean time for filling out one point of the final product inspection. The costs that are saved depend on the number of checkpoints on both the final and cross check. It has been estimated to an annually amount of around 41000 € per device group. On the other hand, the costs needed to implement such an automated digital inspection system consists of the material needed to build the inspection garage, the cameras and developer kit using the object detection technique as well as the labour costs to plan, build and validate such a model. The costs of material are in the range of 2500 €. Considering the ability of scaling the inspection system on to medical devices of all sorts, the benefits in terms of quality assurance and minimising waste outweigh the costs of development by far.

4 Conclusion

In conclusion, this paper presents an approach to establish a digitized final and cross product check and the economical and environmental benefits of this approach for companies deploying the system. A LabVIEW 2016 version was used to create an interface that allows the operator to have clear work instructions using the command lines and a direct transfer of data without interacting with the MES. This digitized checklist can be filled with any sort of parameters making it a universal tool of data transfer. The software was validated using the operational qualification and will be used in combination with an edge AI optimized device for object detection. Furthermore an inspection garage was designed and constructed. Future test results will show the automation of the final inspection using the combination of edge AI, digital checklist and inspection garage.

Acknowledgement

The work has been carried out at Philips Medical Systems DMC GmbH, Hamburg Germany. It has been supervised by Dr. rer. nat. Jinghua Groppe, Institut für Informationssysteme, Universität zu Lübeck.

Author's Statement

Authors state no conflict of interest.

5 References

[1] recall index, *stericycle recall index 2020*. Available: https://www.stericycleexpertsolutions.com/product-recall-index/ [last accessed on 2021-01-17].

[2] FDA, *Medical Device Recalls*. Available: https://www.accessdata.fda.gov/scripts/cdrh/cfdocs/cfres/res.cfm [last accessed on 2021-01-17].

[3] M. Lichtenhagen, *Utilizing Embedded Deep Learning-based Object Detection for Visual Inspections of Medical Devices*. Luebeck University of Applied Sciences, Luebeck, 2021.

[4] Liker, Jeffrey K, *The Toyota Way: 14 Management Principles from the World's Greatest Manufacturer*. McGraw-Hill, 2004.

[5] FDA, *Corrective and Preventive Actions (CAPA)*. Available: https://www.fda.gov/corrective-and-preventive-actions-capa [last accessed on 2021-01-19].

[6] Label, *Example of symbols used on medical device Labels*. Available: https://medicaldeviceregulations.home.blog/2019/07/31/mdr-rules-for-information-supplied-on-the-labels/ [last accessed on 2021-01-21].

Provision of sensitive clinical and biobank data for research in compliance with data protection regulations

Friedrich Simon [1], Ann-Kristin Kock-Schoppenhauer [2], Hannes Ulrich [2], Martina Oberländer [3], Regina Maushagen [3], Friedemann Flügge [3], and Josef Ingenerf [4]

[1] Medical Informatics, Universität zu Lübeck, f.simon@student.uni-luebeck.de
[2] IT Center for Clinical Research, Lübeck, {annkristin.kockschoppenhauer,h.ulrich}@uni-luebeck.de
[3] Interdisciplinary Center for Biobanking-Lübeck, {f.fluegge,martina.oberlaender,regina.maushagen}@uni-luebeck.de
[4] Institue of Medical Informatics, Universität zu Lübeck, josef.ingenerf@uni-luebeck.de

Abstract

The Interdisciplinary Center for Biobanking-Lübeck is a centralized biobank operating at the Campus Lübeck. They provide a clinical research infrastructure which enables a researcher to search for patient and sample data in pseudonymized form. An approved data protection concept exists for the process and is in routine use. The established process is time-consuming and requires many manual steps. Extensions and necessary adaptations on the process are difficult due to the implemented architecture and techniques. The aim of this project is to renew and improve the process of provision of pseudonymized data to researchers, without the need to change the data protection concept. The first step was to analyse and describe the existing process in detail. Next resulted in a Selection, Pseudonymisation and Synchronisation Pipeline (SPSP), which extends the existing infrastructure and fulfils all aspects of the data protection concept.

1 Introduction

Biobanks usually collect project-related biospecimens that are then retrieved for a specific research project. At the Interdisciplinary Center for Biobanking-Lübeck (ICB-L), bio material is also collected for future research projects. As a hospital-integrated biobank, there is access to clinical data. At hospital stay, the patient agrees by signing a broad consent that his/her clinical data and also his/her samples will be made available for clinical research. The clinical data are transferred from the hospital information system (HIS) into the biobank information and management system (BIMS). The IT Center of Clinical Research (ITCR-L) is responsible for the configuration and technical administration of the BIMS. The aim of the biobank is to make biosamples (sources of the genotype) in combination with clinical data (phenotype) available for research, mainly by correlating genotype and phenotype data from many patients. Due to the increasing networking of biobanks and research platforms, it is advantageous for the biobank to make its sample inventory visible. Since the data is sensitive, direct identification is prevented by removing and pseudonymising [1] direct identifiers and also obfuscation of other attributes. Furthermore, researchers agree in a data usage contract not to attempt depseudonymisation and require an explicit research project to gain access. On the other hand, re-identification of patients and biospecimens is necessary to feed research data back into the internal system and also to identify specimens for shipment. This task currently has to be done manually by administrators and trustees.
The research system is set up as an extra instance. Data from the Internal System are transferred to the research system on a regular basis. During the transfer, identifying data are omitted and other necessary data are obscured. This process consists of many individual manual steps and requires in-depth understanding of system processes and storage structures of the BIMS. When this process was defined, existing interfaces in the BIMS were not yet sufficient. In particular, software updates and new data elements require intensive maintenance and constant improvements.
The integration of an seperate trustee service should be supported flexibly. These and other innovations planned for the future would be difficult to implement in the existing architecture. In the course of the project, we therefore decided to question the existing architecture and technologies - but not the degree of pseudonymization. On the contrary, transparency and effectiveness will have a positive impact on the data protection concept. At the end of the project the SPSP was implemented as a prototype with in the envisioned environment to show how the process of data provision at ICB-L could work.

2 Material and Methods

Right at the beginning, the project was divided into two sections. First, the existing internal data transformations had to be thoroughly analyzed. Furthermore, it was discussed with the stakeholders which features should be considered currently and also in the future. All steps were examined and evaluated in detail. The second part consisted of applying the findings from the first part and implementing them

in a new process. The key technologies used were extensively evaluated in a test environment and implemented as prototype. At ICB-L, the CentraXX [2] software solution from the company Kairos is used. CentraXX is used both as an internal system for documentation and, in a separate instance, as a research system. The system stores all data on the samples, as well as quality characteristics such as time stamps, storage temperatures, and results of analytics. All samples are clearly assigned to a patient. In addition to the sample data, clinical data from the hospital information system (HIS) AGFA Orbis are transferred to CentraXX based on HL7-standardized interfaces [3]. Only the sample data, as well as explicit clinical data of the patients, are intended for the transfer of the data to the research system.
The transfer of this data is currently realized by batch scripts that mainly execute SQL commands in several iterative steps. Therefore, the whole process depends on the actual database schema. It was developed when the system had only insufficient interfaces. The scripts were developed and implemented in cooperation with the manufacturer of the BIMS software. All documentation related to the development was reviewed and re-evaluated. Further, the scripts were analyzed in detail and the possibility for further development and/or partial reuse was discussed. It concerns 7 script files, as well as a variable file, as well as 14 SQL scripts. The data in the system is distributed over about 1000 tables, including audit tables. Nowadays, the system offers a Extensible Markup Language (XML) format described by a XML Schema Definition (XSD) with about 8800 lines of code. There is also an almost full Representational State Transfer (REST) interface, as well as a Fast Healthcare Interoperability Resources (FHIR) interface [3].

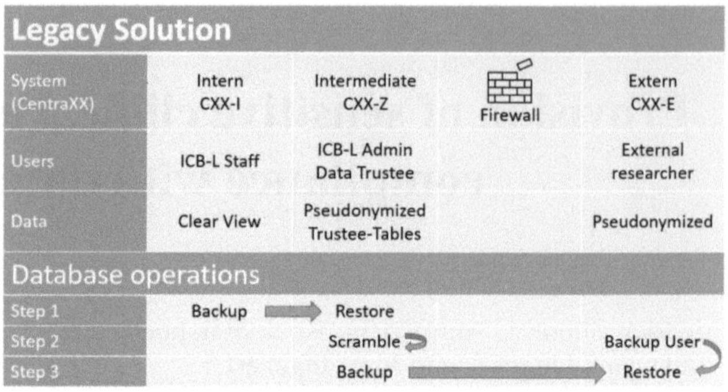

Figure 1: ICB-L's legacy solution architecture. CXX-I is the internal system on which the ICB-L staff works directly, located in the secure network of the clinic. CXX-Z is an intermediate instance on which the validation of data for the external system takes place. The trust tables are also located in the database on this server. That is also located in the secure network. CXX-E is the external system in the demilitarized zone of the clinic. CXX-E is used by eligible researchers from all over the world. The steps for providing data for research is shown in the lower part of the table. The database operations in Step 1 copy the entire database of the Internal System to CXX-Z. In Step 2, the entire pseudonymisation is carried out on the CXX-Z database. In Step 3, the pseudonymised data set is copied from CXX-Z to CXX-E.

2.1 Legacy Solution

An application purpose-bound division of the systems is necessary to separate data items for the different use cases. During data transmission, data is specifically excluded and others are obscured. To accommodate multi-level pseudonymization, several trust tables were created on the database. With the help of these tables, a re-identification from the research system (CXX-E) to the internal system (CXX-I) is possible. The transfer was realized at database level. Almost with every update of the system, an adaptation of this process was also necessary. Newly added data also had to be critically checked to determine whether it could be transferred. The solution, developed by the BIMS vendor, is based on the architecture shown in the figure (Fig. 1). Shown are the CentraXX instances Internal(I), trust tables and External(E). The user groups and the view of the data are also described. The analysis of the existing solution is shown in the bottom part of the figure.

2.2 Data vs Metadata in SPSP

The data elements in CentraXX can be extended dynamically without adapting the basic SQL database schema. These data elements are defined separately as metadata conforming to the so-called Entity-Attribute-Value (EAV) model [4]. This allows the database to be flexibly adapted to the needs. Changed or new metadata in the source system must be transferred to the target system. Otherwise, the data can not be imported properly. Note that this is not a problem by copying the entire database (Legacy Solution). When selectively copying via the newly developed interface, however, it must be ensured that the corresponding metadata are available on the target system.

2.3 Trust Service in SPSP

In this project, a trust service is used to exchange IDs through a pseudonym via an interface. In the same way, the original ID can be requested from the trust service with the pseudonym. Both pseudonym and original ID are known only to the trustee. The *Mainzelliste* [5] was used as a suitable candidate for such a trustee service, as it is already successfully used and recognised in many funded projects. The trustee can also access the trustee service via a web interface. This would eliminate the need for a system administrator with database access for re-identification.

2.4 Communication Server in SPSP

A communication server is needed to orchestrate message flows. In this project, Mirth Connect [6] was used for test purposes. Mirth Connect is also fondly referred to as the Swiss Army Knife of healthcare. Processes are configured as channels in Mirth Connect. A channel always has one input and any number of outputs. The system can be interactively used via a web interface. Mirth already supports many common formats in healthcare such as HL7, XML and JSON. Predefined connectors are provided using access methods like database queries, file reader as well as REST/FHIR [3] interfaces. Through Javascript integration, processes can be customized as desired. Especially interesting is the monitoring and reporting function. This helps to keep an overview and to generate automated messages in case of problems.

3 Results and Discussion

First, an extensive analysis of the existing system led to a systematic recording of all constraints and technical requirements. Further, it was discussed with the stakeholders which features are desired. This resulted in a specification for the implementation. A process architecture was created and examples were used to show how data provision could work in the specific use case of ICB-L following the existing data protection concept and architecture. The two biggest challenges with the current solution are the extraordinary high maintenance effort for updates of the BIMS and the non-persistent trust tables - these are overwritten with every process run. This also results in the manual process of transferring research data from the research system back to the internal system. To solve the two biggest problems, copying the entire database was discarded in the first step. This made it necessary to additionally address the metadata transfer, but has the huge advantage that we can specify exactly which data should be transferred. To address the problem of the trust tables and to increase the usability for the trustee, a trust service was added. This creates and manages a new pseudonym for each patient and each sample from the pseudonymised ID of the internal system. This new pseudonym is persistent and can be requested from the trustee service again and again. Data elements that are to be transferred are entered in a so-called white list. It is also possible to disguise these data elements if they are too specific. For instance, dates are changed to 01.01 of the year. In turn, information that is required by the research system is concealed by masks. For example, specific storage location information of the biobank is irrelevant for the researcher. All other data elements that are not specified in the white list are discarded.
The newly created problem of keeping the metadata and configuration up to date on the target system was also solved by the white list. Since all data elements that are transferred are known, the corresponding metadata can be specifically requested from the source system. This is done in a so-called initialisation phase before the SPSP runs. The SPSP is a modular pipeline for transferring desired or incrementally new data records from the internal system to the external system with pseudonymized data. In the other direction, changes and additions to the pseudonymised data could in principle be fed back into the internal system via the trustee. The Selection, Pseudonymisation and Synchronisation Pipeline (SPSP) was exemplary realised with current available tools in a test environment (Fig. 2).
Initialisation: Before starting with the SPSP, the initialization ensures that the metadata is updated beforehand. In two steps, the data elements (DE) are selectively requested from the source system and sent to the target system.
Selection: The first step is to identify patients in the internal system who have had an update. Of these patients, certain patients are excluded from the transfer by means of a blacklist. Subsequently, pseudonymised exports are requested selectively for each patient via the REST interface. These exports are simply pseudonymised, but still contain all additional data elements defined in the system.
Pseudonymisation: In step 3, the already pseudonymised IDs of the patients and biospecimens are pseudonymised again and exchanged via a trust service. In step 4, the remaining data is raised to the higher pseudonymisation standard of the ICB-L. Only data elements explicitly defined in a white list remain in the message or are further obfuscated. Data specified and required by the system are masked. For example, the explicit storage location of a sample is reduced to a dummy value. All other undefined data is discarded.
Synchronisation: In step 5, the pseudonymised data set of this patient is sent to the CXX-Z system and is ready for validation by the ICB-L staff. After successful validation of the entire CXX-Z system, a copy is made available as CXX-E. This procedure is necessary to remain close to the data protection concept. It would certainly also be conceivable to dispense with this additional instance as soon as the system has proven itself to be trustworthy.

With the SPSP prototype, exemplary test data sets could be translated in the sense of the data protection concept. Fictitious patients with typical clinical and biobank data were created in a CXX test environment. These data were successfully pseudonymised with the SPSP in accordance with data protection.

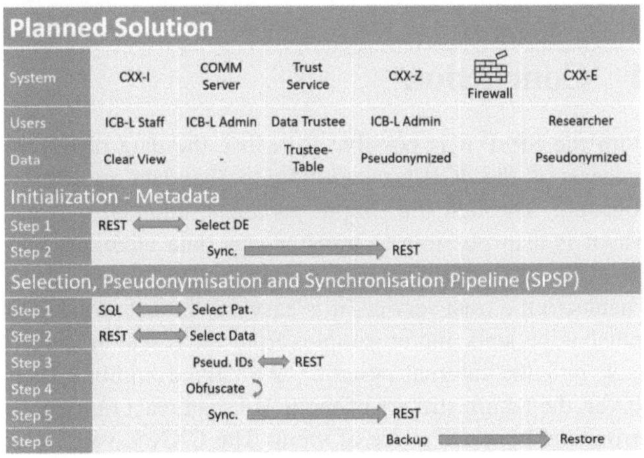

Figure 2: The table shows a summary of the planned architecture and the communication of the systems. Compared to the legacy solution, the communication server (COMM Server) and the trust service have been added.

3.1 An Example

The example (Fig. 3). is intended to show what happens to the various data elements in the SPSP. The name and date of birth are basic elements of the BIMS. This is removed or concealed during the pseudonymised query of the patient data. The white list data element is transmitted unchanged. The obfuscate data element is also on the whitelist, but is obfuscated accordingly. All other data elements are not transmitted (and do not exist as metadata on the target system). The Trust Service is not aware of any of this data. All that is stored at the Trust Service is whether it is a patient or a sample, as well as an internal ID and an external ID. A researcher with access to CXX-E only has a view of the pseudonym ID, which is not known in CXX-I or the trust service.

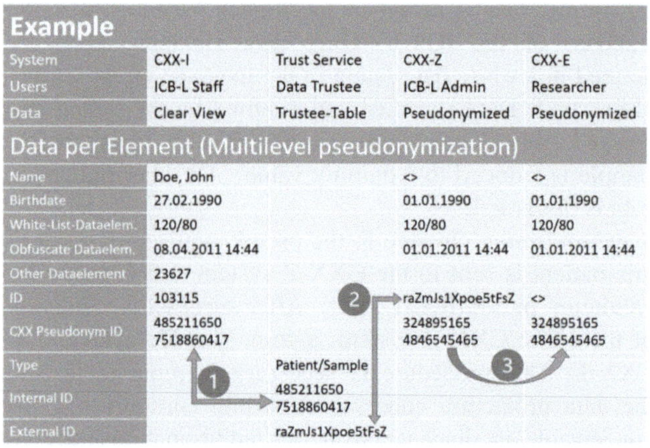

Figure 3: The systems on which data is stored can be seen in the upper part. In the lower part, selected data elements are listed on the left and the values in the respective system are shown in the individual cells. Empty cells do not exist in the respective system, and <> means that no value is entered. Furthermore, the steps of the ID pseudonymisation are marked with the numbers 1-3.

4 Conclusion

With the SPSP it is possible to realise the data provision process of the ICB-L according to the data protection concept. Through the simple parametrisation of a white list, it is also possible to transfer new data elements into the research system in a disguised or complete manner. Thanks to the trust service, it is easy for the data trustee to translate patients and/or samples from the research system back into the internal system. With the communication server, the administrators of the ICB-L can react quickly to errors and be made aware of them. The CXX-Z validation system also ensures (as with the legacy solution) that only validated systems are accessible to researchers. Patient data on the research system is still highly sensitive and must be protected. This is achieved with ICB-L through strict rules for researchers and their access to the system.

With more and more new requirements for research systems and networked research based on the communication server, as well as the trust service, it will be possible to meet these requirements. It is relatively easy to adapt the existing SPSP to provide data sets for other networked research platforms. Current requirements are very relevant, for example, with regard to a data integration center (DIC) in the context of the Medical Informatics Initiative (MII) [7], where an IHE-based Master Patient Index (MPI) is used for pseudonymization. To connect the CentraXX system to such a DIC, only the currently integrated tool Mainzeliste needs to be replaced by the MPI service in view of the SPSP.

Acknowledgement

The project was carried out in close cooperation with the Interdisciplinary Center for Biobanking Lübeck and the IT Center of Clinical Research Lübeck. The work was supervised by the Institute of Medical Informatics, Universität zu Lübeck.

Author's Statement

Conflict of interest: Authors state no conflict of interest.

5 References

[1] E. U. A. for Network and I. Security., *Recommendations on shaping technology according to GDPR provisions: an overview on data pseudonymisation.* Publications Office, 2018.

[2] Kairos. (2020-12-01) Centraxx basic. [Online]. Available: https://www.kairos.de/produkte/centraxx/

[3] T. Benson and G. Grieve, *Principles of Health Interoperability*. Springer International Publishing, 2021.

[4] C. A. Brandt, R. Morse, K. Matthews, K. Sun, A. M. Deshpande, R. Gadagkar, D. B. Cohen, P. L. Miller, and P. M. Nadkarni, "Metadata-driven creation of data marts from an EAV-modeled clinical research database," *International Journal of Medical Informatics*, vol. 65, no. 3, pp. 225–241, nov 2002.

[5] M. Lablans, A. Borg, and F. Ückert, "A RESTful interface to pseudonymization services in modern web applications," *BMC Medical Informatics and Decision Making*, vol. 15, no. 1, feb 2015.

[6] G. Bortis, "Experiences with mirth," in *Proceedings of the 13th international conference on Software engineering - ICSE '08*. ACM Press, 2008.

[7] S. Semler, F. Wissing, and R. Heyder, "German medical informatics initiative," *Methods of Information in Medicine*, vol. 57, no. S 01, pp. e50–e56, jul 2018.

Market analysis of ENT Equipment – on the Iranian market–

Termeh Juyandeh [1] and Naeimeh Razavirad [1]
[1] Medizinische Ingenieurwissenschaft, Universität zu Lübeck, {termeh.juyandeh naeimeh.razavirad}@student.uni-luebeck.de

Abstract

This paper focuses on the market analysis of Ear, Nose & Throat (ENT) Medical Devices in Iran. In addition to the establishment, the export of ENT treatment units from the company HEINEMANN Medizintechnik GmbH (Kaltenkirchen Germany) to the country is also being investigated. The market term is fundamental for such a market analysis. In addition, it is crucial which marketing strategies must be used and what the influencing factors are to bring a product successfully to the market. With the help of a field study, the current state of the art in Iran and the possibility of a new product launch are examined. The current political situation in Iran and the relationship between Iran and Germany are also considered because this has a strong influence on the potential for a successful trade (import and export). The aim of this work is to develop a strategic concept for the company HEINEMANN in order to conquer the market with their products.

1 Introduction

To successfully establish a product on the market, it requires a detailed market analysis which must be carried out before it is launched. The identification and analysis of the market is a crucial step to prepare the company for the introduction of the product and to establish the product successfully in the market. For an optimal preparation, the purchasing behavior of customers must be carefully considered. *"After all, the worm must taste good to the fish and not to the angler"* [1]. As newcomer in the Iranian market companies must always clarify which requirements must be met for the products from the marketing and from the customer's perspective. The aim of this paper is to develop a strategic solution concept for the company HEINEMANN Medizintechnik GmbH (Kaltenkirchen Germany). The needs and requirements of the customers must be considered in the Ear, Nose & Throat (ENT) area to both quantitatively and qualitatively have an opportunity for establishment of the products in Iran to be able to. The following key questions can be derived from the objective:

- How large is the need for ENT units?
- Which technical requirements are needed to be fulfilled?
- Which services are to be expected?
- What are the customer and price requirements?
- Which international manufacturers are already integrated in the market?
- Does a local manufacturer exist?
- How realistic is the possibility for HEINEMANN to conquer a new market?

Further, the current political situation in Iran and the relationship between Iran and Germany must be considered at this has an huge impact on the potential for a successful trade (import and export). The embargo against Iran that has existed for many years has restricted and made the import, export, and transport of goods more difficult. These restrictions also affect the financial transfer [2]. A detailed consideration of the political situation in Iran is not possible within the scope of this paper. Only a needs analysis of the ENT market with consideration of the trade restrictions due to Iran Embargo is examined and analyzed here. To be able to gain a detailed insight into the state of the ENT technology on the Iranian market, a field study is carried out firstly. This should provide the answers to the key questions mentioned above, enable a detailed and comprehensive analysis. Based on the analysis, it is discussed what influence the current political situation in Iran has on the import and export of the products.

2 Material and Methods

2.1 Product launch concept

As part of the market launch concept, strategic and operational sub-concepts are necessary in order to be able to guarantee a successful market launch. The decision to launch a new product on a market requires a correct planning process and a comprehensive analysis of the entire market, which Guido Call has defined as a strategic sub-concept [3][4]. As part of this strategic decision, the following aspects must be analyzed and discussed:

- Performance concept in terms of the product and correlating service

- Information about customer experience and the experience of competitors
- Consider company-relevant data
- Determine relevant product segments
- Define the target group for the new product

Moreover, it must be decided how the product should be positioned and which marketing mix adapted to the product (e.g. market entry point) should be chosen. In corporate objective decisions a complete market strategy must be defined based on product segment, target group, positioning, marketing mix and market entry date. This definition is important, because it must be implemented in an operational sub-concept [3][4]. The strategic and operational sub-concepts have the following hierarchical structure:

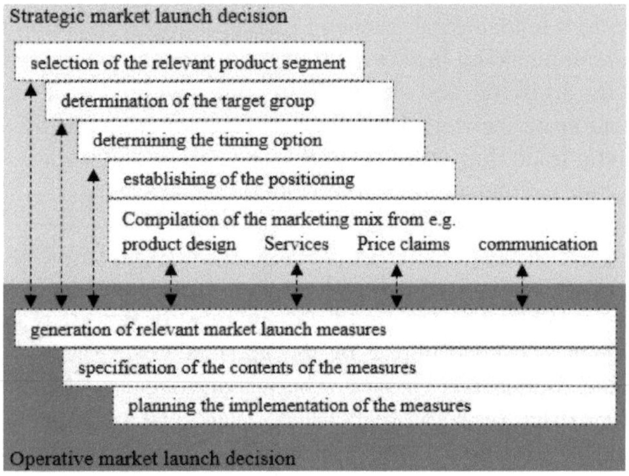

Figure 1: Strategic and operational sub-concepts as part of a market launch decision [4].

2.2 Market analysis

A good strategy is important in order to gain market share. This is the only way to guarantee a successful product launch. To be able to analyze the current situation of the Iranian ENT market in detail, a field study was carried out on site. This is the first step to receive comprehensive information about the existing conditions in the ENT area and, if necessary, to identify and fill the gaps.

2.3 Field study

A correct analysis includes a study of the current status of all possible existing and known ENT devices from different manufacturers and countries. As part of a field study survey, medical device dealers and ENT specialists (doctors, medical device manufacturers, salespeople, buyers, service employees) in Iran were asked to answer few questions. These questions aimed at finding out to what extent ENT units are already established on the Iranian market. The following questions were asked to 20 participants:

1. Which ENT companies are known in Iran and from which company and which brand (international companies) is the purchase of ENT units preferred?
2. Which characteristics are important for making a purchase decision?
   - ☐ Price-performance
   - ☐ Quality
   - ☐ Functional requirement
   - ☐ Service performance
   - ☐ Image
3. In which company is the price-performance ratio appropriate?
4. Which company has the highest quality?
5. Which company meets customer requirements (Iran)?
6. Which company has a better service after purchase?
7. Which company has the best image in Iran?
8. Are ENT treatment units produced in Iran (Made in Iran)?
   - ☐ yes
   - ☐ no
9. Are domestic local or foreign products preferred? (With regard to all medical devices, especially the ENT treatment units)

Figure 2: Field study survey (own representation).

3 Results and Discussion

The presented study shows that the following manufacturers are represented in Iran:

- Atmos MedizinTechnik GmbH & Co. Kg (Germany)
- Mega Medical Co., Ltd. (Korea)
- Chammed Co., Ltd. (Korea)
- Dantschke Medizintechnik GmbH & Co. Kg (Germany)
- Happersberger Otopront GmbH (Germany)

For all participants of the study, the Decisive facts for buying a product are especially the price and further the functionality and the quality. After the product has been sold, the service must respond to the requirements, needs, and the wishes of the customer. This also includes that the services are provided during the offered guarantee period. For most of the participants, an effective guarantee period is more important than a longstanding guarantee period. Half of all participants say that the reputation of the offering company is decisive in making a purchase decision. For the majority the title "Made in Germany" stands for quality, functionality, performance and above all for trust. However, some of the participants focused on the importance of the label "Made in Germany", whereby they also mentioned the importance of supporting local manufacturers if all the expected requirements are met on the Iranian market. The Iranian market is also preferred for this reason, as it is very difficult or impossible to get to foreign products due to the sanctions. With several intermediary, the price-performance ratio will no longer be appropriate. In the following diagram, the meaning of various features that are important for a purchase decision are compared.

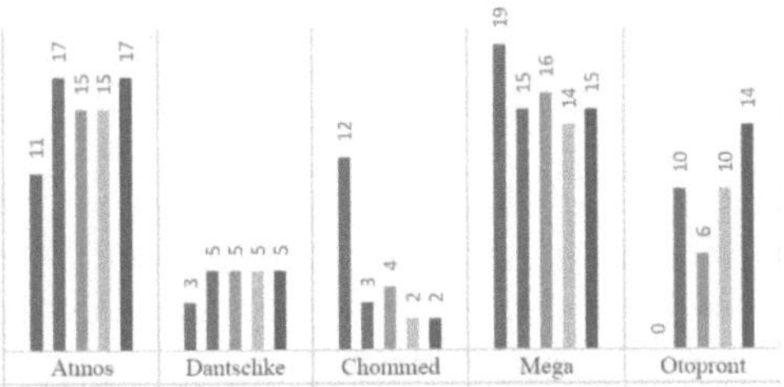

	Atmos	Dantschke	Chommed	Mega	Otopront
price-performance	11	3	12	19	0
quality	17	5	3	15	10
functional requirement	15	5	4	16	6
service	15	5	2	14	10
reputation	17	5	2	15	14

Figure 3: Company comparison-field study (own representation based on private communication with business experts during interview - Numbers present the number of respondents (20 participants))

The above figure shows that the best-selling units on the Iranian market come from the manufacturers Atmos Medizintechnik , Chommed and Mega Medical. 19 out of 20 participants who took part in this study stated that the Mega brand (C31 Economy, S61 Servant – intermediary: X-Ray Iran Co) indicated good price-performance ratio - which means reasonable prices for good quality. Atmos, a German company (Limited NET-3000A, Grand NET-3000C, Advanced NET-3000D, Multi NET-600A, Mobile NET-1100), sells one of the oldest units known in Iran and enjoys a high reputation. Since the units meet these requirements, many Iranians are willing to pay a higher price for these products. In addition, German manufacturers offer an effective guarantee period. The participants in the field study knew the producer Happersberger Otopront GmbH, but they thought the company was no longer actively represented in the market. In a conversation with an Iranian medical device salesman, who worked with Otopront himself in the past, it emerged, however, that Otopront continues to actively participate in the market. The company now focuses almost exclusively on existing customer contacts. Incidentally, the company is HEINEMANNs greatest competitor in many countries. The reasons are on the one hand the increased prices, problems with dealers in Iran and, on the other hand, the increasing active competitors. The field study has shown that in addition to the manufacturers already mentioned in the study, there is a local manufacturer called Pishro Teb Karan Asia Co. The units of this brand are often purchased by customers with small capital. Another point of sale for these units is that there are different opinions in Iran regarding imported products. On the one hand, there are some Iranians who oppose the importation of foreign currency into their country. This group believes that the foreign goods have no business in Iran, because there are many potential engineers in Iran who can produce and develop these products themselves. Accordingly, Iran should not be dependent on any other country. On the other hand, there is the opinion that the local manufacture of medical products, especially in the ENT area, is still in development and growth phase. Although medical technology is one of the most innovative Iranian industries, the need for imports remains high. The context of the field study shows that there are enough potential engineers in Iran for manufacturing and production, but due to the lack of an international CE mark, it is difficult for local manufacturers to develop and expand internationally.[6]

Managing the market launch in a new country also means taking the current situation into account, as the political situation can change positively or negatively at any time. In order to be prepared to avoid possible problems in advance and to observe their influence on imports and exports. The embargo against Iran began on December 23, 2006 following the resolution of the United Nations [7]. Since 16. January 2016 (Implementation Day), the UN and EU have relaxed and partially lifted the existing economic and financial sanctions against Iran, which were implemented as a result of the Iranian nuclear program [8]. The Iran embargo was to be relaxed in two phases, however, could not come about due to the unilateral withdrawal of the United States of America from the Joint Comprehensive Plan of Action (JCPoA) on 8. May 2018 [9]. What will happen in the next months, years and cannot be forecasted in advance. Although medical devices have never been banned so far for humanitarian reasons (for example, drugs and medical devices) [10], the access to the international financial market and the transfer of funds are becoming more difficult, with the aim of isolating Iran from the global financial market [9]. As a result of this contradictory coordination, many medical device manufacturers, are leaving the Iranian market behind. Sanctions against Iran have brought many disadvantages for the country, but perhaps also the advantage that Iranian manufacturers have moved in the direction of development and production more than before. However, as the study results show, it is difficult for the local manufacturer to get an international CE mark. Therefore, the import demand remains high at the same time.

4 Conclusion

Summarizing this paper answered the question, if and how a launch in a new market is possible, which measures must be observed and which problems can occur. The following factors are important for introducing a product to a new market [5]:

- Risk theory
  The purchase of a product is associated with risk and uncertainty for the buyer. For example, the degree of novelty of a product has a large effect on the market launch.
- Advantage of the product or product property
  What advantage does the product compared to prod-

ucts that are already on the market? These can for example refer to the price or the use of a guarantee.

- Early product announcement
- Focused alignment on specific consumer groups

For a long term success, the HEINEMANN company has to show a high performance in quality and quantity. In addition to that, it has to provide new designs in order to stand out from the competition. A reasonable price-performance ratio and a mature marketing strategy are also important. At the same time, it is important to always keep an eye on the development of local manufacturers. For the future it is important that the company looks for an intermediary with good contacts in Iran. These contacts are important, if the unstable political situation changes. Because with direct connections to Iran it is easier to supply the Iranian market. It is advisable for the company to present the units at the next important trade fairs with the help of selected intermediaries. These important contacts should be made through discussions with customers. Before entering the market, all new sales channels abroad should also be carefully considered and analyzed. When exporting to countries outside the EU, certain regulations and conditions must be taken into account. When exporting from Germany to Iran, an export control must be carried out. This is one of the most important tasks that the "Bundesamt für Wirtschaft und Ausfuhrkontrolle" (BAFA) must fulfill. BAFA is an administrative and licensing authority that decides whether a delivery of goods may be exported and imported [11].
Another important conclusion of the study is that it only reflects a small fraction of the opinions held in Iran. Surveys are generally limited in their informative value to the number of people, who participated and it is difficult to reflect the opinion of an entire country. In order to be able to achieve a meaningful presentation of the opinion of all ENT specialists in the country, the access to a significantly larger part of the population would have been necessary, which would have gone beyond the scope of this paper.

Acknowledgement

This work has been carried out at HEINEMANN Medizintechnik GmbH (Kaltenkirchen, Germany) and supervised by the Institute of Biomedical Optics, Universität zu Lübeck. Informed consent has been obtained from all individuals included in this study.
I would like to thank Christin Babbick my paper for proofreading.
I also thank all participants who tooked part in the survey.

Author's Statement

Authors state no conflict of interest.

5 References

[1] Thoma T. , *Erfolgreiche Markteinführung*. Available: https://www.zitate.eu/autor/prof-dr-helmut-thoma-zitate/190904 [last accessed on 2021-01-26].

[2] Hohmann Rechtsanwälte, *Iran-Embargo*. Available: https://hohmann-rechtsanwaelte.de/iran-embargo.html [last accessed on 2021-01-26].

[3] Geiss M., *Marketing-Konzeption zur Rückgewinnung ausgewählter Einzelhandelskunden: Ein Relatiopnship Management Ansatz am Bsp des deutschen Buchhandels*. Springer Gabler, 2016.

[4] Call G., *Entstehung Und Markteinführung Von Produktneuheiten*. Gabler, 1997.

[5] Kuhn J., *Markteinführung neuer Produkte*. Auflage1, Deutsche Universität Verlag 2007.

[6] Privat communication with business experts during field study-interview

[7] Zoll, *Embargomaßnahmen*. Available: https://www.zoll.de [last accessed on 2021-01-26].

[8] Melchio O., *Implementation Day: Iran-Embargo gelockert-nicht aufgehoben*. Available: https://www.luther-lawfirm.com/fileadmin/user_upload/PDF/Presse/News/Iran_Embargo.pdf [last accessed on 2021-01-26].

[9] SPECTARIS e.V., *SPECTARIS-Standpunkt*. Available: https://www.spectaris.de[last accessed on 2021-01-26].

[10] Federal Register, *Verhängung von Sanktionen*. Available: https://www.federalregister.gov/documents/2020/01/14/2020-00534/imposing-sanctions-with-respect-to-additional-sectors\-of-iran [last accessed on 2021-01-26].

[11] Bundesamt für Wirtschaft und Ausfuhrkontrolle. Available: http://www.bafa.de/DE/Aussenwirtschaft/Ausfuhrkontrolle/Embargos/Iran/iran_node.html [last accessed on 2021-01-26].

Extend a Test Automation Framework with a Performance Logger

Till Wittenborg [1], Michael Voelker [2], and Steffi Jannasch [2]

[1] Biomedical Engineering, Luebeck University of Applied Sciences, till.wittenborg@stud.th-luebeck.de

[2] Drägerwerk AG & Co. KGaA, Lübeck, {michael.voelker, steffi.jannasch}@draeger.com

Abstract

When executing automated tests on Dräger medical devices using the framework *RTF*, it must be possible to reconstruct the test result from the information of the generated log files. In this work, the *RTF* is extended by the *Performance Logger* to record the hardware performance of the tested device in a file. The performance data can be requested via a network connection to the device. The Test Driven Development approach was used to achieve the high-quality requirements demanded by the *RTF* when adding the *Performance Logger*. A module named *Performance Analyser* was developed to visualize the performance data of a test execution in graphs and to add it to the *RTF* result database. The result database contains information about all test executions which are now extended by three tables for the performance data. The entries of the database can be analysed to compare the data over many test executions.

1 Introduction

Test Automation ensures the quality of a product and has great importance in all larger developments. For Drägerwerk as a medical manufacturer with highest quality standards the Test Automation is of particular importance. Automated tests at *Dräger* are executed using an internally developed framework, the *Remote Test Framework* (*RTF*), implemented in *Python*. The *RTF* is used during development and for official verification tests. The tests are autonomously executed without an observation through a person. Therefore, potential issues must be reconstructed from the log files. The *RTF* provides several different logger, each of which creates a log file for a different analysis purpose. Most issues during a test are either caused by an observed deviation of the DUT from its requirements, a bug in the test itself, or an issue during the test execution, like network problems. The log files are essential for the success of automated test execution.

The *Performance Logger* is implemented as an additional logger in the *RTF* to record the hardware performance of the DUT during the test execution in a log file. The recorded performance data includes the memory usage and the CPU load. These parameters can indicate performance issues of the DUT, like a linearly increasing allocation of memory blocks. Furthermore, an additional package, the *Performance Analyser*, is implemented to visualize the result file of the *Performance Logger*. A visualisation eases the analysis of the raw data. The *Performance Analyser* can also insert the most important indicators (maximum, minimum, mean) of the raw data into a database of the *RTF*. This allows comparing performance data between test executions.

2 Material and Methods

This chapter describes the applied implementation method Test Driven Development (TDD) and its influence on the code quality and the requirements of the *Performance Logger* and the *Performance Analyser*.

2.1 Requirements

The requirements were developed with the users and maintainers of the *RTF*. The *Performance Logger* is the actual logger integrated in the *RTF*. The *Performance Analyser* is a *Python* package to process the result file and is not integrated in the *RTF*, because the extension of the *RTF* shall be as small as possible. The desired structure is shown in figure 1.

2.1.1 Requirements Performance Logger

The *Performance Logger* should periodically request the performance data from the Medical Information Bus (MIB) nodes of the DUT, format them and write them to a result CSV file. The MIB is defined in ANSI/IEEE 1073 [1] and is a communication system for health care. The performance data of the DUT can be requested via the MIB nodes.
The *RTF* must meet high-quality requirements, as it is used for the verification and international certification of medical devices according to, among others, the Medical Device Regulation. The *Performance Logger* modules added to the *RTF* have to fullfil these requirements. The *Performance Logger* shall not influence the test execution with the *RTF* in any way. This must be proven by performance and unit tests.

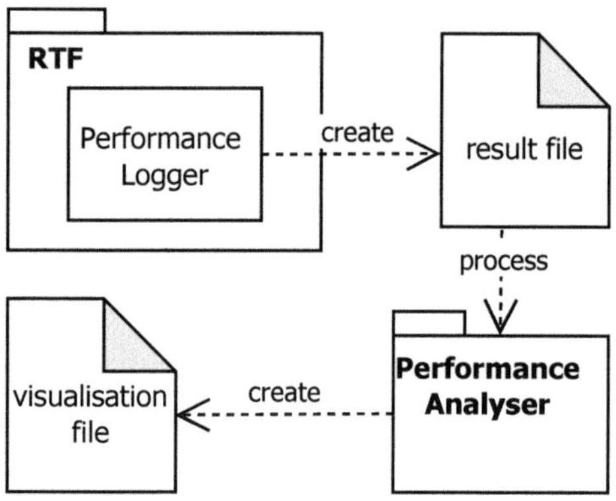

Figure 1: This figure shows the *Performance Logger* as one module of the *RTF* and the *Performance Analyser* as separate package. The result file is created by the *Performance Logger* and processed to the visualisation file by the *Performance Analyser*. The (other) modules of the packages are not shown.

The *RTF* configuration file defines all settings for test execution. The *Performance Logger* should be controlled with two settings in the *RTF* configuration to enable or disable the *Performance Logger* and to control the interval between records. The created result file should contain the time stamp as the first column and the measured data in the following columns.

2.1.2 Requirements Performance Analyser

The *Performance Analyser* should visualize the raw data of the result file in graphs. The graphs shall be stored together with the most important information of the test execution in a visualisation file. For each recorded performance parameter, there should be one graph with the time on the x-axis and the values on the y-axis. It shall be possible to add trends to the graphs.
The most important indicators (maximum, minimum, mean) for every parameter shall be inserted in the already existent *RTF* result database. The database must be extended with suitable tables to store the data.

2.2 TDD Application

Test Driven Development (TDD) was used during the implementation of the *Performance Logger*. TDD is a development methodology focused on testing during the implementation. The special aspect is that unit tests are written before the corresponding product code. This initially slows down the implementation progress, but results in unit tests that cover almost the entire product code. With a high test coverage, new errors introduced due code changes can be located quickly. The earlier an error is detected, the easier and cheaper it is to correct [2]. [3]
Another advantage is that the developer must define the expected behaviour of the feature to implement in the test. The test serves as executable documentation of the product code [3]. The requirements for the *Performance Logger* include a high test coverage that can be intuitively reached with the application of TDD. Another reason for the usage of TDD, also for the *Performance Analyser*, is that TDD improves the quality and the maintainability of the code. [3]

3 Results and Discussion

This section describes the *Performance Logger* to generate the result file, the *Performance Analyser* to further process the result files after a test execution and the extension of the *RTF* result database.

3.1 Performance Logger

The *Performance Logger* is activated in the *RTF* via the configuration file of test execution. Then, an extra thread to request, format, and log the performance data is started.
The MIB nodes of the DUT providing the performance data have an address and can be requested with an already existent *RTF* module via a network connection. Requesting a MIB node with its address returns a string containing one or many performance values. For instance, a MIB node could return a string containing the CPU loads of four kernels. The single values must be extracted from the strings and are then written into the CSV file. This is one record. The names of the performance parameters are written as column headers in the first row of the file and the single performance values are then assigned to the corresponding column. The DUT can be a ventilator, anaesthesia device or another type of device which is supported by the *RTF*. The device types have different hardware (e.g. number of CPU-kernels) and therefore, different MIB nodes returning different strings. Therefore, special handling is implemented for every device type. The processing of the returned strings is error prone and therefore is tested by numerous unit tests for every device type.
Two new settings are added to the configuration file to control the *Performance Logger*. The first setting enables the *Performance Logger* when set to True and the second setting takes an integer determining the interval between the requests. For a smaller interval, the resolution of the performance data gets higher at the cost of increased network traffic. Too high network traffic might influence the test execution and should be avoided. Therefore, the resolution is restricted to maximum of one request per second. The activation of the *Performance Logger* via the configuration has the benefit, that no testcase must be adapted to enable performance logging. Test executions for official verification can disable the *Performance Logger* simply via the configuration file, if the performance data are not required for this.
The requesting, formatting and writing of the performance data in the *RTF* is done within the separate thread *SystemHealthThread* that is started, when the *Performance Logger* is enabled. The *Python threading* package [4] is used for its implementation. Multithreading has the big advantage, that the main logic of the *RTF* is executed in parallel to the *SystemHealthThread* which lowers the risk of an influence significantly.

As required, the potential influence of the *Performance Logger* on the test execution was analysed. The two biggest risks of an influence are delays in the test execution due to increased network traffic and termination of the test execution due to an error in the modules of the *Performance Logger*. The duration of test execution with and without the *Performance Logger* was compared to check if the increased network traffic through the *Performance Logger* slows the test execution. As a result, the duration was not affected by the *Performance Logger*. Furthermore, the time of an active *Performance Logger* thread was compared with the total execution time. The result is a share of significantly less than one percent on the total execution time. The high unit test coverage reduces the risk of errors in the *Performance Logger* and a unit test focusing on the performance of the string processing was passed. In conclusion, it was proven that the *Performance Logger* does not influence the test execution. The performance analysis, unit tests and code reviews lead to an approval of the integration of the *Performance Logger* into the *RTF*.

3.2 Performance Analyser

The *Performance Analyser* aims to further process the raw data from the result file. The *Performance Analyser* can process a result file "locally" to create a visualisation file with graphs for all parameters at the local PC or "globally". Processing the result file "globally", creates the visualisation file in a public directory available for all users of the *RTF* and inserts the key performance values (maximum, minimum, mean) of each parameter to the *RTF* result database. The *RTF* database is a *MySql* database that stores information about every test execution. Figure 2 shows the two processing options. The visualisation file is generated with the *Python* package *plotly* [5]. Figure 3 shows an example graph of the visualisation file in HTML format that can be opened with every browser. It is possible to add linear trends to the graphs to forecast workload problems, such as when the maximum available memory blocks will be reached.

The local or global processing is started by executing the *Performance Analyser* with the path to the result file as an argument. When the argument is a directory, all found result files in the directory are processed. Other options, like adding trends, can be controlled by additional arguments. The local processing is made available as windows executable file (exe) to ease the usage and to remove the dependency on a properly configured *Python* environment. The local processing can be used for a fast check of the performance data after test execution. The global processing is suitable to store the results in the long term and publicly. When many performance results are processed globally, the database will contain many performance key values and the device performance between many test executions on different software versions of the products can be compared. The database contains only the key performance values which might be insufficient for a further investigation of one test execution. To allow a detailed view of one specific test execution, the result file and the visualisation file are copied to a public directory where all users of the *RTF* have access to. The path to the public directory is inserted in the database.

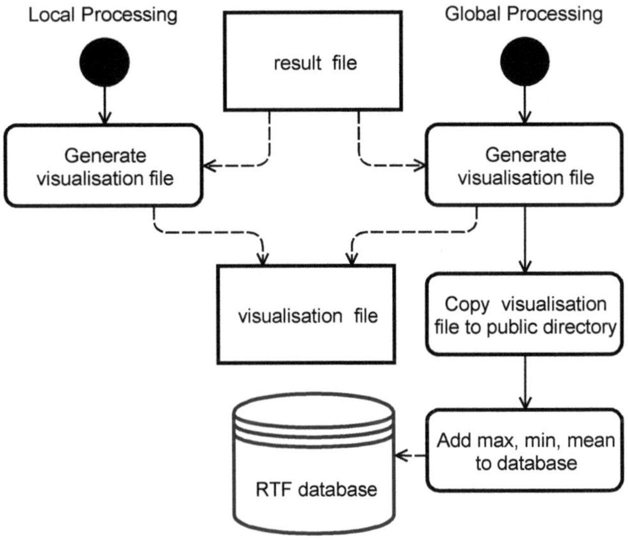

Figure 2: Activity diagram showing the local and global processing options to create a visualisation file containing graphs for every parameter from a result file. The global processing additionally adds the key figures to the *RTF* result database and makes the visualisation file available for all *RTF* users.

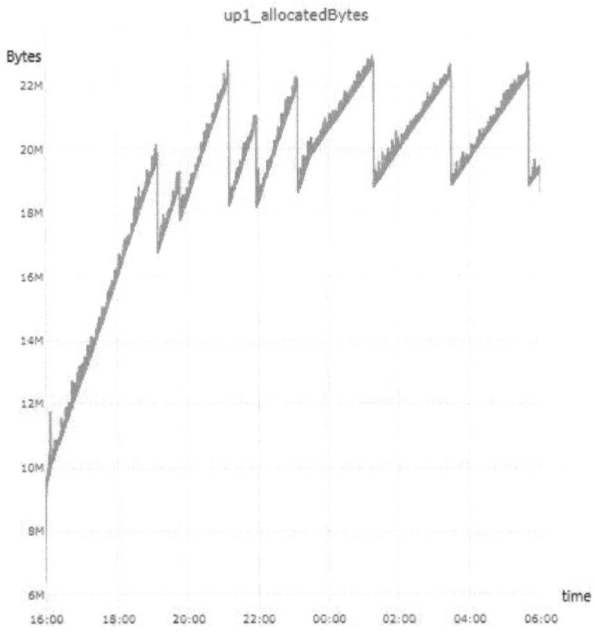

Figure 3: One graph of the visualisation file generated by the *Performance Analyser* opened in a browser. It can be seen, how the memory blocks are more and more allocated until they are released again. The x-axis shows the time and the y-axis the allocated memory bytes.

3.3 Database Extension

The *RTF* result database contains entries of millions of test executions. Much information about a test execution is stored in this database, for instance the start time, the duration and the result. Every test execution has the unique key *testExecutionID*. The performance data should be linked as additional information to test execution. Three new tables are added to the database and linked to the corresponding test execution using the *testExecutionID* key. The *RTF* result database can not store all information of the result file, because one file contains thousands of values. Therefore, only the maximum, minimum and mean value for every parameter are inserted in the database.

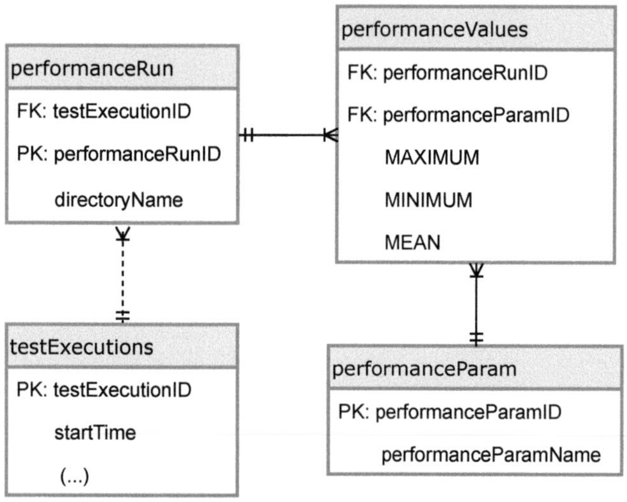

Figure 4: Excerpt of the *RTF* result database showing the three added tables for the performance data. The *testExecutions* table has the primary key *testExecutionID* that is unique for every added test execution. Three tables necessary are to avoid any redundancy. *PK* means primary key and *FK* foreign key.

Figure 4 shows the three added tables to store the performance information. There are three tables required, because otherwise redundant values would occur. The directory path had to be added in a table to the *testExecutionID*, because it is unique for every test execution. For every DUT type, there is a set of different performance parameter (for every CPU and memory usage) independent of the test execution. Therefore, the table *performanceParam* is independent of the *testExecutionID* in the database. The *performanceValues* depend on the test execution and the parameter. So, the table *performanceValues* also depends on the foreign keys *performanceParamID* and *performanceRunID*. The *performanceRunID* is coupled to the *testExecutionID* via the *performanceRun* table. The queries to extend the database, to insert data and to get data are developed in *Python* scripts using the *MySqldb* package [6] and are part of the *Performance Analyser*. As the *RTF* result database already contains a large amount of valuable data, it is important to not affect the database with the extension for the performance data. All queries had to be reviewed properly and were tested on a local backup of the production database before being applied to the production database.

4 Conclusion

The *Performance Logger* has been implemented successfully and is enabled for most test executions, because no additional hardware is required. Furthermore, it was proven that no negative influence on the *RTF* happens. The graphs with linear trends of the visualisation file ease the analysis. With the support of the *Performance Logger*, one issue in a device has already been identified. The *Performance Analyser* has been extended to support visualization of data from different file formats. Therefore, the *Performance Analyser* is not restricted to visualize data of the *Performance Logger*. This extension was possible due to the clearly structured programming of the *Performance Analyser* through the application of TDD. Global processing is not used as frequently as local processing, yet. The more performance data of a product is stored in the database, the more valuable this data becomes. The global processing must be promoted to be automatically executed as part of the automated test execution for all products using the simple interface of the *Performance Analyser*.

Acknowledgement

The work has been carried out at Drägerwerk AG & Co. KGaA and supervised by Professor Mertins, Institute for Signal Processing, Universität zu Lübeck.

Author's Statement

Conflict of interest: Authors state no conflict of interest. Informed consent: Informed consent has been obtained.

5 References

[1] M. Glass, *ANSI/IEEE 1073: Medical Information Bus (MIB)*, Health Informatics Journal 4.2, pp. 7283 1998

[2] J. Gregory and L. Crispin., *Agile Testing*, Pearson Education, 2009

[3] R.C. Martin, *Clean Code*, Pearson Education, Inc., 2009

[4] Python Software Foundation, *threading Thread-based parallelism*, https://docs.python.org/3.7/library/threading.html, , [Accessed: 25-January-2021]

[5] Plotly, *Plotly Python Open Source Graphing Library*, https://plotly.com/python, [Accessed: 25-January-2021]

[6] Andy Dustman, *MySqldb Documentation*, https://mysqlclient.readthedocs.io/user_guide.html, [Accessed: 25-January-2021]

Development and Evaluation of a digital shop floor board in an administrative quality department

Jan Dieker [1]

[1] Biomedical Engineering, Luebeck University of Applied Sciences, jan.dieker@stud.th-luebeck.de

Abstract

The objectives of performance increase, utilization of workers‘ complete potential and reduction for waste are ongoing topics for the production. In the production departments shop floor management is used to reach these objectives. In administrative departments the use of shop floor management is presently uncommon. Therefore, the aim of this paper is to develop and evaluate a digital shop floor board in an administrative quality department. The development was aligned with the Darmstadt shop floor model on a digital shop floor board. The use of shop floor board shows opportunities in administrative quality departments. In connection with shop floor meetings it can lead to the optimization of Key-Performance-Indicators. Further evaluation is needed to prove the system's performance.

1 Introduction

Current challenges in manufacturing systems are increasing global competition, rising number of product variants and shorter product lifecycles. An answer to face these challenges is lean production. Lean production is a common model for nowadays companies. The goals of lean production are efficient design of value creation, reduction of hierarchy depth and shorter communication channels. [1]

These goals are closely connected to the shop floor management (SFM). SFM can be described as "Leading at the actual production place". The idea is to solve problems directly at the shop floor. Besides, the mentioned advantages of lean production, SFM addresses the objectives of utilization of workers‘ complete potential and optimization of Key-Performance-Indicators (KPIs). [2]

State of the art of SFM is on an analog basis. A new development is the digital SFM. The digital SFM provides several advantages compared to the analog management. A major advantage is the reduction of collection time for the visualisation of the shop floor board and reduction of preparation time for meetings [3]. Further advantages of digital shop floor management are the visualization of KPIs with automatic color coding, matching of tasks directly in the system or automatic reminder of next steps [4].

The advantages of SFM in production departments are widely known. However, the use of SFM in administrative departments is little investigated in the literature so far. This paper describes the development and evaluation of a digital SFB in a supplier quality assurance (SQA) department. The SQA is assigned with administrative quality topics. The range of tasks in the SQA extends over the entire life cycle of a product. Tasks include processing of claims and processing of First Article Inspections (FAIs). [5]

2 Material and Methods

2.1 Darmstadt shop floor management model

The objectives and topics about SFM are differently described in the literature. A model to systematize the SFM is the Darmstadt SFM. The Darmstadt SFM is a systematic approach for SFM with objectives, requirements and activities. The model is shown in Fig. 1. It is built up from a control cycle with different phases. [6]

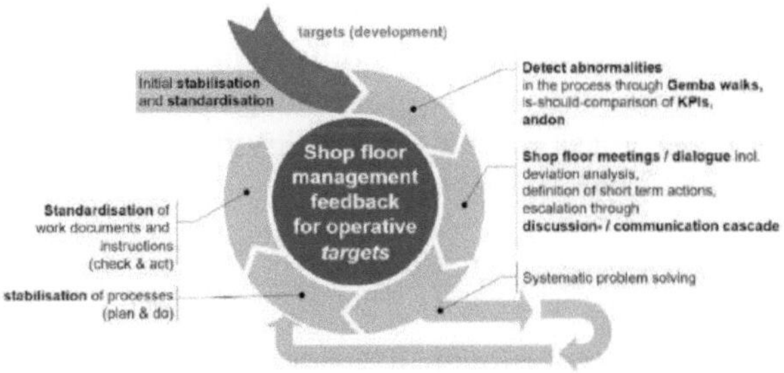

Figure 1: Darmstadt shop floor management model. The model describes a systematic approach to install an SFM.

Phase zero is not a part of the control cycle itself. It enables through an initial stabilisation of processes and standardisation of work instructions, that the shop floor management is not overwhelmed with problems. Additionally, objectives of the related department are defined. The first phase in the model is the detection of abnormalities. This can be done with Gemba walks or is-should-comparison of KPIs on a shop floor board (SFB). The SFB is a collection of visualisations of the regarding KPIs. It enables a quick and easy understanding of the current situation. The second phase in-

cludes shop floor meetings. The meetings include deviation analysis, definition of short term actions and escalations. During the meetings the SFB is used as well. The following phase is outside of the control cycle and is defined through systematic problem solving. Defined measures or solutions for the original problem are planed and tackled in the next phase. The final phase is the stabilisation of processes and standardisation of work instructions.
The Darmstadt SFM model is used to implement the SFB in the SQA.

2.2 Definition of Targets and KPIs

In a first step, the KPIs and the targets are defined for the SFB.

Supplier Failure Rate
Goal: Reduce the number of defective parts delivered from supplier in order to ensure undisturbed production and devices according to the specification.

$$KPI[ppm] = \frac{Sum\ of\ defective\ quantity}{Sum\ of\ total\ received\ goods} * 1.000.000 \quad (1)$$

Target: Target value for the KPI is 400 ppm.

Supplier Claim - on time closed
Goal: Ensure the prompt processing of supplier claims.

$$KPI[\%] = \frac{No.\ of\ closed\ claims\ in\ 28\ days}{No.\ of\ claims\ due\ in\ 28\ days} * 100 \quad (2)$$

Target: Target value for the KPI is 80 %.

First article inspection - first time right
Goal: Reduce the number of repeating FAIs passes to ensure R&D project timelines and undisturbed series production and lifecycle-management.

$$KPI[\%] = \frac{No.\ of\ approved\ FAI}{Sum\ of\ FAI\ performed} * 100 \quad (3)$$

Target: Target value for the KPI is 80 %.

First article inspection – on time closed
Goal: Ensure the prompt processing of supplier claims.

$$KPI[\%] = \frac{No.\ of\ performed\ FAIs\ in\ 28\ days}{No.\ of\ FAIs\ due\ in\ 28\ days} * 100 \quad (4)$$

Target: Target value for the KPI is 80 %.

An initial standardisation and stabilisation does not have to be performed, since the processes of claims handling and FAIs are already sufficiently described.

2.3 Implementation

For the development of the shop floor board the business intelligence software *Power BI* from *Microsoft* is used. Power BI enables wide possibilities regarding the definition of KPIs, sources of data imports, visualisations and interactivity.

2.3.1 Data transformation

The data import flow can be seen in Fig. 2. It starts with the export of the relevant data via transactions from the companies enterprise resource planning (ERP) system. The ERP system is used for electronic process handling and contains all relevant information needed for the evaluation. The exported data is saved as excel format in a *Sharepoint* cloud. The approach has the advantage, that the SFB will be located at the Sharepoint cloud too, so that a high performance regarding loading times can be achieved. In the last step, the data is loaded with an automated scheduled refresh in the board.

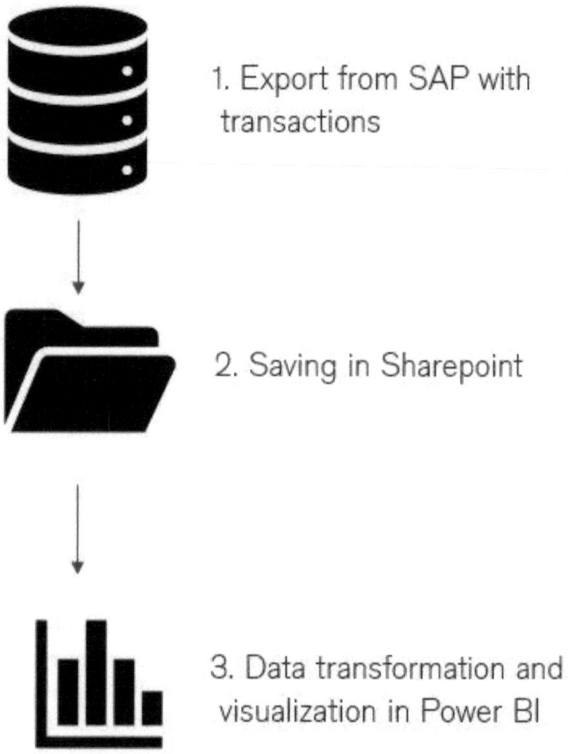

Figure 2: Data import flow of the SFB

The exported data need to be transformed, so that it can be used in the SFB. One possible feature in the transformation of data is connecting several excel files of the same transaction into one table. This enables a continuous update of data without exporting the complete period from the ERP system. Furthermore, the data is cleaned and prepared for visualisations. The preparation includes the creation of additionally needed columns.

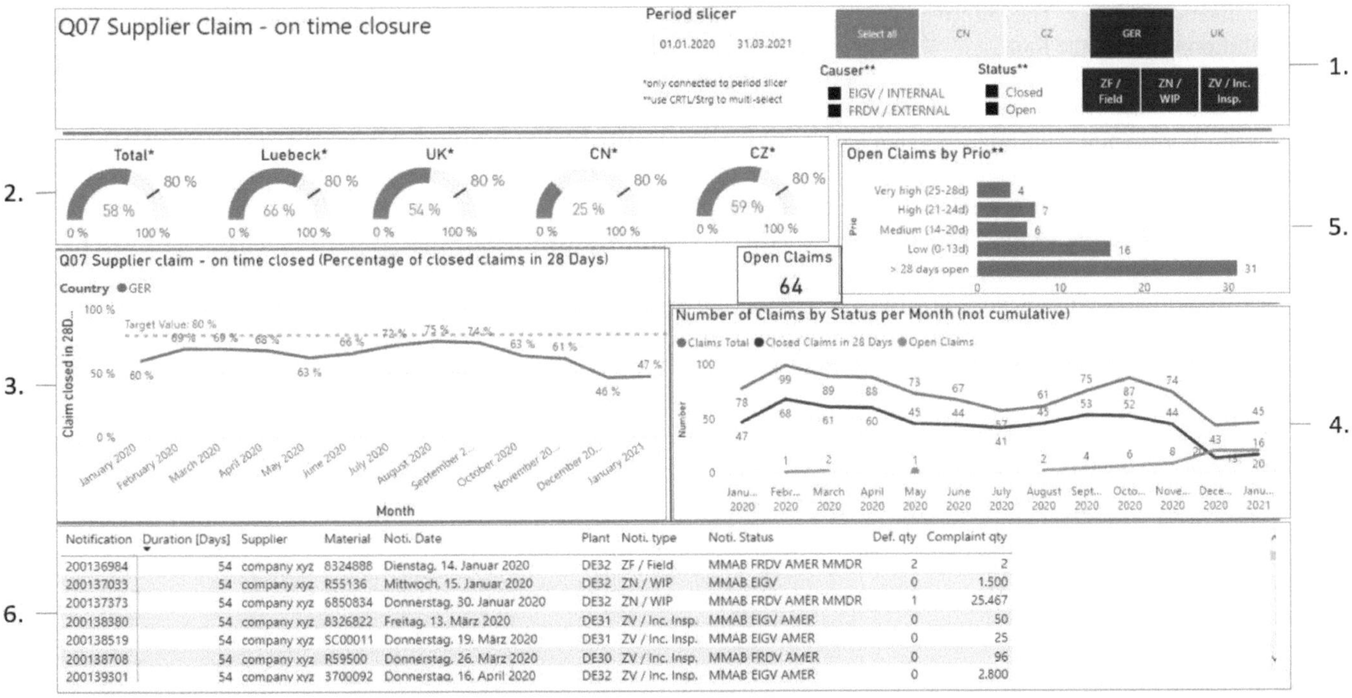

Figure 3: Visualisations of the report page: Supplier claim - on time closed. The report page is filled with different visualisations, which fulfill the main purpose to increase the performance of claim handling. The first area is filled with slicer and main information. The second area shows the overall KPI in different countries. The third chart shows the KPI by month. The fourth chart shows the number of claims in total numbers. the fifth chart shows the claims binned in different categories of prioritisation. The sixth area displays a detailed view of the included notifications.

2.3.2 Visualisation

For every KPI a separate Power BI report page is built. In Fig. 3 the visualisations of the KPI *Supplier claim - on time closed* is exemplary shown. The report pages for the other KPIs have a similar structure. The layout of the report page follows a hierarchic order. In the first section general information about the report page and possible settings for the visualisations are displayed. The report can be filtered regarding the period, country, origin of claim, causer of claim and processing status. Outside of the report view further settings can be done regarding supplier and material.

The second group of visualisations shows the KPI in gauge charts. Gauge charts have a main advantages, that is-should comparisons can be easily done with the underlying color coding. In the shown report it is easy to recognize, that none of the branches reach the target.

The third visualisation shows the KPI on a timeline. Trends and performance can be supervised over a longer period of time. The fourth visualisation displays the number of claims by status per month. The fifth visualisation shows the open claims ordered in a bar chart. The claims are grouped regarding their processing time into different prioritization groups. With the prioritization of claims the SFM can focus on claims, which are almost closely to the target border.

The sixth section is a matrix with the listed notifications including all relevant data. Besides the settings and filters, the report offers a high degree on interactivity. All visualisations are connected, so that on a selection of a data point, the other visualisations react to this. For example, if the label "Very high (25-28d)" is chosen, the matrix shows the associated notifications.

3 Results and Discussion

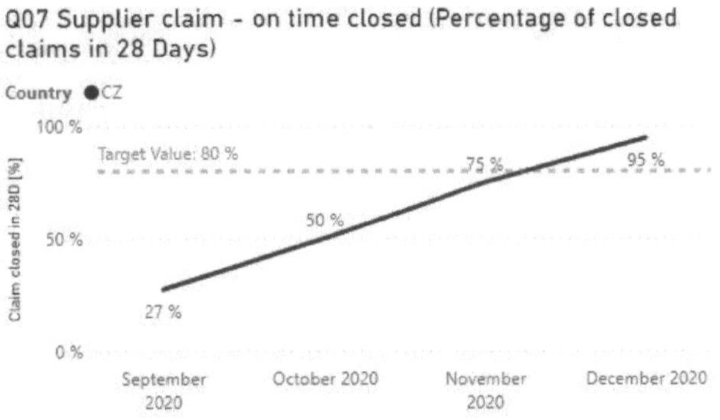

Figure 4: Visualisation of the KPI: Supplier claim - on time closed in Czech Republic. The chart shows an increase in performance from 27% to 95% within three months.

All in all, the established SFB is used on a regular basis in the plants in Luebeck and UK. Due to the reason, that the KPIs are calculated on the same basis, a comparability between the different plants is given. The proposed solution is used as a support during shop floor meetings with the

visualisation of KPIs. The intuitive implementation reduces inhibitions against the tool.
The implementation as a digital SFB is a major advantage because meeting participants do not have to be physically present. Furthermore, the boards do not have to be prepared and are available all the time.
Shop floor meetings in connection with the digital SFB were established in October 2020 in a department for processing claims in a Czech plant. Particularly, the report page for *supplier claim - on time closed* was used during these meetings. As shown in Fig. 4, the efficiency of the claim processing increased from 27% in September 2020 to 95% in December 2020.
The design of the proposed method allows direct systematic problem solving, due to the variety of visualisations and exported calculated data. During shop floor meetings measures for continuous improvement were discussed and are currently in the realization.

4 Conclusion

This paper has presented the development of a digital shop floor board in an administrative quality department and evaluated the result. It has been shown, that the digital shop floor board is a useful model in an administrative quality department. To gather the full potential of SFM further evaluation is needed.

Acknowledgement

The work has been carried out at Dräger Safety AG Co. KGaA, Luebeck and supervised by Prof. Dr. Wen-Huan Wang, Department of Applied Natural Sciences, Luebeck University of Applied Sciences.

Author's Statement

Conflict of interest: Authors state no conflict of interest.

5 References

[1] R. Koether and K. Meier, *Lean Production für die variantenreiche Einzelfertigung. Flexibilität wird zum neuen Standard.* Springer Gabler, München, 2020.

[2] B. Leyendecker and P. Pötters, *Shopfloor Management. Führen am Ort des Geschens.* Carl Hanser Verlag, München, 2018.

[3] A. Grundnig and S. Meitinger, *Produktionscockpit 4.0 als Shopfloor Management der Zukunft.* In: ZWF, vol. 113, no. 12 pp. 873–877, 2018

[4] A. Meißner, F. Grunert and J. Metternich, *Digital shop floor management: A target state.* In: Procedia CIRP, vol. 93 pp. 311–315, 2020

[5] H. Brüggemann and P. Bremer, *Grundlagen Qualitätsmanagement. Von den Werkzeugen über Methoden zum TQM.* Springer Vieweg, Wiesbaden, 2020.

[6] C. Hertle, M. Tisch, J. Metternich and E. Abele, *Das Darmstädter Shopfloor Management-Modell.* In: ZWF, vol. 112, no. 3, pp.118–121, 2017.

7

Sensor Data Analysis

From sEMG based Gesture Classification towards Regression

Kamran Mohammad-Zadeh [1], Philipp Koch [2], Mark Dreier [3], and Alfred Mertins [2]

[1] Medical Engineering Science, Universität zu Lübeck, kamran.mohammadzadeh@student.uni-luebeck.de
[2] Institute for Signal Processing, Universität zu Lübeck, {ph.koch, alfred.mertins}@uni-luebeck.de
[3] Institute for Signal Processing, Universität zu Lübeck, mark.dreier@student.uni-luebeck.de

Abstract

The regression of hand movements based on sEMG data becomes more and more relevant. Therefore this work aims at getting a deeper understanding of the regression problem and the corresponding data as well as developing new training approaches as the choice of the loss function appears to be a critical factor for training the networks. First the possibility of using hand-tracking data to classify hand gestures has been evaluated. For this a RNN was used to predict the hand gesture on the basis of the hand-tracking data reaching an accuracy of 88%. After that the classification performance of a classifier using hand-tracking data regressed by a regressor has been evaluated. Lastly a pre-trained classifier is used to generate the loss needed for the optimization of the regressor leading to an accuracy of 88%.

1 Introduction

Commercially available hand prosthesis only allow for a limited number of hand gestures. The unintuitive control of these hand prostheses leads to a high rejection rate. A study from the American Academy of Orthotists and Prosthetists [1] shows that the unintuitive control and the limited amount of possible hand gestures of prostheses represents one of the major points of criticism.

Advancements in research of artificial intelligence enable a prediction of hand gestures using signals acquired by surface Electromyography (sEMG) [2], [3], [4], which allows for a more intuitive control and a larger amount of hand gestures.

In [5] it has been shown that recurrent neural networks (RNN) are able to classify a fairly large amount of hand gestures using sEMG-signals.

The classification only offers a limited and predefined set of hand gestures for the user. For a more intuitive and more flexible hand prothesis control a regression of the hand position is desired.

As shown in [6] RNNs are capable to regress the hand position using sEMG signals.

This paper examines the possibility of classifying hand gestures using hand-tracking data. The hand-tracking data was collected using a cyber glove and will be referred to as glove data. Preliminary experiments have shown that the loss function has a huge influence on the regression results. Therefore, the aim of this work is to start with investigations leading towards new strategies to train the networks. First, it was investigated whether it is possible to predict the hand gestures based on the glove data. A RNN receives the glove data as input and predicts the corresponding hand gestures. As a second step, it was investigated whether the classification of hand gestures can also be done on the basis of regressed glove data. For this purpose a regressor first predicts the glove data using the sEMG data as input. Then a classifier uses these predicted glove data to predict the corresponding hand gestures. The last experiment is designed similar to the second. Again a regressor predicts glove values which are then used by the classifier to predict the corresponding hand gestures. This time the classifier is pre-trained and its weights are no longer updated. The regressor now uses the loss of the pre-trained classifier to update its weights.

2 Problem definition

To clarify the different problem definitions dealt with in this paper they will be briefly introduced in the following.

2.1 Classification

Classification is the mapping of the feature space onto a set of class labels. In our case this corresponds to the prediction of the hand gesture using the glove data. The resulting classification can be described as

$$\mathcal{C} : \mathbf{y}_t \in \mathbb{R}^D \rightarrow z_t \in \mathbb{L} \tag{1}$$

with $\mathbf{y}_t$ being the glove data and z_t being the class label at time step t, respectively. D is the number of channels of the glove data and $\mathbb{L}$ is the set containing all possible hand gestures.

2.2 Regression

Regression is the mapping of the feature space onto another continuous space. In our case this corresponds to predicting

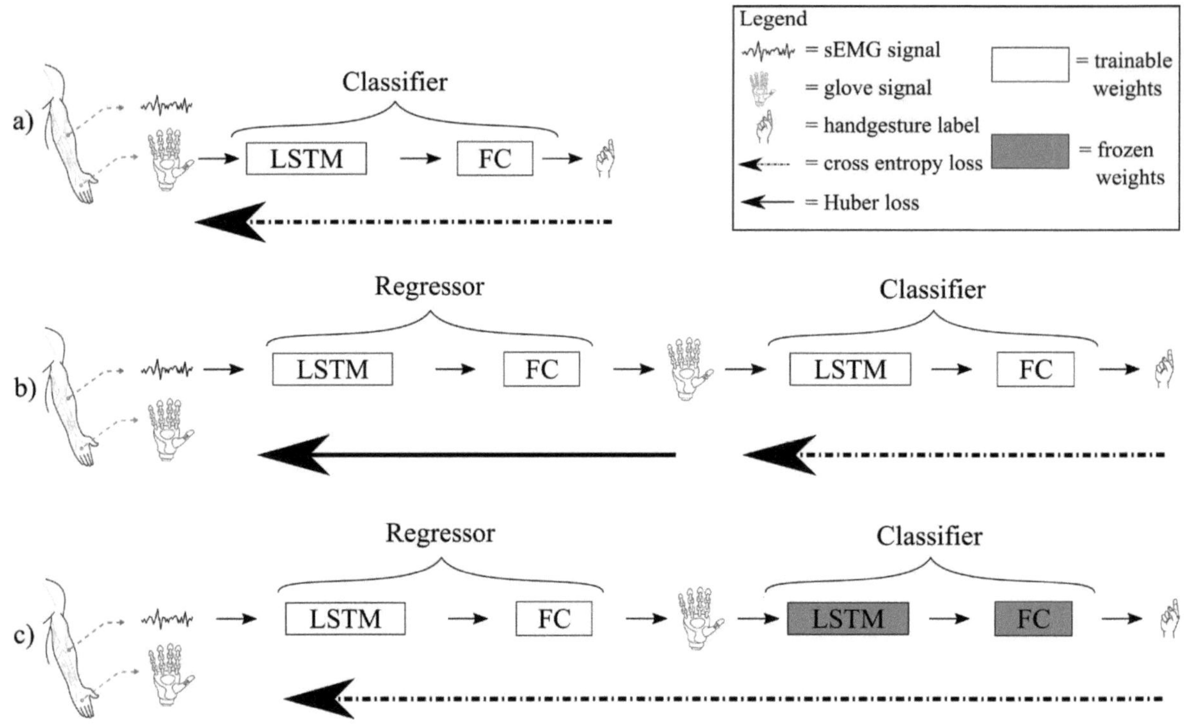

Figure 1: Presentation of the different network architectures and training processes. (a) Classification of the hand gestures using the glove signal. The parameters of the classifier are optimised by minimising the cross entropy loss. (b) Classification of the hand gestures using the regressed glove signal by the regressor. The regressor predicts the glove signal using the sEMG signal. The parameters of the regressor are optimised by minimising the Huber loss while the parameters of the classifier are optimised by minimising the cross entropy loss. (c) Classification of the hand gestures using a pre-trained classifier which takes the glove signal predicted by the regressor as input. While the parameters of the classifier are no longer updated the parameters of the regressor are updated by minimising the cross entropy loss.

the hand position represented by the glove data using the corresponding sEMG signal. Thus the regression problem can be formulated as

$$\mathcal{R} : \mathbf{x}_t \in \mathbb{R}^C \rightarrow \mathbf{y}_t \in \mathbb{R}^D \quad (2)$$

with $\mathbf{x}$ being the sEMG signal and $\mathbf{y}$ being the glove data. C corresponds to the number of electrode channels.

2.3 Combination

In this work we propose the combination of the regression and classification problem. First, the regression problem is solved analogous to (2). Then the classification problem is solved based on the results of the regression. The proposed combination of the regression and classification task can therefore be described as

$$\mathcal{RC} : \mathbf{x}_t \in \mathbb{R}^C \rightarrow \mathbf{y}_t \in \mathbb{R}^D \rightarrow z_t \in \mathbb{L}. \quad (3)$$

3 Material and Methods

In this paper different network architectures and training procedures are proposed which will be described in the following.

3.1 Network architectures

All network architectures in this work are based on RNNs in form of Long-Short-Term-Memory (LSTM) cells [7] as feature extractors. Fully-connected (FC) layers followed by a softmax layer are used as classifier or without the softmax activation function in case of the regressor .

Fig. 1 shows a schematic overview of the three different network architectures and training procedures. The first architecture Fig. 1(a)is used to solve the classification problem described in (1). The LSTM cell takes the glove data as input and the FC layer uses the extracted feature to predict the class label. The classifier networks weights θ_c are optimised by minimising the cross-entropy loss

$$E(\theta_c \mid \mathbf{y}_t, z_t) = -z_t \log(\hat{z}_t(\theta_c \mid \mathbf{y}_t)). \quad (4)$$

Here $\mathbf{y}_t$ represents the glove data, z_t the class label and $\hat{z}_t$ the predicted class label.

The second architecture Fig. 1(b) is used to solve the combined regression and classification problem described in (3). The first part can be viewed as the regressor which takes the sEMG signal $\mathbf{x}_t$ as input and predicts the glove values $\hat{\mathbf{y}}_t$. The weights θ_r of the regressor network are updated by minimising the Huber loss. With $q := (\theta_r \mid \mathbf{x}_t)$ the Huber loss is given by

$$E(q, \mathbf{y}_t) = \begin{cases} \frac{1}{2}(\mathbf{y}_t - \hat{\mathbf{y}}_t(q))^2 & \text{for} \mid \mathbf{y}_t - \hat{\mathbf{y}}_t(q) \mid \leq \delta \\ \delta \mid \mathbf{y}_t - \hat{\mathbf{y}}_t(q) \mid - \frac{1}{2}\delta^2 & \text{otherwise} \end{cases} . \tag{5}$$

The hyperparameter δ has been set to one. The classifier then takes the predicted glove values as input and predicts the class label. The weights θ_c of the classifiers are again optimised by minimising the cross-entropy loss described in (4).

The third network architecture Fig. 1(c) is similar to the second. Again the problem described in (3) is solved, but the classifier is pre-trained identical to the first architecture (a) and the weights are then frozen. Now the weights of the regressor θ_r network are updated by minimising the cross entropy loss

$$E(\theta_r \mid \hat{\mathbf{y}}_t, z_t) = -z_t \log(\hat{z}_t(\theta_r \mid \hat{\mathbf{y}}_t)). \tag{6}$$

Each LSTM cell consists of 128 hidden neurons while the FC layers of the regressor and classifier consist of D and L neurons, respectively. D stands for the number of glove channels and L for the number of different class labels.

4 Experiments

In this section, the dataset used and the data preprocessing are presented.

4.1 Dataset

The dataset [8] used in this paper belongs to the ninapro project which provides various datasets which are used to benchmark the results of various tasks regarding hand prostheses control such as regression and classification. The database contains 20 able bodied subjects and two amputees. For the data acquisition, the subjects were shown a video of the hand movement to be performed, which they were asked to imitate. Each of the 40 hand gestures was repeated six times. The sEMG data was acquired using 14 surface electrodes while the hand position was tracked using a cyber glove. Only the 20 able bodied subjects have been considered as only they provide meaningful glove data.

4.2 Data preprocessing

The data set was divided into training and test set as recommended in [8]. The sEMG data as well as the glove data have been subject to a channel-wise standardisation. The mean and standard deviation of each of the D glove channels and C sEMG channels are computed using the training dataset. The standardisation was achieved by subtracting by the corresponding mean and dividing by the corresponding standard deviation. This results in a mean of zero and a standard deviation of one for the training set.

To create the training data, the sEMG data as well as the glove data are divided into one-second windows. This is followed by a subdivision of the windows into 200 segments of length 5 ms. This process is shown schematically in Fig. 3. Unlike the training data, the test data is not divided into windows. In the test case, a repetition of a hand movement is transferred to the network as a complete sequence. This sequence is also divided into 5 ms segments. In the test, the network predicts again a hand movement for each of these segments.

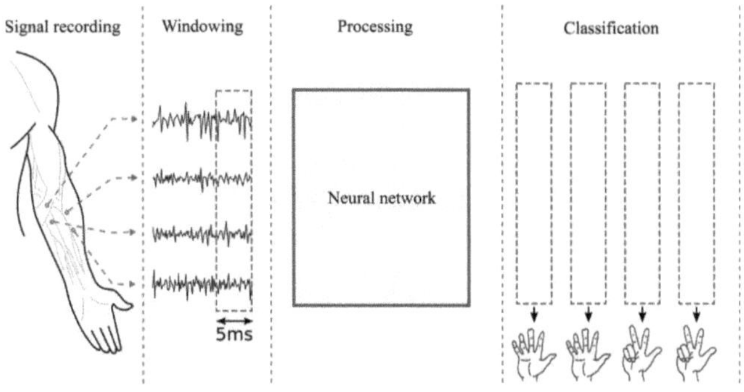

Figure 2: Schematic processing of the windowing of the sEMG signal and the following classification. First the sEMG signal is devided into 5 ms window segments. These window segments are then fed into a neural network which predicts a hand gesture for each segment.

5 Results

For the evaluation of the three proposed network architectures and training procedures, the classification accuracy P on the testing set has been used. It denotes the ratio of the number of correctly classified hand movements N_{correct} to the total number of hand movements included in the testing set. Thus P is given by:

$$P = \frac{N_{\text{correct}}}{N_{\text{total}}} \cdot 100\%. \tag{7}$$

In the Fig. 2 the course of the testing accuracy P over the ten training epochs is shown. The full line corresponds to the setup in Fig. 1(a) while the dashed and dotted lines represent the approaches in Figs. 1(b) and 1(c), respectively. The first architecture starts with an accuracy of 86.6% and rises slightly to a final accuracy of 88.0%. The second architecture starts with an accuracy of 76.4% which rises to a final accuracy of 87.3%. The last setup starts with a lower accuracy of 73.5% which continues to rise to a final accuracy of 86%. Thus, the first architecture achieves the highest accuracy, while the second and third approaches achieve an accuracy lower by 1% and 2%, respectively.

The results show that glove data based classification is possible and that regressed glove data can also be used for classification. The use of a pre-trained classifier for loss generation led to a deterioration of the classification results.

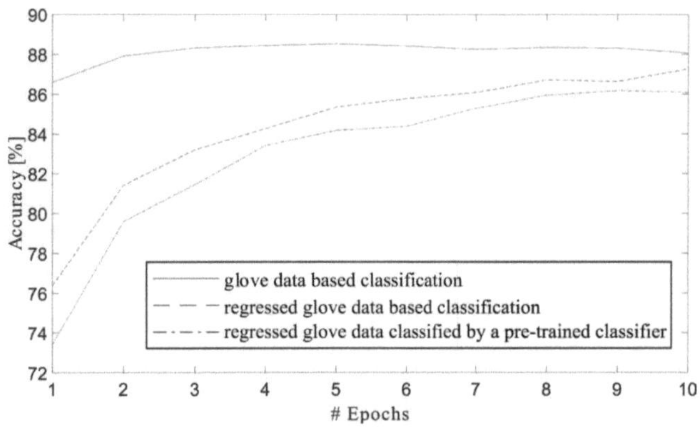

Figure 3: Course of the test accuracy over the epochs for the presented network architectures and training procedures. In green the classification based on the glove data is shown. Red represents the classification based on the regressed glove data. Lastly blue shows the course of the accuracy of the classification using the pre-trained classifier.

6 Conclusion

In this work the possibility of predicting hand gestures using the glove data has been explored. Three network architectures and training procedures have been tested. It has been shown that glove data based classification is possible and that using the regressed glove values leads to a good classification results. The approach of using a pre-trained classifier to train the regressor resulted in slightly worse classification results.

Acknowledgement

The work has been carried out at and supervised by the Institute for Signal Processing, Universität zu Lübeck.

Author's Statement

Conflict of interest: Authors state no conflict of interest.

7 References

[1] D. J. Atkins, D. C. Heard, and W. H. Donovan, "Epidemiologic overview of individuals with upper-limb loss and their reported research priorities," *Jpo: Journal of prosthetics and orthotics*, vol. 8, no. 1, pp. 2–11, 1996.

[2] X. Zhai, B. Jelfs, R. H. Chan, and C. Tin, "Short latency hand movement classification based on surface emg spectrogram with pca," in *2016 38th annual international conference of the IEEE engineering in medicine and biology society (EMBC)*. IEEE, 2016, pp. 327–330.

[3] I. Kuzborskij, A. Gijsberts, and B. Caputo, "On the challenge of classifying 52 hand movements from surface electromyography," in *2012 annual international conference of the IEEE engineering in medicine and biology society*. IEEE, 2012, pp. 4931–4937.

[4] M. Zia ur Rehman, A. Waris, S. O. Gilani, M. Jochumsen, I. K. Niazi, M. Jamil, D. Farina, and E. N. Kamavuako, "Multiday emg-based classification of hand motions with deep learning techniques," *Sensors*, vol. 18, no. 8, p. 2497, 2018.

[5] P. Koch, H. Phan, M. Maass, F. Katzberg, and A. Mertins, "Early prediction of future hand movements using semg data," in *2017 39th Annual International Conference of the IEEE Engineering in Medicine and Biology Society (EMBC)*. IEEE, 2017, pp. 54–57.

[6] P. Koch, M. Dreier, A. Larsen, T. J. Parbs, M. Maass, H. Phan, and A. Mertins, "Regression of hand movements from semg data with recurrent neural networks," in *2020 42nd Annual International Conference of the IEEE Engineering in Medicine & Biology Society (EMBC)*. IEEE, 2020, pp. 3783–3787.

[7] S. Hochreiter and J. Schmidhuber, "Long short-term memory," *Neural computation*, vol. 9, no. 8, pp. 1735–1780, 1997.

[8] A. Krasoulis, I. Kyranou, M. S. Erden, K. Nazarpour, and S. Vijayakumar, "Improved prosthetic hand control with concurrent use of myoelectric and inertial measurements," *Journal of neuroengineering and rehabilitation*, vol. 14, no. 1, p. 71, 2017.

Detection of glycemic abnormalities based on continuous glucose measurements

Dominik Klein [1], Oliver Witt [2], Marcin Grzegorzek [3]
[1] Medical Informatics, Universität zu Lübeck, dominik.klein@student.uni-luebeck.de
[2] Perfood GmbH, Lübeck, oliver.witt@perfood.de
[3] Institute of Medical Informatics, Universität zu Lübeck, grzegorzek@imi.uni-luebeck.de

Abstract

The aim of this study was to evaluate the capabilities of machine learning models to detect glycemic abnormalities by means of raw continuous glucose measurements using diabetes and prediabetes as examples. A model for classifying people with these diseases was built and trained on a glucose measurements dataset with corresponding labels predicted in a previous step. For the main task of the prediction, based on glucose measurements, a support vector machine (SVM) achieved the best classification performance at about 0.739 area under the receiver operating characteristic curve using simple features extracted from the glucose measurements. The study demonstrates that machine learning modeling is a promising classification approach for detecting people with glycemic abnormalities such as diabetes and prediabetes based on continuous glucose measurements. To our knowledge, this is the first report that a machine learning approach can be successfully used to detect diabetes and prediabetes based on continuous glucose measurements.

1 Introduction

Much scientific work is being done in the field of diabetes mellitus. Especially the detection of diabetes, as well as other diseases, is treated quite frequently. However, the prediction is usually based on questionnaire data [1], [2]. Rather few work is done in the analysis of continuous glucose monitoring data in the context of diabetes mellitus, although blood glucose is obviously directly related to the disease. Only some work on predicting the future glycemic status of patients with diabetes mellitus is based on these continuous measurements [3]. But there are just a few studies available on the diagnosis of diabetes mellitus based on continuous glucose measurement (CGM) data. One reason for this could be the lack of large datasets containing CGMs combined with information on glycemic abnormalities such as diabetes. To solve this problem, a machine learning system has been developed to label a large dataset of CGMs (about 2200 observations) based on questionnaire data. This system was built using data from the National Health and Nutrition Examination Survey. Next, on the basis of these labeled CGM data, a classifier for the prediction of diabetes and prediabetes was developed. The aim of this approach was to investigate whether it is possible to predict glycemic abnormalities, using the example of diabetes and prediabetes, from raw continuous blood glucose measurements without additional information.

2 Material and Methods

Figure 1 shows the workflow of the entire system, which has two stages. Each stage consists of 1) Data Mining, 2) Model Development and 3) Model Evaluation. In the first part of the system a dataset from the National Health and Nutrition Examination Survey was used to develop and evaluate different supervised machine learning models for predicting individuals with diabetes and prediabetes. This classifier was used in the second part to label the given CGM data. This made it possible to create a new model capable of predicting the assigned labels based on features extracted from the CGMs. In the following, the data, models and methods used are described in more detail.

2.1 Machine learning models

During the two stages, different models of supervised machine learning were investigated. In the training process, the machine learning algorithm gets both the data (feature vectors) and the assigned labels for the respective observations. Thus the algorithm can build a model that can predict a label for given new unseen data. In the following, the models that were used during the research are briefly explained:

- The *k nearest neighbor* (KNN) assigns a label based on the most similar samples observed in the training data by searching for k nearest training points in the feature space and selecting the most frequent class.
- *Support vector machine* (SVM) is a classifier that builds a hyperplane in a high dimensional feature space to separate the observations with different class

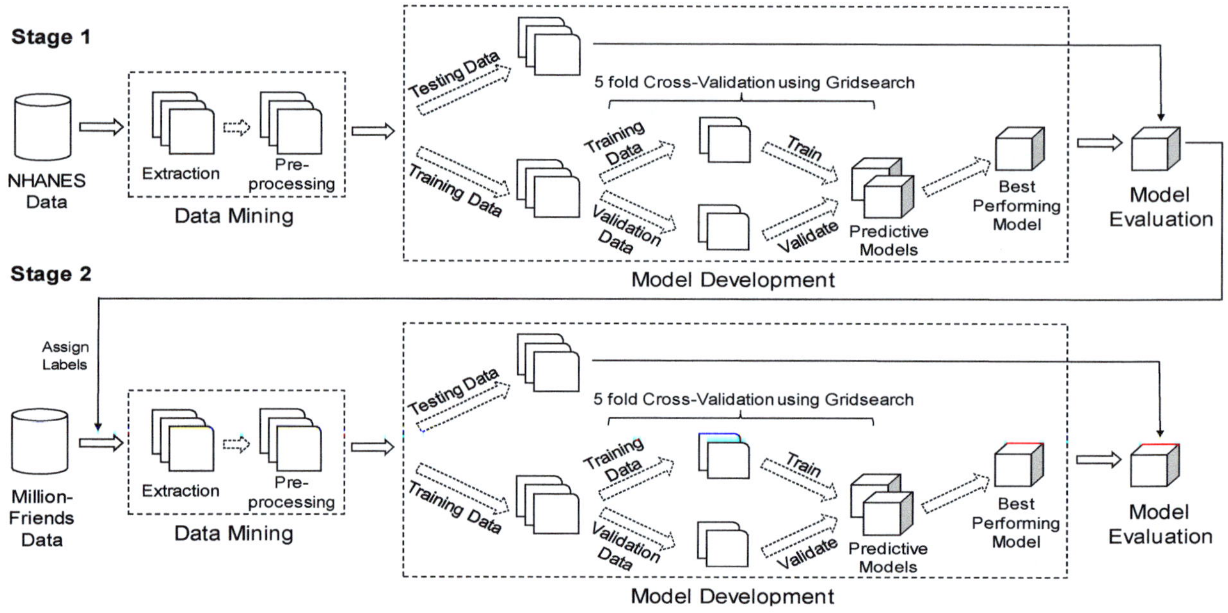

Figure 1: Systematic representation of the dataflow in the two stages - 1.) Classification based on questionnaire data 2.) Classification based on glucose measurements.

labels. The optimization of the model leads to a hyperplane that has the largest distance to the observations closest to the hyperplane, the so-called support vectors.

- *Ensemble methods* combine the results of multiple individual classifiers, which can lead to better performance than the single results of the models.
  - A *random forest* (RF) classifier consists of a large number of decision trees, whose class predictions are combined to an overall prediction of the model.
  - An *AdaBoost classifier* is made up of many decision stumps, each of which depends on a single variable for its class prediction, which in turn are combined to give an aggregated class prediction. The classifier focuses more on hard-to-learn examples by assigning more weight to misclassified samples.

2.2 Data sources

To develop a classifier that can predict diabetes and prediabetes based on questionnaire data, datasets from the National Health and Nutrition Examination Survey (NHANES) from 2011 to 2018, which are freely available through the *Center for Disease Control and Prevention*, were collected. The NHANES program is designed to determine and document the general health and nutritional status of people in the USA. The dataset includes survey interviews, physical examinations and laboratory tests. The survey data covers economic, demographic, nutritional and health-related questions. As in [1] and [2], the NHANES dataset was limited to non-pregnant individuals between 18 and 79 years of age to focus on predicting type II diabetes and exclude other types such as gestational diabetes and type I diabetes, which is usually developed by children. In addition, data were limited to people without insulin medication and to the specific ethnic *non-Hispanic White* category of NHANES to increase comparability with the cohort present in the continuous glucose monitoring dataset.
Another dataset used in this work is taken from the *MillionFriends* program of the company Perfood and comprises continuous glucose monitoring data of about 2200 people. The data combines CGMs with an anamnesis containing basic information such as age, body mass index (BMI), or cumulative weekly activity. Glucose values were recorded over 14 days with a *FreeStyle Libre* glucose sensor, which measures glucose levels in the interstitial fluid every five minutes.

2.3 Stage 1

2.3.1 Data Mining

The Data Mining included the extraction of the data from the NHANES database, the labeling and the feature generation. In order to apply supervised machine learning, labeling of each observation was necessary. Labels were created using the existing laboratory data (including fasting glucose and 2-hour oral glucose tolerance test), by applying the diagnostic guidelines of the German Diabetes Society and some diabetes-specific questions that were present in the NHANES dataset. For the purpose of this study, people with diabetes (diagnosed or undiagnosed) and prediabetes were grouped in one class and all healthy people in the other class. The labeled dataset was processed further to generate feature vectors used for training. As the classifier needed to be applied to the CGM dataset in the next step, the selection of possible usable features was limited due to the content of the anamnesis included in the MillionFriends program.

It was only possible to extract the following features: age, sex, weight (current and previous year), height, BMI, waist circumference, occurrence of diabetes of a close relative, high blood pressure, smoking behavior, cumulative weekly activity and regularity of alcohol consumption. The necessary questionnaire answers were extracted and processed. Selected features, like age and weight were normalized to values between 0 and 1. Ordinal features, such as smoking habits or cumulative weekly activity were mapped to values between -1 and +1. Moreover, missing values were replaced using mean imputation and observations with too many missing values were excluded. After exclusion and labeling, around 5000 samples remained in the dataset.

2.3.2 Model Development

Before training the model, 30% of the dataset was excluded for evaluation. The rest of the data was used to train the classifier models. A grid search was used for hyperparameter tuning and a 5-fold cross validation was performed for each hyperparameter combination to ensure the robustness of the trained model. After the best hyperparameter combination was found, a final classifier was trained on the entire training dataset and the performance was evaluated using the unseen testing dataset.

2.4 Stage 2

2.4.1 Data Mining

The resulting classifier of the previous stage was applied to the anamnesis of the continuous glucose monitoring dataset to assign a label to each person. After labeling the data, different features have been extracted from the raw glucose measurements. For each person in the dataset, different characteristics based on glucose values were extracted for each day of the 14 measurement days. On the one hand, simple parameter describing the time series such as mean, minimum, maximum, standard deviation, time over mean and skewness were calculated for each day. On the other hand, the glucose-specific parameter mean amplitude of glycemic excursion (MAGE) [4] and the glycemic variability metric low blood glucose index (LBGI) [5] were calculated. For each of these characteristics which were extracted for each day, the maximum, minimum, mean and standard deviation were calculated and used as features for the classification. Additionally to these features, an estimated glycated hemoglobin ($eHbA_{1c}$) was calculated. Nathan et. al. proposed a formula for deriving the estimated average glucose $\bar{g}_e$ from the glycated hemoglobin (HbA_{1c}) [6]. Since we have glucose measurements and an average glucose $\bar{g}$, the formula can be adapted to derive an $eHbA_{1c}$:

$$eHbA_{1c} = 0.0348 \cdot \bar{g} + 1.627 \quad (1)$$

Then, the extracted features have been normalized by removing the mean and scaling to unit variance. The normalized feature vectors, combined with the assigned labels, were used to train the new classifier models.

2.4.2 Model Development

As shown in Figure 1 the models were trained and evaluated the same way as in the first stage. One difference to the first model development stage was the handling of the imbalanced class distribution (only 10% with glycemic abnormality). To handle this, a stratified sampling was used to split the data into testing, training and validation data. Since many classifiers have empirically shown better performance when trained on a balanced dataset [7], an adaptive synthetic sampling approach (ADASYN) was used to create synthetic observations by linear interpolation between observations of the minority class. While creating observations, ADASYN uses density distributions to determine the areas of boundary between two classes to create more "harder-to-learn" observations [8]. The resampling coefficient, which regulates how many observations are generated, was also optimized during training of the entire system. Subsequently, random undersampling was applied, where observations of the majority class are randomly removed to obtain an equal class distribution during training.

3 Results and Discussion

The performance achieved in the first stage of the system (the classification based on questionnaire data) is presented in Table 1. The support vector machine performed with 0.798 ROC AUC and 73.6% balanced accuracy best in terms of overall discriminatory ability. Other works had similiar results (0.732 ROC AUC) using a SVM [1]. Although direct comparisons are difficult due to the use of different NHANES datasets and a slightly different classification scheme, the discriminatory power in both studies appears to be equivalent, while using slightly different features. This underlines the potentially useful work of machine learning to detect glycemic diseases such as diabetes and prediabetes without information about laboratory values using just simple variables.
In the second stage, the support vector machine was used to label a large dataset of CGMs. This newly labeled dataset was used to train different machine learning models for the detection of diabetes and prediabetes based on 14-day raw glucose measurements. The performance evaluation for the second stage can also be seen in Table 1. The SVM- and RF-classifier achieved the best results with an overall classification discrimination ability of 0.739 and 0.725 ROC AUC. The two differed mainly in the higher positive predictive value (PPV) of the SVM and the higher sensitivity of the RF, respectively. In contrast, the KNN-classifier could not achieve satisfactory results due to the low PPV (0.145) and the AdaBoost classifier due to a low sensitivity (0.067). When evaluating the outcome, it is important to remember that the ground truth labels for these classifiers were based on a previously trained classifier. This means that the absolute level of accuracy of these results should be evaluated with caution.

	Stage 1						Stage 2					
Classifier	B. Acc.	AUC ROC	Sens.	Spec.	PPV	NPV	B. Acc.	AUC ROC	Sens.	Spec.	PPV	NPV
KNN	0.673	0.729	0.611	0.735	0.650	0.703	0.600	0.679	0.625	0.582	0.145	0.930
RF	0.703	0.773	0.711	0.695	0.681	0.762	0.667	0.725	0.609	0.726	0.249	0.944
SVM	0.736	0.798	0.761	0.711	0.689	0.767	0.658	0.739	0.419	0.879	0.318	0.948
AdaBoost	0.724	0.791	0.658	0.790	0.715	0.744	0.530	0.651	0.067	0.998	0.601	0.905

Table 1: The performance of the classifier. The balanced accuracy (B. Acc.), the area under the receiver operating characteristic (AUC ROC), sensitivity (Sens.), specificity (Spec.), positive predictive value (PPV) and negative predictive value (NPV) were evaluated [10].

4 Conclusion

In this study we investigated the detection of glycemic abnormalities based on CGMs using diabetes as an example. The results of the second stage demonstrate that it is possible to distinguish people with glycemic abnormalities such as diabetes and prediabetes from healthy people based on raw glucose measurements.

The positive predictive value for the SVM- and RF-classifier does not appear to be very high. This could be caused by the low prevalence of diabetes and prediabetes in the cohort under research. Moreover the sensitivity, especially of the SVM, seems to be rather low. But if the HbA_{1c}, which is also used as a laboratory parameter for diagnosis and as a screening tool, is compared with the laboratory parameters (plasma fasting glucose and oral glucose tolerance test) used in the first stage for labeling, it also achieves a high specificity of 0.992 and a low sensitivity of 0.249 in the diagnosis of diabetes and a specificity of 0.855 and sensitivity of 0.316 in the diagnosis of prediabetes [9]. A look at these results for the individual diseases shows that even medical tests used in this area can have a low sensitivity.

Since the approach does not require any additional information than the raw glucose values, it is easy to use by simply wearing a glucose sensor for a few days. Together with other phenotypic information, such as the anamnesis information, the performance of the approach could be improved and also be used as a screening tool. In any case, our study provides useful proof-of-principle by demonstrating the predictive power of machine learning, especially of SVM and RF, with a set of features extracted from raw CGMs without further knowledge about the subject. This approach can be extended to include other or more complex features, more complex preprocessing and more reliable training labels. Furthermore, an analysis of the importance of the features used would be conceivable. To our knowledge, this is the first report that a machine learning approach can be successfully used to detect type II diabetes and prediabetes based on continuous glucose measurements.

Acknowledgement

The work has been carried out in the company Perfood in Lübeck, which provided the glucose data and was supervised by the Medical Data Science team of the Institute of Medical Informatics at the University of Lübeck.

Author's Statement

Conflict of interest: Authors state no conflict of interest.

5 References

[1] W. Yu, T. Liu, R. Valdez, M. Gwinn and M. Khoury, *Application of support vector machine modeling for prediction of common diseases: the case of diabetes and pre-diabetes*. In: BMC Medical Informatics and Decision Making, 2010.

[2] J. Semerdjian and S. Frank, *An Ensemble Classifier for Predicting the Onset of Type II Diabetes*. In: ArXiv e-prints, 2017.

[3] E. Dassau, F. Cameron, H. Lee, B. W. Bequette, H. Zisser, L. Jovanovič, et al., *Real-Time Hypoglycemia Prediction Suite Using Continuous Glucose Monitoring*. In: Diabetes Care, 2010.

[4] P. A. Baghurst, *Calculating the Mean Amplitude of Glycemic Excursion from Continuous Glucose Monitoring Data: An Automated Algorithm*. In: Diabetes Technology & Therapeutics, vol. 13, no. 3, 2011.

[5] J. P. Le Floch and L. Kessler, *Glucose Variability: Comparison of Different Indices During Continuous Glucose Monitoring in Diabetic Patients*. In: Journal of Diabetes Science and Technology, vol. 10, 2016.

[6] D. M. Nathan, J. Kuenen, R. Borg, H. Zheng, R. Heine, et al., *Translating the A1C Assay Into Estimated Average Glucose Values*. In: Diabetes Care, 2008.

[7] G. M. Weiss and F. Provost, *The Effect of Class Distribution on Classifier Learning: An Empirical Study*. In: Technical Report ML-TR-44, Department of Computer Science, Rutgers University, 2001.

[8] H. He, Y. Bai, E. A. Garcia and S. Li, *ADASYN: Adaptive Synthetic Sampling Approach for Imbalanced Learning*. In: IEEE International Joint Conference on Neural Networks, 2008.

[9] F. Guo, D. R. Moellering and W. T. Garvey, *Use of HbA1c for Diagnoses of Diabetes and Prediabetes: Comparison with Diagnoses Based on Fasting and 2-Hr Glucose Values and Effects of Gender, Race, and Age*. In: Metabolic Syndrome and Related Disorders, 2014.

[10] M. Hossin and M. N. Sulaiman, *A Review on Evaluation Metrics for Data Classification Evaluations*. In: International Journal of Data Mining & Knowledge Management Process, 2015.

Test Automation of Auto-tuning of Velocity and Position Robot Controllers and Verifying Actual Stability

Sameed Quais[1], Petr Lukin [2], Achim Schweikard [3]

[1] Robotics and Autonomous Systems, Universität zu Lübeck, sameed.quais@student.uni-luebeck.de

[2] Controls Engineering, Synapticon GmbH, plukin@synapticon.com

[3] Institute of Robotics and Cognitive Systems, Universität zu Lübeck, schweikard@rob.uni-luebeck.de

Abstract

Automatic Tuning (AT) is defined as the process of obtaining efficient gains of the PID controller based on the performance requirements. The AT engine is already implemented for Synapticon servo nodes but due to the possible uncertainties in the firmware or software, an automated verification process is needed to assert that the system remains stable in practice as well after tuning. To create an automatic verification of the AT engine, we created an automated test using the Pytest automation tool and integrated it into Continuous Integration (CI) test bench, which is composed of multiple robot axis chains. The automatic verification is performed by confirming through Fast Fourier Transform (FFT) analysis on test signals after tuning. We achieved a stability threshold of $0.7\frac{N.m}{sec}$ for both velocity and position controllers under which our test ensures the proper tuning of the system with a smooth profile.

1 Introduction

Continuous Integration (CI) is a process in which different developers of a company incorporate their contributions frequently into a common shared repository. Every merging process can afterward be confirmed by automated tests. The automated testing is a practice that verifies if the software is working properly and fulfilling the requirements before its public release. This method of testing of software uses a sequence of scripted commands that are implemented by the testing tools. The automated tools for testing examine the firmware or software, generate log reports, and then compare the results against the standard values.

In the Python ecosystem, there are various testing automation tools including PyUnit, Python Robot Framework, Pytest, and others. PyUnit is appropriate for simple tests as it needs a lot of code to be written to achieve the minimum functionality. In Synapticon, Pytest is used because of its advantage of being open-source, well online documented, and its support for more compact test suites. It stores all result values inside test cases and gives information about which calculated values have asserted the stated conditions, and which one of them failed along with making tests simpler to write and understand with the use of fixtures to cover various combinations of parameters without rewriting test cases.

Synapticon servo node's controllers are based on Proportional-Integral-Derivative (PID) control structure. The process of selecting the appropriate gains of the controllers is known as tuning of the controller and if this process is done automatically then it is also known as Automatic Tuning or Auto-tuning (AT). It is an important task in setting up a motion control system.

In this paper, we checked the proper software functionality of the cascaded position and velocity PID controller auto-tuning engine for motion control services. This is performed by implementing the auto-tuning engine in Pytest using Python bindings and integrating it into the CI test bench which replicates robot axis chains in industries. Then, the automated test is verified by observing the actual stability of the system through Fast Fourier Transform (FFT) analysis. The aim is to make sure that if there is some misbehaviour of firmware or software, the PID controller does not get over-tuned and this can be reflected in FFT analysis, hence causing the automated test to raise an error.

2 Material and Methods

For the automatic verification of the AT engine in the firmware, we first set up a single robot axis chain on which testing is performed. Then, the respective control structure is selected. The AT engine for the position and velocity controller is implemented in Pytest for the automated testing. The tuned system is then given an input signal and the stability analysis is performed to obtain the stability threshold for the automated verification of the test. The test is integrated into the CI test bench for the daily testing of the software on the multiple robot axis chains.

2.1 Physical Setup

The multiple robot axis chain, on which CI Testing is conducted, contains a single EtherCAT network with multiple simple axes. Each simple robot chain axis represents 1-Degree of freedom (DOF) of the robot and is composed of a SOMANET hardware, a Brush-less DC (BLDC) motor paired appropriately to the Servo Node, encoders for commutation and/or for motion control, and optional static load. First, the testing is performed on the single robot axis chain and then verified on CI Test Bench. The implementation is carried on different types of SOMANET hardware: SOMANET Node, SOMANET Circulo, and Customized SOMANET Nodes. Synapticon's OBLAC Drives Box is a physical machine or a master that is connected to the SOMANET servo node and gives command to it. OBLAC Box supports access over WiFi or local area network to connect to PC and is connected via Ethernet LAN to SOMANET servo drives as shown in Fig. 1.

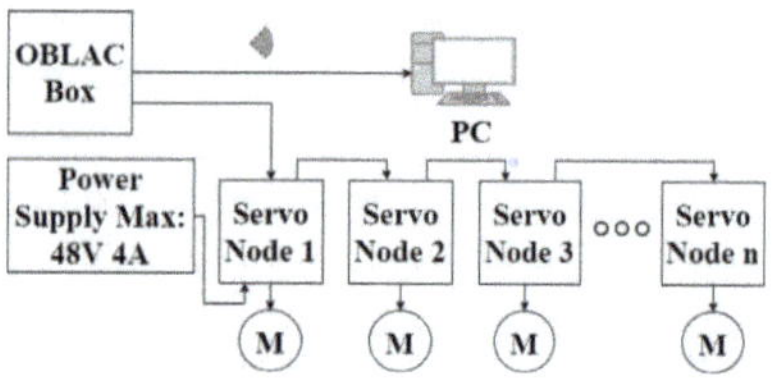

Figure 1: Connection of SOMANET Oblac Box with PC and SOMANET Servo Nodes connected in chain.

2.2 Control Architecture

The overall control structure comprises a torque control loop, velocity control and the cascaded position control loop is shown in Fig. 2. The cascaded position controller comprises of two PID feedback loops. The purpose of the outer loop is to compare the target position (current position set point) with the actual position value. The PID controller calculates a target velocity from this difference. The inner loop compares this target velocity with the currently measured velocity and feeds this difference to the torque PID controller that calculates a target torque. This target torque is then controlled by the torque/ current control loop. Generally, no derivative gains are used in the cascaded controller and the two integral gains are used only alternatively, not together. This reduced control structure is a combination of one P controller and one PI controller: PI-P or P-PI.

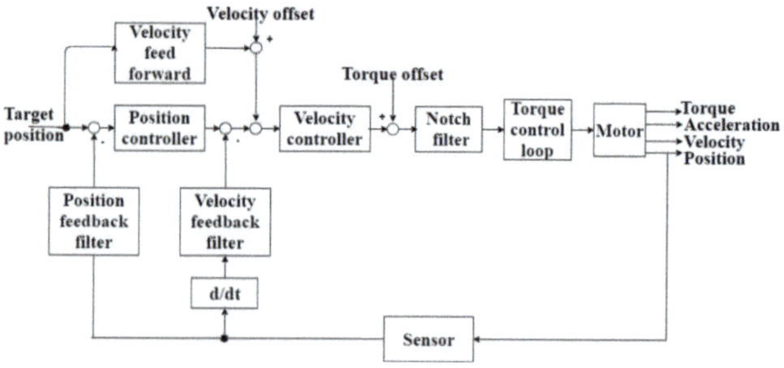

Figure 2: Cascaded Position Control Loop.

2.3 Pytest and CI

SOMANET Drives are configured with the help of browser-based OBLAC application which runs on the docker containers. It helps to set up and test the motor, encoder and EtherCAT bus. All the parameters can be easily read and can be downloaded. DevOps is an approach that combines Development team (Dev) and the operations team's (Ops) work with shared tools and practices. In short, the basic aim of DevOps can be described as to automate everything. Synapticon's CI uses Jenkins as a built tool that runs automated tests on the actual hardware connected to the robot axis chain. Jenkins is a DevOps tool that is open source and automates the part of the software development process. Master-Slave architecture is used by Jenkins to run distributed builds.

2.4 Velocity and Position Controller AT

System Identification is considered as the prerequisite for the automated verification of AT engine. The system identification generates the transfer function of an electromechanical system from a frequency response which is used for calculating gains in the test. The sensors for the desired motion control modes are configured by initializing as a Pytest fixture which makes sure that for every test, the configuration of sensors is checked.

The goal of the velocity AT (VAT) engine is to search for a set of PID controller gains so that the system reaches maximum bandwidth while maintaining the specified stability margins. For this purpose the AT engine uses the identified mechanical model from the system identification process and drive configurations to design the model of the whole velocity control loop. Six different configurations are chosen as shown in Table 1 to design the model of the control loop from which PID gains are calculated. By default the torque controller is tuned for a settling time of 1000 micro-seconds, velocity feedback filter and notch filter are disabled. The drive configuration set 1 has enabled velocity low pass filter with 200 Hz set as cut-off frequency. Similarly, the drive configuration set 2 checks for the effect by enabling $2nd$ order low pass filter. For the drive configuration set 3, the torque controller is tuned for large settling time as compared to default to check for the effect of slower systems. The drive configuration set 4 checks for the effect of enabling the notch filter. The drive configuration set 5 and 6 checks for the combined effect of enabling the velocity low pass filter of 1st order and the notch filter at different cut-off frequencies. This model obtained is used to compute the optimal velocity PID controller gains. The drive configuration and calculated velocity gains are used to initialize the transfer function of the velocity controller, velocity feedback low pass filter, notch filter, torque controller and combine these mathematical models to generate an open loop and a closed loop model of the whole system. From the open loop transfer function, the stability margins values are obtained. When at least one stability boundary is violated, sharpening is reversed.

A limit on maximum bandwidth produced by AT engine

Table 1: Different drive configurations for velocity AT

Element	1	2	3	4	5	6
Velocity Low Pass Filter Order	1	2			1	1
Velocity Low Pass Filter Cut-off Frequency(Hz)	200	200			200	1000
Torque Controller Settling Time			15000		10000	2000
Notch Filter Status	Disabled	Disabled	Disabled	Enabled	Enabled	Enabled
Notch Filter Center Frequency				300	300	1000
Notch Filter Rejection Band				200	200	600

should be there as a higher value of bandwidth indicates less settling time which makes the system react faster. This is theoretically possible but practically, there are some limitations of using extremely high bandwidth. This is limited due to the supplied current to the system as for quick response more torque is needed which means the system will draw more current from the supply. For continuous integration purpose the current supplied is limited to maximum of 4 amperes. The other physical problem could be due to improper mechanical assembly of the drive, additional mass attached to the drive which has not been taken into account in the system identification process. After performing multiple experiments and observing the physical behavior of drives the value of the maximum bandwidth limit was set to be 50 Hz. With the updated demanded bandwidth the new velocity controller gains are obtained. The simulated step response of the system is also calculated from the derived mathematical model of the system to verify that the system reaches steady state.

The basic aim of position auto-tuning (PAT) process is to calculate the efficient gains for the cascaded position controller so that minimum settling time is reached while remaining within the described stability boundaries. Same as for velocity AT testing, for cascaded position AT seven different configurations are considered which are similar to velocity AT. All the default conditions are also the same as velocity AT along with position feedback filter and velocity feed-forward filters are disabled and follows the same procedure as the velocity AT. A limit on minimum settling time produced by cascaded position AT is set to be 80 ms, as less settling time makes the system reacts much faster.

2.5 Actual Stability Analysis of Tuned System

The controller gains produced by the AT engine in 2.4 are provided to the servo node through Oblac drive. These efficient gains obtained are based on the mathematical modeling which confirms that the modeled system is stable. But this modeling is the approximation of the real system and does not cater other uncertainties such as attached mass to the drive, poor mechanical assembly issues and noisy measurements through the encoder. Due to these issues, our system might behave noisy on the tuned controller gains, known as over-tuning, as these uncertainties can not be assumed in the mathematical modeling and vary from device to device. Therefore, an actual stability test must be performed to ensure that system does not get over-tuned and validate our automated test.

Most of the stability analysis methods involve the use of the mathematical model (transfer function) of the system. The bode plot is a vital method for the stability analysis of the system as it is based on calculating the amplitude and phase angle for the open loop system transfer function [1]. Based on the AT engine, the closed loop system was already designed stable with conservative margins. But for practical applications, we need to check stability from the data of the actual response of the system as it includes the effect of all irregularities present in the system. The target signal is a trapezoidal response in our test. The trapezoidal waveform can be considered as a combination of two ramp response as shown in Fig. 3. The demanded torque value is recorded during the whole profile for further analysis.

The Fourier series can be defined as the way of representing complicated signals or waves in terms of the sum of sine and cosine waves. The Fourier transform (FT) splits a complicated signal into the frequencies and the relative amplitudes of its component signals which makes it applicable for our test [2]. Fast Fourier Transform(FFT) algorithm can be said as the fast implementation of Discrete Fourier transform (DFT) technique [3]. FFTs are helpful for measuring the frequency content from data acquired in time-domain. FFTs gives the average frequency content of acquired time-domain signal. Therefore, FFTs are used in cases where only the average energy at each frequency line is required [4]. For this reason, frequency sampling is considered as 1 kHz which is the frequency of data collection through EtherCAT. The FFT of the demanded torque is computed in our test. Considering the nyquist theorem [5], only the first half cycle is considered. The data from 20 Hz to 300 Hz is considered for further analysis as shown in Fig. 4. The area under the FFT curve denotes the power stored in

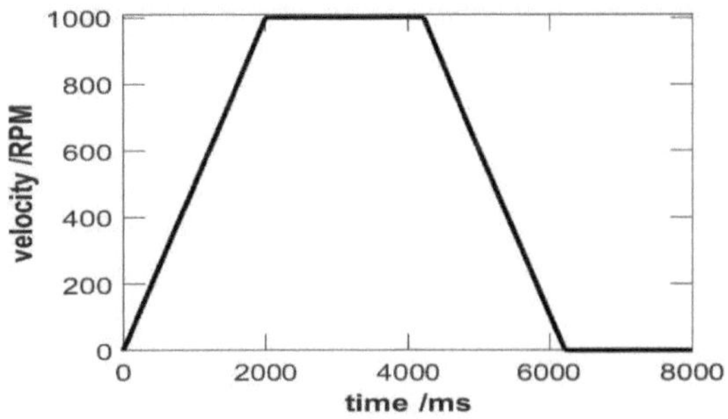

Figure 3: Trapezoidal velocity response showing the acceleration time, sustain time, and deceleration time.

the system within the specified frequency range.

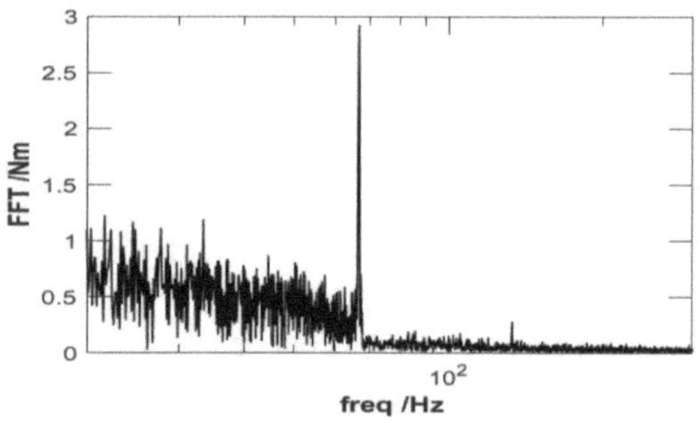

Figure 4: FFT curve of demanded torque from 20-300 Hz. The x-axis is a logarithmic scale and the y-axis has been standardised for ease.

3 Results and Discussion

The mean result of area under the FFT curve within 20-300 Hz for different drive configurations is shown in Table 2. It can be observed that the values obtained are less than 0.7 $\frac{N.m}{sec}$. Therefore a threshold of 0.7 is set for automated verification of our test. After the CI is configured and the AT engine can give reliable default tuning for different setups we can detect misbehavior of the firmware and software by simply observing the value of area under the FFT curve larger than the set threshold which is shown in Fig. 5. It can be observed that for a cascaded position PI-P controller the calculated area under the FFT is 0.35 $\frac{N.m}{sec}$ but when an unwanted feature was enabled in the firmware we can directly observe the spikes in the FFT curve at different frequencies and the calculated area is 18.45 $\frac{N.m}{sec}$ which is outside our calculated stability threshold and our automated test will fail in this case due to *Assertion Error*.

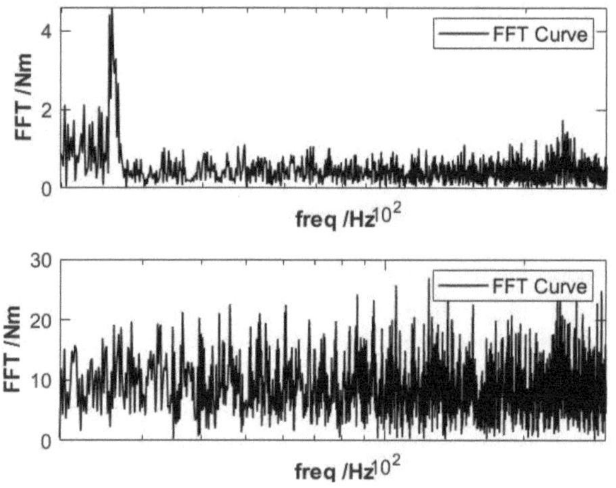

Figure 5: FFT curve for a PI-P cascaded position controller (top). FFT curve for a PI-P cascaded position controller with an unwanted feature enabled showing spikes at different frequencies (bottom).

Table 2: Results of area under the FFT curve from 20-300 Hz for six drive configurations for velocity AT and seven drive configurations for position AT.

	1	2	3	4	5	6	7
VAT	0.15	0.13	0.45	0.11	0.37	0.27	-
PAT	0.3	0.35	0.4	0.33	0.56	0.34	0.52

4 Conclusion

An automated test for the velocity and the cascaded position PID controller's auto-tuning has been designed for the Synapticon CI Test bench along with the automatic verification of the AT engine through verifying the stability threshold obtained from FFT analysis. This response to the unexpected problem in firmware or software of AT engine if the results do not assert the defined threshold.

Acknowledgement

The work has been carried out at Synapticon GmbH and supervised by Prof. Dr. Achim Schweikard, Institute of Robotics and Cognitive Systems, Universität zu Lübeck.

Author's Statement

Conflict of interest: Authors state no conflict of interest.

5 References

[1] J. Hann, T. Edison, T.F. Edgar, *A note on stability analysis using bode plot.* In: Chemical Engineering Education; pp. 208-211;2001.

[2] T. A. Gallagher, A.J. Nemeth and L.Hacein-Bey, *An Introduction to the Fourier Transform: Relationship to MRI.* In: American Journal of Roentgenology;Volume 190; Issue 5;pp.1396-1405;2008.

[3] H. J. Nussbaumer, *The Fast Fourier Transform* In: Fast Fourier Transform and Convolution Algorithms. Springer Series, Berlin, 1981.

[4] M. Cerna, A.E. Havery *The Fundamentals of FFT-Based Signal Analysis and Measurement.* National Instruments Application Note; 041; pp 01;2000

[5] R. Oshana, *Overview of Digital Signal Processing Algorithms.* In: DSP Software Development Techniques for Embedded and Real-Time Systems;pp. 59-121; 2006

Soft Actor Critic for Mapless Navigation in Warehouses

Benedikt Hein [1, 3], Honghu Xue [2], Elmar Rückert [2] and Bengt Abel [3]

[1] Robotics and Autonomous Systems, Universität zu Lübeck, benedikt.hein@student.uni-luebeck.de
[2] Institute for Robotics and Cognitive Systems, Universität zu Lübeck, {xue,rueckert}@rob.uni-luebeck.de
[3] Technology and Innovation, Still GmbH, {benedikt.hein,bengt.abel}@still.de

Abstract

We aim to explore the benefits of Deep Reinforcement Learning in the field of intralogistics. The main purpose of our work is to present a mapless navigation model, trained from scratch by the Soft Actor-Critic algorithm, and investigate its strengths and weaknesses. Reinforcement Learning revolves around the learning from interaction between an agent and its environment. We consider the agent to be a vehicle that is typically used in intralogistics, a Transport Robot in this case. The used environment consists of five different warehouse-like test scenarios, which our model learns to solve. We use the Nvidia Isaac SDK as well as the IsaacSim Unity3D and its access to a variety of sensors, actuators, robots and comprehensive 3D simulation environments.

1 Introduction

Intralogistics is in a constant state of change, and this can be seen in the layout of department stores. Pallets can be at different places every day, and entire rows of shelves can be moved. Therefore, purely map-based navigation may lead to problems. Modifications in the warehouse layout can lead to continuous updates of a global map. For many operations that involve navigation, a reliable localization method is required. Mapless navigation, on the other hand, works without a global map and in the best case still works with a non-stationary environment.

Deep Reinforcement Learning (DRL) has been explored in a wide variety of fields. Successful applications can be found in solving Atari games [5], manipulation tasks and mobile robotics [6] [2]. Previous publications in the field of mapless navigation based on DRL, address the use of a Double Deep Q-Network (DDQN) as means to train a model for navigation using local sparse laser observations and a target position [2]. Other works even go further and aim to provide an end-to-end navigation method for multi-robot systems [1], trained by a Parallel Deep Deterministic Policy Gradient (PDDPG) algorithm, which incorporates relative target distance and angle as a additional input. The work [4] points out a way to learn a control policy of a differential drive mobile base in simulation. Based on visual inputs they effectively implement Object Navigation, without using additional target guiding information. In our application, a robot navigates solely based on LiDAR data and our goal is to navigate the robot into a target area. Similar to [4], we apply the state-of-the-art off-policy learning algorithm Soft Actor Critic (SAC) to a mapless navigation task. Our approach assumes the goal state to be unknown, whereas many other works incorporate explicit goal knowledge into the state design. Compared to their settings, our application is completely independent of any form of map and uses minimal to none labeling strategies. Our main contribution is the formulation of the mapless navigation task as a DRL problem with little to no information on the goal state. Furthermore, we implement a software-technical combination of OpenAI Gym [8] and Isaac SDK [7].

2 Background knowledge and simulation environment

In this section we briefly introduce our simulation environment and the used learning method. For more details regarding the SAC algorithm we kindly refer to [3].

2.1 The Reinforcement Learning Problem

A Reinforcement Learning (RL) problem deals with the interaction between a learning agent and its environment. The agent can take an action a_t at every time-step t. These actions affect the environment and the agent is able to detect changes in the environment by making observations s_t. A policy denoted as $\pi(a_t|s_t)$ is a function that chooses an action a from the action space A based on a state s from the state space S. As a result, a reward signal $r(t)$ is then received by the agent on each time-step t. The RL problem can thus be described as a policy search in a Markov decision process (MDP), defined by a tuple (S, A, p, r). With the state dynamic being characterized by a unknown distribution $p(s_{t+1}|s_t, a_t)$. The goal of the RL agent is the

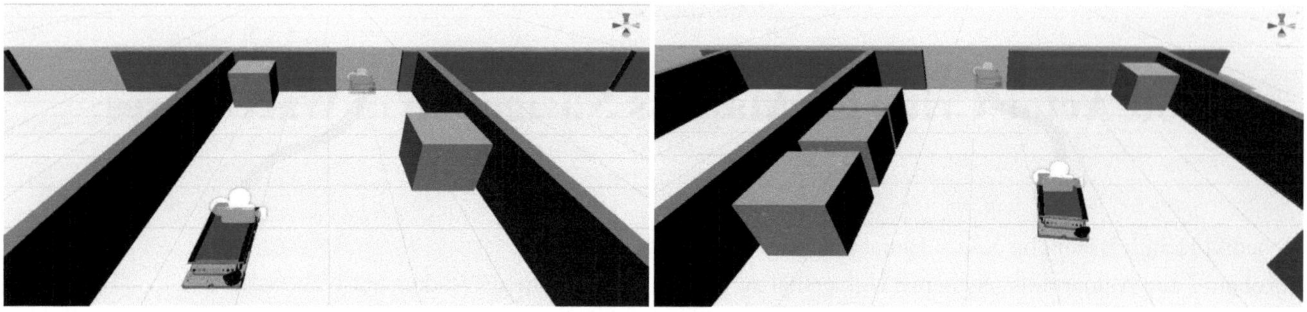

Figure 1: Illustration of two successfully driven trajectories performed by a fully trained LiDAR navigation model

maximization of the expected sum of rewards at any time t:

$$\sum_t \mathbb{E}_{(s_t,a_t)\sim\rho_\pi}[r(s_t,a_t)], \quad (1)$$

where ρ_π denotes the state marginals of the trajectory distribution generated by $\pi(a_t|s_t)$. The goal of the SAC is thus to learn a policy $\pi(a_t|s_t)$ that maximizes this objective.

2.2 Soft Actor Critic

The Soft Actor Critic is an off-policy algorithm that is usually used with continuous action and observation spaces. The major characteristic of SAC is that it generalizes the expected return RL objective [3]. In contrast to maximizing rewards, SAC also aims to maximize the policy entropy. High policy entropy can be interpreted as encouraging exploration. Therefore, SAC often overcomes the parameter brittleness problem by encouraging the policy network to explore unknown subsets of the action space when no best action can be found. This is done by not assigning a striking high likelihood to any possible action. State-of-the-art implementations feature a policy π_ϕ and two Q-functions $Q_\theta, Q_{\overline{\theta}}$ to mitigate maximization bias, as well as an entropy regularization coefficient α that is varying throughout training [3]. The main functions of the DRL problem, i.e. the state-action function Q which assigns a value for to a state-action pair, and the policy function π_ϕ are soft function approximators implemented by neural networks with the parameter sets (i.e. weights) $\theta, \overline{\theta}$ and ϕ. As described in [3], in the SAC algorithm we utilize a RL framework called maximum entropy learning, resulting in the following objective:

$$\pi^* = arg\ \max_\pi \sum_t \mathbb{E}_{(s_t,a_t)\sim\rho_\pi}[r(s_t,a_t)+ \alpha\mathcal{H}(\pi(\cdot|s_t))] \quad (2)$$

The soft Q-function parameters can be trained to minimize the soft Bellman residual:

$$J_Q(\theta) = \mathbb{E}_{(s_t,a_t)\sim D}\Big[\frac{1}{2}\big(Q_\theta(s_t,a_t) - \big(r(s_t,a_t)+ \gamma\mathbb{E}_{s_t+1\sim\rho}[V_{\overline{\theta}}(s_{t+1})]\big)\big)^2\Big], \quad (3)$$

where the value function $V_{\overline{\theta}}(s_{t+1})$ is implicitly parameterized through the soft Q-function parameters $\overline{\theta}$, and the discount factor $\gamma \in [0,1]$ ensures that the sum of the expected rewards (and entropies) is limited. The policy network parameters are trained by minimizing the following error:

$$J_\pi(\phi) = \mathbb{E}_{s_t\sim D}\Big[\mathbb{E}_{a_t\sim\pi_\phi}\big[\alpha\ log(\pi_\phi(a_t|s_t))- Q_\theta(s_t,s_t)\big]\Big] \quad (4)$$

Finally we compute the α gradients with the objective:

$$J(\alpha) = \mathbb{E}_{a_t\sim\pi_t}\big[-\alpha\ log\pi_t(a_t|s_t) - \alpha\overline{\mathcal{H}}\big], \quad (5)$$

where $\overline{\mathcal{H}}$ is a desired minimum expected entropy.

2.3 Simulation environments

For the simulation of the environment as well as the robot, its sensors and actuators, and the communication between algorithm and simulation environment, we rely on the robotics application software Isaac SDK from Nvidia [7]. This is a powerful toolkit providing the building blocks and tools to easily develop robotic applications. The simulation is IsaacSim Unity3D which is a part of the Isaac SDK. As an interface between Isaac SDK and our SAC algorithm we rely on the OpenAI framework [8].

3 Problem definition and Results

In this section we introduce our experimental setup and the chosen RL problem definition as introduced in section 2.1.

3.1 Experiments (Arena setup)

The used robot is part of the assets included in the IsaacSim Unity3D called STRv4, it comes equipped with two horizontally oriented LiDAR sensors placed in the front-left and back-right corner of the robot, a differential drive and a RGB-D Camera. The robot navigates in an arena with a surface area of $63m \times 15m$, which in itself is sectioned into five smaller scenarios with an average surface area of $8m \times 7m$ to generalize the learned policy. Two of the five sub-scenarios can be seen in Fig. 2. Four of those arenas are

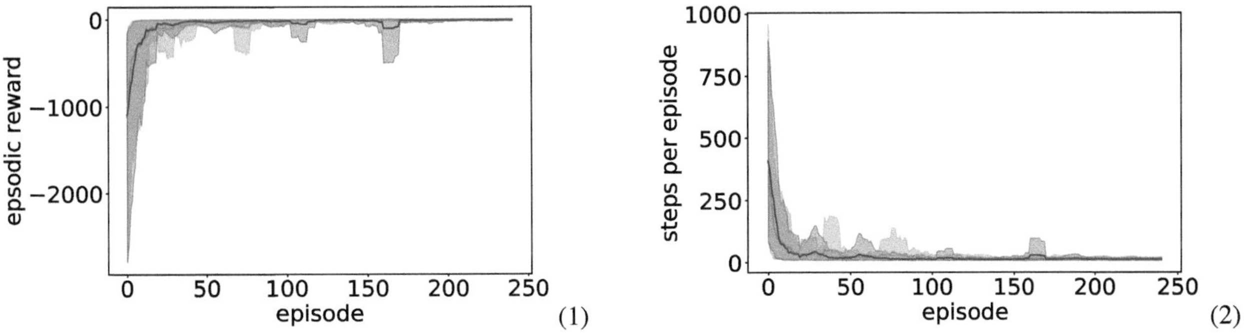

Figure 2: Plotted mean and variance of the episodic rewards (1) and the steps per episode (2), of the mapless LiDAR based navigation task, averaged over 5 experiments. The orange curve shows the results obtained with the use of goal-directed rewards r_l and r_{ad} and the blue curve shows it without the use of r_l and r_{ad}.

used for training and testing. A fifth arena called the "Impossible Test" is used to test the limits of the learned policies. Furthermore, up to five box-like obstacles are placed on fixed positions in each of the individual arenas. The goal of the robot is to reach the gray area outside the arenas, which can only be reached by driving through the openings in the arena walls. These openings are of different sizes and relative position to the robot's starting positions and can therefore only be reached by targeted navigation.

3.2 Formulation of the navigation problem as an RL problem

For the LiDAR-based navigation, we use two horizontally aligned LiDAR sensors with 18 measuring beams each. We set the maximum range of the sensors to $20m$, since a maximum distance (corner to corner) of approx. $12.5m$ is reached within the arenas to be solved. The goal state can be inferred from the LiDAR readings as soon as one of the LiDAR beams passes through an opening. Our state definition for the LiDAR use case is therefore defined as: $\vec{s_l} \in \mathbf{R}^{36}$. The continuous action space is described by $\vec{a} = [v_l, v_a]$ with $v_l, v_a \in \mathbf{R}^1$ in the interval $[-1, 1]$. Here v_l and v_a are linear and angular target velocity inputs to a Isaac SDK module called Unity Differential Base Simulation. The actions are performed for at least 0.4 seconds. To encourage exploration the start positions of the robot are randomized in x-y coordinates ($-0.5m$ to $0.5m$), as well as in yaw angle ($-90°$ to $90°$) according to a uniform distribution. For the design of the reward function we decided to use a combination of the following components:

$$r(t) = r_{ad} + r_{s_t} + r_c + r_l + r_g, \tag{6}$$

with: $r_{ad} = -0.3$ a negative reward for a high Euclidean distance between two successive actions , $r_{st} = -1$ a negative reward for each step, $r_c = -5$ a negative reward for collisions with obstacles or walls, r_l a positive reward of $\frac{1}{19}$ for each front-facing LiDAR beam detecting a distance above $19.6m$ (pointing towards the goal) and $r_g = 10$ a positive reward for successfully solving the navigation task. In a second set of experiments, we exclude r_{ad} and r_l to further reduce goal information. When one of the wheels of the robot reaches the gray target area, the episode is successfully completed. Our policy network and the two Q networks have two hidden layers with 64 nodes each, and we use a Leaky ReLU as activation function.

Note that we do not give any explicit information about the target position. Therefore the model has to infer target information from the input data based on the reward function and the experience buffer, which is a clear difference from many other RL navigation tasks.

3.3 Results LiDAR

From Fig. 2, we can learn that a robust policy is achieved after 250 episodes, even if the two goal-related rewards r_{ad} and r_l are excluded. The total number of interactions is about 9000 which corresponds to approx. 45 minutes of training. We also observe that no unnecessary turns are made and collisions are effectively avoided. However, if there is a very close approach to an edge or object, a short backward movement is performed by the robot. Due to the continuous action space, we also see hardly any over or understeering. In Fig. 2 we see two exemplary trajectories, these are without sharp curves and lead to the destination without detours. Fig. 2 additionally displays the effect of a not target aligned initialization, i.e. the robot must be driven in a curve to reach the goal. We have also encountered a limitation of the learned policy. In Fig. 3 we can see that the robot moves in the direction of high LiDAR measurement points when no target hitting Lidar measurement points exist. From the middle part of Fig. 3 we learn that the robot almost comes to a standstill as soon as no clear direction can be deduced from the sensor data. This inevitably leads to failure of the task. However, if an opening appears (part (3) in Fig. 3), the robot will pass through it correctly.

3.4 Future work

Camera-based navigation, unlike LiDAR navigation, relies on only one sensor instead of two. We use the Depth Camera script of the Isaac SDK to generate a 1280×720 pixels RGB-D image which is then normalized and re-scaled to 84×84 pixels. The camera is centered on the front of the

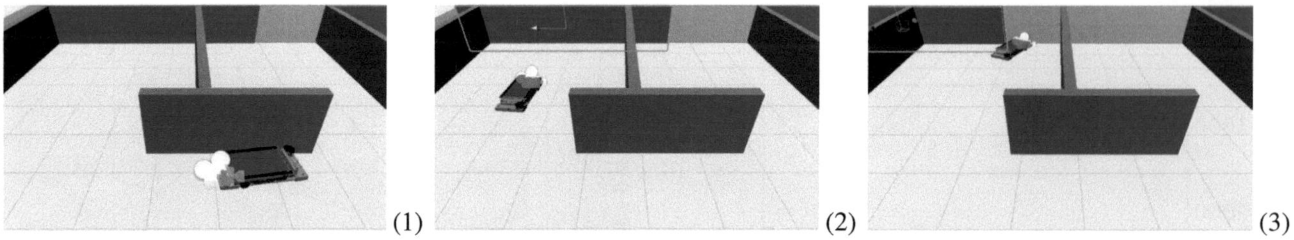

Figure 3: Display of an interrupted path in the "Impossible Test" scenario. (1) shows the starting position in which none of the LiDAR sensors can see the target opening. (2) shows the successfully bypassed edge and the "wait and avoid" situation. (3) illustrates the successful solution of the task after a suitable opening has been manually created.

mobile robot and has a field of view (FOV) of 180°. In our experiments, we only use depth information and set a maximum detectable depth of $20m$. To counteract the problem of partial observability, we use a method called frame stacking. In this technique, the latest four camera images are combined in a stack. A state in the camera-based navigation use case can therefore be summarized as: $s_c \in R^{4\times84\times84}$. Early results shown in Fig. 4 seem to be promising.

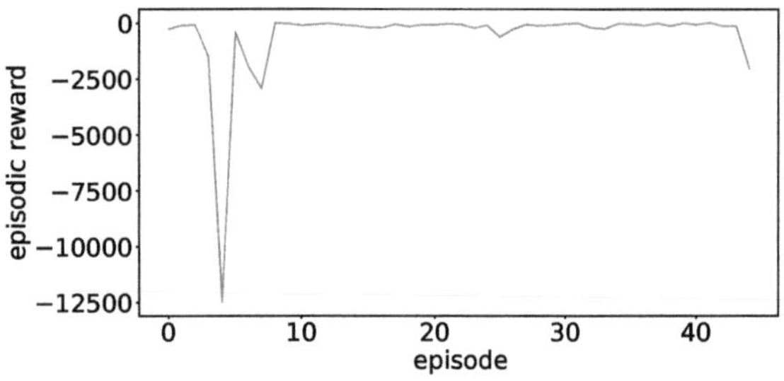

Figure 4: Plot of episodic rewards for mapless navigation based on visual input

4 Conclusion

Based on our results, it is evident that the SAC algorithm can be successfully applied to mapless LiDAR-based navigation. In particular, it demonstrates the sample efficiency and asymptotic training performance mentioned in [3], which we witness from the fast convergence to a robust policy. The shown trajectories further suggest that it is possible to create a goal-directed trajectory without the use of explicit goal-directed inputs, which would require knowledge about the environment. However, with the learned policy, solving our task will only be possible if the model can infer target guidance based on the received sensor information. It is also interesting to note that the target is immediately approached as soon as the goal position can be inferred. Further, we conclude that the arenas were not memorized, but a generalized policy was learned since the "Impossible test" was not part of the training and is nevertheless solved if a goal is dynamically added. We conclude that our definition of the navigation problem as an RL problem leads to a usable policy for mapless navigation based on LiDAR data. In a future work we will compare a policy based on RGB-D data with the results presented here.

Acknowledgement

The work has been carried out at STILL GmbH, D-22113 Hamburg and was supervised by the Institute for Robotics and Cognitive Systems, Universität zu Lübeck.

Author's Statement

Conflict of interest: Authors state no conflict of interest.

5 References

[1] W. Chen, S. Zhou, Z. Pan, H. Zheng and Y. Liu, *Mapless Collaborative Navigation for a Multi-Robot System Based on the Deep Reinforcement Learning*. Applied Sciences. 2019; 9(20):4198.

[2] E. Marchesini and A. Farinelli, *Discrete deep reinforcement learning for mapless navigation*. In: 2020 IEEE International Conference on Robotics and Automation (ICRA) IEEE, 2020

[3] T. Haarnoja, A. Zhou, K. Hartikainen, G. Tucker, S. Ha, J. Tan, V. Kumar, H. Zhu, A. Gupta, P. Abbeel and S. Levine, *Soft Actor-Critic Algorithms and Applications*, 2018.

[4] A. Wahid, A. Stone, K. Chen, B. Ichter and A. Toshev, *Learning Object-conditioned Exploration using Distributed Soft Actor Critic*, 2020.

[5] V. Mnih, K. Kavukcuoglu, D. Silver, A. Graves, I. Antonoglou, D. Wierstra and M. Riedmiller, *Playing Atari with Deep Reinforcement Learning*, 2013.

[6] A. Singh, L. Yang, K. Hartikainen, C. Finn and S. Levine, *End-to-End Robotic Reinforcement Learning without Reward Engineering*, 2019.

[7] NVIDIA, 2020. ISAAC SDK, release: 2020.1, Available at: https://developer.nvidia.com/isaac-sdk.

[8] G. Brockman, V. Cheung, L. Pettersson, J. Schneider, J. Schulman, J. Tang and W. Zaremba, *OpenAI Gym*, 2016.

Camera Test for Distance Measurement by Laser Triangulation

Josefine Lekon [1]

[1] Medical Engineering Science, Universität zu Lübeck, josefine.lekon@student.uni-luebeck.de

Abstract

For the determination of a distance with a pilot laser by using a camera, the behavior of the camera is important, especially the behavior at multiple measurements. By repeated measurements at different heights the camera was checked under different conditions. The camera has a motorized focus, so its behaviour was tested too because deviations can occur if the same focus value is approached several times. By adding an illumination, the accuracy of the detected pixel position could be increased significantly. In addition, it is important to let the camera run for awhile before the measurement and keep the illumination stable during the measurement, this also increase the stability. In order to obtain knowledge about the behaviour of the camera the temperature must be examined.

1 Introduction

Using a camera to measure distances is a good way to determine the distance between a camera and a measuring point without contact. The application is economical, it is possible to react quickly to changes in the working distance. Furthermore, cameras can be manufactured in a space-saving manner, so they can also be installed in small components. The calculation of the working distance can be done by triangulation. Finally, the distance measurement is supposed to be introduced in a laser marking system. For this distance measurement, a camera with a motorized focus was used. It is particularly important that the camera always takes the same images during use, since even slight differences caused by the camera can lead to a deviation in the calculation of the distance. This paper explores whether a selected camera meets the requirements for distance measurement, especially regarding resolution.

2 Material and Methods

In chapter 2, the basic principles of triangulation and detection of the laser point are described. Furthermore, the methods for verification of the behaviour of the camera at multiple measurement will be explained.

2.1 Triangulation

A laser beam, the pilot laser, is directed on the measuring plane with an angle, here denoted with β. A camera detects the reflection of the laser light. If the distance between the camera and the measuring plane changes, the position of the reflected laser spot on the detector changes as well [1]. The position of the laser beam is specified in (x,y) coordinates. Due to the change on the detector the change of the work distance can be calculated with Fig. 1:

$$\alpha = tan\left(arctan\left(\frac{x}{f}\right) + \beta\right) \cdot c \tag{1}$$

with x:

$$x = \sqrt{(x-x')^2 - (y-y')^2} \cdot 2.2\,\mu m \tag{2}$$

The distance between two points on the detector will be calculated by multiplying the distance between the two pixel values by the distance of two adjacent pixels which is 2.2 µm. Where the coordinates [x,y] are the measured coordinates at the unknown distance and the coordinates [x',y'] are the point where the laser dot is exactly perpendicular to the detector, in figure 1 denoted as viewing point of the camera. This setup results in a theoretically calculated resolution. The resolution decreases with increasing working distance like Fig. 2 shows. The resolution indicates by how many pixels the laser dot on the camera detector shifts for a change of one millimeter in the working distance. For the desired application, it is required that the work distance can be resolved to an accuracy of 0.5 mm.

2.2 OpenCV simpleblobdetection

To determine the exact position of the laser dot on the detected image, a function provided by OpenCV 'simpleblobdetection' was applied, since it determines a sufficient detection of the blobs. OpenCV is an open source library that provides algorithms for image processing [2]. The blobs were detected by converting the taken image into binary images. For this several thresholdfilter are applied from minThreshold to maxThreshold with a set distance between neighboring thresholds. With the help of findContours connected components are extracted, center is calculated. The

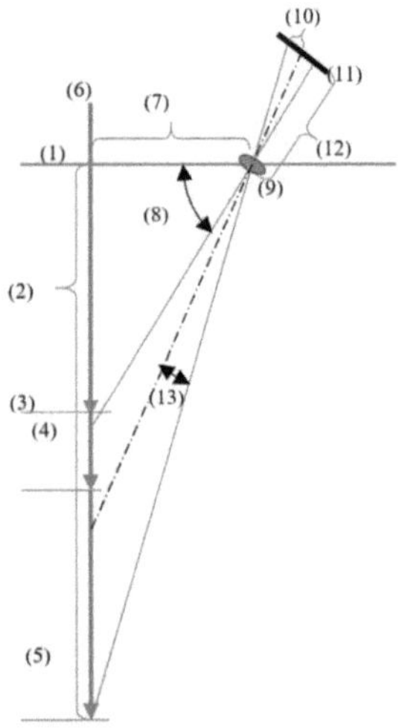

(1) 0 mm (2) working distance (3) minimal working distance (70 mm) (4) viewing point of the camera (5) maximal working distance (180 mm) (6) pilot laser (7) distance between pilot laser and detector (c = 30 mm) (8) angle β (9) lens of the camera (10) distance on the detector between the coordinates [x,y] and [x',y'] (x) (11) detector (12) focal distance (f = 1.6 mm) (13) angle ϵ 80°

Figure 1: The determination of the working distance takes place by the principle of triangulation in which the unknown quantity is calculated with the help of a known distance, a known angle and a measured angle.

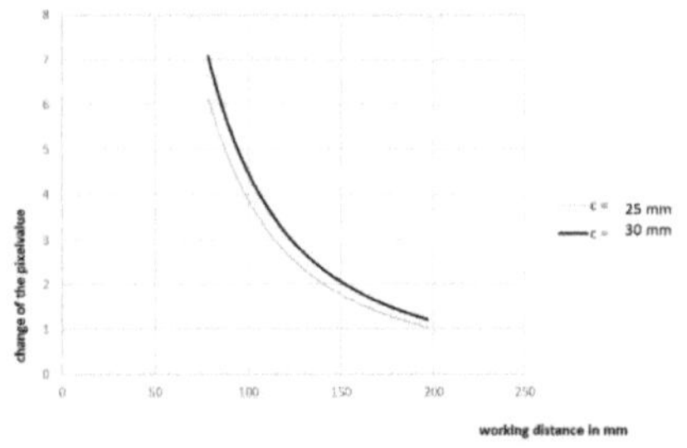

Figure 2: The theoretically possible distance resolution depends primarily on the distance between the camera and the pilot laser: The longer the distance, the higher the resolution. Calculated with Eq. (1). The working range in which the distance is measured, is between 90 mm and 180 mm.

centers of several binary images are grouped by their calculated coordinates.. The function returns the coordinates and the size of the blobs. The parameters are adapted to the given circumstances. To prevent structures from the background being incorrectly detected as blob, an image of the background is first taken without the pilot laser switched on. Then the images are taken with the pilot laser and the images are subtracted. Because the laser spot creates a crown around the actual spot, it is removed by a threshold filter and other artefact like scatter removed by morphological operators [3], [4], so that only the actual spot is detected and no other structures in the images affect the center point. Afterwards, the returned center point is used (1) to calculate the working distance.

2.3 Construction distance measurement

In order to test the camera requirements experimentally, a simplified setup was created in which the dimensions are similar to the planned dimensions of the prototype. In addition, the test setup can be easily modified if necessary. For instance, changes are made to the design of prototype. The camera with the laser is attached to a horizontal item aluminum profile which in turn is attached to a measuring device. Thus, the ITEM aluminum profile can be adjusted in height with a crank and the height can be read with millimeter precision without remeasuring. The angle of the laser and the camera can be changed independently of each other, shown in Fig. 3. In addition, the distance between camera and laser is infinitely adjustable. The control of camera takes place via a raspberry pi [5]. The setup was placed in a lab so the environmental conditions have remained identical during all measurements.

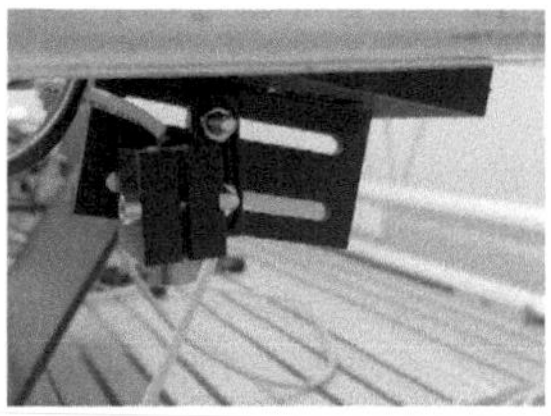

Figure 3: The angle of the camera to the laser beam and the distance between the camera and the laser beam can be adjusted as required. In addition, the height of the setup can be changed.

2.4 Multiple measurements

First, the stability of the pixels is measured at constant focus value. For this purpose, 100 images were taken in a row with the setup and the environmental conditions remaining identical. Subsequently, the blob on the recorded images were detected and the pixel values determined. In order to obtain the correct focus value for the chosen working distance, the autofocus program already provided by the camera's manufacturer was used. The focus value was fixed in advance to prevent deviations in the pixel position caused by a different focus value. Then, the difference between the maximum pixel value and the minimum pixel value was determined in the measurement and thus the largest possible deviation in the worst case. In order to exclude the influence of external disturbing factors, such as an unstable behaviour of the laser as well as an insufficient illumination, the measurement was repeated with an illumination as well as a stationary marking in the form of a painted point on the marking plane. At different heights the deviation is not allowed to become larger, since the computational resolution decreases with increasing distance. Therefore, the measurement was performed at different heights and the respective deviations in the pixel position were determined. Measurements were made in steps of ten mm. It is important that the camera outputs the same pixel values in every situation.

2.5 Focus value change

The used camera is equipped with a motorized focus. This means that the focus can be set automatically by the camera. To test the precision of the motor or whether the camera delivers the same results when the same focus value is approached several times. Here again the optimal focus value for the selected height was determined by the autofocus program of the camera and fixed manually, because it cannot be excluded that the autofocus finds small differences in the optimal focus value when applied several times and thus this source of error is excluded. Likewise, these images were taken with external illumination, as well with a painted dot instead of the pilot laser. Since deviations from the previous measurements are known, the first 15 exposures are not considered, and the following 35 values are averaged to determine the focus value. During the measurement there was a change in the pixel values over the time. It had to be specified more precisely how significant this change was. In addition, it was necessary to see after which measurement period a stable value occurred. For this purpose, the measurement was carried out over a longer period time. For each measurement, 50 images were taken. The measurement was repeated 150 times. Since the average duration for 50 exposures is about 40 seconds, a camera run time of about two hours was tested.

2.6 Various working distances

Subsequently, it was necessary to test how the pixel deviations changes at different heights. It is important to know if there is any change with increasing working distance.

3 Results and Discussion

In the following, the result of the various tests of the camera are described, compared with the given requirements and the possible causes are discussed.

3.1 Distribution of pixel values

The first measurement for the stability of the pixel values was performed at a working distance of 100 mm. The calculated pixel values lie between 1103.6 and 1103.01 for the x-coordinates values. For the y-coordinate, the minimum value is 839.08 and the maximum value is 839.99. This results in a pixel deviation for the y-coordinate of 0.83. Since only the accuracy is calculated at this moment, the absolute pixel value is not relevant, only the change. The calculated theoretically possible resolution is three pixels change per 1 mm change of the working distance. A deviation of 0.8 pixel is therefore 0.24 mm inaccuracy in the determination of the working distance. Possibilities for the deviation of the pixel position are interfering factors like vibrations which are transmitted by other devices in the laboratory and thus cause a vibration of the setup. Other possible causes for the deviation are the irregular illumination on the marking plane due to shadows caused by the ceiling illumination, so continuous illumination was added to the setup and the measurement was repeated. The illumination used significantly increased the accuracy of the blob detection. Thus, on average, there was a deviation at x-coordinate of 0.13 and at y-coordinate 0.26. Due to the illumination, the images were taken at a working distance of 120 mm. It was found that the deviations were highest for the first 15 shots these were not taken into account when calculating the maximum pixel deviation. It is assumed that the camera needs this time to finish the focus adjustment.

3.2 Behaviour focus value change

When starting the focus value several times, it was found that the calculated pixel values reject larger deviations during the first measurements. In addition, the pixel values wander. After about four measurements, the pixel values converge to one value and do not change much from this point on. This finding is particularly important for later use, since the camera must first perform several test measurements before reproducible values can be obtained. The curve shown in Figure 4 is reproducible.

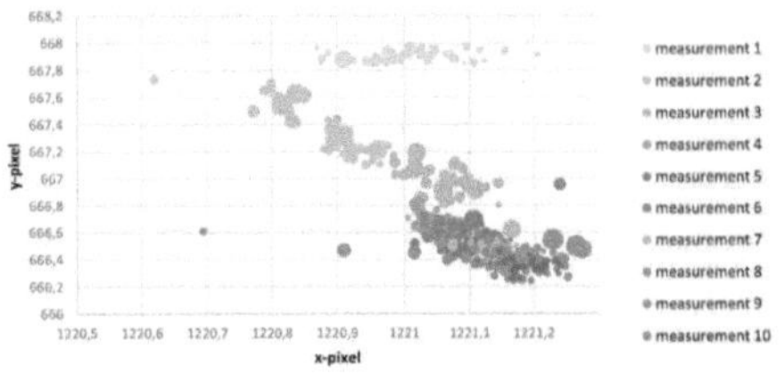

Figure 4: Multiple measurements: between each measurement the focus was set to a random value and then to the original one and 50 exposures were taken. The measurements were performed successively.

The results of the long-term measurement were as improved. At the beginning of the measurements, there were larger deviation in the pixel position, up to one pixel. With a longer running time of the camera the points approach more and more to one value and deviate around this with a deviation approximate 0.1 - 0.2, shown in Fig. 5. It can be assumed that the camera supplies stable values from this time on. The causes for the deviations at the beginning of the measurement are not yet clarified, the assumption is close that the temperature is the main cause: the camera becomes warm by the longer running time. After 2500 images, the camera gives off as much heat to its environment as the camera produces, which means that the temperature is stable and further fluctuations occur.

3.3 Behaviour at different working distances

In order to determine how the deviation of the pixel values behaves as the working distance increases, a few test

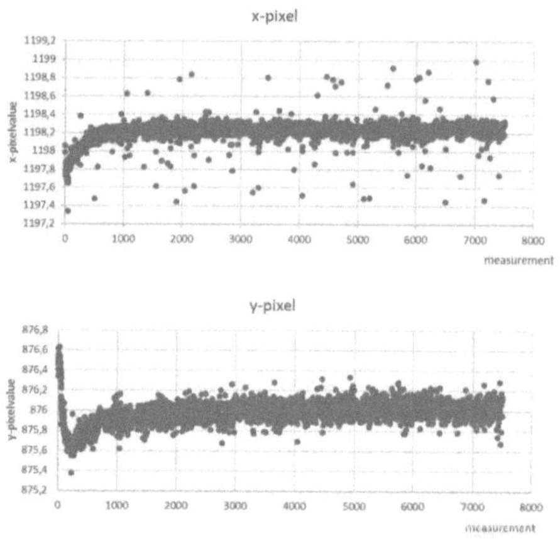

Figure 5: Stable pixel values are output after approximately 1000 exposures. The strong outliers can be neglected because they occur directly after the focus is adjusted and are not taken into account when calculating the pixel position. No cause could be found for the stronger deviations in the y-pixel value yet.

shots were first taken to ensure that the camera produces stable values, as described previously. The deviation in the pixel position remained approximately the same even with increasing working distance, the fluctuations between the different working heights are most likely not related to the changed working distance but to the other possible causes for the vibrations. Therefore, the camera provides the necessary resolution even at a higher working distance. Thus, a deviation of the pixel position at a working height of 150 mm means an error of 0.12 mm in the determination of the working distance.

Table 1: resolution depending on the working distance

working distance in mm	x-pixel value	y-pixel value
120	0.13	0.2
125	0.12	0.22
130	0.09	0.19
135	0.12	0.25
140	0.10	0.20
145	0.11	0.21
150	0.10	0.21

4 Conclusion and Outlook

The measurements confirm that the camera can be used for the laser marking systems. The achieved resolution is sufficient to determine the working distance between the pilot laser and the marking plane. By averaging several images, the pixel position of the laser dot on the marking plane can be reproduced sufficiently to allow accurate determination of the working distance. To avoid large deviations, the camera must take several test shots before starting the measurement. By introducing an external illumination, the deviation in pixel position reduced from 0.8 to 0.2. This corresponds to an improvement in resolution was reduced from 0.24 mm accuracy to 0.03 mm accuracy at a height of 110 mm. At a height of 150 mm, the accuracy was improved from 0.27 mm in determining the working distance to 0.07 mm accuracy. In order to be able to further specify the behaviour of the camera, further factors must be checked. On the one hand, it must be tested from which point in time the camera delivers stable images and how this time can be influenced. Secondly, it must be checked whether other cameras of the same type exhibit the same properties. Furthermore, the behaviour at higher temperatures must be checked, since temperature changes can also lead to different behaviour. Thus, the camera is able to meet the requirements that the working distance should be determined to an accuracy of 0.5 mm. To further increase the accuracy, adjustments could be made to the blob detection algorithm. On the one hand, the parameters of the blob detection algorithm can be further adjusted, on the other hand, other blob detection algorithms could achieve better results. Since the current measurements were still performed with the provisionally painted dot, this has to be replaced by the pilot laser, where further adjustments might be necessary. As soon as the results of further tests are sufficient, the camera can be used for distance measurement.

Acknowledgement

This work has been carried out at the ALLTEC GmbH, Selmsdorf and was supervised by the Institute of Biomedical Optics at the Universität zu Lübeck.

Author's Statement

Conflict of interest: Authors state no conflict of interest.

5 References

[1] E. Westkämper and H.-J. Warnecke, *Einführung in die Fertigungstechnik.* Springer-Verlag, 2010.

[2] J. Cicolani, "An introduction to opencv," in *Beginning Robotics with Raspberry Pi and Arduino.* Springer, 2018, pp. 297–341.

[3] B. Jähne, *Digitale Bildverarbeitung.* Springer-Verlag, 2013.

[4] K. S. Choi, E. Y. Lam, and K. K. Wong, "Source camera identification using footprints from lens aberration," in *SPIE*, vol. 6069, 2006, pp. 172–179.

[5] I. Culjak, D. Abram, T. Pribanic, H. Dzapo, and M. Cifrek, "A brief introduction to opencv," in *2012 proceedings of the 35th international convention MIPRO.* IEEE, 2012, pp. 1725–1730.

8

Auditory Technology

Development of a measurement setup for the transmission behavior of a Hearing Contact Lens®

Philipp Kohlhauer [1,2], Hendrik Husstedt [2], Florian Denk [2] and Volker Steenhoff [3]
[1] Auditory Technology, Universität zu Lübeck, philipp.kohlhauer@student.uni-luebeck.de
[2] Deutsches Hörgeräte Institut GmbH, Lübeck, h.husstedt, f.denk@dhi-online.de
[3] Vibrosonic GmbH, Mannheim, volker.steenhoff@vibrosonic.de

Abstract

Despite technological advancements of hearing aids, acceptance can be improved. In order to make the wearing of hearing aids more comfortable, methods like the direct excitation of the eardrum through a vibration transducer are under investigation. An advantage of direct excitation is the broadband frequency transmission, which improves speech understanding compared to conventional hearing aids that excite the eardrum via air. We here present first work towards the design of a measurement setup that enables a repeatable and robust testing of a vibroacoustic hearing aid, here the Hearing Contact Lens®. To this end, a coupler is used to measure acoustic pressure caused by small motion excitations emitted from the HCL®. First results demonstrate that this measurement principle is functional. Further work is needed to consider all middle ear impedances for this principle to become an accepted test method.

1 Introduction

Studies in Europe show that 30 % of men and 20 % of women under 70 years have a hearing loss of 30 dB or greater, and 55% of men and 45% of women over 80 years [1]. Speech understanding problems associated with hearing loss can lead to reduced quality of life for those affected, as people isolate themselves from conversations and/or avoid social activities. Among other things, this can lead to impaired health, a cognitive decline and even depression [2].
The primary solution to compensate for a hearing loss are hearing aids. The average first-time hearing aid user is 74 years old, and they have been suffering from hearing loss for an average of 10 years [3]. However, despite hearing loss and the potentially associated risks not everyone with a hearing aid indication wears a hearing aid [4]. This is often attributed to the difficulty of inserting the hearing aids, poorer speech understanding in noise, and hearing one's voice louder (occlusion effect) due to a closed ear canal by an earmould [5]. However, studies show that wearing a hearing aid improves the quality of life. Thus, in terms of communication in relationships, cognitive abilities, and emotional stability, the goal should be to provide hearing aids to as many people as possible who have a hearing aid indication [6].
Hearing aids compensate for a hearing loss by amplifying signals. In general, conventional hearing aids consist of three different main components. First, one or more microphones pick up the acoustic signal and convert it into an electrical signal. Second, the electrical signal is passed through a digital signal processor (DSP). For example, the modern DSPs can amplify signals frequency-dependent, and reduce noise or feedback. Third, the modified electrical signal is emitted into the ear canal by a miniature loudspeaker.
However, the hearing aid is limited in its transmission behavior. For example, the loudspeaker of the hearing aid only allows for a reduced mean bandwidth, and hearing aids usually suffer from acoustic feedback problems due to a coupling between the loudspeaker and microphone, which affects the performance. Closing the ear canal with an earmold can improve these factors, but has a negative effect on wearing comfort.
Various technologies are being tested, which are intended to make wearing hearing aids more comfortable for the hearing impaired. For example, one method is the direct excitation of the eardrum using vibrations, such as the EarLens™ system [7]. An advantage of this is the broadband frequency transmission, which improves speech understanding compared to conventional hearing aids in quiet and noisy environments [8]. Another recent example is the hearing contact lens® (HCL) from Vibrosonic GmbH. The HCL® is a nonsurgical investigational outer-ear hearing device shown in Fig. 1. The HCL® sitting in contact with the tympanic membrane (TM) and stimulates the umbo directly by mechanical signals. This HCL® is connected to a behind-the-ear (BTE) unit, as with other hearing aids.

However, hearing aids based on direct stimulation of the ear drum lack standardized measurements as there is no suitable artificial middle-ear coupler testing this system. In general, couplers are used to evaluate the performance of

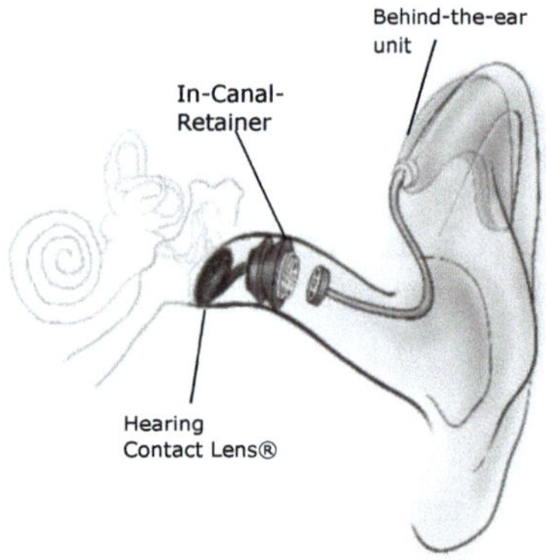

Figure 1: The hearing contact lens® (HCL) is a non surgical investigational hearing device consisting of three components: a behind-the-ear (BTE) unit for charging the in-canal retainer (ICR) that processes incoming sound and transforms it into an amplified electrical signal. The ICR-unit sends the electrical signal to the HCL®, a piezoelectric actuator, that stimulates directly the middle ear through contact with the umbo.

hearing aids. For example, a widely used coupler among hearing aid specialists is the 2 cm³ coupler according to the norm IEC 60318-5:2006-08. They are designed to emulate the ear canal and are the acoustic connection between the hearing aid receiver and the measurement microphone. A coupler offers the advantages of having both high mechanical and temperature stability, as well as high reproduction accuracy.
To be able to analyze the transmission behavior of the HCL® by measurement, we here present first work towards the design of a measurement setup that enables a repeatable and robust evaluation of the HCL®. Also, the essential properties of the measurment setup can be adapted so that the TM with coupler middle and inner ear, e.g., spring stiffness and mass of the TM, are mechanically emulated. Through the coupler it should be possible to measure very small motion excitations generated by the vibrations of the HCL®. These small vibrational excitations are converted into acoustic signals by the resulting acoustic pressure in the coupler.

2 Material and Methods

2.1 Vibro-acoustic coupler design

The 0.4 cm³ coupler is to be the basis of the measurement setup, shown in Fig. 2a. It is possible to measure acoustic pressure caused by very small motion excitations with it. A membrane similar to the TM is first clamped in the coupler. To emulate the impedances of the middle ear, a glass plate is placed on the membrane. In addition, a bending beam is placed underneath the membrane. A motion excitation of the membrane due to the HCL® leads to an increase or decrease of the coupler volume. Due to this an over- and underpressure is generated in the coupler by the vibration excitation of the HCL®. The resulting pressure variation is picked up and processed by the measuring microphone. An optomechanical measurement setup, shown in Fig. 2b, was put together to hold the coupler and HCL® in position and can be adjusted accurately to within a few micrometers for a precise setting.
For the current measurement setup, the 3D printed bending beam and the glass plate have not yet been installed and are therefore not taken into account.

As mentioned in the introduction, the aim is to emulate the middle ear with its mechanical impedances. The parameters for the middle ear were derived from values in the literature [9].
The middle-ear stiffness (K_{TM}) of 1300 N/m will be emulated with a 3D printed bending beam. The synthetic material „medicalprint clear“ (Detax GmbH & Co.KG) with a youngs modulus of 2000 MPa will be used for 3D printing. For a defined volume change and to emulate the mass of the TM, a glass plate with a diameter of 5 mm, and a thickness of 0.13 - 0.16 mm will be used. For the emulation of the

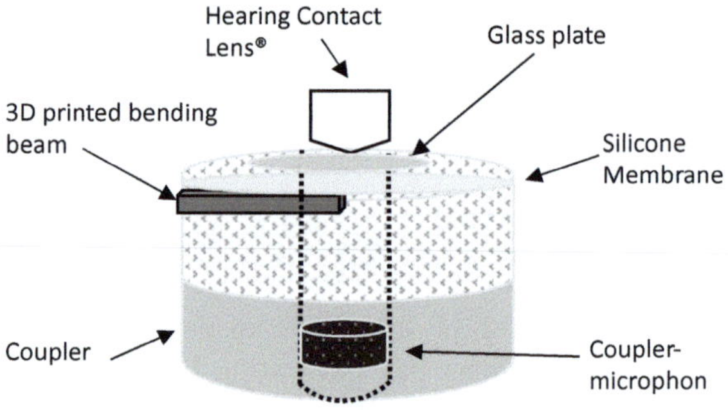

(a) Schematic structure of the coupler

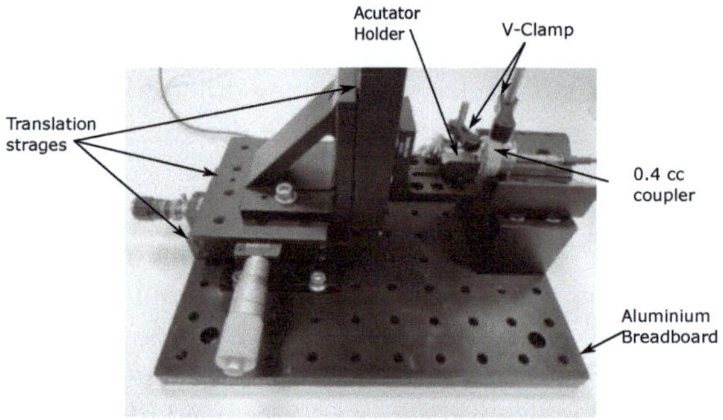

(b) Measurement Setup

Figure 2: a) The HCL® is clamped separately and touches the glass plate, which lies on the silicone membrane. The glass plate is intended to emulate the stiffness of the tympanic membrane. The silicone membrane is fixed in front of the measurement microphone. Underneath the silicone membrane is the 3D printed bending beam. The measurement microphone records the acoustic pressure generated by the membrane change.
b) The measurement setup is mounted on an aluminum breadboard. With the translation stages, the actuator holder which is held in the small V-Clamp can be adjusted within a few micrometers. The coupler is fixed by another V-Clamp.

TM a silicone membrane (Invotec International Inc) with a thickness of 130 μm is employed, which is normally used for tympanoplasty.

2.2 Coupler selection

As described in the previous section, a coupler can be used to measure pressure changes. For the selection of the appropriate coupler a rotational trapezoid is considered, which describes the volume change due to vibroacoustic tympanic excitation. The volume calculation is obtained by considering a cone with cutted peak, with an outer radius r_o (= half the coupler diameter), an inner radius r_i (= half the glass plate diameter) and height Δx (due to vibration excitation). The volume change is linearly dependent on the motion excitation Δx and can be simplified to

$$\Delta V = C_v \Delta x \text{ with } C_v = \frac{1}{3}\pi \frac{r_o^3 - r_i^3}{r_o - r_i}. \quad (1)$$

Because of the volume change, the volume of the coupler decreases, and the pressure increases. This can be described by an adiabatic compression

$$p_0 V_0^\kappa = p_1 (V_0 - \Delta V)^\kappa \quad (2)$$

this is valid for the atmospheric pressure p_0 (1013 hPa), the coupler volume V_0 and the adiabatic constant κ (for air = 1.4).
Solving for the pressure difference $p = p_1 - \Delta p$, we find

$$p = \left(\left(\frac{V_0}{V_0 - C_V \Delta x} \right)^\kappa - 1 \right) p_0. \quad (3)$$

Equation (3) can be linearized around $p = 0$ using a first-order Taylor expansion

$$p(\Delta x) = \left. \frac{\partial p}{\partial \Delta x} \right|_{\Delta x = 0} p \approx \frac{\kappa C_v p_0}{V_0} \Delta x. \quad (4)$$

The error due to linearization lies within 0.1 dB up to Δx = 100 μm. As an example, Fig. 3 shows sound pressure levels inside cavities of the generated pressures from a 0.4 cm³, 0.8 cm³, and 2 cm³ coupler depending on the membrane displacement. This calculation shows that the smaller the volume of the coupler, the more sensitive it is. For the present work, the 0.4 cm³ coupler was selected since motion excitations down to 30 pm are still measurable with this coupler, smaller excitations would be superimposed by the noise of the measurement microphone. The larger the pressure changes in the coupler due to the membrane movements become, the larger deviations due to linearization are created. Therefore, the upper limit is given by the linearity of the pressure in the coupler due to the larger membrane movements.

2.3 Measurements

The measurement was performed at Deutsches Hörgeräte Institut GmbH (Lübeck). Signals were controlled by an RME Fireface 802 (RME Audio) sound card. This sound card is connected to an HCL® preamplifier with unity gain (Vibrosonic GmbH). For the calibration of the output signals, a hand-multimeter Voltcraft VC960 (Conrad Electronic AG) was used.
The generated pressure change was measured in a GRAS RA0252 1/4" 0.4cc High Frequency Coupler (GRAS Sound & Vibration) by a GRAS 40BD 1/4" Prepolarized Pressure Microphone. This measurement microphone is supplied by a GRAS 12AL 1-Channel CCP Power Module.
The measurement was automated in dhiAudio with custom software written for MatLAB R2020b (MathWorks, Natick, MA) running on a PC (64-bit Windows 10 Professional).
The measurements to this point have been performed with a 0.4 cm³ coupler and a clamped silicone membrane. Therefore, the effects of bending beam (spring stiffness) and glass plate have not yet been taken into account. The resulting transfer function describes the ratio of measured sound pressure to the HCL® driving voltage at each frequency. This transfer function was measured using a sweep signal with a duration of 10 seconds, a frequency range from 18 Hz up to 22000 Hz, and a output voltage RMS (V_{rms}) of 0.1 [10].

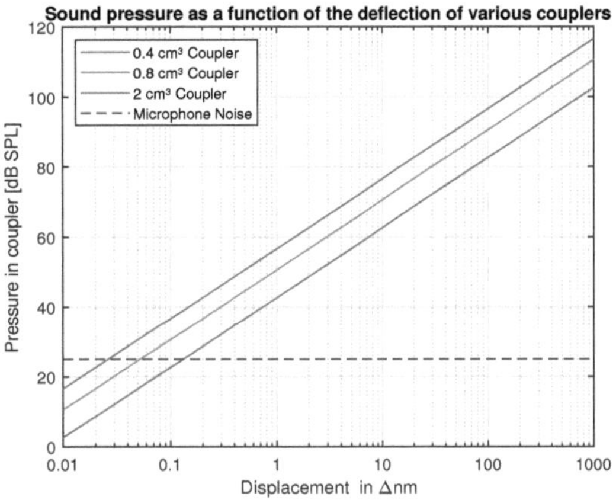

Figure 3: Calculated pressure in the coupler as a function of the membrane displacement.

3 Results and Discussion

Fig. 4 shows the measured transfer function of pressure due to the vibrations of the HCL®. The membrane excitation by the HCL® and the resulting pressure is shown in the curves „1st Measurement: HCL® in contact“ and „2nd Measurement: HCL® in contact“. Other measurements („1st Measurement: HCL® no contact“ and „2nd Measurement: HCL® no contact“) are shown where the HCL® was not in contact with the silicone membrane but close to the it.
The measurements show a higher pressure in the coupler due to the excited membrane especially in the lower frequency range < 1 kHz. The resonance frequency at about 2 kHz is characteristic of the transmission behavior of the HCL®. The fact that the measurement without contact shows an attenuation compared to the touched curve, in-

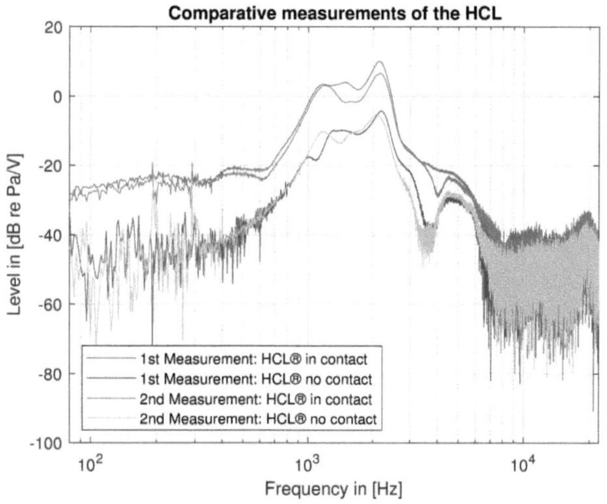

Figure 4: Comparing of the transfer functions when the HCL® touched the silicone membrane(„1st Measurement: HCL® in contact") and the HCL® did not touch the silicone membrane („1st Measurement: HCL® no contact"). After disassembling and re-assembling the setup, a second measurement run was performed.

dicates that the HCL® does not send sound pressures but transmits mainly information about vibrations. This measurement only served to check the functionality of the selected principle.
This article does not cover the measurement reproducibility because the middle ear properties have not yet been considered since the bending beam and glass plate are still missing.

4 Conclusion

The project's overall goal is to create a robust and repeatable setup to verify the transmission behavior of the HCL®. Therefore, a method is in development to emulate the middle ear's mechanical impedances to perform realistic HCL® measurements. A coupler was designed that transforms vibroacoustic excitations of a membrane emulating the TM to pressure changes in a cavity that can be measured with a microphone.
The measurements show that larger pressure differences can be measured while the HCL® is in contact with the silicone membrane, which are caused by vibrations of the HCL®. The measured transfer functions show a larger pressure difference per volt when the HCL® touches the silicone membrane. In comparison, the curves („1st Measurement: HCL® no contact" and „2nd Measurement: HCL® no contact") are damped, which suggests that the pressure signal is mainly dominated by touch excitation and not by generated sound pressure of the HCL®.
However, the impedances such as spring stiffness of the middle ear have not yet been taken into account and there in the future the measurement setup needs to be supplemented and extended to become an accepted test method for future vibroacoustic tympanic membrane measurements.

Acknowledgement

The work was conducted and supervised at Deutsches Hörgeräte Institut GmbH, Lübeck. In addition, this work was supported by Vibrosonic GmbH, Mannheim.

Author's Statement

Conflict of interest: Authors state no conflict of interest.

5 References

[1] Roth, T.N., Hanebuth, D. and Probst, R., *Prevalence of age-related hearing loss in Europe: a review*, Eur Arch Otorhinolaryngol 268, 1101–1107, 2011.

[2] Mener D.J., Betz J., Genther D.J., Chen D. and Lin F.R., *Hearing loss and depression in older adults*, J Am Geriatr Soc., 61(9):1627-1629, 2013.

[3] Davis A., Smith P., Ferguson M., Stephens D. and Gianopoulos I., *Acceptability, benefit and costs of early screening for hearing disability: a study of potential screening tests and models*, Health Technol Assess, 11(42):1-294, 2007.

[4] World Health Organization (WHO) 2016, *Deafness and hearing impairment*, Fact sheet No. 300. Available: https://www.who.int/en/news-room/fact-sheets/detail/deafness-and-hearing-loss [last accessed on 2020-12-23]

[5] Brooks D.N., *Factors relating to the under-use of postaural hearing aids*, Br J Audiol, 19, 211 – 217, 1985.

[6] McCormack A. and Fortnum H., *Why do people fitted with hearing aids not wear them?*, Int J Audiol, 52(5):360-8, 2013.

[7] Perkins, R., Fay, J.P., Rucker, P., Rosen, M., Olson, L., and Puria, S., *The EarLens system: new sound transduction methods. Hearing research*, 263(1-2), 104–113, 2010.

[8] Struck C.J. and Prusick L., *Comparison of real-world bandwidth in hearing aids vs Earlens light-driven hearing aid system.* Hearing Review., 24(3):24-29, 2017.

[9] Puria S., Maria P.L., Perkins R., *Temporal-Bone Measurements of the Maximum Equivalent Pressure Output and Maximum Stable Gain of a Light-Driven Hearing System That Mechanically Stimulates the Umbo.* Otol Neurotol., 37(2):160-6, 2016.

[10] Müller, S. and Massarani, P., *Transfer-function measurement with sweeps*, Journal of the Audio Engineering Society 49.6: 443-471, 2001.

Audiovisual integration during speech recognition in cochlear implant listeners with contralateral acoustic hearing

Peter Ihly [1,4], Hartmut Meister [2], Daniela Hollfelder [3] Karl-Ludwig Bruchhage [3], and Tim Jürgens [4]
[1] Auditory Technology, Universität zu Lübeck, peter.ihly@student.uni-luebeck.de
[2]Jean-Uhrmacher-Institute for Clinical ENT-Research, University of Cologne, hartmut.meister@uni-koeln.de
[3]Klinik für HNO-Heilkunde, Universitätsklinikum Schleswig-Holstein, Lübeck, {daniela.hollfelder, karl-ludwig.bruchhage}@uksh.de
[4] Institut für Akustik, Technische Hochschule Lübeck, tim.juergens@th-luebeck.de

Abstract

This study investigated the audiovisual benefit in speech intelligibility in cochlear implant (CI) users with contralateral acoustic hearing. Nine CI users (seven bimodal, two single-side deaf) and six normal-hearing listeners (as controls) were tested using the HSM sentence test in noise with and without time-aligned visual stimuli. The "bimodal benefit" was assessed by presenting the stimuli either binaurally or monaurally to each ear (and masking the opposite ear). The results indicated an audiovisual benefit of 11.1 % over all conditions in CI users and an audiovisual benefit of 10.8 % in the normal-hearing listeners. For the CI users, a significant bimodal benefit of 16.8 % in comparison to acoustic-only listening was observed. Furthermore, there was no significant interaction between the factor modality (monaural or binaural) and the factor visual information. This indicates that the audiovisual benefit is independent of the benefit that each listener obtains from the access to acoustic information contralateral to the CI.

1 Introduction

In times of Covid-19 pandemic, face-covering masks have become daily routine. While [6] examined the acoustic effects of several face masks on speech signals, [7] showed that audiovisual cues can support a higher speech intelligibility for normal hearing listeners as well as for hearing impaired listeners. This study focused on the effects of audiovisual stimuli on speech intelligibility in noise in cochlear implant users with and without access to contralateral acoustic hearing. These listeners obtain speech intelligibility improvements from "binaural" access to acoustic hearing and it is investigated whether or not this bimodal benefit is independent from the audiovisual benefit. Further investigations focused on the question whether bimodal listening leads to a higher speech intelligibility than acoustic-only listening in CI users.

2 Material and Methods

2.1 Subjects

Nine unilateral, postlingually deafened cochlear implant listeners aged 26 to 69 years (mean age 48,3 years, four female, five male) participated in this study. All subjects were native German speakers with normal or corrected-to-normal visual acuity. Seven subjects were using a hearing aid in addition to the cochlear implant on the contralateral side (bimodal subjects). Hearing impairment on the contralateral side ranged from mild to profound hearing loss. Two subjects had normal hearing on the contralateral side (i.e., these participants were implanted after single-sided deafness (SSD)). Additionally, six normal hearing subjects (mean age 30,5 years, 3 female, 3 male) were tested as controls using the same procedure.

2.2 Stimuli

2.2.1 Auditory Target Stimuli

This study used the Hochmair-Schulz-Moser (HSM) test [1] as auditory target stimuli which contains everyday sentences spoken by a male talker. 15 test-lists with 20 sentences each were used for presentation to the subjects. Every sentence had a length of three to eight words.

2.2.2 Noise

Two types of noise were used for presentation simultaneously to the target stimuli. One was the stationary CCITT noise (Comité Consultatif International Téléphonique et Télégraphique). The second one was the "International Speech Test Signal" (ISTS), representing a fluctuating background noise with all important characteristics of real speech, but being unintelligible [2]. At the beginning and at the end of each presentation, a fade-in and fade-out of 500 ms was applied to each noise type.

2.2.3 Visual Stimuli

For each sentence of the 15 HSM test-lists a visual stimulus was generated using the MASSY (articulation model for audiovisual speech synthesis) [3]. Fig. 1 shows the MASSY while presenting the vocal “U”.

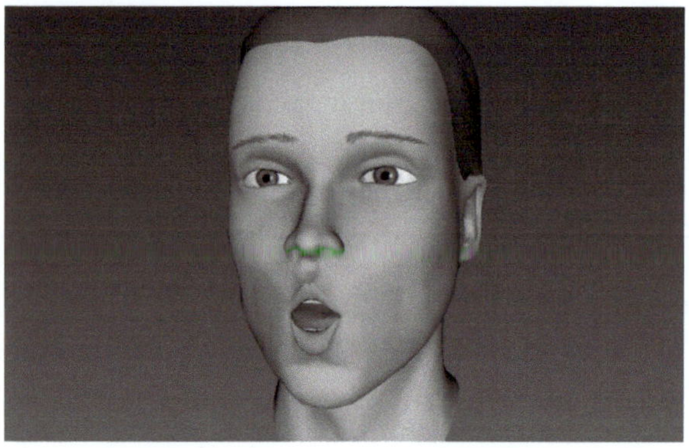

Figure 1: MASSY during the presentation of the vocal "U".

The presentation of auditory target stimuli and visual stimuli was time-synchronous with an accuracy of less than 5 ms.

2.3 Aparatus

Subjects were seated in a double-insulated sound-proof-booth. Auditory and visual stimuli were presented via a loudspeaker (Genelec 2080A, 50W) and a 24-inch flatscreen monitor in a distance of 100 cm frontal to the subjects. D/A conversion and signal routing was done with the external audio interface RME Fireface UC. Signal calibration was done using a level meter (Type 2250) which was integrated in an artificial head. The CCITT signal was played for ten seconds over free field in a distance of 100 cm to the loudspeaker and the RMS of the CCITT signal was altered to generate a constant level of 65 dB(A). The ISTS signal and all acoustic stimuli of the HSM-test were set to the same RMS value as the CCITT signal at 65 dB(A).

2.4 Test Procedures

2.4.1 Familiarization

Before testing started, every participant took part in a training session to get familiar to the procedures and the auditory and visual stimuli. Subjects were instructed to listen to the sentences carefully and repeat them as good as possible. Three out of 15 test-lists were randomly picked for familiarization. Presentation level was set to 65 dB(A) for the auditory target stimuli as well as for the two types of noise, resulting in a SNR of 0 dB. familiarization was performed binaurally (i.e., participants used both of their ears/devices). At first, 10 HSM sentences were presented in quiet without visual stimuli, followed by 10 sentences with synchronous presentation of visual stimuli. The second test-list added background noise to the HSM sentences, the first 10 sentences with CCITT noise, the last 10 with ISTS noise. Half of the sentences with CCITT noise and ISTS noise included the presentation of the MASSY. The third test-list of the session was used to determine the point where 50% of the words were repeated correct (SRT50) in a condition with CCITT background noise and without visual stimuli. Starting with an SNR of 0 dB, the SNR changed after presentation of five sentences by raising or lowering the target speech volume, collecting speech recognition scores at these different SNRs. Using linear interpolation, the SRT50 was calculated and rounded to the nearest higher value. After completing the training session all participants had a mandatory five minutes break before continuing with the speech recognition test session.

2.4.2 Speech recognition test

The speech recognition test for CI users included two monaural and one bimodal condition where subjects were instructed to use either both devices or only the CI (electric) or only the contralateral ear (acoustic). In monaural condition where bimodal participants used the hearing aid only, SSD participants were instructed to perform with their normal hearing ear only. All three conditions were tested with CCITT and ISTS background noise, once with visual stimuli given and one time without visual stimuli. This made a total of 12 test conditions. Normal hearing subjects were tested in monaural and binaural condition, both conditions once with ISTS and once with CCITT noise. One time without visual stimuli and one time with visual stimuli given, normal hearing subjects performed eight conditions. All conditions and sentences in each test list were presented in randomized order. Subjects were instructed before each condition about the following stimuli and which hearing device to use. For conditions where subjects were instructed to use only the CI, CCITT noise at 65 dB(A) was presented to the contralateral ear with in-ear headphones in order to mask the contralateral ear. The same procedure was done with the normal hearing subjects in monaural conditions. Subjects were instructed to use their left ear only for listening while the right ear was wearing in-ear headphones with CCITT noise at 65 dB(A).

2.5 Statistical Analysis

Subject scores for each condition were measured in percent correct. To make the acquired data more suitable for statistical analysis, percentages were transferred into rationalized arcsine units (RAU, [4]). The RAU-transferred datasets were analysed for normal distribution with the Shapiro-Wilk Test. For analysis of variance the dataset of the CI subjects was splitted into a ISTS and a CCITT dataset to perform a 3x2 repeated measures ANOVA analysing the factors modality (acoustic-only, electric-only, bimodal) and visual information (audio-only (A), audiovisual (AV)). A 2x2 repeated measures ANOVA was performed on the normal hearing listeners datasets with the factors modality (monaural, binaural) and visual information (audio-only, audiovisual). Multiple comparisons were performed using Bonferroni's correction at the level of $\alpha = 0.05$.

3 Results and Discussion

3.1 Results of normal hearing listeners

Fig. 2 shows the mean speech intelligibility scores and standard error for all normal hearing subjects in all tested conditions.

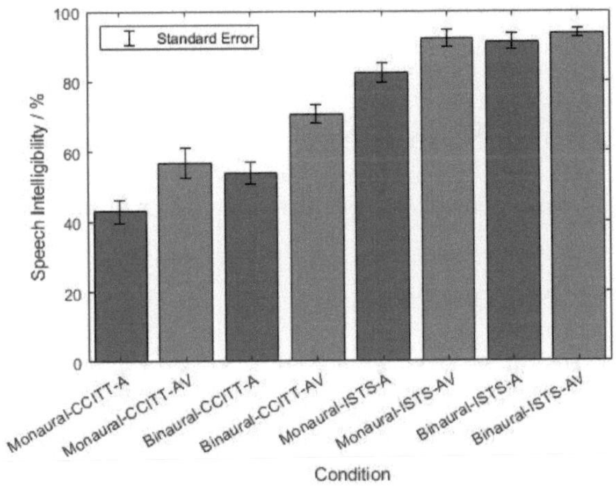

Figure 2: Mean speech intelligibility of normal hearing subjects for all conditions.

The Shapiro-Wilk Test displayed a normal distribution of the data for all conditions ($p > 0.050$). Data analysis with the 2x2 ANOVA revealed for conditions using CCITT noise a significant influence of the factor modality ($p = 0.040$, $F = 7.62$) and visual information ($p = 0.001$, $F = 40.63$) on speech intelligibility but no significant interaction between both factors ($p = 0.782$, $F = 0.09$). Conditions with ISTS noise also showed a significant influence of the factors modality ($p = 0.020$, $F = 11.28$) and visual information ($p = 0.039$, $F = 7.74$) with no significant interaction between both factors ($p = 0.252$, $F = 1.68$).

3.2 Results of CI users

Fig. 3 shows the mean speech intelligibility scores and standard error for all CI users in all tested conditions.

The Shapiro-Wilk Test revealed a normal distribution of the data for all conditions except the condition "Acoustic-CCITT-AV" ($p = 0.041$). Data analysis using the 3x2 ANOVA for the CCITT noise conditions showed that speech intelligibility was significantly influenced by the factors modality ($p = 0.009$, $F = 6.36$) and visual information ($p < 0.001$, $F = 36.37$). There was no significant interaction between both factors ($p = 0.505$, $F = 0.71$). Conditions with ISTS noise also showed a significant influence of modality ($p < 0.001$, $F = 15.58$) and visual information ($p = 0.008$, $F = 12.56$) on the speech intelligibility without significant interaction between both factors ($p = 0.134$, $F = 2.29$).

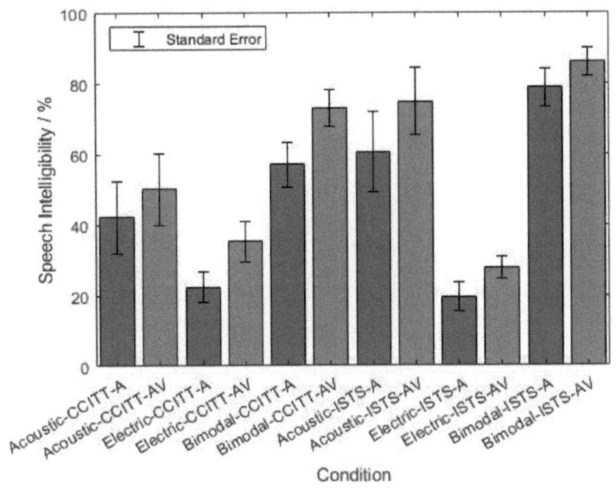

Figure 3: Mean speech intelligibility of CI subjects for all conditions.

3.2.1 Audiovisual Benefit

Audiovisual benefit was defined as the individual difference in speech intelligibility score between the audio-only and audiovisual conditions. Fig. 4 shows the mean audiovisual benefit of CI and NH subjects for all test conditions.

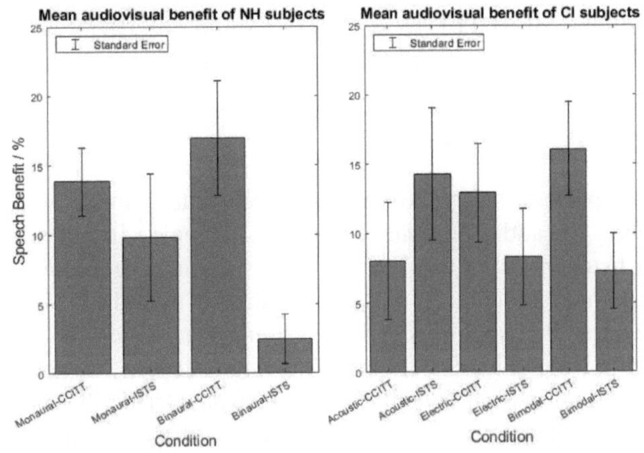

Figure 4: Mean audiovisual benefit of CI and NH subjects for all conditions.

Cochlear implant users showed an audiovisual benefit of 11.2 % and normal hearing listeners of 10.8 % averaged across conditions. Data analysis using Bonferroni's Multiple Comparisons Test delivered significant speech benefits for CI users in the conditions Electric-CCITT ($p = 0.012$), Bimodal-CCITT ($p = 0.002$), Acoustic-ISTS ($p < 0.001$) and Electric-ISTS ($p = 0.037$). The conditions Acoustic-CCITT and Bimodal-ISTS showed no significant results. Normal hearing listeners showed a significant audiovisual benefit in the condition Binaural-CCITT ($p = 0.040$).

3.2.2 Bimodal Benefit of CI-usage

Fig. 5 displays the mean bimodal benefit of the CI users, which was defined as the difference in speech intelligibility between the bimodal and better-ear-only conditions. In this study the better ear was either normal hearing (two participants) or the aided hearing-impaired ear (seven participants).

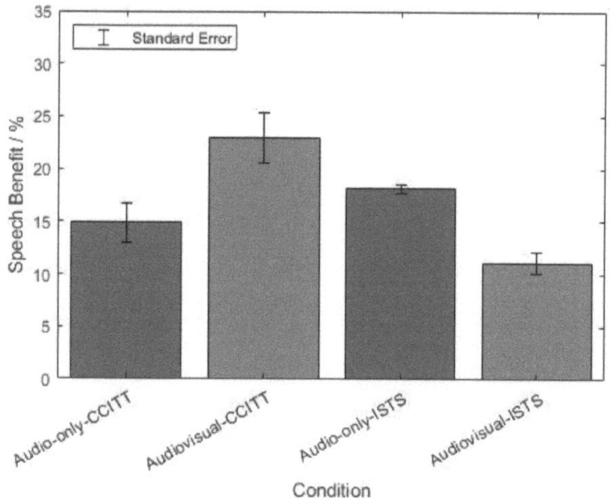

Figure 5: Mean bimodal benefit of CI users for all conditions.

Multiple comparisons analysis comparing the acoustic conditions with the bimodal conditions delivered significant results for the conditions Audio-only-CCITT ($p = 0.003$), Audiovisual-CCITT ($p < 0.001$), Audio-only-ISTS ($p < 0.001$) and Audiovisual-ISTS ($p = 0.030$).

3.3 Discussion

The present study compared speech intelligibility (SI) scores for audio-only and audiovisual listening in bimodal CI listeners using two different types of background noise and three modalities (acoustic, electric, bimodal). The mean audiovisual benefit for CI users over all tested conditions was 11.2 %. Normal hearing listeners showed a mean audiovisual benefit of 10.8 %. Considering that normal hearing listeners showed a mean speech intelligibility score of over 80 % in all ISTS conditions even without visual stimuli, ceiling effects could have been a limiting factor on the audiovisual benefit. However, ceiling effects only had a small impact on CI users scores, although one participant showed a speech intelligibility score of 100 % in one audiovisual condition. The audiovisual benefit of 11.2 % supports the findings of [5] who simulated the effects of bimodal CI listening using a vocoder during presentation of audio-only and audiovisual speech. The improvements in SI of bimodal listening compared to monaural listening suit to the findings of [8] who proved several benefits (including SI) of bimodal CI listening.

4 Conclusion

Findings suggest that audiovisual stimuli lead to a higher speech intelligibility than audio-only stimuli in CI listeners as well as in normal hearing listeners. Furthermore, CI listeners seem to benefit significantly from the usage of the CI additional to a contralateral hearing aid. No significant interaction between the factors modality and visual information in CI users was found, indicating that the audiovisual benefit is independent from the benefit that CI users obtain from binaural listening in contrast to monaural listening.

Acknowledgement

The work has been carried out and supervised by the Institute of Acoustics, Technische Hochschule Lübeck.

Author's Statement

Conflict of interest: Authors state no conflict of interest.

5 References

[1] I. Hochmair-Desoyer, E. Schulz, L. Moser, M. Schmidt, "The HSM sentence test as a tool for evaluating the speech understanding in noise of cochlear implant users", The American Journal of Otology, Vol. 6, pp. 83, 1997

[2] I. Holube, S. Fredelake, M. Vlaming, B. Kollmeier, "Development and analysis of an International Speech Test Signal (ISTS)", International Journal of Audiology, Vol. 49, pp. 891-903, 2010

[3] S. Schreitmüller, M. Frenken, L. Bentz, M. Ortmann, M. Walger, H. Meister, "Validating a method to assess lipreading, audiovisual gain and Integration during speech reception with cochlear-implanted and normal-hearing subjects using a talking head", Ear and hearing, Vol. 39, pp. 503-516, 2018

[4] G. A. Studebaker, "A "rationalized" arcsine transform", Journal of Speech and Hearing Research, Vol. 28, pp. 455-462, 1985

[5] M. Engler, H. Meister, T. Jürgens, "Audiovisual Integration during Speech Reception with Simulated Bimodal Cochlear Implant Users", BioMedTec Studierendentagung, Vol. 1, 2019

[6] R. M. Corey, U. Jones, A. C. Singer, "Acoustic effects of medical, cloth, and transparent face masks on speech signals", The Journal of the Acoustical Society of America, Vol. 148, pp. 2371-2375, 2020

[7] M. B. Winn, A. E. Rhone, M. Chatterjee, W. J. Idsardi, "The use of auditory and visual context in speech perception by listeners with normal hearing and listeners with cochlear implants", Frontiers in Psychology, Vol. 4, pp. 824, 2013

[8] E. Wallhäusser-Franke, T. Balkenhol, S. Hetjens, N. Rotter, J. J. Servais, "Patient benefit following bimodal CI-provision: Self-reported abilities vs. hearing status", Frontiers in Neurology, Vol. 9, pp. 753, 2018

Evaluation of Impulse Noise Reduction in Hearing Aids

Wiebke Hilgerdenaar [1,2], Simone Wollermann [2], and Hendrik Husstedt [2]
[1] Auditory Technology, Universität zu Lübeck, wiebke.hilgerdenaar@student.uni-luebeck.de
[2] Deutsches Hörgeräte Institut GmbH, s.wollermann@dhi-online.de, h.husstedt@dhi-online.de

Abstract

Disturbing impulse noises frequently occur in everyday life. Hearing impaired people can benefit from an impulse noise reduction in hearing aids, as it reduces the hearing effort. This study deals with the effect of impulse noise reduction on different impulse sounds, at different sound pressure levels and the dependence on other hearing aid features. Different impulse sounds were presented to an artificial head equipped with hearing aids at different sound pressure levels and using different hearing aid feature settings. The results show that the impulse noise reduction of the tested hearing aids does not depend on other features. Furthermore, impulse noise reduction was more reliable and stronger in lowering impulsive noise (up to 18 dB reduction), as the general noise reduction showed no effect (just 1-2 dB reduction) and maximum power output had a limited effect (about 8 dB reduction).

1 Introduction

In everyday life, people are exposed to a wide variety of sounds, which can have psychological and physical effects [1]. One type of noise is impulse noise, such as a bursting balloon or hammering. Such noises are characterized, among other things, by their short duration and high peak sound pressure level. An impulsive signal increases by at least 40 dB per 0.5 seconds, which results in a steep leading edge. Impulse noise causes significantly different effects on hearing compared to continuous noise [2]. According to Pfander (1975), the hearing damage risks of impulse sound in Germany are assessed based on the threshold elevation still present in 95% of the persons involved 24 hours after termination of the sound exposure [1].

To characterize impulse noise, the standard ISO 10843:1997 has defined some parameters [3]. For instance, three types of durations are named to describe an impulse. The A, B and C duration, which are shown in Figure 1, define the rise time of an impulse as well as different ways of describing the decrease. In an idealized signal, such as a gunshot, the A duration is the shortest and the B duration is the longest duration. For everyday impulse sounds, this type of characterization has been sparsely examined in the literature.

In the life of a hearing aid user, impulse noise is omnipresent and often the trigger for not wearing hearing aids. Chalupper (2007) describes that about one third of the annoying noise in the daily life of a hearing aid user consists of impulse noises [4].

The general noise reductions (NR) for hearing aids have been developed to reduce noise exposure. However, these were not able to detect and reduce impulsive noise. Thus, impulse noise reduction (INR) had to be developed. In the past, this was controlled by automatic gain control or peak clipping. However, these not only suppressed impulsive noise, but also reduced speech intelligibility [6]. Nowadays, the input signal is analyzed temporally and spectrally and the impulse noise is lowered above a defined trigger threshold [4]. Various studies have shown that no significant difference in speech intelligibility results from impulse noise reduction, and instead improves listening comfort [4] [6] [7] [8].

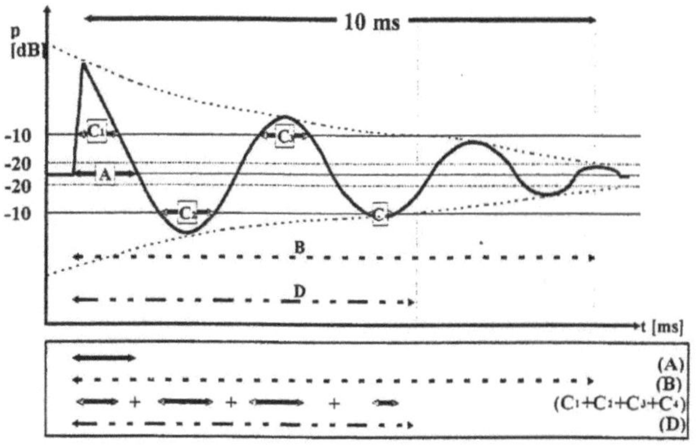

Figure 1: [5] Shown are the A, B, C and D durations of an idealized impulse noise. (The ISO 10843:1997 standard ignores the D duration). The A and C durations use the time signal and the B an D durations use the envelope. For the B duration, the duration between the start of the signal and peak - 20 dB is determined. (D duration start to peak - 10 dB)

In this study, the effect of the impulse noise reduction in hearing aids was investigated for different types of impulsive noise. In addition, the effects of the noise reduction (NR) and the maximum power output (MPO) were analyzed. For this purpose, realistic impulse sounds were recorded and the impact of hearing aids with different settings was compared.

2 Material and Methods

2.1 Recording impulse noise

Initially, various impulse sounds were recorded in an anechoic chamber. Therefore, a Brüel and Kjaer Falcon 1/4" Condenser microphone was positioned at a distance of one meter from the sound event. Nine different sounds from everyday life were selected. The recordings were repeated several times and the C-weighted peak sound pressure levels were averaged for each signal. The respective signal recording with the smallest deviation from the C-weighted peak sound pressure level mean was selected for further investigation. For each signal, the C-weighted peak sound pressure level (see table 1) and the three durations A, B and C (see table 2) were determined.

Table 1: Peak sound pressure levels (SPL) in dB(C) of the recorded signals

Signal	Peak SPL
bursting balloon	128
clattering cutlery	82
closing book	99
rattling dishes	92
tapping a knife against a glass	86
putting down a glass on a table	100
cutting with knife on a plate	96
falling keys	109
choke valve	133

Table 2: Durations of the recorded signals in ms.

Signal	A	B	C
bursting balloon	0.5	2.4	0.9
clattering cutlery	15.8	49.8	4.3
closing book	1.2	4.2	0.9
rattling dishes	4.1	23.9	4.0
tapping a knife against a glass	1.8	80.3	15.6
putting down glass on table	1.2	12.9	2.5
cutting with knife on plate	2.1	35.9	6.3
falling keys	17.5	37.3	5.9
choke valve	0.1	2.6	0.2

2.2 Investigation of the impulse sound reduction

The test setup for the investigation of the hearing aid features on the different impulse signals is shown in figure 2. Hearing aids were fitted fully occluded with foam plugs to an artificial head GRAS KEMAR Head and Torso (KEMAR) and a Genelec loudspeaker of type 8351A was placed at a distance of one meter. For monitoring the measurements, a reference microphone was positioned above the KEMAR (Figure 2).

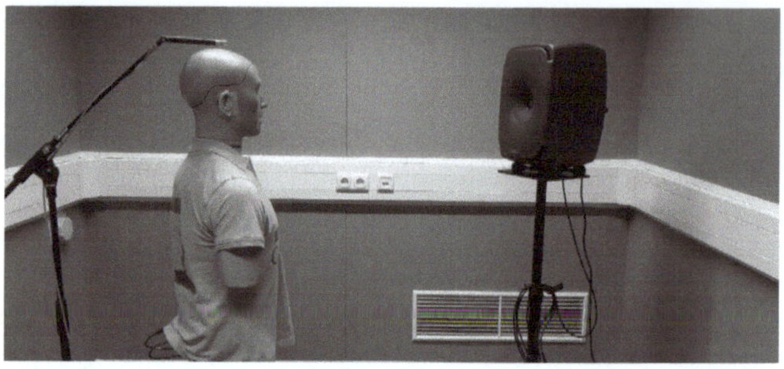

Figure 2: Measurement setup with KEMAR, hearing aids, loudspeaker and reference microphone.

The high-end behind the ear hearing aids were fitted for an N3 hearing loss according to ISO EN 60118-15:2012 [9]. This is a moderate hearing loss with slightly decreasing thresholds towards higher frequencies. All adaptive features were deactivated and the microphones were set to omnidirectional mode. The features impulse noise reduction (INR), noise reduction (NR) and maximum power output (MPO) were investigated on their own and in combination. Therefore, as shown in table 3, eight different conditions were tested. Feature "on" indicates a maximum setting of the feature and feature "off" a deactivated, or minimal setting.

Table 3: Hearing aid conditions

	INR	NR	MPO
1	on	on	on
2	on	on	off
3	on	off	off
4	on	off	on
5	off	on	on
6	off	on	off
7	off	off	on
8	off	off	off

Each impulse signal was presented with three different peak sound pressure levels. In addition to the measured sound pressure level, the signals were also presented with 6 dB more or 6 dB less to simulate a larger or smaller distance to the signal source. However, the maximum allowed sound pressure level was set to 120 dB, so that two signals (bursting balloon and starter flap) were reduced in sound pressure level and additionally presented with -6 and -12 dB.

To create a situation as realistic as possible, the impulse sounds were combined with the international speech test signal (ISTS) before playback. Each test signal had a length of 35 s. After 19 s of ISTS, there was a pause of 100 ms, followed by the impulse signal and ending with ISTS again. As shown in figure 3, each test signal was presented in sequence for all three sound pressure levels.

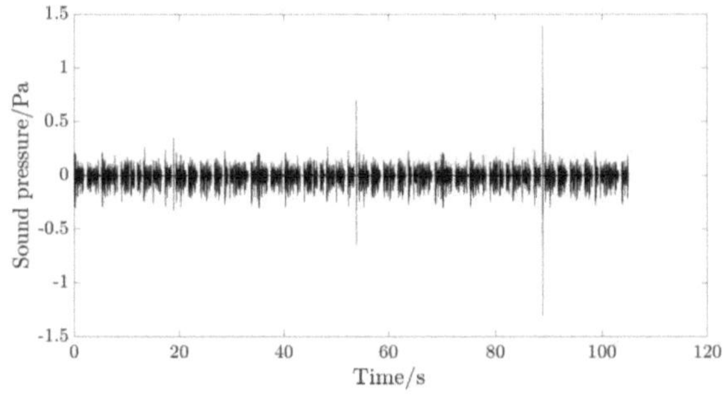

Figure 3: Time signal of the clattering cutlery signal with ISTS.

3 Results and Discussion

The impulse signals processed by the hearing aids were extracted from the KEMAR recordings and analyzed. All peak sound pressure levels were compared with the peak sound pressure levels of the hearing aid condition "all features off". In figure 4 the oscillograms of the sound "falling key" for the conditions "all features off", 'INR", "MPO" and "NR" on are compared. Especially the first peak of the signal was reduced clearly by the INR. Also the second part of the noise at around 170 ms is visibly attenuated with the feature impulse noise reduction on. The MPO reduced the peak only slightly and the NR had almost no effect.

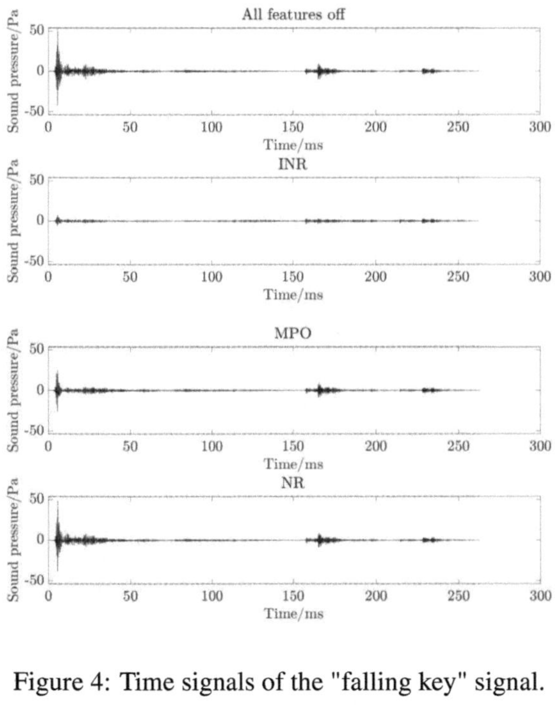

Figure 4: Time signals of the "falling key" signal.

In Figure 5, the gain processed by the hearing aids for all conditions are compared depending on the input peak sound pressure level. The higher the input sound pressure level, the lower the amplification of the hearing aid in general. This gain reduction to higher levels is increased by the MPO.

The MPO reduces the gain by about 7 dB at lower sound pressure levels and by about 10 dB at higher levels. The NR, on the other hand, only reduces the gain by about 1 dB. The maximum gain reduction of about 18 dB is achieved by the INR at lower input sound pressure levels. At higher input sound pressure levels, the attenuation is reduced to 15 dB.

It is clearly shown, that the MPO causes a reduction in the peak sound pressure level. However, this is less pronounced than in the combination with impulse noise reduction or in the sole use of impulse noise reduction. The noise reduction, on the other hand, shows no effect on the impulsive noise. A dependence of the features on each other cannot be seen either.

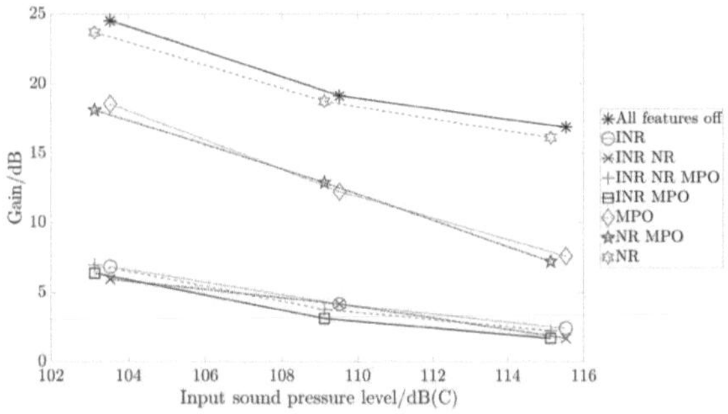

Figure 5: Comparison of the eight hearing aid feature settings. Gain of the impulse peak in relation to the input sound pressure level for the "falling key" signal.

With the condition "MPO", a stronger dependence of the gain reduction on the input sound pressure level than in the case of impulse sound reduction can be observed. This can be seen especially with the signal "knife cuts on plate" in Figure 6. Here, a triggering threshold for the MPO can be seen from approx. 100 dB input sound pressure level. Thus, the MPO is not suitable for reducing softer impulse noise. No trigger level can be identified for impulse sound reduction in the sound pressure level ranges investigated.

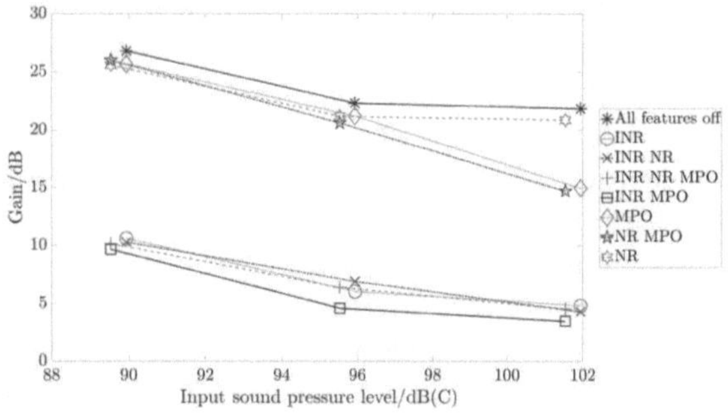

Figure 6: Comparison of the eight hearing aid feature settings. Gain of the impulse peak in relation to the input sound pressure level for the signal "knife cuts on plate".

An overview of the reduction of the absolute peak sound pressure level in relation to the hearing aid condition "all features off" is shown in Figure 7. Each box shows the pooled distribution across all signals and all levels. The op-

timal reduction of impulse noise is also visible here for all conditions with INR. Thereby 75% of the test signals were reduced by more than 13 dB in the peak and 25% even more than 16 dB. Since the reduction of the sound pressure level is in a very similar range, the INR feature alone seems to be decisive for the greatest reduction. The other features do not seem to add any value for impulse noise reduction.
An independence of the features from the test signals can be observed. Only one signal falls out a bit here. The outliers in figure 7 represent the quietest recorded signal. This was significantly less attenuated than sounds played at a very similar sound pressure level. This could be an indication of a limit of the impulse detection of the impulse noise reduction. However, further research is needed to understand these findings.

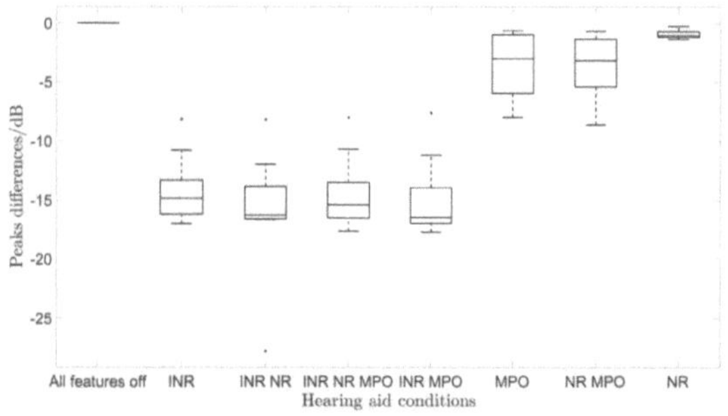

Figure 7: Differences of the peak sound pressure level for the eight hearing aid conditions to the condition "all features off".

4 Conclusion

Impulse noise reduction is essential to reliably detect impulse noise and reduce it to a minimum. The maximum gain reduction was around 18 dB and is largely independent on the type of noise. However, further investigations may be useful for this purpose. In particular, impulse noise with a lower sound pressure level is attenuated by impulse noise suppression, while other features such as MPO deliberately take effect only at a higher triggering threshold. The NR shows no influence on impulse noise, which allows for a specific decision which types of noise should be attenuated and which should not.
In this study, only one pair of hearing aids were investigated so far. Therefore, further investigations with other hearing aid manufacturers are to follow. A review of the different signal processing strategies of the manufacturers for different processing of the impulse sounds would be interesting. Furthermore, the psychoacoustic effects of impulse sound reduction should be evaluated. The perception of impulsive noise by hearing aid users is important in the selection of a signal processing strategy in impulse noise reduction. Impulse noises that are not perceived as annoying do not necessarily have to be reduced. Likewise, it is interesting to study the subjective perception of the effectiveness of the INR. A comparison to the perception of a normal hearing person without hearing aids would also be interesting to investigate.

Acknowledgement

The work was conducted and supervised at Deutsches Hörgeräte Institut GmbH, Lübeck.

Author's Statement

Conflict of interest: Authors state no conflict of interest.

5 References

[1] F. Pfander, H. Bongartz and H. Brinkmann, *Das Knalltrauma, Analyse, Vorbeugung, Diagnose, Behandlung, Prognose und Begutachtung*. Springer-Verlag, Berlin Heidelberg GmbH, 1975.

[2] M. Spreng, S. Leupold and P. Firsching, *Gehörschäden durch Impulsgeräusche, Vorschlag für ein gehörschadensrichtiges Impulsbewertungssystem*. Schriftenreihe der Bundesanstalt für Arbeitsschutz, Dortmund, 1991.

[3] ISO 10843:1997(E) *Acoustics - Methods for the description and physical measurement of single impulses or series of impulses*. 1997.

[4] J. Chalupper and T. A. Powers, *New algorithm is designed to take the annoyance out of transient noise*. The Hearing Journal, vol. 60, no. 7, pp. 42-48, 2007.

[5] H. H. Brinkmann, *Techniques and Procedures for the Measurement of Impulse Noise*. Defense Technical Information Center Compilation Part Notice, ADPO10340, 2000.

[6] H. Liu, H. Zhang, R. A. Bentler, D. Han and L. Zhang, *Evaluation of a Transient Noise Reduction Strategy for Hearing Aids*. Journal of the American Academy of Audiology, vol. 23, no. 8, pp.606-615, 2012.

[7] K.-H. Dyballa, P. Hehrmann, V. Hamacher, W. Nogueira, T. Lenarz and A. Büchner, *Evaluation of a transient noise reduction algorithm in cochlear implant users*. Audiology Research, vol. 5:116, pp. 44-49, 2015.

[8] J.J. DiGiovanni, E. A. Davlin and N. K. Nagaraja. *Effects of Transient Noise Reduction Algorithms on Speech Intelligibility and Ratings of Hearing Aid Users*. American Journal of Audiology, vol. 20, pp. 140-150, 2011.

[9] ISO EN 60118-15:2012, *Akustik – Hörgeräte – Teil 15: Methoden zur Charakterisierung der Hörgeräte-Signalverarbeitung*. 2012.

Comparison of an open source hearing aid prototype with commercially available hearing aids

Lukas Jürgensen [1], Hendrik Husstedt [2], Florian Denk [2]

[1] Auditory Technology, Universität zu Lübeck, lukas.juergensen@student.uni-luebeck.de

[2] Deutsches Hörgeräte Institut GmbH, Lübeck, {h.husstedt, f.denk}@dhi-online.de

Abstract

As medical devices, hearing aids compensate for a hearing loss but they also consist of several interacting features such as directional microphones, noise reductions or feedback reductions. To facilitate the process of developing such features, the open master hearing aid (openMHA) has recently been made available as an open source tool. In combination with a miniature computer and realistic hearing aid headsets, the openMHA can be used as a hearing aid prototype. In this work, the performance of the feedback reduction as well as frequency-dependent gains and latencies of the aformentioned are evaluated and compared to a recent commercial device operated in two technology levels. The results show that the performance of the prototype is comparable to the commercial system, as the feedback reductions were functional in both cases, while the maximum provided gain was 10 dB higher and the latencies were 4 ms longer for the prototype.

1 Introduction

Hearing aids are medical devices, made to compensate for a hearing loss. For this purpose, modern hearing aids capture the acoustic signal with up to two microphones, split it up into different frequency channels and modify it with different features. Examples for basic features are the automatic gain control (AGC), which applies a frequency- and input level-dependent gain to the signal or a feedback reduction, which prevents or reduces the occurance of a whistling noise (critical feedback), caused by sound returning from the hearing aid output to the microphone inlets [1]. The processed channel signals are recombined to a single output signal, which is then played back by a receiver. The number of channels, as well as the number and/or the performance of other features, increases with the technology level of the hearing aid. The latency, caused by the signal processing of the hearing aid, leads to a decrease in sound quality, as the interference of the processed and the unprocessed signal in the ear canal causes comb filter effects. Thus latencies are only tolerable up to 20 ms in general [2].

The development and evaluation of new signal processing algorithms in hearing aids is a timeconsuming and expensive process. To facilitate this process, the open Master Hearing Aid (openMHA) has been developed by the Carl von Ossietzky University Oldenburg and Hörtech GmbH, Oldenburg. The openMHA is an open source, PC-based software platform, on which the entire development and evaluation of hearing aid features can be performed [3]. It offers real-time audio signal processing with standard PC hardware and software and allows for the testing of new hearing aid features, embedded in a set of interacting signal processing features, rather than in isolation. The single hearing aid features are realized with plugins for the openMHA (e.g. one plugin for the noise reduction, one plugin for the feedback reduction, etc.). By combining and arranging several plugins in the desired way, the complete signal processing of a hearing aid can be simulated. There is a set of already existing plugins available, but own plugins can also be created considering certain rules.
In this work the performance capability of the openMHA in a standard configuration combined with openly available hardware was evaluated. For this purpose, frequency-gain-curves, frequency-dependent latencies and the performances of the feedback reductions were measured. The results achieved with the openMHA setup were then compared to those measured with commercial hearing aids.

2 Material and Methods

2.1 Experimental Setup

All measurements were performed inside an anechoic test box (Brüel & Kjær, Type 4232), that included one loudspeaker, one coupler-microphone and one reference-microphone (both Brüel & Kjær, Type 4192). The coupler-microphone was inserted into a 2cc-coupler with the adaptor (Type 4946) for in-ear devices. The test box was controlled with a laptop that was connected to it via a RME FIREFACE UC sound card. The exact experimental setup for the measurement of the feedback reduction is shown in Fig. 1. For all other measurements the setup was the same, but without the additional feedback tube.

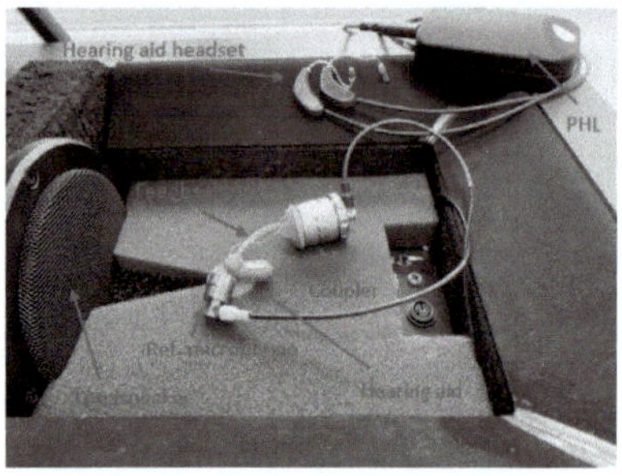

Figure 1: Experimental setup for the measurement of the feedback reduction. A commercial hearing aid is attached to the 2cc-coupler. An additionally inserted tube allows for provoking feedback [1]. For an optical comparison, the hearing aid prototype is also shown in the top right corner.

2.2 Hearing Aids

The openMHA was used with a standard configuration (generic-hearing-aid, openMHA version 4.12). A reduced diagram of the resulting signal processing for one ear is shown in Fig. 2. It consists of two microphones that allow processing to create a desired directivity. In 5 channels a binaural coherence filter attenuates frequency bands with a low coherence between left and right ear signals, which is usually the case for signals like feedback, noise and reverberation. The automatic gain control applies an input level- and frequency dependent gain to the signal, which is then shifted to higher frequencies by a small amount to reduce feedback and played back by a speaker.

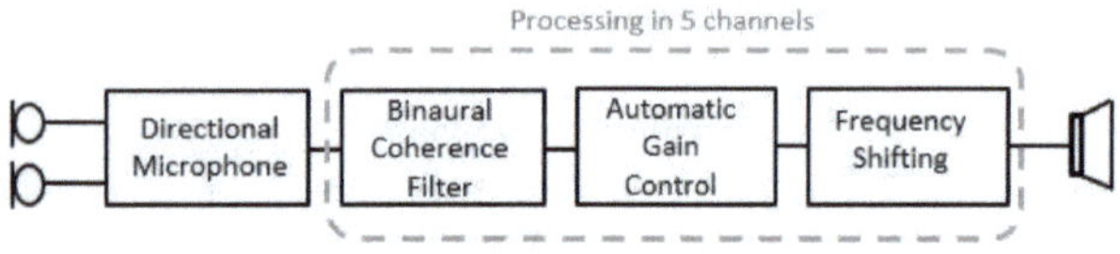

Figure 2: Strongly simplified schematic layout of the openMHA signal processing.

The hardware used for the openMHA in this work, was the Portable Hearing Lab (PHL), which is shown in Fig. 1. It is based on a portable miniature PC (Beagle Bone Black) with a 6-channel audio interface [4]. Due to its small size and the opportunity to connect realistic hearing aid headsets, it enables the openMHA to be tested mobile, as well as being tested identically to a commercial hearing aid. Additionally, a WiFi connection offers control via a remote computer or smartphone. The hearing aid headsets were Behind the Ear (BTE) designs with external Receivers In the ear Canal (RIC). In one setup, the external receivers had the strength *S* (Small), in another one their strength was *M* (Medium), whereby the M-speakers offer a higher power output than the S-speakers. In the following these combinations of openMHA, PHL and hearing aid headsets will be referred to as *Protype S* and *Prototype M*. For a comparison, two technology levels (second lowest and second highest) of a commercial hearing aid series (released 2019) were used with M-speaker RICs. Those devices will be called *HA Low* and *HA High* hereafter.

2.3 Measurement Procedures

2.3.1 Frequency-Gain-Curves

The frequency-gain-curves, i.e. the Sound Pressure Level (SPL) in 1/3 octave bands at the coupler microphone, relative to those at the reference microphone, were measured with 2 different gain-configurations of the hearing aids. The first configuration was a flat 0 dB gain-setting, the second one was a full on gain (FOG) setting, which means all gain configurators were set to the maximum value. In both cases, the output limiter was set to minimum impact, all accessable features were disabled and the input signal was the International Speech Test Signal (ISTS) [5]. It was presented to the hearing aid inside the test box at 70 dB SPL for the 0 dB-setting and 50 dB SPL for the FOG-setting. Each time the signal duration was 45 seconds, but only the last 30 seconds of the recordings were used to compute the 1/3 octave levels at the coupler and reference microphone. By subtracting the reference microphone level and the Coupler Response for Flat Insertion Gain (CORFIG) [6] values from the coupler microphone levels, an estimate of the gain across frequency provided by the inserting hearing aid in a real ear is obtained.

2.3.2 Latencies

For the measurement of frequency dependent latencies caused by the signal processing of the hearing aid, a pink noise at 70 dB SPL was presented to the devices over a period of 5 seconds inside the test box. Both the signal measured by the coupler microphone (processed, delayed signal) and the signal measured by the reference microphone (undelayed signal) were then filtered in 1/3 octave bands. For each 1/3 octave band, the cross-correlation between the processed and the unprocessed signal was computed. The resulting difference in samples from the peak of the cross-correlation to the zero point was then converted to a time in ms. To investigate the effect of certain signal processing algorithms on the frequency dependent latencies, this procedure was performed for various combinations of activated and deactivated hearing aid features. The hearing aids were programmed to a neutral setting, i.e., a broadband gain of 0 dB, no compression and the output limiter was set to minimum effectiveness.

2.3.3 Feedback Reduction

As a measure for the efficiency of the feedback reduction the Added Stable Gain (ASG) was considered. The ASG was measured based on the IEC 60118-16 draft [1]. According to this method the hearing aid was attached to the coupler with an additional sound tube to provoke feedback as shown in Fig. 1. The device was configured with a broadband 1/12 octave band gain of 10 dB and all other features available in the fitting software were disabled. A pink noise with a 1/12 octave band level of 44 dB SPL was presented to the hearing aid in cycles. After each cyle the 1/12 octave band gain was increased by 5 dB, until a critical feedback condition occured. This was the case when the measured gain increased disproportionately due to positive feedback, usually around a single frequency. Contrary to [1], for this work the last gain increase was then undone and the gain was increased in steps of 1 dB again to capture the starting point of the critical feedback condition more precisely. The feedback reduction was then turned on and the measurement procedure was repeated. The ASG was calculated by subtracting the gain that lead to a critical feedback condition with activated feedback reduction from the corresponding gain with activated feedback reduction.

For the hearing aid prototypes the measurement was done for the binaural coherence filter and the frequency shifting activated separately and both features activated simultaneously. For the comercial systems the two possible configurations for the feedback reduction (min and max) available in the fitting software were measured.

3 Results and Discussion

3.1 Frequency Curves

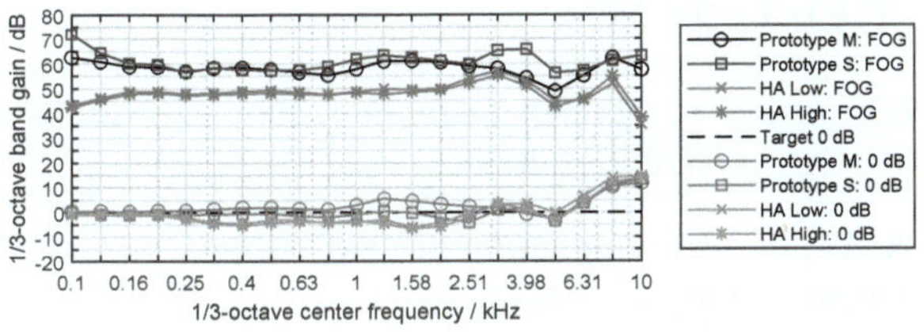

Figure 3: Frequency-gain-curves for two different gain-configurations. The grey curves depict the results for a full on gain setting, the black curves show those for a flat 0-dB-gain setting,

The measured frequency-gain-curves for two different hearing aid configurations are shown in Fig. 3. The configuration with flat 0 dB gain was chosen to see how precise the devices match a certain adjustment made in the fitting software. All 4 devices matched the 0 dB-target well for frequencies below 250 Hz. In the frequency range between 250 Hz and 5 kHz, there were deviations of approximately ±5 dB. At higher frequencies the deviations increased for all 4 devices up to 15 dB at 10 kHz.
The frequency-gain-curves measured in the FOG setting showed similar results for both technology levels of the commercial hearing aid with a maximum 1/3 octaveband gain of approximately 55 dB. Compared with this, both openMHA setups achieved a maximum 1/3 octave band gain of approximately 65 dB.
All in all, the devices showed similar deviations from the programmed gain targets. However, the openMHA setups were able to provide a higher gain.

3.2 Latencies

Fig. 4 shows the 1/3 octave band latencies of all devices. When all features were deactivated, both prototypes showed almost constant latencies of 10 ms for frequencies above 400 Hz and deviating latencies for frequencies below 400 Hz. Activating all features resulted in two effects for the prototypes. The first effect was a change in latency below 400 Hz. The second effect was a very steep increase of latency from 2 kHz onwards for both prototypes. The second effect can be well explained with the here used method of feedback reduction and the measuring procedure. The shifting of the signal components from a certain frequency on to higher frequencies, led to a loss of correlation between the unprocessed and the processed signal at the affected 1/3 octave bands. Consequently, computing the cross-correlation between those 1/3 octave bands was no longer expedient to get the latencies. Measurements with only single features being activated indicated that the increase in latency at low frequencies can be related to the directional microphone. The other features did not result in any changes regarding the latencies.
The latencies for the two technology levels of the commercial hearing aid were identical and are shown exemplary for HA Low. It provided constant latencies of 6 ms for almost the complete frequency range. With all features activated, there was a steep ascend of latency from 1,6 kHz onwards. Just like it was the case with the prototypes, this effect disappeared, as soon as the feedback reduction was deactivated. It is therefore likely, that the measured commercial systems do also use the method of frequency shifting to reduce feedback. All other configurable features available in the fitting software did not effect the measured latencies.
In conclusion, both the prototypes and the commercial systems provided almost the same latency across all frequencies. These latencies lay within a tolerable range [2]. Nervertheless, they cause artifacts and reduce the sound quality. As the latencies of the prototypes were longer, the decrease in sound quality is also expected to be greater.

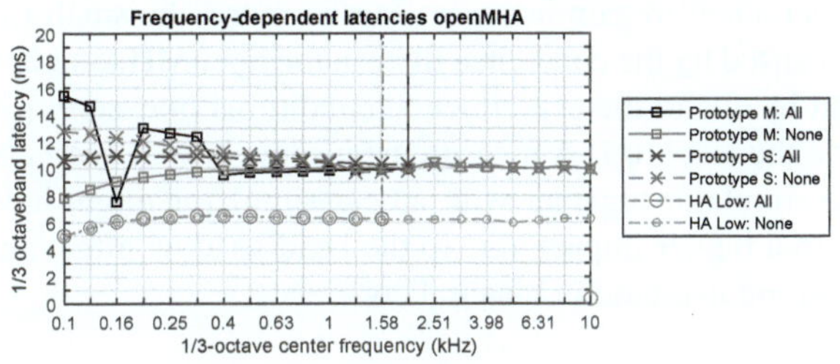

Figure 4: Frequency-dependent latencies of all devices, measured for one condition with all features being activated (All) and another one with all features being deactivated (None). The results for *HA High* are identical to those of *HA Low* and thus not included in the graphic.

3.3 Feedback Reduction

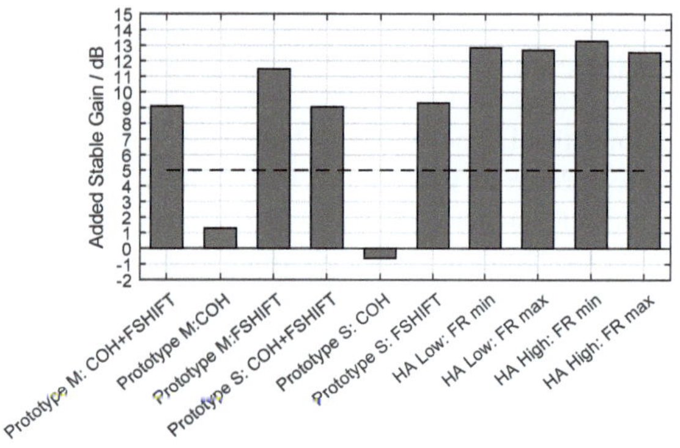

Figure 5: Measured added stable gain for all devices and all possible feature configurations. The dashed line at 5 dB ASG indicates the threshold for proven functionality of the feedback reduction according to [1].

The measured ASG for all hearing aids and configurations is shown in Fig. 5. For both prototypes, the ASG was to a large extent effected by the frequency shifting and reached its maximum value at approximately 9 dB with the S-speaker headset and 11,5 dB with the M-speaker headset. In comparison the coherence filter, when activated alone, caused an ASG of only slighly above 1 dB (Prototype M) and could even produce a negative effect as measured with Prototype S. When both features were activated, the ASG was equal to (S-speaker headset) or 2,5 dB lower (M-speaker headset) than the frequency shifting only configuration.

For the commercial hearing aids neither the technology level nor the configuration-level of the feedback reduction, chosen in the fitting software, had a noticeable effect on the measured ASG, which lay at values between 12,5 and 13,3 dB in all cases.

The functionality of a feedback reduction is considered to be proven, when the ASG is 5 dB or more [1]. This was clearly the case for both prototypes and the commercial hearing aids. Nevertheless, the performance was better with the commercial systems, as the achieved values for the ASG were higher in all configurations. It has to be mentioned that there was a measurement uncertainty of 1 dB, as this was the increment in gain increase. Furthermore, the small impact caused by the coherence filter in the openMHA-setups, might be due to the experimental conditions (measurement inside the test box). A measurement setup with a head and torso simulator together with an ear simulator might have lead to a bigger impact, due to the head shadow effect and a resulting decrease in binaural coherence.

4 Conclusion

In comparison to the observed commercial hearing aids, the openMHA setup was able to provide 1/3 octaveband gains that were approximately 10 dB higher with equal accuracy to the programmed gain. In terms of the frequency dependent latencies, the results were about 4 ms higher for the openMHA setups, but still within a tolerable range [2].

The feedback reductions of all 4 devices were proven to be functional, but with ASGs that were up to 4 dB higher, the commercial systems showed a better performance. However, this difference in ASG might be caused by the test box setup used here, and in real conditions with hearig aids worn on the ear, the binaural coherence filter might contribute to feedback reduction as well.

All in all the openMHA setups performed on a comparable level as the commercial systems. For further evaluations, more complex experimental setups would be nessecary, as the performance of essential features like directional microphones, noise reductions and hearing aid channels has not been included in this work.

Acknowledgement

The work has been carried out at Deutsches Hörgeräte Institut GmbH, Lübeck. Furthermore, we would like to thank Bat&Cat Sound Labs, Palo Alto, USA for providing the PHL hardware with hearing aid headsets.

Author's Statement

Conflict of interest: Authors state no conflict of interest.

5 References

[1] IEC 60118-16 (draft). *Definition and verification of hearing aid features*, 2020.

[2] H. Dillon, *Hearing Aids*. Second edition, pp. 35-36. Thieme. Stuttgart, 2012.

[3] G. Grimm, T. Herzke, D. Berg and V. Hohmann, *The Master Hearing Aid: A PC-based Platform for Algorithm Development and Evaluation*. ACTA ACUSTICA UNITED WITH ACUSTICA,vol. 92, pp. 618-628, 2006.

[4] C. Pavlovic, H. Kayser, R. Kassayan, T. Herzke and V. Hohmann, *A High-Fidelity Portable Platform for Development of Novel Algorithms for Assistive Listening Wearables*. Presented at AAS annual meeting, 2020.

[5] I. Holube, S. Fredelake, M. Vlaming and B. Kollmeier, *Development and analysis of an International Speech Test Signal*. International Journal of Audiology, 49:12, pp. 891-903, 2010.

[6] M.C. Killion, and E.L. Monser, *CORFIG: COUPLER RESPONSE FOR FLAT INSERTION GAIN*. In: Studebaker GA, Hochberg I. (eds): Acoustical Factors Affecting Hearing Aid Performance, pp. 147-168, 1980.

Evaluation of Noise Reduction Algorithms in Hearing Aids in Multi-Talker Conversations

Larissa Jäger [1], Marlitt Frenz [2] and Hendrik Husstedt [2]

[1] Auditory Technology, Universität zu Lübeck, larissa.jaeger@student.uni-luebeck.de
[2] German Institute of Hearing Aids, {m.frenz, h.husstedt}@dhi-online.de

Abstract

Adaptive single- and multichannel noise reduction algorithms are important features of hearing aids to improve the signal-to-noise ratio providing a better and easier understanding of speech. For an objective evaluation of these features in a situation with multiple sound sources, the phase inversion method has been used. In previous works, primarily static sound scenes have been considered. As realistic acoustic scenes behave more dynamic (e.g. dialogues), this work applies the extended phase inversion method to evaluate a multi-talker conversation. To this end, a setup with 8 loudspeakers and an artificial head (KEMAR) was used. Various adaptive noise reduction settings of two state-of-the-art behind-the-ear hearing aids (BTE) were measured. The results show that the modified extended phase inversion method can be applied for an evaluation of adaptive noise reduction algorithms. Further considerations need to be made to test the robustness of the method.

1 Introduction

The ability to focus a target source while filtering out negligible sources is reduced for hearing impaired people. In general adaptive parameters in hearing aids such as noise reduction algorithms (NR) shall increase the signal-to-noise ratio (SNR) and thus provide a better and easier understanding of speech [1]. Noise reduction algorithms enhance the SNR by first estimating various parameters of the noise signal such as the frequency spectrum, the level or the modulation and then reducing noise while keeping the speech signal as it is. Directional microphone characteristics use the spatial separation of sounds in an acoustic scene to amplify target signals from certain directions and reduce noise coming from other directions. Therefore hearing aids use microphone arrays to create different beamforming patterns [2]. These features need only a few milliseconds to adapt to changes within an acoustic environment. Additionally, binaural coupling between two hearing aids can draw a benefit as, every microphone can be used to analyze the acoustic scene and adapt the signal processing accordingly [3]. Some hearing aid manufacturers use asymmetrical directional settings, where one hearing aid is omnidirectional and monitors the environment and one hearing aid is directional to focus on the sources in front of the listener [4].
In order to investigate noise reduction algorithms, a measurement setup is created that emulates realistic listening situations. To this end, the phase inversion method by Hagerman and Olofsson can be used [5]. Thereby two uncorrelated signals are superimposed at the microphones of the hearing aid. The processed signals can be separated and evaluated independently, if prior knowledge exists. However, two signals do not describe hearing situations in sufficient detail. To this end, the phase inversion method can be extended for the separation of an arbitrary number of signals [6]. In previous studies, the extended phase inversion method was used to investigate digital hearing aids in static acoustic setups with multiple sound sources [6, 7]. In order to assess adaptive features in hearing aids, a changing acoustic environment is required. A realistic scene could be a conversation in front of the listener with ambient noise. The purpose of this work is to define an acoustic scene, which includes two sound sources and multiple uncorrelated noise scources. Within this setup, two state-of-the-art hearing aids were assessed with different settings of adaptive noise reduction and directional microphones, and the results are visualized in polar plots.

2 Material and Methods

2.1 Modified Extended Phase Inversion Method

In this work, $N = 9$ signals are used to define the acoustic scene. To extract the individual signals of the mixture, the extended phase inversion method is used. For the application of this method, the input signals $(s_1,...,s_N)$ are assigned with different phase relations and represented as superpositions (x_1,...,x_N) by a matrix-vector multiplication

$$\underbrace{\begin{pmatrix} x_1 \\ x_2 \\ \vdots \\ x_N \end{pmatrix}}_{x} = \underbrace{\begin{bmatrix} -1 & 1 & \cdots & 1 \\ 1 & -1 & \cdots & 1 \\ \vdots & \vdots & \ddots & \vdots \\ 1 & 1 & \cdots & -1 \end{bmatrix}}_{\mathbf{A}} \underbrace{\begin{pmatrix} s_1 \\ s_2 \\ \vdots \\ s_N \end{pmatrix}}_{s} \quad (1)$$

where the system matrix **A** includes the phase information and has a condition number of $\kappa = 3.5$. The entries of the system matrix are either +1 or -1 so that the signals are not amplified or attenuated. Additionally, the columns of the system matrix define the phase inversion of each signal, as each row describes the superposition of every signal in one measurement cycle. As 9 signals are used, 9 measurement cycles are needed. All superpositions are presented one after the other with 5 seconds pause each and recorded at the KEMAR microphones. It is assumed that the different phase relations do not change the signal processing of the hearing aid and thus the phase relations between the input signals (x_1,...,x_N) and the recorded output signals (y_1, ..., y_N) are the same. The recorded signals $\mathbf{y} = (y_1, ..., y_N)^T$ are multiplied with the inverse of **A**

$$\mathbf{A}^{-1} = \frac{1}{2(N-2)} \begin{bmatrix} -(N-3) & 1 & \cdots & 1 \\ 1 & -(N-3) & \cdots & 1 \\ \vdots & \vdots & \ddots & \vdots \\ 1 & 1 & \cdots & -(N-3) \end{bmatrix} \quad (2)$$

to determine the processed signals (s'_1,...,s'_9) of the hearing aids. Afterwards, their acoustic characteristics (e.g. level or frequency spectrum) can be evaluated independently. Additionally the signal-to-noise ratio (SNR) can be calculated and compared with defined measurement setup.
The conversation can be defined as a superposition of the speech signal with a step function for each desired azimuth. The step function has two conditions. In a defined time interval $[t_a, t_b]$ the function is 1 and otherwise the speech signal is attenuated by $C_{att.}$.

2.2 Setup

The measurements were performed in a room with a background noise level below 30 dB SPL. Here, an artificial head was placed at the center of a measurement circle with a radius of 1 m. 8 loudspeakers are positioned on a circular path with an equidistant step size of 45° beginning at 0°, as shown in Fig. 1. A measurement tool was programmed in MATLAB to automize all measurement and to analyze the results.
Eight uncorrelated noise signals were presented from all directions with a sum level of 67.5 dB. The noise signals have been created from the International Speech Test Signal (ISTS), so that the long term spectrum of each noise signal is similar to the ISTS. To simulate a conversation, the ISTS was presented alternately from +45° and -45° with a level of 70 dB for 30 seconds each. It is to note, that an attenuation of C_{att} = -20 dB is defined as shown in Fig. 2. All signals had a total length of 60 seconds.

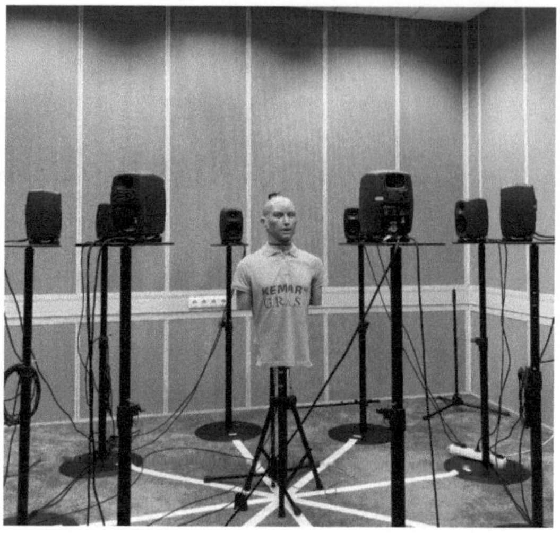

Figure 1: Measurement setup consisting of eight loudspeakers in equidistant intervals of 45° and a KEMAR directed to the speaker at 0°. The circle has a radius of 1m.

For the measurements two state-of-the-art behind-the-ear (BTE) hearing aids were placed at the KEMAR according to IEC 60118-15 [8]. The ear canals were occluded using foam plugs with sound tubes. The occluded gain (with deactivated hearing aid) was intended to be below -10 dB between 100 Hz and 10.000 Hz. NAL-NL2 was used as the fitting rule and a frequency independent gain of 20 dB with a compression ratio of one was programmed. All adaptive parameters, which are not investigated in this work were deactivated.

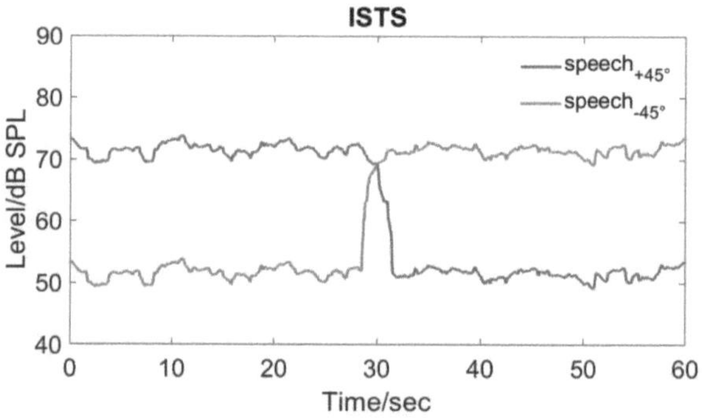

Figure 2: Fading of the ISTS as a function of time with a speaker change after 30 seconds for the directions 45° and -45°.

Four test settings are analyzed within this work:
1. omnidirectional microphone with noise reduction off (omni, NR off)
2. omnidirectional microphone with noise reduction on (omni, NR on)
3. adaptive directional microphone with noise reduction off (adaptive, NR off)

4. adaptive directional microphone with noise reduction on (adaptive, NR on).

3 Results and Discussion

The processed noise signals at the output of the left hearing aid for each direction are visualized in Fig. 3. To this end, the root mean square levels (RMS) were calculated for a window length of 5 seconds and 50% overlap. The levels of three test settings (1. omni, NR on, 2. adaptive, NR off and 3. adaptive NR on) are shown in relation to the omnidirectional setting. The first subplot of Fig. 3 shows the results for an activated noise reduction in the omnidirectional microphone mode (omni, NR on), while the second and third subplot visualize the adaptive microphone setting with noise reduction turned off (adaptive, NR off) and on (adaptive, NR on).

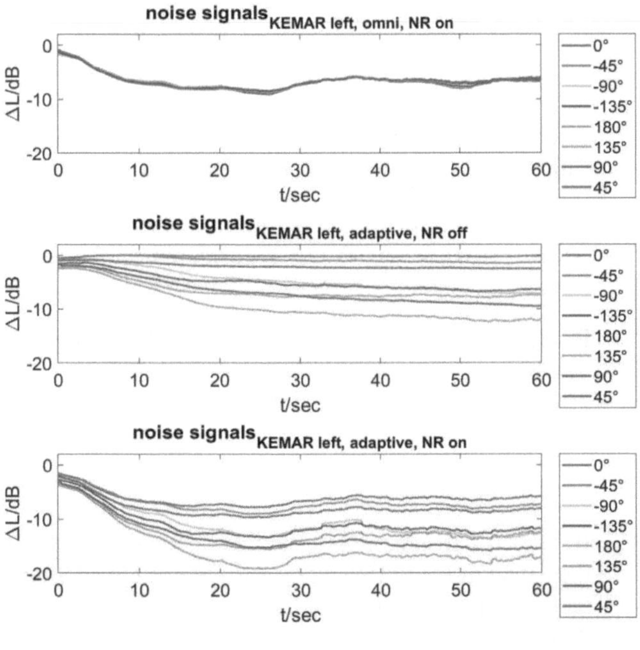

Figure 3: Noise signals at the left hearing aid for each direction (0°,45°,...,-45°) with three test settings (omni, NR on), (adaptive, NR off) and (adaptive NR on). The levels of all test settings are shown in relation to the omnidirectional test setting (ΔL).

The first subplot shows, that an activation of the NR causes an overall attenuation of about 8 dB regardless of the direction. This can also be recognized while comparing subplot 2 and 3. The second and the third diagram visualize that the noise signals in the rear area between -90° and 90° are attenuated in comparison to the omnidirectional microphone setting. Thus, the azimuth interval between 45° and -45° reveals less attenuation. This indicates a microphone directionality centered around 0°, e.g. cardioid. As the target speech changes between 45° and -45°, a cardioid microphone directionality focuses both sources simultaneously. Additionally, the results in all diagrams show an attack time of the hearing aid in the first 15 seconds. The attack time needs to be taken into account in further evaluations. The time-dependent representation indicates a fluctuation and thus shows modifications of the output signal over time due to the adaptive signal processing.

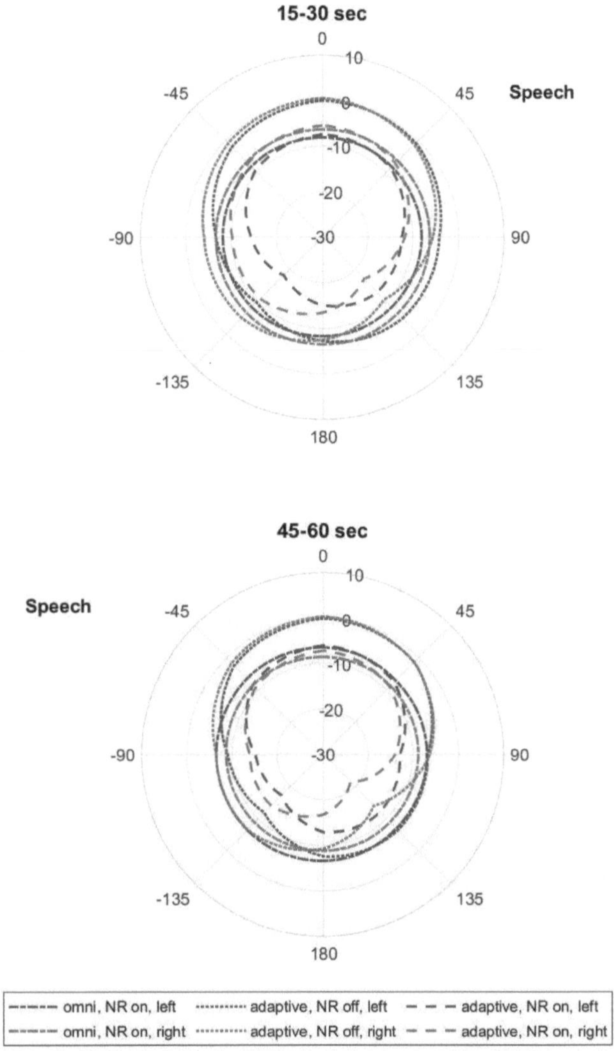

Figure 4: RMS levels of the adaptive directional microphone setting (adaptive) in relation to the omnidirectional test setting for noise reduction activated (NR on) and deactivated (NR off) at the left and right hearing aid. The top polar plot shows the RMS values for the time frame of 15-30 seconds with speech from 45° and the bottom plot shows the RMS values for the time frame of 45-60 seconds with speech from -45°.

To represent the modifications spatially, polar diagrams of the output signals are shown for two time intervals. For this purpose, time frames of 15 seconds to 30 seconds and

45 seconds to 60 seconds are taken into account. Within this time frame the sound pressure level for each azimuth is calculated and interpolated with a step size of 1°. Fig. 4 shows the difference between the settings omni, NR on, adaptive, NR off and adaptive, NR on to the setting omni, NR off. The left hearing aid is represented in blue and the right hearing aid is plotted in red, while the line styles represent the results for each test setting.

The results in the first polar plot of Fig. 4 show minor differences between the left hearing aid and the right hearing aid for the test settings omni, NR on and adaptive NR off. The noise signals of the adaptive directional microphones are attenuated in the rear area between 45° and -45° compared to the omnidirectional test setting, which outlines a microphone directivity to the front. When comparing the curves for NR off and NR on, an average attenuation of approximately 8 dB can be seen for each direction due to the activation of the noise reduction. This overall attenuation can also be recognized in the bottom plot of Fig. 4, where speech was presented from -45°. A comparison of the curves for speech coming from 45° and speech coming from -45° shows that the behavior of noise reduction algorithms stays the same and reduces the noise signal equally from all directions. The adaptive microphone directionality of the left hearing aid doesn't change while the right hearing aid attenuates noise coming from 90° to 165° and amplifies sounds from -45° to 165°. An explanation could be, that the hearing aid manufacturer may define the left hearing aid as a dominant side which keeps the directivity setting and the hearing aid on the other side chooses a directivity depending on the current listening situation. Overall, slight differences due to the modified direction of the speech signal over time can be presented in this work. However, the results visualize that the microphone directionality changes adaptively depending on the acoustic scene. This effect may be enhanced by noise reduction settings that use binaural coupling, which need to be analyzed in further studies. In addition the effects may increase by using other directions of speech such as 90° and -90° or 0° and 180°.

4 Conclusion

This work intended to define a realistic acoustic scene considering a conversation with two speakers and multiple uncorrelated noise sources. Within this acoustic scene, the modified phase inversion method was intended to be used for analyzing adaptive noise reduction algorithms in hearing aids. To this end, measurements with two state-of-the-art BTE hearing aids were made in a setup with 8 speakers and various noise reduction settings. The results have been visualized as functions of time on the one hand and as directional polar plots on the other hand. Both visualizations show an average attenuation for each direction due to the single-channel noise reduction. The results for the initial setup showed minor differences between the directivity of the left and the right hearing aid. A different digital signal processing can be found according to the direction change of the target speech. It can be expected that measurements with other signal setups and noise reduction algorithms using binaural connectivity between both hearing aids increase the observed effects. To this end, further studies with binaurally coupled hearing aids and other directions of speech signals need to be made to get insight into the performance of adaptive and binaural noise reduction algorithms.

Acknowledgement

The work has been conducted and supervised at the German Institute of Hearing Aids GmbH, Lübeck.

Author's Statement

The authors declared no potential conflicts of interest with respect to the research, authorship, and/or publication of this article.

5 References

[1] K. Chung, "Challenges and Recent Developments in Hearing Aids. Part 1. Speech Understanding in Noise, Microphone Technologies and Noise Reduction Algorithms," *Trends in Amplification*, vol. 8, no. 3, 2004.

[2] H. Dillon, *Hearing Aids*, ser. Thieme Publishers Series. Boomerang Press, 2012. [Online]. Available: https://books.google.de/books?id=594YLgEACAAJ

[3] R. Herbig and M. Froehlich, "Binaural Beamforming: The Natural Evolution," *Hearing Review*, vol. 22, no. 5, 2015.

[4] J. Nelson, "ReSound's directional philosphy," *Audiology Online*, 2016.

[5] B. Hagerman and A. Olofsson, "A method to Measure the Effect of Noise Reduction Algorithms Using Simultaneous Speech and Noise," *Acta Acustica united with Acustica*, vol. 90, pp. 356–361, 2004.

[6] M. Frenz, A. Mertins, and H. Husstedt, "Evaluation of Noise Reduction in Digital Hearing Aids in Situations with Multiple Signal Sources," in *6th International Symposium on Audiological and Auditory Research.* International Symposium on Audiological and Auditory Research ISAAR, 2017.

[7] L. Johannsen, "Examination of Microphone Directivity of Hearing Aids in Situations with Multiple Speech Signals," 2018, Undergraduate Thesis, University of Applied Sciences Lübeck.

[8] IEC 60118-15, "Electroacoustics - Hearing aids - Part 15: Methods for characterising signal processing in hearing aidswith a speech-like signal (IEC 60118-15)." Geneva, Switzerland, 2012.

Are Sound Emissions of the Harbour Porpoise Replicable Using Acoustic Lenses?

Larissa Scheller [1], Jürgen Tchorz [2], Silke Anders [3], and Christoph Waldmann [4]

[1] Auditory Technology, Universität zu Lübeck, Larissa.Scheller@student.uni-luebeck.de
[2] Applied Sciences, Luebeck University of Applied Sciences, Juergen.Tchorz@th-luebeck.de
[3] Center of Brain, Behavior and Metabolism, Universität zu Lübeck, silke.anders@neuro.uni-luebeck.de
[4] MARUM - Center for Marine Environmental Sciences, University of Bremen, waldmann@marum.de

Abstract

Marine mammals, especially the harbour porpoise, are often studied. These animals still remain a mystery in certain aspects of their physiology and scientists can only speculate about the reasoning behind their doing. This work is a compilation of the most repetitive findings in regards to echolocation sounds while also analyzing different acoustic lenses to decipher if those findings could be rebuild in a device that provides reliable information without specifically needing the animal. The results showed that acoustic lenses do not quite yet meet all needs for such a device, alternative methods like microphone arrays appear to provide more flexibility to meet the most important needs. Though acoustic lenses have gained more interest and new developments and possibilities, meaning do not rule the acoustic lenses out for a harbour porpoise replication completely. They might be the best option in a few years.

1 Introduction

The harbour porpoise (Phocoena phocoena) uses echolocation signals for various situations. It allows them to locate prey and generally orientate themselves under water. The signals fall within the range of the narrow-band echolocation and are short-ranged and of high-frequency [1].

The emitted sounds, usually a certain amount of clicks with different duration and succession, vary in frequency range and sound pressure level. Scientists indicate different frequency ranges for these signals, though the most reappearing tend to be sounds around 130 kHz with a range of 100 kHz - 160 kHz and an approximated sound pressure levels of for example 178 to 205 dB re 1 µPa at a distance of 1 m [2]. The varying echolocation signals are hypothesized to be created with the *phonic lips*, though there are different opinions and results in regards to if both phonic lips create clicks, or if only one of them creates them. From the phonic lips, the signal traverses through the fatty tissue at the front of the head called *melon* and performs a narrow-band beam [3]. This enables returning signals from up to a few tens of meters [4].

The ultimate goal of this project is to build a device that can recreate the emitted sounds of the harbour porpoise as accurately as possible. To achieve this, the sometimes vague data of the sound emission and properties needs to be compiled, as well as possible sound output options theoretically checked for compatibility. The following paper will show a compilation of relevant data and take a look at the possible use of systems labeled *acoustic lenses* in the sense of manipulating the input sound for certain frequencies in specific angles one way or another. Furthermore, the practical application of these systems is analyzed.

2 Material and Methods

2.1 Harbour Porpoise

One of the most common marine mammals is the harbour porpoise. Though they are fairly common, quite a lot of data gathered by scientists is speculation based. For example, the specified frequency ranges of the echolocation signal vary from 100 kHz - 160 kHz to 120 kHz - 160 kHz, whereas 160 kHz appears to be a common peak cut-off frequency due to physical limitations of the animal. 130 kHz is often referenced as center frequency [3] [5]. This means that the planned device should be able to cover a frequency output of 100 kHz - 160 kHz to avoid losing possible valuable information. As most of the analyzed systems are passive devices, this feature falls back to a suitable loudspeaker used with the device. Sound pressure levels are also of importance. It has been shown that harbour porpoises living in captivity tend to use lower echolocation sound source levels with up to 30 dB than their wild counter parts. This is speculated to be due to too loud returning signals during the echolocation [2] [4]. It suggests the planned device either cover these varying sound pressure levels, or it should be build for captive or wild research only.

Recent results take a closer look at how the beam-forming performed by harbour porpoises is being influenced by

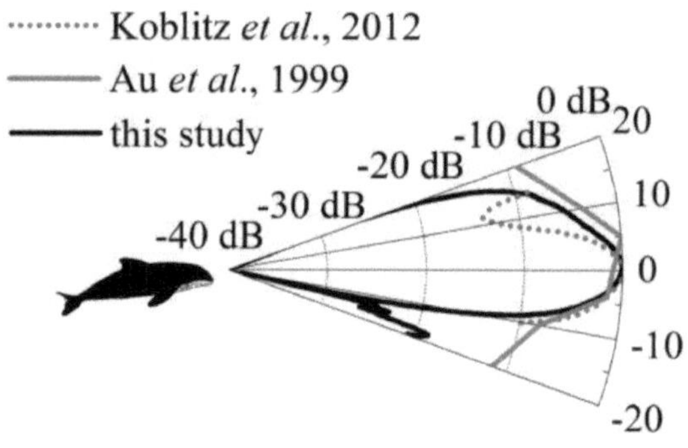

Figure 1: This image shows the vertical beam-forming comparison of sound reduction in dB and angle in degree from Wei et al. (2017) using the solid black line, with Au et al. (1999) as the solid grey line and Koblitz et al. (2012) as the dotted red line [5].

anatomical properties, as well as comparing their findings about the angle of the beam-forming to already existing results (Fig. 1) [5]. The findings indicate a certain pattern, which should be recreated in regards to beam-width and angle with the planned device.

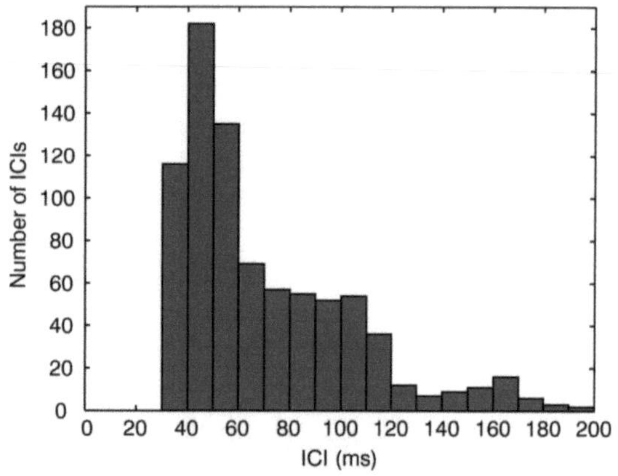

Figure 2: The duration of the inter-click interval is compared to the amount of inter-click intervals by Villadsgaard et al. [2]. A peak at 50 - 60 ms can be seen.

The sounds emitted by the harbour porpoise usually is a series of narrow-band clicks. These clicks are speculated to be too high in frequency to be used for elaborate social communication and might be evolutionary to avoid predators from picking up on the echolocation. The clicks can be classified as low-repetition rate calls (100 - 600 clicks per second), high-repetition rate calls (800 - >1000 clicks per second) and buzzes [6]. It also showed that all measured individuals emitted low-repetition rate calls, whereas only a few emitted high-repetition rate calls. These clicks and the spacing between should also be considered when designing a device to copy the echolocation sounds. Villadsgaard et al. (2007) plotted the inter-click intervall (ICI) as a histogram that indicates a most common ICI at 50 ms (Fig. 2) [2].

2.2 Acoustic Lens

Acoustic lenses have been successfully used for underwater imaging sonar for years. The main advantage is no complex beam-forming [7]. Thus, the question arises if the beam from the harbour porpoise can be recreated using an acoustic lens. The echolocation beam itself could be, purely optical speaking, described as an envelope (Fig. 1). This envelope would be the ideal shape of the possible output sound. Researching acoustic lenses provided a lot of different setups and methods, though not a lot of underwater applications apart from sonar. For this, setups that have been either used underwater, are working with water or are promising in their sound manipulation have been picked. For the passive setups, it is presumed that the actuator provides the necessary frequency and sound pressure level outputs and only influences the setup if explicitly mentioned.

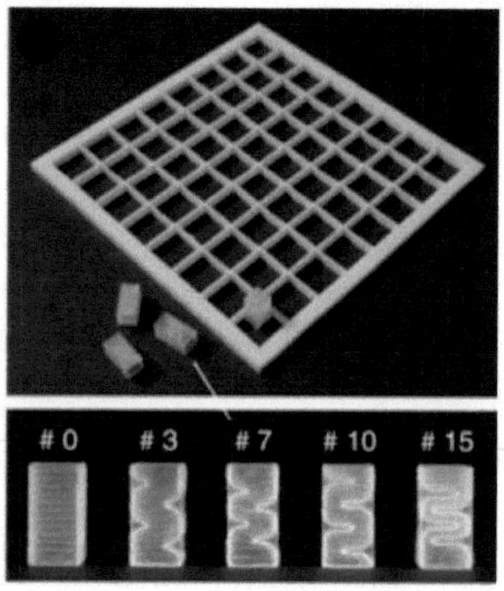

Figure 3: Displayed are a few exemplary bricks of the 16 total variations, as well as the structure they are arranged in to create different acoustic situations [8].

Taking a closer look at the currently used acoustic lenses immediately puts a focus on the research of Gianluca Memoli et al. (2019) [8] [9]. During the last few years, his team focused on optimizing the usage of acoustic lenses as we know them. His idea is to be able to manipulate sound in the same way we are able to manipulate light with the usage of lenses. For this, they created 16 Lego like bricks which influence the direction of the incoming sound of a loudspeaker due to their individual shape. If arranged in a certain way (Fig. 3), these bricks supposedly allow them to direct loudspeaker sound in a specific angle and even split off certain frequencies to different angles at the same time. To accomplish this, they basically created an acoustic prism. Acoustic metamaterials were used and simply printed with a 3D-Printer. This system is also able to form beams in a way the harbour porpoise would create them, making it a possible solid base for the project. Practical application discovered the beam getting narrower the higher the transmitted frequencies, which results in an intensity peak at 30° for 5 kHz, and a significant decrease of sound pressure level afterwards, limiting the applicable frequency range immensely [9]. With the frequency range the harbour porpoise uses for echolocation, this system will need further development in the frequency ranges before it could be considered for the planned device, as current metamaterials might not be able to print detailed enough structures for the bricks to reach the necessary frequencies.

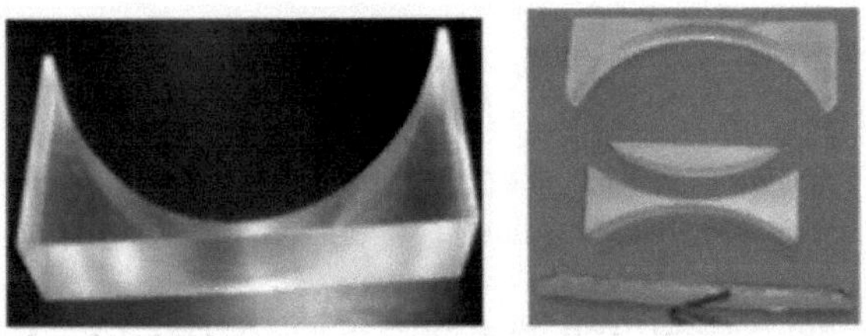

Figure 4: Examples of spherical plano concave acoustic lenses [7].

Another possibility is the acoustic lens in the classical style, meaning for example spherical plano concave acoustic lenses (Fig. 4) in front of a loudspeaker. The specific shape of the lens enables the beam to focus a certain way. A cylindrical lens would be used to produce a line focus, whereas a spherical lens produces a point focus. With this type of lens, the material properties are very important. They influence the quality and functionality of the lens and therefore the beam. Depending on the material, temperature changes could also have a negative influence on the measurements. A problem with the fixed lens for this project would be the frequency range and the influence the shape of the lens has on the sound pressure level. Certain frequencies are providing higher sound pressure levels at certain distances due to the way the lens is formed. Meaning if the lens has been tailored for 120 kHz, other frequency wavelengths will not be manipulated in the same way, as the lens has not been manufactured for them. This can be beneficial as it would mean less electrical power is consumed, but it could also hinder measurements with unplanned sound manipulations for other frequencies. The acoustic lens also depends on the angle of the sound input, meaning the expected results will deviate if the sound output and the lens are not aligned correctly. This could be problematic if the somewhat similar scenario as the harbour porpoise is replicated in an array of phase controlled acoustic lenses. The array would be needed to provide a more realistic manipulation with the classic style acoustic lenses for harbour porpoise echolocation replication [7]. The classic acoustic lens seems to be suitable for working with a fixed frequency, if for example only 120 kHz or 130 kHz are used, it could be a starting point for the project. Though it still does not quite fit the before mentioned requirements for a harbour porpoise replication, at least not in the sense that would be ideal.

The third acoustic lens possibility that appeared promising is an experimental realization of a non linear acoustic lens with a tunable focus. Donahue et al. (2014) created a platform holding an array of 13 independent tubes filled with steel spheres to ensure the non linearity (Fig. 5), (Fig. 6). This setup enables compact focusing and allows individual adjustment of each sound output with the help of the

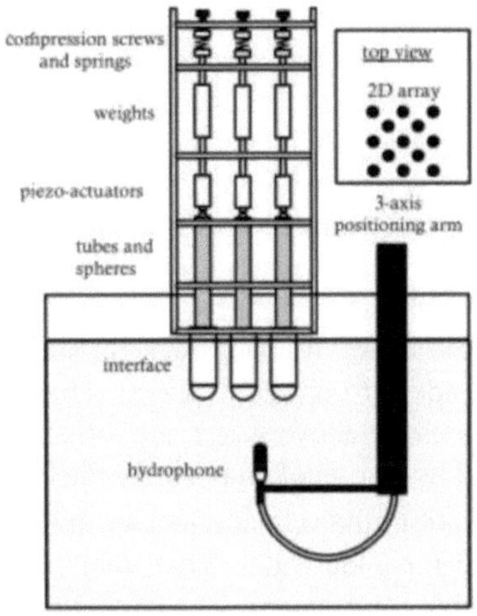

Figure 5: Displayed is the experimental setup from Donahue et al. (2014) [10]. The individual tubes can be adjusted with the screws and springs which allows adjustment of the beam.

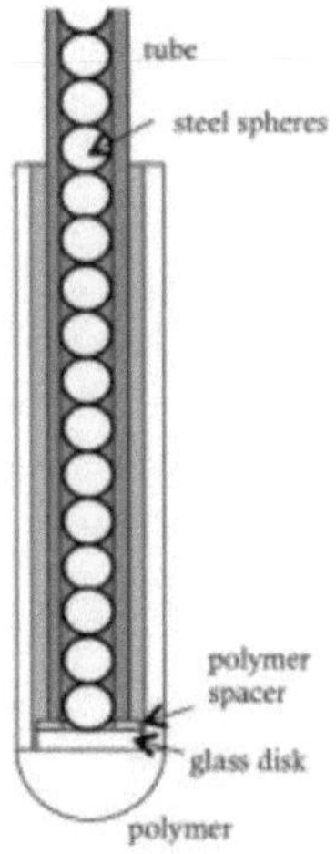

Figure 6: A look at the inside of one of the tubes from (Fig. 5). The steel spheres provide the non linearity. The glass disk and polymer spacer are part of the interface that can influence the wavelength [10].

screws, springs and weights. Donahue pointed out the importance of the interface for this setup. They concluded that softer interface materials mean longer wavelengths and pulse shapes that collide with previously calculated results [10]. Due to this setup depending on being adjustable with springs, screws and weights to ensure the spheres keep in contact and thus ensuring the non linearity, it is not practical for a harbour porpoise replication. It would have to be rotated, which might cause difficulties with the needed specific setup.

3 Results and Discussion

It appears that none of the analyzed acoustic lenses meet all of the necessary requirements just yet. The first option, acoustic metamaterial to create rearrangeable bricks and in turn create the acoustic prism opens up new possibilities for sound manipulation in a certain frequency range and angle, but the necessary frequency range for harbour porpoise sounds can not yet be manipulated as it is barely covering human hearing frequency levels. The influence of the prism appears to cover all necessary sound emission angles and creates the echolocation beam in a way that could come close to the real beam, it is not the right solution. Another current downside for this setup is, that it has only been designed for the usage above water, the influence of water as a medium and not air would have to be analyzed too.

The second option, the acoustic lens in the classical sense, has been used for underwater sonar imaging for years and provides reliable information. Though further investigation resulted in quite a few counterarguments. This specific lens appears to be ideal for a fixed frequency, but could cause difficulties when used with the necessary frequency range for harbour porpoises. If the commonly used click frequency would act as a base for the acoustic lens, certain measurements could probably be performed accordingly, but the frequency range exists for a reason. Picking only one frequency would not replicate the real echolocation signals of the harbour porpoise.

Lastly, the nonlinear acoustic lens with a tunable focus does not allow the necessary setup needed for replicating harbour porpoises. If the setup could be adjusted and more importantly rotated as a whole without disrupting the specific necessary alignment, the non linear acoustic lens would be an interesting candidate for replicating a harbour porpoise.

4 Conclusion

Acoustic lenses do not yet meet all necessary requirements needed for a harbour porpoise replica. Alternatively, microphone arrays could be a good start. Different directional microphones in a certain setup could provide different output angles. The beam-forming can also be adjusted using directional microphones. A specific setup would have to be calculated to avoid accidentally amplifying or erasing the output signal. Though acoustic lenses should not be forgotten. Their continued improvement and research interest could provide an ideal solution fairly soon. Next steps should include an underwater setup of microphone arrays to try and recreate the echolocation beam the harbour porpoise uses. If the idea of acoustic lenses still wants to be pushed, a phase controlled classical acoustic lens setup would be advised for now.

Acknowledgement

The work has been carried out at Universität zu Lübeck and supervised by the Institute of Signal Processing, Universität zu Lübeck. Thank you to my supervisors for their continued support and interest in the topic.

Author's Statement

Conflict of interest: Authors state no conflict of interest.

5 References

[1] W. W. L. Au, *The Sonar of Dolphins*. New York, NY: Springer New York, 1993.

[2] A. Villadsgaard, M. Wahlberg, and J. Tougaard, "Echolocation signals of wild harbour porpoises, phocoena phocoena," *The Journal of experimental biology*, vol. 210, no. Pt 1, pp. 56–64, 2007.

[3] P. T. Madsen, D. Wisniewska, and K. Beedholm, "Single source sound production and dynamic beam formation in echolocating harbour porpoises (phocoena phocoena)," *The Journal of experimental biology*, vol. 213, no. Pt 18, pp. 3105–3110, 2010.

[4] M. Linnenschmidt, P. Madsen, L. Miller, M. Wahlberg, and D. Wisniewska, "The acoustic world of harbor porpoises," *American Scientist*, vol. 103, no. 1, p. 46, 2015.

[5] C. Wei, W. W. L. Au, D. R. Ketten, Z. Song, and Y. Zhang, "Biosonar signal propagation in the harbor porpoise's (phocoena phocoena) head: The role of various structures in the formation of the vertical beam," *The Journal of the Acoustical Society of America*, vol. 141, no. 6, p. 4179, 2017.

[6] P. M. Sørensen, D. M. Wisniewska, F. H. Jensen, M. Johnson, J. Teilmann, and P. T. Madsen, "Click communication in wild harbour porpoises (phocoena phocoena)," *Scientific Reports*, vol. 8, no. 1, pp. 1–11. [Online]. Available: https://www.nature.com/articles/s41598-018-28022-8

[7] G. Suresh, V. Natarajan, and A. Shanavas, "Underwater imaging using acoustic lens," in *Underwater Technology (UT), 2015 IEEE*. IEEE, 2/23/2015 - 2/25/2015, pp. 1–3.

[8] G. Memoli, L. Chisari, J. P. Eccles, M. Caleap, B. W. Drinkwater, and S. Subramanian, "Vari-sound," in *CHI 2019*, S. Brewster, G. Fitzpatrick, A. Cox, and V. Kostakos, Eds. New York, NY: ACM, 2019, pp. 1–14.

[9] G. Memoli, T. J. Graham, J. T. Kybett, and A. Pouryazdan, "From light to sound," in *ACM SIGGRAPH 2019 Talks*, ser. ACM Digital Library. New York,NY,United States: Association for Computing Machinery, 2019, pp. 1–2.

[10] C. M. Donahue, P. W. J. Anzel, L. Bonanomi, T. A. Keller, and C. Daraio, "Experimental realization of a nonlinear acoustic lens with a tunable focus," *Applied Physics Letters*, vol. 104, no. 1, p. 014103, 2014.

Development of a Knowlegde Base and a Learning Content Management System Course for a Medical Measurement Software

Julian Weigert [1], Siegrid Meier [2]

[1] Auditory Technology, Universität zu Lübeck, julian.weigert@student.uni-luebeck.de

[2] Auditory Technology, Akademie für Hörakustik, s.meier@afh-luebeck.de

Abstract

Rapid developments in medicine and medical technology require new ways of knowledge transfer. Medical measuring devices are increasingly being released before they are fully developed and accordingly only mature in practice at the user. E-learning platforms optimize knowledge development, knowledge distribution, knowledge utilization and knowledge retention. Dynamic learning content management systems (LCMS) support this process. In this project, the Moodle course "Otosuite Help" is developed as a knowledge base for the software Otosuite of the company Natus GmbH. Otosuite is a widely used medical measurement software in hearing acoustics. The goal of the knowledge base is to have a learning and teaching tool that includes content and experiences that go beyond a manufacturer's guide. In order to grow the knowledge base, the collaboration and sharing of the users' experiences is essential. Finally, the structure of the knowledge base should be usable for any medical measurement software.

1 Introduction

The use of computers, tablets, smartphones and the Internet is now part of everyday life. The use of digital media has also found its way into all areas of educational institutions, companies and private educational processes, for which corresponding multimedia and Internet-based resources and forms of e-learning are being developed and made available. Modern medical measuring devices regularly pose challenges to the user, so that the manufacturer's guides are often no longer sufficient. First, the operation of measuring devices becomes more demanding as the range of functions increases. Instruction sessions become more extensive and time-consuming. Users need a longer period of time to become experts in operation. Bugs can occur that are not in the manufacturer's manual. Secondly, the quality of measurement and the interpretation of measurement results is an important factor in medicine. These factors should be optimized by using the manufacturer independent and user oriented knowledge base.

A knowledge base for medical measuring devices must meet certain requirements. In addition to the provision of information and data, an exchange between users should also be possible. Moodle is a powerful system that meets these requirements. It is an open source online course management system and learning platform. The software offers the possibilities to support cooperative teaching and learning methods. With a large number of features, Moodle enables the individual design of courses, which is helpful for the creation of the knowledge base.

The Akademie für Hörakustik (afh) and the Bundesoffene Landesberufsschule für Hörakustikerinnen und Hörakustiker (LBS) each already use a Moodle platform for online teaching. Both institutions are responsible for the education and training of hearing care professionals in Germany. Associated exams are taken in the Otosuite software. However, the students are often not trained users of the Otosuite software, so using it is often a problem. A knowledge base should therefore serve as support.

In this project, a knowledge base is to be created for each of the afh and LBS, which are identical in structure. The requirements for a knowledge base for a medical measuring device and the advantages compared to the manufacturer's guide are to be determined. This is to be evaluated by the users with the help of a questionnaire.

2 Material and Methods

2.1 Otosuite

Otosuite is an audiometry software that combines multiple audiological devices into one software surface. It is developed by Natus GmbH, which also offers the matching hardware which is called Aurical. This allows for up to 57 different tests to being performed via one interface. In addition, Otosuite is compatible with Noah 4, one of the most widely used software in hearing care for electronic medical record [1].

Otosuite is most commonly used for audiometry to detect hearing loss. This includes pure tone and speech audiometry. In addition to audiometry, numerous other measurements and functions can be performed. These can be used for: hearing aid fitting, speech mapping, hearing loss and hearing aid simulators, hearing instrument test, video otoscopy, otoacoustic emissions and tympanometry. A large number of these measurements are used to determine the hearing loss more precisely.

2.2 Knowledge Base

The networking of information enables its use in a specific field of action, which can be referred to as knowledge [2]. A knowledge base is used to easily record and edit knowledge objects and establish links between them [3]. With knowledge bases, users have access to this information at any time. Due to the large range of functions of modern medical measuring devices, the operation and evaluation of measurement results is becoming more and more complex for the user, which is simplified by the knowledge base. In addition, users can share experiences and measurement data with other users. For more complex measurements in hearing acoustics, there are not always measurement results that lead to a clear diagnosis. An exchange between different users and the involvement of experts can lead to the correct diagnosis if necessary.
Afterwards, the newly gained knowledge can be recorded in the knowledge base in a wiki or glossary.

2.2.1 Software

For the technical implementation, the LCMS software Moodle is used in each case. LCMS are a hybrid of content management systems (CMS) and learning management systems (LMS). On the one hand, this makes it possible to create, manage and research content (CMS). And on the other hand, learning processes can be tracked and an exchange between users can be enabled (LMS) [4]. The existing Moodle platforms of the afh and LBS are used for this purpose. The platforms are maintained in each case by the technical service. Numerous Features make the LCMS very flexible and customisable according to one's own requirements. The general features can be seen in Table 1 [5].

Table 1: General Features of Moodle

Feature	Explanation
user interface	Designed to be responsive and accessible, the Moodle interface is easy to navigate on both desktop and mobile devices.
dashboard	Display current, past and future courses, along with tasks due.
collaborative tools and activities	Work and learn together in forums, wikis, glossaries, database activities, and much more.
all-in-one calendar	Moodle's calendar tool helps you keep track of your academic or company calendar, course deadlines, group meetings, and other personal events.
convenient file management	Drag and drop files from cloud storage services including MS OneDrive, Dropbox and Google Drive.
simple and intuitive text editor	Format text and conveniently add media and images with an editor that works across all web browsers and devices.
notifications	When enabled, users can receive automatic alerts on new assignments and deadlines, forum posts and also send private messages to one another.
track progress	Educators and learners can track progress and completion with an array of options for tracking individual activities or resources and at course level.

2.2.2 Activities, Resources and Structure

A group of features is called an activity or resource in Moodle. Activities are features to which users actively contribute, such as live chats. Resources are functions for sharing fixed content, such as texts or links. Moodle has 14 basic functions, but these can be extended with plugins. All the functions used are shown in Table 2 [6].

Table 2: Used Activities and Resources of Moodle

Function	Explanation
forum	Allows users to have asynchronous discussions.
URL	Forwarding to additional content on the internet.
web conference	BigBlueButton plugin is used for online video conferences.
glossary	Enables users to create and maintain a list of definitions, like a dictionary.
wiki	A collection of web pages that anyone can add to or edit.

A clear and concise structure is essential for the knowledge base. It must be as easy as possible for users to use. It has been shown that the forums are one of the most important parts of the knowledge base, as they serve the active exchange of information between users. Due to the exchange of discussions, entries in the glossary or the wiki can be created together. Above all, the wiki benefits from a large number of contributing users and for quality assurance of the knowledge base. The completed structure of the knowledge base is shown in Figure 1.

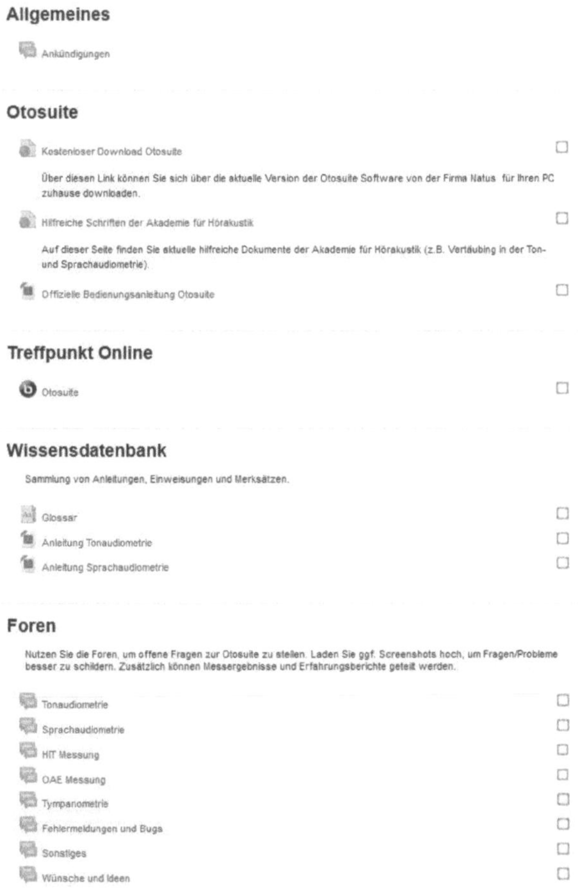

Figure 1: Structure of the Moodle course.

2.2.3 Users

With Moodle, only registered users are granted access to the knowledge base. In this way, roles can be used to control who is allowed to disseminate and modify information. Users of the afh platform are lecturers of the afh and participants of further training courses of this institution. Users of the LBS platform are teachers and students of the vocational school. All users, with a few exceptions of the teachers of the LBS, are hearing care professionals. Instructors and teachers, as well as course participants and students, each occupy a comparable status in terms of knowledge and experience. Lecturers and teachers, as well as continuing training participants and students, each occupy a comparable status in terms of knowledge and experience. The number of participants is shown in Table 3.

Table 3: Number of Users

Role	Number
Lecturers	3
Training participants	27
Teachers	4
Students	3069

Otosuite exams are administered at both institutions. Continuing education participants and students often need to be inexperienced in using the software.

2.3 Questionnaire

To obtain feedback on the knowledge base, a questionnaire consisting of seven questions was developed. The first two questions are single choice. The following four questions have a Likert scale and the last question is an open question. The Likert scale goes from strongly disagree (P1) to strongly agree (P5). The aim of the questionnaire is to clarify the added value of the LCMS knowledge base compared to a manufacturer's manual.. In order to achieve a meaningful result, this questionnaire was digitally transmitted to the students of the LBS. The questions of the questionnaire are shown in Table 4.

Table 4: Questionnaire Questions

Number	Question
1	Have you ever used or looked at the manufacturer's guide?
2	Have you ever used the Moodle course "Otosuite Help"?
3	I would rather look in the Moodle course than in the manufacturer's guide.
4	I can imagine writing a post in the forum if I have a question.
5	If I have worked out a fact sheet or something similar, I can imagine sharing it with others in the Moodle course.
6	A platform for exchange between users (Moodle course) I find better than a static page (manufacturer's guide).
7	In your opinion, what are the advantages of the Moodle course over the manufacturer's guide?

3 Results and Discussion

3.1 LCMS

Content for the knowledge database runs through the content lifecycle. This describes the creation and development of content [7]. An LCMS can manage the entire content lifecycle, from planning to development, structuring, publication, and evaluation.
The first self-created content has already been added to the course and knowledge base. Quick reference guides for sound and speech audiometry are frequently accessed documents. In addition, external content was included, such as the free download for Otosuite and the manual. Self-generated content proved to be very time consuming. External content sometimes needs to be thoroughly vetted and can be costly. Managing this content in the LCMS is user-friendly and easy to learn. The structure and activities described above contribute to the usability of the application. The LCMS can be expanded at any time. Likewise, new users can be added at any time.

3.2 Questionnaire Results

243 students responded to the questionnaire. The percentage responses of the single choice questions are shown in Table 5. The Likert scale questions in Table 6 and the most frequent responses of the open-ended question in Table 7.

Table 5: Single Choice - Results in %

Number	Yes (%)	No (%)
1	13,17	86,83
2	21,41	78,6

Table 6: Likert Scale - Results in %

Number	P1	P2	P3	P4	P5
3	5,35	7,41	28,40	37,04	21,81
4	19,75	23,87	30,45	16,46	9,47
5	14,40	18,52	31,28	24,69	11,11
6	7,00	6,17	30,86	33,33	22,63

Table 7: Open Question - Most Frequent Answers in %

Answer	%
Possibility to ask individual questions	74,65
Interaction between users	72,30
Contents are easier to understand	57,75
Contents can be found faster	44,13

3.3 Discussion

The LCMS has confirmed in practice that it is suitable as a basis for the knowledge base. It offers the necessary flexibility through the many possibilities to retrieve or exchange information. Learning on demand describes the possibilities to retrieve and process content independently of time and place and especially in a targeted manner [8]. The LCMS has further essential advantages compared to many static knowledge bases and manufacturer manuals. Through the interaction of the users with each other, not only the actively discussing users benefit, but also the passive readers. The student survey has shown that users prefer an LCMS to the manufacturer's guide. Above all, the exchange between users is highlighted as a positive feature. This includes the possibility to ask individual questions or to share measurement data with other users. The willingness to share finished content with other users, on the other hand, is assessed differently.

In a further investigation, the success of the LCMS-based knowledge base needs to be verified. It must be verified whether users gain knowledge faster through the knowledge base and become expert in operating the measurement system and interpreting the measurement results faster. In relation to evidence-based medicine, the quality of the measurements is a decisive factor.

4 Conclusion

The existing research question whether a knowledge base on a medical measuring device based on a LCMS can be successful can be answered with yes. It is important that the interest of the users is high to ensure the build-up and maintenance of the knowledge base. The quality and scope of the knowledge database is strongly dependent on the activity of the users. Only with information and experiences of the users the knowledge base shows its advantages compared to a classical manufacturer manual.

Instructions, as required by the Medical Device Directive, can be carried out digitally and, if necessary, subsequently verified by a test. Measurement conditions and results can be compared and discussed. These factors can ultimately lead to better results in medical technology.

Acknowledgement

The work has been carried out and supervised by the Akademie für Hörakustik.

Author's Statement

Conflict of interest: Authors state no conflict of interest.

5 References

[1] Natus GmbH, *Otosuite*. Available: https://hearing-balance.natus.com/de-de/produkte-loesungen/otosuite [last accessed on 2020-01-18].

[2] G. Probst, S. Raub and K. Romhardt, *Wissen Managen: Wie Unternehmen ihre wertvollste Ressource optimal Nutzen*, vol. 7, p. 16, 2012.

[3] M. Springmann, *Definition und Aufbau einer Wissensdatenbank mit Intranettechnologie*, p. 18, 2001.

[4] P. Arnold, L. Kilian, A. Thillosen and G. Zimmer, *Handbuch E-Learning*, vol. 4, pp. 87-88, 2015

[5] Moodle, *General Features*. Available: https://docs.moodle.org/310/en/Features [last accessed on 2021-01-19].

[6] Moodle, *Acitivites*. Available: https://docs.moodle.org/310/en/Activities [last accessed on 2021-01-20].

[7] Innovatia, *Content Lifecycle Management*. Available: https://www.innovatia.net/content-lifecycle-management [last accessed on 2021-01-24].

[8] E. Trondsen, K. Vickery, *Learning on Demand*, Journal of Knowledge Management, Vol. 1 Iss 3 pp. 169 - 180, 1997

Determination of the source parameters of a balanced-armature driver for modelling the individual sound propagation in the human ear canal

Nils Odenwald [1], Florian Denk [2] and Hendrik Husstedt [2]

[1] Auditory Technology, Universität zu Lübeck, nils.odenwald@student.uni-luebeck.de

[2] Deutsches Hörgeräte Institut GmbH, {f.denk, h.husstedt}@dhi-online.de

Abstract

The auditory canal represents an important part in the process of hearing aid fitting. The anthropometric characteristics of the auditory canal can differ significantly between individuals. Current methods to compensate for this are complex and time consuming. This work deals with the first steps for setting up a system, where only a single measurement for one ear is necessary and the test effort is considerably reduced. The change of the sound propagation path e.g. by modifying the earpiece or venting can then be simulated by an acoustical computer model.This first part of the project describes how to determine the source parameters (Source Flux $\underline{q}_s$ and Source Impedance $\underline{Z}_s$) of a driver that is intended to be used in the measurement probe. Measurements are made with a $0.4\,\text{cm}^3$ coupler and additional volume extensions as known load volumes. By a matrix calculation based on the load models and the measurements made with the different volumes, the source parameters are obtained. With these source parameters the sound propagation through new unknown loads can be predicted.

1 Introduction

For the fitting process of hearing aids, the acoustic properties of the propagation chain from the hearing aid driver to the eardrum have to be considered. Since all human ears are unique, the sound propagation from the end of the earpiece through the auditory canal to the tympanic membrane also varies. In order to compensate for these individual properties and the impact from the earpiece, common methods need a measurement of the sound pressure close to the eardrum with a probe microphone. However, if after the fitting process the propagation chain is changed by e.g. adjustment of venting or length of the earpiece, this compensation has to be repeated. This is time consuming and expensive.

Thus it is desirable to have a method, that only requires one measurement per ear and that can predict the effect of further modifications. This could be done by a measuring probe consisting of a driver and a microphone inside an anthropometric earpiece described by [1]. Additionally a computer model of the physical properties is necessary to simulate the effect of changes.

This paper deals with the initial step of determining the source parameters (Source Flux $\underline{q}_s$ and Source Impedance $\underline{Z}_s$) of the driver. For this various load volumes are needed. The theory described by Kirchhoff [2] explains the propagation of sound in one-dimensional acoustic ducts that is used here. The physical model of the cylindrical duct can then be translated into an electro-acoustic circuit as shown by Balkenhol [3]. The length l and the cross-sectional area A_{cr} determine the load of a duct. The method of the linear equation model described by Blau et al. [4] allows for the calculation of the source parameters $\underline{Z}_s$ and $\underline{q}_s/u_s$ from the calculated loads and the measured sound pressure at the microphone, with u_s as the source voltage. These source parameters of the driver can then be used to predict the sound field of new models.

2 Material and Methods

2.1 Electro-acoustic model

The acoustical properties of a cylindrical duct as shown in Figure 1 can be mathematically described by

$$\begin{pmatrix}\underline{p}_s\\ \underline{q}_s\end{pmatrix} = \begin{pmatrix}a_{11} & a_{12}\\ a_{21} & a_{22}\end{pmatrix}\begin{pmatrix}\underline{p}_m\\ \underline{q}_m\end{pmatrix}, \tag{1}$$

with sound pressure $\underline{p}_s$ and sound flux $\underline{q}_s$ of the source and $\underline{p}_m$ and $\underline{q}_m$ of microphone respectively. The sound flux $\underline{q}$ describes the amount of volume per time unit that is transmitted through a reference area. The acoustic impedance is obtained by $\underline{Z} = \underline{p}/\underline{q}$. In general the sound propagation through a tube is determined by its length l and cross-

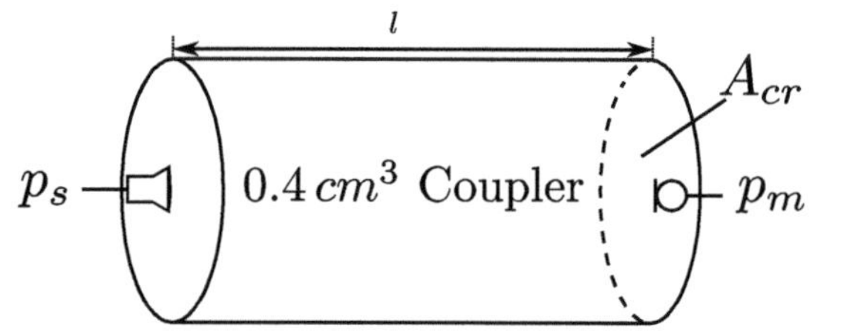

Figure 1: Schematic chain of the physical model with source pressure p_s, coupler volume and the microphone pressure p_m.

sectional area A_{cr} as mentioned by Kirchhoff [2].
The electro-acoustical model corresponding to Figure 1 is shown in Figure 2 according to Balkenhol [3] with

$$A = \begin{pmatrix} cos(kl) & \frac{Z_0}{A_{cr}} j sin(kl) \\ \frac{j A_{cr}}{Z_0} sin(kl) & cos(kl) \end{pmatrix}. \quad (2)$$

$Z_0 = \rho c$ is the characteristic impedance and $k = (2\pi f)/c$ or $k = \omega/c$ is the wave-number.
The given coupler with the driver and microphone attached can be assumed to be closed on both ends. In this case the impedance at the microphone will be infinite ($\underline{Z} = \infty$) resulting in a source flux of zero ($\underline{q} = 0$).
In Figure 2 $\underline{p}_m/u_s$ describes the sound pressure at the microphone and shows where the source flux is $\underline{q} = 0$ as described before. The block labelled A describes the sound propagation though the rigid tube. The left hand side of the model consists of the driver circuit with the source pressure $\underline{p}_s$, source flux in relation to the source voltage $\underline{q}_s/u_s$ and the source impedance $\underline{Z}_s$. The source is powered by a constant voltage of 0.05 V. In order to determine the unknown source parameters ($\underline{Z}_s$, $\underline{q}_s$) for a given volume, the method described by Blau et al. [4], (3) is used. This method requires a set of measurements with different volumes. Therefore volume extensions are Computer Aided Designed (CAD) and 3D printed, with keeping the diameter (9.4 mm) of the coupler constant. The extensions are printed from UV-curing resin.

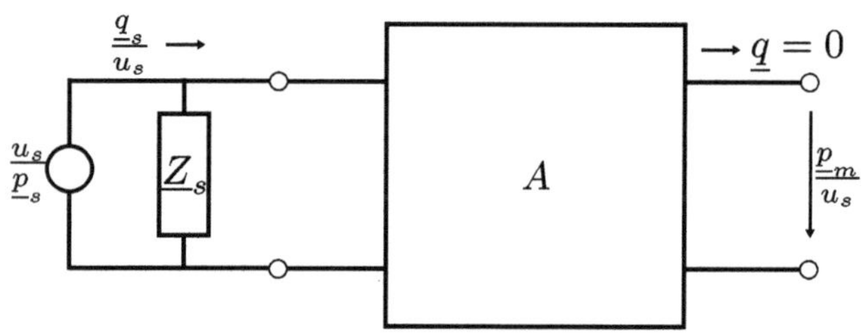

Figure 2: Electro-acoustic circuit of the physical model as shown in Figure 1.

In

$$\begin{pmatrix} -a_{21_1} & \frac{u_s}{\underline{p}_{m_1}} \\ \vdots & \vdots \\ -a_{21_n} & \frac{u_s}{\underline{p}_{m_n}} \end{pmatrix} \cdot \begin{pmatrix} \underline{Z}_s \\ \frac{\underline{q}_s}{u_s} \underline{Z}_s \end{pmatrix} = \begin{pmatrix} a_{11_1} \\ \vdots \\ a_{11_n} \end{pmatrix}, \quad (3)$$

n corresponds to the number of measurements with different volumes. The matrix equation (3) is of the shape $Ax = b$ and is solved with the Moore-Penrose Pseudoinverse $x = A^+b$. For calculating the unknown source impedance $\underline{Z}_s$ and source flux $\underline{q}_s/u_s$ as a minimum two equations (measurements) are necessary. To achieve a more reliable result more measurements are made and accordingly more equations are obtained. For solving the resulting indefinite equation system the method of least squares is used. The measurements as well as the model and matrix calculations are performed with MATLAB.

2.2 Set-Up with the 0.4 cm³ Coupler

For the experiment the 0.4 cm³ coupler (GRAS 43BA-3 1/4") is used as a cylindrical duct. The CAD modelled and 3D-printed extensions, extend the total volume to 0.5, 0.6, 0.7, 0.8, 0.9 and 1 cm³. So in total 7 different volumes are used for the source parameter calculation. For the set-up as

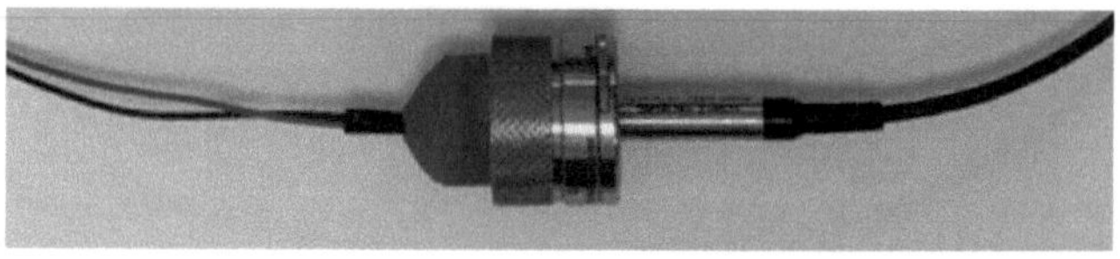

Figure 3: Measuring set-up of the coupler with 3D-printed extension and mounted driver.

depicted in Figure 3 the balanced armature driver (Knowles fk-23451-000) is mounted flush with the beginning of the extensions, followed by the volume load, ending with a 1/4" microphone provided by the coupler.
For each tube model i, the volume load (a_{21_i} and a_{11_i}) and the corresponding measured pressure at the coupler microphone ($u_{s_i}/\underline{p}_{m_i}$) make up one row of (3).

2.3 Measurements

For the measurements a 10 seconds exponential sine sweep is used as input signal and played back from the armature driver with the predefined voltage amplitude of 0.05 V. From the recording of the signal at the microphone p_m the impulse response (IR) is calculated as described by Farina [5]. The IR is then cut to a length of 0.05 seconds to improve the signal-to-noise ratio. In general the IR characterizes the behaviour of a linear time-invariant system for all frequencies. For each load volume, five measurements with remounting the driver after each measurement are made to take variations into account. In total 5 repetitions and 7 conditions are considered resulting in 35 measurements and in $n = 35$ rows in (3). The means of the five measurements

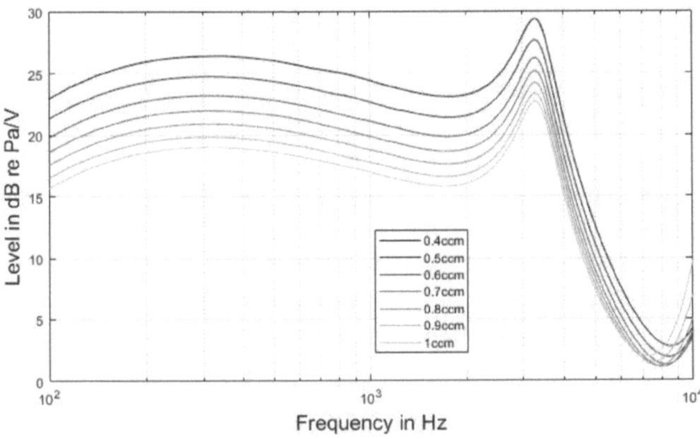

Figure 4: Sound pressure level at microphone for the different volumes. Each averaged from five measurements.

(IRs) for each of the seven calibration volumes are depicted in Figure 4 in the frequency domain.

3 Results and Discussion

3.1 Evaluated Data

The results of solving the equation system (3) is shown in Figure 5. As can be seen in the upper graph, the source Impedance $\underline{Z}_s$ decreases with higher frequencies and shows a notch at a frequency around $3,300\,\text{Hz}$. In the lower graph the source flux $\underline{q}_s$ is shown in dependence of the source voltage u_s. It increases with higher frequencies and shows a resonance peak at around $3,300\,\text{Hz}$. Comparing the two graphs of $\underline{Z}_s$ and $\underline{q}_s$ the course of the lines are almost counter-proportional to each other. The area at around $3,300\,\text{Hz}$ indicates the resonance frequency of the driver

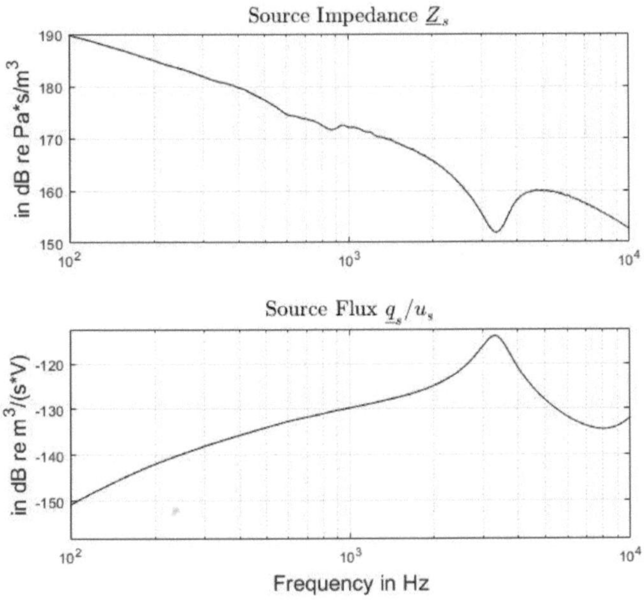

Figure 5: Source impedance $\underline{Z}_s$ and source flux $\underline{q}_s$ of the balance armature driver, depending on the frequency range of 100 to $10,000$ Hz.

membrane, at which the least energy is needed to generate sound pressure. At this resonating point, the impedance shows the lowest value.

3.2 Statistical Analysis

In order to find out where the different volumes influence the quality of the measured results and to check the reproducibility, the standard deviations of the repeated measurements have been calculated. As depicted in Figure 6 the standard deviation in the most cases is at around or below $0.1\,\text{dB}$ except the measurements made with the $0.5\,\text{cm}^3$ extension (highest remount deviation of the driver in the setup). Even though for smaller volumes remount deviations are expected to be greater than for larger volumes, such a trend is not clearly visible. The greatest deviations for all volumes are right before and after the driver resonance at $3,300\,\text{Hz}$. Overall, the deviations can be neglected. In order to check the reproducibility of the data, all possible combinations, summing up to $78,125$ of one measurement from each calibration volume are taken to calculate the source parameters. Meaning each combination calculates the source parameters by 7 measurements without having measurements of a calibration volume twice.
Finally the mean of all solutions as well as the minimum and maximum deviating results are calculated. This is illustrated in Figure 7. The printed lines are almost identical, expect in the area of the resonance where the maximum deviating results shows a strong spike of $+50\,\text{dB}$ and the minimum shows a drop of around $-5\,\text{dB}$ shortly below the resonance. The averaged data line q_{mean} matches the calculated curve from all measurements $\underline{q}_s/u_s$ shown in Figure 5.

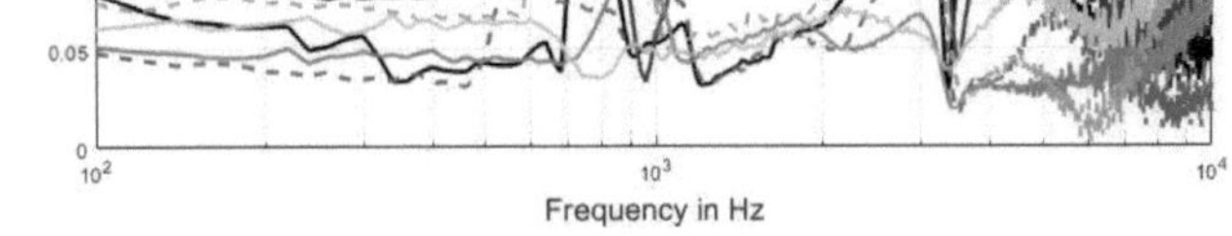

Figure 6: Standard deviation of the sound pressure transfer functions from the five repeated measurements for each condition.

3.3 Prediction of behaviour of an unknown load volume

For testing the model, a measurement with an additional volume extension of $2\,\text{cm}^3$ is used. The diameter of the

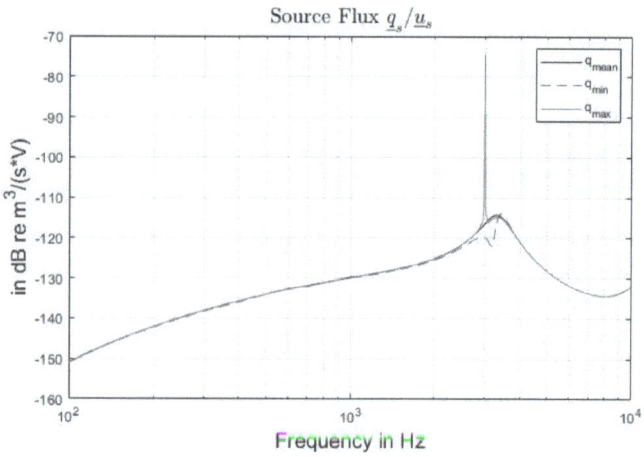

Figure 7: Mean, minimum and maximum transfer functions of the source flux determined by the 78, 125 combinations.

coupler remains the same, the length is extended. The reason for modelling a new volume is, that for testing purposes an unknown load volume should be used. From (1) and $\underline{q}_m = 0$ we get:

$$\underline{p}_m = \underline{q}_s \cdot \frac{1}{a_{11}/(\underline{Z}_s + a_{21})}. \tag{4}$$

This allows us to calculate the sound pressure at the microphone for any load volume. The resulting transfer function is now compared to the estimated data calculated with (4) and visualized in Figure 8. The comparison shows a good match. The -difference- line in the lower part of the graph shows a deviation of 4.8 dB at the first resonance frequency at 5, 900 Hz for the 2 cm^3 volume. At the other frequencies the deviation is below 1.2 dB. The results show, that the method used to determine the source parameters gives reliable results.

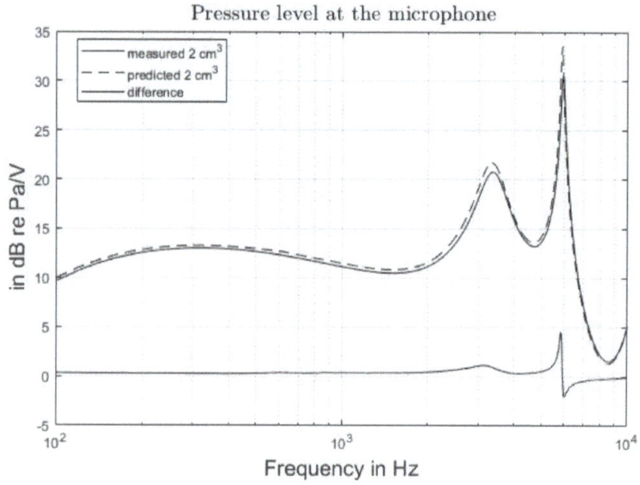

Figure 8: Measured vs. predicted transfer function of the sound pressure at the microphone of a 2 cm^3 volume.

4 Conclusion

The paper points out how an acoustical system can be described as a circuit model to determine the source impedance and the source flux of an unknown driver. This driver can then be used within new models with known parameters to determine the unknown loads to predict e.g. the sound pressure at the end of different load volume.

During the calculations all physical quantities such as volume (length and diameter), temperature, voltage and sound pressure have to be precisely recorded to obtain useful results. In order to reduce deviations caused by remounting as depicted in Figure 6 the socket for mounting the driver may should be optimised.

The next step will be to find a way to create a model representing the individual auditory canal to predict the sound pressure at the ear drum as done by Hudde [6]. With a customised earpiece based on [1] including the driver as described and a probe microphone, the acoustic properties of the human ear should be modelled so that the acoustic behaviour can be predicted.

Acknowledgement

The work has been carried out at Deutsches Hörgeräte Institut GmbH, Anschützstr. 1, Lübeck.

5 References

[1] F. Denk, F. Brinkmann, A. Stirnemann, B. Kollmeier, (2019), *The PIRATE: an anthropometric earPlug with exchangeable microphones for Individual Reliable Acquisition of Transfer functions at the Ear canal entrance.* doi = 10.5281/zenodo.2574395.

[2] C. Kirchhoff, (1868), *Über den Einfluss der Wärmeleitung in einem Gase auf die Schallbewegung.* Pogg. Ann. 134, 177–193.

[3] T. Balkenhol, (2009), *Adaptive Digitalfilter für die aktive Schalldämpfung in Röhrensystemen. Dissertation.* Universität Paderborn.

[4] M. Blau, T. Sankowsky, P. Roeske, H. Mojallal, M. Teschner and C. Thiele, (2010), *Prediction of the Sound Pressure at the Ear.* Acta Acustica United with Acustica, Vol. 96 554-566.

[5] A. Farina, (2000), *Simultaneous Measurement of Impulse Response and Distortion with a Swept-Sine Technique.* Audio Engineering Society Convention 108.

[6] H. Hudde, (1998), *Measuring and Modeling Basic Properties of the Human Middle Ear and Ear Canal. Part II: Ear Canal, Middle Ear Cavities, Eardrum, and Ossicles.* Acta Acustica United with Acustica Vol. 84 894-913.

Comparison of different sound pressure level measurement systems for industrial facilities

Katharina Schlecht [1], Björn Heichen [2] and Miriam Sparr [2]

[1] Auditory Technology, Universität zu Lübeck, katharina.schlecht@student.uni-luebeck.de
[2] LAIRM Consult GmbH , Bargteheide, {heichen,sparr}@lairm.de

Abstract

Measurements are carried out to record noise in physically measurable quantities. Various measurement systems are available for this purpose. The measuring systems have different technical specifications depending on the manufacturer. Whether this aspect has an effect on the execution of measurements and on the measurement results was investigated in this project. For this purpose, the a-weighted sound pressure levels of a diesel locomotive were measured under free-field conditions with two measuring systems from different manufacturers using the enveloping surface method of accuracy class 2 according to DIN EN ISO 3744:2011-02 in order to subsequently determine the sound power level. The results from measurements at 14 firmly defined measuring points show that deviations in the measurement results can be attributed to device-specific presettings for determining the measured values.

1 Introduction

Noise is an ever-increasing, omnipresent disturbance factor in our society due to advancing mechanization and globalization. The term noise covers all sounds that have a disturbing or stressful effect on people and the environment. The perception of sounds as noise depends on individual, subjective factors and perceptions as well as on physically measurable variables such as sound pressure level, pitch, tonality and impulsiveness [1].

Despite subjective noise perception, there are assessment options that allow conclusions to be drawn about the annoyance caused by sound events. First of all, it is necessary to distinguish between different types of noise, such as road traffic, rail traffic, aircraft noise, industrial noise, construction noise, recreational noise or sports noise. The assessment of noise pollution takes place for each of these noise types individually, since each noise type differs in its annoyance, its temporal behavior and its local occurrence. In order to do justice to these types of noise with their different characteristics, assessment procedures have been developed and summarized in corresponding rules and regulations, which must be observed when finding solutions to noise problems. A special law that explicitly regulates the protection against noise does not exist in this form. However, the Federal Immission Control Act plays an overriding role, the purpose of which is to generally protect the environment from harmful effects such as noise [2].

This project deals with the industrial noise of a siding near a residential area requiring protection. Residents complain about the noise of the diesel locomotives passing by and partly parking on the track. In contrast to electric locomotives, the diesel locomotives used on the track are the main emitters of noise, as they generate significantly higher emission levels due to the design of the diesel units (internal combustion engines) used.
By using different metrological methods, these quantities can be recorded and evaluated. The question arises whether, when using different technical measuring systems with a different number of measured values per second, the same or different measurement results are obtained using the same metrological procedure. In order to address this question, measurements of emission levels were carried out in the test setup on a diesel locomotive in the specified operating state using two different measurement systems from the manufacturers Sinus [1] and Brüel & Kjaer [2] in order to be able to determine their sound power levels. To ensure the comparability of the measurement results, the measurements were carried out in parallel, using the enveloping surface method according to DIN EN ISO 3744:2011-02 of accuracy class 2 in order to create an equal and consistent starting/measurement situation for both systems [3].

2 Material and Methods

2.1 Measurement systems

For the emission level measurement of the diesel locomotive during warm-up on the siding, calibrated measuring systems were used which corresponded to the same technical standard of accuracy class 1 [4]. The measurement systems used are, on the one hand, a four-channel measurement device from the manufacturer Sinus with the designation "Soundbook MK2 4LG [1]" and, on the other hand, a single-channel measurement device "Noiselogger Type 2250-N-D02 [2]" from the manufacturer Brüel & Kjaer. Both systems were configured as comparable as possible in their settings for the measurement runs with the possibilities of the respective measurement systems. By calibrating the microphones of both systems before and after the measurement, it was ensured that the sensitivity of the microphones was consistent over the entire measurement period.

The calibration of the microphone belonging to the Soundbook was done with the calibrator RION-NC 74. The microphone of the Brüel & Kjaer measuring system Type 2250 was calibrated with the calibrator type 4231.

2.2 Measurement procedure

The measurements were carried out on a diesel locomotive on an exposed siding in order to avoid the influence of reflections from nearby objects. Ambient noise occurring during the measurement processes, such as general operating noise on the site, was taken into account in the measurement evaluation. The diesel locomotive was measured to determine the microphone positions. With dimensions of 16.4 meters in length, 3.14 meters in width and 4.6 meters in height, measurement positions were marked at a distance of 2 meters from each other for the placement of the microphones on a previously defined cuboid measurement surface. Using DIN EN ISO 3744:2011-02, a measurement area of 509.18 m² was calculated as Table 1 shows [3].

Table 1: Calculation of the measurement area.

Measurement area		
Length		16.40 m
Width		3.14 m
Height		4.60 m
Measurement distance		2.00 m
Measurement area	a	10.20 m
according to	b	3.57 m
DIN EN ISO 3744:2011	c	6.60 m
Measurement area		509.18 m²

The set-up was carried out in parallel at a total of 12 positions on the long sides and with one position in front of and one behind the diesel locomotive. Fig. 1 shows an exemplary arrangement of the measurement setup.

The microphone of the Soundbook and the microphone of the measuring system Type 2250 were fixed at a height of 2.5 meters along the measurement path, since the ventilation inlets of the diesel units are located at this height,

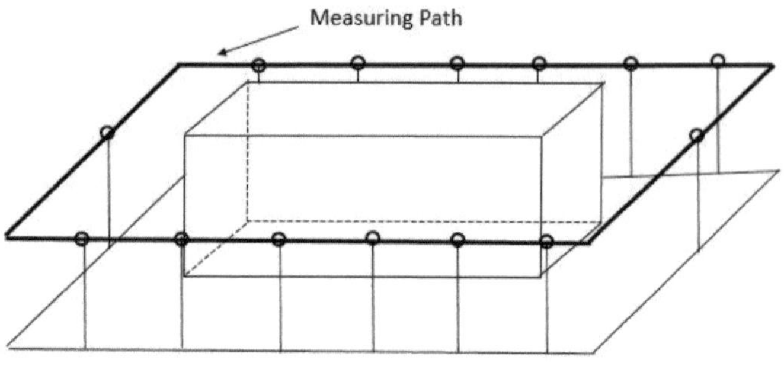

Figure 1: Exemplary representation of the measuring area and the microphone positions (measuring path) for the diesel locomotive.

from which subjectively the loudest noise emissions can be heard. To avoid possible mutual interference between the microphones during the measurement processes, a distance of four inches was selected between the microphones at each measurement position. Furthermore, each of the microphones was equipped with a microphone windscreen to protect the microphones from occurring wind noise thus not to falsify the measurement results.

Before starting the measurements, the microphones were calibrated and set up at the first measurement position at the respective heights in the direction of the diesel locomotive. The first measurement run involved starting the diesel locomotive followed by a transition to the specified operating state (warm-up of the diesel units). The measurement systems were started simultaneously and stopped simultaneously after a measurement period of five minutes at each of the 14 measurement points in order to document the time-averaged sound pressure level over the typical operating cycle of the diesel locomotive. In order to guarantee a comparable level-time curve between the individual measuring positions for the evaluation of the emission levels, the starting as well as the stopping of the diesel aggregates for operating the diesel locomotive were not included. Fig. 2 shows the evaluation of an exemplary level-time curve documented by the Type 2250 measuring system at the fourth measuring position.

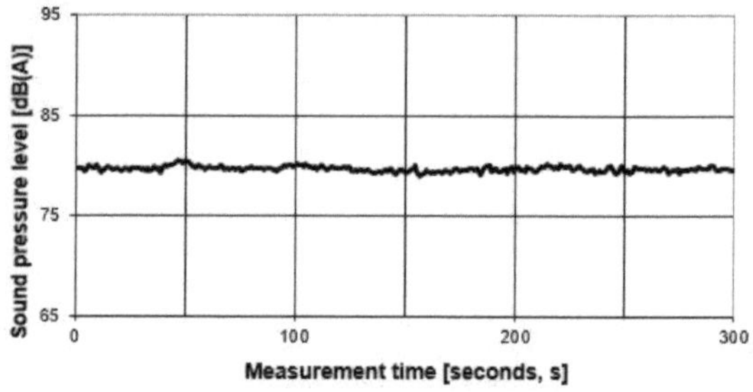

Figure 2: Exemplary evaluation extract of a level-time curve documented by the Type 2250 measuring system at the fourth measuring position.

After completion of the last measurement, the microphones were calibrated again in order to be able to determine possible deviations in the microphones during the measurement processes.

3 Results and Discussion

All recorded measurement data were evaluated under the enveloping surface procedure described in DIN EN ISO 3744:2011-02 [3]. Consideration of the extraneous noise and ambient correction as well as the measurement uncertainty were included in this procedure. Table 2 shows the a-weighted equivalent continuous sound pressure level from the 14 measurement positions from the Soundbook and the Type 2250 measurement systems.

The evaluation of the measurement from the Soundbook resulted in an a-weighted equivalent continuous time-averaged sound pressure level of 77.5 dB(A). The Type 2250 measurement system, on the other hand, whose microphone was fixed at the same height of four meters as that of the Soundbook, produced an A-weighted time-averaged measurement area sound pressure level of 77.0 dB(A) during the measurement evaluation. No differences were found between the measurement systems during the measurement procedure with regard to the handling and operation of the systems.

Comparing the time-averaged measurement area sound pressure levels of the two different measurement systems with the fixed microphone height at four meters results in a small negligible deviation of 0.5 dB(A), which is correspondingly within the measurement accuracy of Class 2 of the measurement devices [5]. The A-weighted sound pressure level difference of 0.5 dB(A) can be attributed to the manufacturer-specific setting options of the systems. The Soundbook from the manufacturer Sinus is configured in such a way that the measured sound pressure level is acquired and recorded every 0.005 seconds. Accordingly, the system records 12.000 sound pressure level values in one minute. The Type 2250 measurement system from Brüel & Kjaer, on the other hand, records one sound pressure level value every second. This results in 60 recorded sound pressure level values in one minute. The time-averaged measurement area sound pressure level of 77.5 dB(A) of the Soundbook measurement system can be considered more accurate in relation to the measurement result of the 2250 measurement system due to the finer presetting.
The determination of the sound power level, which is determined according to the applied enveloping surface method of accuracy class 2, also shows, as in the previously measured sound pressure levels of the two measuring systems used, a difference of 0.5 dB(A) between the two systems, which also differ from each other.

The sound power level, calculated from the a-weighted equivalent continuous time-averaged sound pressure level shown in Table 2, is 104.6 dB for the four-channel measurement system and 104.1 dB for the single-channel measurement system. Since the time-averaged A-weighted sound pressure levels and the area of the measurement surface serve as the basis for calculating the sound power level in the enveloping surface method described in DIN EN ISO 3744:2011-02, the sound power level of the single-channel system is 0.5 dB higher than that of the dual-channel system [3]. As a result, the sound power level to be determined depends on manufacturer-specific presettings in the measurement accuracy and recording of the systems.

Table 2: A-weighted equivalent continuous sound pressure level [dB(A)] from the 14 measurement positions (MP) of the two measurement systems Type 2250 and Soundbook.

MP	Type 2250	Soundbook
1	74.4	75.7
2	78.4	78.4
3	79.1	79.9
4	79.7	80.2
5	77.3	77.7
6	67.3	67.4
7	73.4	73.1
8	74.4	75.7
9	78.4	78.4
10	79.1	79.9
11	79.7	80.2
12	77.3	77.7
13	67.3	67.4
14	73.4	73.1
Ø	77.0	77.5

4 Conclusion

The question posed in the project as to whether the same or different measurement results are obtained when using different technical measurement systems using the same metrological procedures could be investigated by applying the enveloping surface method according to DIN EN ISO 3744:2011-02 of accuracy class 2 on a diesel locomotive with subsequent evaluation and comparison of the measurement results. It was found that almost identical measurement results were obtained when a comparable technical standard was applied to the measurement systems used and when the standard-compliant performance was taken into account. The measuring system to be used could therefore be selected on the basis of the object size to be measured or the amount of work involved.

Acknowledgement

The work has been carried out at LAIRM Consult GmbH, Bargteheide and supervised by Prof. Dr. rer. nat. Jürgen Tchorz, University Lübeck, Lübeck.
The company LAIRM Consult GmbH contributed to the design and implementation of the research and to the analysis

of the results.

Author's Statement

Conflict of interest: Authors state no conflict of interest.

5 Manufacturer information

[1]SINUS Messtechnik GmbH, Leipzig,
Measurement system: Soundbook MK2 4LG
Available: https://sinus-leipzig.de/de/ [last accessed on 2021-01-23]

[2] Hottinger Brüel & Kjaer, Darmstadt,
Measurement system: Noiselogger Type 2250-N-D02
Available: https://www.bksv.com/de-DE [last accessed on 2021-01-23]

6 References

[1] J. H. Maue, H. Hoffmann and A. Lüpke, *0 Dezibel + 0 Dezibel = 3 Dezibel, Einführung in die Grundbegriffe und die quantitative Erfassung des Lärms* . Erich Schmidt Verlag GmbH & Co., 2. Auflage, Berlin, Januar 2009.

[2] Bundes-Immissionsschutzgesetz (BImSchG), *Gesetz zum Schutz vor schädlichen Umwelteinwirkungen durch Luftverunreinigungen, Geräusche, Erschütterungen und ähnliche Vorgänge*, in der Fassung der Bekanntmachung vom 17. Mai 2013 (BGBI. I S. 1274), das zuletzt durch Artikel 13 der Verordnung vom 19. Juni 2020 (BGBI. I S.1328, 1340) geändert worden ist.

[3] DIN EN ISO 3744:2011-02, *Akustik - Bestimmung der Schallleistungs- und Schallenergiepegel von Geräuschquellen aus Schalldruckmessungen - Hüllflächenverfahren der Genauigkeitsklasse 2 für ein im Wesentlichen freies Schallfeld über einer reflektierenden Ebene (ISO 3744:2010).* Deutsche Fassung EN ISO 3744:2010. Beuth Verlag GmbH, Berlin, Februar 2011.

[4] DIN EN 61672-1:2014-07, *Elektroakustik - Schallpegelmesser - Teil 1: Anforderungen (IEC 61672-1:2013)* . Deutsche Fassung EN 61672-1:2013. Beuth Verlag GmbH, Berlin, Juli 2004.

[5] DIN EN ISO 3740:1998-12, *Akustik - Bestimmung der Schallleistungspegel von Geräuschquellen - Leitlinien zur Anwendung der Grundnormen (ISO:DIS 3740:1998)* . Deutsche Fassung prEN ISO 3740:1998. Beuth Verlag GmbH, Berlin, Dezember 1998.

9

Signal Processing

Breathing Rate Estimation during Sleep using Capacitive ECG Electrodes

Leonie Basso [1], Martin Oehler [2], Marcin Grzegorzek [3]
[1] Medical Informatics, Universität zu Lübeck, leonie.basso@student.uni-luebeck.de
[2] Capical GmbH, Braunschweig, m.oehler@capical.de
[3] Institute of Medical Informatics, Universität zu Lübeck, grzegorzek@imi.uni-luebeck.de

Abstract

Breathing rate (BR) is a key physiological parameter and often measured by invasive and intrusive sensors e.g. nasal cannula. BR can also be estimated from the electrocardiogram (ECG). The use of capacitive electrodes enables a comfortable monitoring trough textile. ECG data is recorded during sleep using capacitive electrodes integrated in a bed sheet. An algorithm for the estimation of BR from amplitude, frequency and baseline modulation is presented. The extraction of respiratory signals, estimation of BRs, and fusion of BRs are implemented. The resulting algorithm and reference algorithms are evaluated on capacitive ECG signals from one subject. Overall, good results were achieved with both the proposed and reference algorithms. The lowest relative error of 5.82% was achieved by the implemented baseline method. The use of fusion methods such as temporal fusion improves the results. Further work is required to evaluate algorithms on a more diverse dataset.

1 Introduction

Breathing rate (BR) is an important parameter for various conditions and is often used in diagnostics and prognosis. Respiratory monitoring also provides valuable information about the health status of patients from home [1]. Direct measurement of respiration is possible with various sensors, which measure e.g. the change in chest circumference with a breathing belt or the airflow through the nose with a cannula. However, these are invasive sensors that interfere with natural breathing and lead to high costs with low comfort [2]. Such measurements are particularly unpleasant during sleep.

Another possibility is the indirect measurement of breathing via the electrocardiogram (ECG). The ECG is modulated due to changes in the electrodes position relative to the heart axis and changes in the electrical impedance of the thorax [3]. The modulation is also caused by the respiratory sinus arrhythmia (RSA), which is the increasing and decreasing of the heart rate during inspiration and exhalation. Several algorithms for ECG-derived respiration (EDR) have been proposed in literature [2], [4]. Electrodes connected directly to the body are usually used to measure the ECG. The use of wearables such as wristbands is also increasingly being investigated [4], [5]. The mentioned sensors are directly attached to the body surface, which may be uncomfortable and may affect the sleep of a subject. The development of unobtrusive systems is pursued to raise acceptance and avoid data distortion due to abnormal behavior.

The use of capacitive electrodes allows a comfortable measurement. Capacitive electrodes offer the same access to the human electrocardiogram as galvanic electrodes. They use the change of the charge on the body surface by the body potentials. These charge shifts influence the charge on a conductive textile area near the body, which does not require direct electrical skin contact. Therefore, the measurement of the capacitive ECG is also possible through layers of clothing [6]. Capical GmbH has developed a bed pad with capacitive ECG electrodes, which enables a permanent ECG measurement during sleep. New challenges arise for EDR-algorithms due to a higher susceptibility to movement artifacts and varying modulation magnitudes.

In this work, the possibility of estimating the BR using capacitive ECG electrodes during sleep is investigated. Different methods are implemented and their performance is tested.

2 Material and Methods

2.1 Dataset

The ECG data is recorded with a bed sheet consisting of capacitive electrodes developed by the Capical GmbH. 15 differential leads are available from six coupled electrodes. The dataset consists of ten recordings from one healthy volunteer. The duration ranges between 17 and 60 minutes (50 $\pm$ 16). Measurements were performed during sleep.

Reference respiration data is obtained with a resistive respiration belt (TMSI, Oldenzaal, Niederlande). The chest belt measures the circumference of the chest through an electrical resistance. All signals were acquired at a sampling rate of 560 Hz.

2.2 Preprocessing

ECG. The raw channels are first filtered in two different ways to obtain certain properties for later processing.
(1) A Butterworth bandpass filter with cutoff frequencies of 15 - 30 Hz is applied to the channels. This removes low-frequency fluctuations and highlights the QRS complexes, which contain the high R-peak. The filtered signal is later used for QRS detection.
(2) A notch filter for 50 Hz and 100 Hz is used to eliminate mains hum. A Butterworth bandpass filter with cutoff frequencies of 0.05 - 20 Hz is applied to eliminate frequencies irrelevant to breathing and high-frequency noise. This signal is later used to extract the baseline fluctuation.
The leads are calculated from the differences of the filtered channels. Since the electrodes have no direct skin contact and people often move during sleep, the capacitive ECG signals are particularly affected by movement artifacts. Therefore an artifact detection is performed using a sliding window and a historical minimum over the maxima of the previous windows as a threshold. One lead, that contains a visible respiration modulation and little noise, is manually selected for evaluation.
Respiration. Low-frequency fluctuations are determined with a moving average filter and subtracted from the signal to normalize it to an average value of zero. High-frequency signal components are removed by applying a low-pass filter with a cut-off frequency of 0.5 Hz. Below this frequency are the frequencies relevant to breathing during sleep. The signals are downsampled to a sampling rate of 5 Hz. Artifacts contained in the signal are detected and removed.

2.3 Algorithm for BR Estimation from ECG

The algorithm for BR estimation consists of three steps: (1) Extraction of respiratory signals, (2) Estimation of BRs, and (3) Fusion of BRs.

2.3.1 Extraction of Respiratory Signals

Three types of respiration-induced modulation are extracted from the ECG: (1) Amplitude Modulation (AM), (2) Frequency Modulation (FM), and (3) Baseline wander (BW), which are displayed in Fig. 1.
(1) To extract the AM of the ECG, the R-peaks are detected using a QRS detector, that is based upon the algorithm of Pan and Tompkins [8] and specially adapted for capacitive ECG data. For each R-peak the corresponding Q-wave is detected as the minimum value in the neighborhood. From this, the amplitude differences of the R- and Q-wave are calculated for each QRS complex. The values of the amplitudes are interpolated with a piecewise cubic interpolation to obtain a regular sampled signal.
(2) The FM is extracted as the length of the RR-intervals. The distances between R-peaks are calculated as differences between the indices of two adjacent R-peaks. The values of

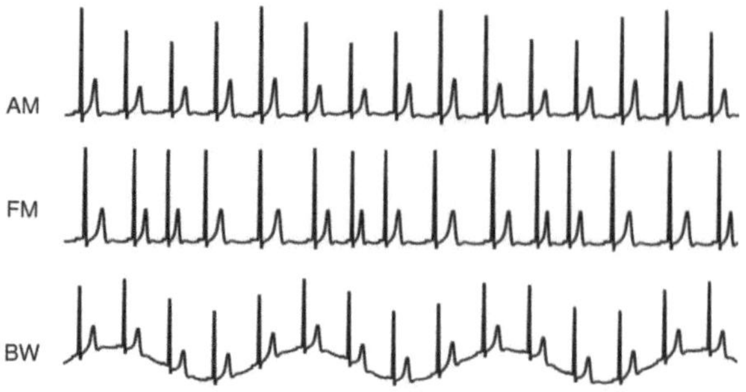

Figure 1: Simulation of the way respiration modulates the amplitude (AM), frequency (FM), and baseline (BW) of the ECG. Adapted from [7] (CC BY 3.0: https://creativecommons.org/licenses/by/3.0/).

RR-intervals are interpolated with a piecewise cubic interpolation as well.
(3) The BW is calculated by a moving average filter over a 2 s window.
The obtained respiration signals of all modulation types are normalized to mean zero. A Buttwerworth bandpass with cutoff frequencies of 0.1 Hz - 0.75 Hz is applied to eliminate non-breathing frequencies. The signals are downsampled to 5 Hz.

2.3.2 Estimation of BRs

To estimate the BR, the time intervals between the individual breaths must be determined. The breaths are detected as peaks of the modulation signal with a minimum distance of 2s and the differences between the peaks are calculated. The final BR is computed from the sampling rate F_s and the n differences d with $\mathrm{BR}_i = \dfrac{60 \cdot F_s}{d_i}, i = 1, ..., n$.

2.3.3 Fusion of BRs

A combination of different BR estimates can increase robustness. The fusion can be performed temporally within one estimate or between different modulation types.
Lázaro, Gil, Bailón, *et al.* proposed a Temporal Fusion method, in which neighboring values are included within a BR estimate [9]. As shown in (1), the BR at a point k is calculated based on the estimate $\mathrm{BR_{est}}$ and the previous value at $k-1$ with $\alpha = 0.8$. This results in a smoothing of the final estimated BRs.

$$\mathrm{BR}(k) = (1-\alpha) \cdot \mathrm{BR_{est}}(k) + \alpha \cdot \mathrm{BR}(k-1) \quad (1)$$

The several BR estimates from AM, FM and BW can be combined to achieve a better result. One method is Smart Fusion by Karlen, Raman, Ansermino, *et al.* [10], which was developed for estimating BR from photoplethysmography (PPG) signals. First, a quality check of the estimates is performed, removing areas with artifacts or low signal quality. The final BR is estimated as the mean, but only if the standard deviation between the estimates is ≤ 4 breaths per minute (bpm). Otherwise no BR output is given. This method may increase the robustness [7].

3 Results and Discussion

3.1 Experiments

To evaluate the performance of the implemented methods, reference algorithms are executed on the capacitive ECG data. For this purpose the RRest-toolbox [11] is used, which was developed by Charlton *et al.* as an open source platform to support the development of new algorithms.
The originally used QRS detector performs poorly due to a high occurrence of artifacts in capacitive ECG signals. Precalculated indices were used instead, which were detected with an algorithm specially adapted for capacitive ECG data. This ensures comparability between the EDR-algorithms. The presented algorithm and reference algorithms are executed on the test dataset with the same pre-computed BR as reference.

3.2 Error Metrics

Metrics are needed to evaluate the agreement between the estimate of the algorithm y^{alg} and the reference data y^{ref}. A mean BR estimate was calculated for each 32s window of all recordings. The absolute error AE is given by the difference $y^{\text{alg}} - y^{\text{ref}}$ between the results of the algorithm and the reference. The performance of the algorithms was assessed using the root-mean-square error RMSE and the relative error RE. For N windows they are given by:

$$\text{RMSE} = \sqrt{\frac{1}{N}\sum_{i=1}^{N}(\text{AE}_i)^2}, \text{RE} = \frac{100}{N}\sum_{i=1}^{N}\left(\frac{\text{AE}_i}{y_i^{\text{ref}}}\right). \quad (2)$$

3.3 Results

The error values of the implemented algorithms are shown in Table 1. BW achieves the best results, with a RMSE value of 2.01 bpm by comparison to over 3 bpm at the AM and FM methods and a RE half as high. The use of Smart Fusion did not improve the results.

Table 1: Mean μ and standard deviation σ of RMSE in bpm and RE in % for BR-estimation with proposed methods.

Algorithm	RMSE		RE	
	μ	σ	μ	σ
AM	3.05	0.78	13.06	4.74
FM	3.00	0.90	11.8	4.58
BW	**2.01**	0.66	**6.11**	2.00
Smart Fusion	2.40	0.60	9.80	3.08

The use of Temporal Fusion leads to a visible improvement of the results (Table 2). The RMSE values are reduced by up to 1 bpm and the RE by sometimes more than 4%. The included smoothing also reduces the standard deviation of the error values. The improvements are particularly evident in the methods AM and FM. As a result, the Smart Fusion also achieves better performance and the overall lowest RMSE of 1.59 bpm.

Table 2: Mean μ and standard deviation σ of RMSE in bpm and RE in % for BR-estimation with proposed methods using Temporal Fusion.

Algorithm	RMSE		RE	
	μ	σ	μ	σ
AM	2,11	0,47	8,88	2,62
FM	2,12	0,61	8,06	2,76
BW	1,75	0,51	**5,82**	1,16
Smart Fusion	**1,59**	0,43	6,29	1,85

The results of the top-five reference algorithms are displayed in Table 3. Each algorithm consists of a method for three steps of estimating the BR: (1) Extraction of respiratory features, (2) BR estimation, and (3) Fusion of BR estimates. The toolbox implements other methods for the extraction of the baseline shift. BW1 computes the mean amplitude of Q-waves and proceeding R-peaks, and BW2 the mean signal value between consecutive Q-waves. BRs are estimated for 32.87% of all available windows. The remaining are discarded due to low quality.
Overall, good results were achieved with RMSE values below 2 bpm and RE below 7%. All of the top-five methods use peak detection (PD) for breath detection. Again, the use of fusion methods improves the results visibly. The lowest RMSE is achieved when using Smart Fusion, which merges the methods AM, FM, and BW2 by averaging. This leads to lower error measures compared to the individual estimates. All of the five best algorithms use Temporal Fusion for smoothing the BRs.

Table 3: Mean μ of RMSE in bpm and RE in % for BR-estimation with reference algorithms, top-5 sorted after μ.

Algorithm			RMSE	RE
Features	BR est.	Fusion	μ	μ
AM, FM, BW2	PD	Temporal, Smart F.	**1.69**	6.54
BW1	PD	Temporal	1.72	**6.42**
BW2	PD	Temporal	1.85	7.24
FM	PD	Temporal	1.94	7.57
AM	PD	Temporal	1.95	7.97

Overall, good results were achieved with both the implemented algorithm and reference algorithms. The lowest RE was achieved by the implemented BW method. The use of Temporal Fusion improves the results visibly. The use of Smart Fusion from AM, FM and BW leads in this case to the lowest RMSE of all tested algorithms. Without Temporal Fusion, however, no improvement can be observed with Smart Fusion because of worse AM and FM estimates.

3.4 Discussion

One advantage of Temporal Fusion is the ability to be performed online, because subsequent values are not included in the calculation. It is assumed that the BR is not subject to strong fluctuations within a short period of time. Single incorrect values have a smaller effect. However, this could also make it more difficult to detect abrupt changes or spontaneous breathing stops.

The implementation of the AM and FM methods from the RRest-toolbox achieved better results than from the proposed algorithm. The extraction of respiratory signals is based on the same principles. Therefore, the adaptation of the pre- and post-processing could be investigated for further improvement. This includes the use of other filter parameters or methods.

For the estimation of the BR good results could be achieved with a simple peak detection. To correct erroneous peaks other methods with thresholding can be used. However, due to strong amplitude fluctuations in the modulation signals, these have so far led to a less accurate detection. Possibly an adaptation of the used thresholds to the use of capacitive data may result in an improvement.

For the results of the reference algorithms, only about one third of the available recording time was used. The rest was discarded due to low quality. Thus, a trade-off between correct estimates of BR and estimation for as many sections as possible is evident.

The results are subject to some limitations. The available dataset comprises only one subject and is therefore very small. For more meaningful results an evaluation with different test persons is necessary. The characteristics of the modulations differ e.g. in age [11] and the sleep position.

The extraction of AM and FM depends on correct QRS detection. Incorrect positions include incorrect amplitude and time intervals, which affects the respiratory signals. The filter-based BW method, however, is independent of this. For a comparable evaluation of the methods the correctness would have to be ensured.

Some available algorithms were not included in the reference algorithms or could not be executed. Another possible method to extract the respiratory signals is based on the slope of the QRS complex and the angle of the R-peak [12]. This has shown good results in a recently published comparative study [2].

Future work may also include other methods to increase the robustness of BR estimation. In this work, one ECG lead was selected for estimating the BR. A combination of different leads is possible by e.g. correction of outliers [3].

4 Conclusion

In this work, an algorithm for the estimation of the BR from ECG signals was presented and evaluated. It was shown that it is possible to estimate the BR using capacitive ECG electrodes during sleep without large deviations. This can already be achieved with relatively simple methods such as the extraction of the baseline with a moving-average filter and temporal fusion. Further work is required to evaluate EDR-algorithms on a diverse dataset.

Acknowledgement

The work has been carried out at Capical GmbH, Braunschweig and supervised by the Institute of Medical Informatics, Universität zu Lübeck.

Author's Statement

Authors state no conflict of interest.

References

[1] P. Bonato, "Wearable sensors and systems," *IEEE Eng. Med. Biol. Mag.*, vol. 29, no. 3, pp. 25–36, 2010.

[2] C. Varon *et al.*, "A comparative study of ECG-derived respiration in ambulatory monitoring using the single-lead ECG," *Sci. Rep.*, vol. 10, no. 5704, 2020.

[3] R. Bailón, L. Sörnmo, and P. Laguna, "A robust method for ECG-based estimation of the respiratory frequency during stress testing," *IEEE Trans. Biomed. Eng.*, vol. 53, no. 7, pp. 1273–1285, 2006.

[4] P. H. Charlton *et al.*, "Breathing rate estimation from the electrocardiogram and photoplethysmogram: A review," *IEEE Rev. Biomed. Eng.*, vol. 11, 2018.

[5] J. Lazaro *et al.*, "Electrocardiogram derived respiratory rate using a wearable armband," *IEEE Trans. Biomed. Eng.*, pp. 1–1, 2020.

[6] M. Oehler, M. Schilling, and H. D. Esperer, "Capacitive ECG system with direct access to standard leads and body surface potential mapping," *Biomed. Eng.*, vol. 54, no. 6, pp. 329–335, 2009.

[7] P. H. Charlton *et al.*, "An assessment of algorithms to estimate respiratory rate from the electrocardiogram and photoplethysmogram," *Physiol. Meas.*, vol. 37, no. 4, pp. 610–626, 2016.

[8] J. Pan and W. J. Tompkins, "A real-time QRS detection algorithm," *IEEE Trans. Biomed. Eng.*, vol. BME-32, no. 3, pp. 230–236, 1985.

[9] J. Lázaro, E. Gil, R. Bailón, A. Mincholé, and P. Laguna, "Deriving respiration from photoplethysmographic pulse width," *Med. Biol. Eng. Comput.*, vol. 51, no. 1-2, pp. 233–242, 2013.

[10] W. Karlen, S. Raman, J. M. Ansermino, and G. A. Dumont, "Multiparameter respiratory rate estimation from the photoplethysmogram," *IEEE Trans. Biomed. Eng.*, vol. 60, no. 7, pp. 1946–1953, 2013.

[11] P. H. Charlton *et al.*, "Extraction of respiratory signals from the electrocardiogram and photoplethysmogram: Technical and physiological determinants," *Physiol. Meas.*, vol. 38, no. 5, pp. 669–690, 2017.

[12] J. Lázaro *et al.*, "Electrocardiogram derived respiratory rate from QRS slopes and R-wave angle," *Ann. Biomed. Eng.*, vol. 42, no. 10, pp. 2072–2083, 2014.

Development of Breath Phase Detection Algorithms for the Performance Measurement of an Emergency Ventilator

Annika Multusch [1] and Anke Ihnken[2]

[1] Medical Engineering Science, Universität zu Lübeck, annika.multusch@student.uni-luebeck.de
[2] Weinmann Emergency Medical Technology GmbH + Co. KG, Hamburg, A.Ihnken@weinmann-emt.de

Abstract

Breathing phase detection is an important part of the performance measurement of a ventilator, which is helpful to improve the effectiveness of the development process of ventilators. To measure the performance of an emergency ventilator, Weinmann Emergency Medical Technology GmbH + Co. KG developed a live-data-analysis in which several parameters are determined from the airway pressure and flow provided by the ventilator and compared to target values. Since many of these parameters are time-dependent and should be determined at the beginning or end of inspiration or expiration, a reliable detection of respiratory phases is required. In this work, three algorithms for breathing phase detection were introduced and compared for three groups of patients. Results have shown, that using a combination of the inspiratory flow and airway pressure cause reliable phase-detection that can be used in performance measurement.

1 Introduction

Reliable and exact detection of respiratory phases is the basis to measure the ventilation performance of a ventilator. The performance measurement is a useful tool to check how well the control of the ventilator works, or how successfully a patient would be ventilated. By integrating this into the rapid control prototyping process, device development can be made more efficient and the control of the ventilator can be improved, resulting in better patient ventilation.

To evaluate the performance of a ventilator, several parameters like the inspiratory pressure, the PEEP (positive end expiratory pressure) or inspiratory volume are determined from the airway pressure and flow that are generated by the ventilator and compared to target values. Since most of these parameters are time-dependent and should be determined at the beginning or end of inspiration or expiration, a reliable detection of breathing phases is required.

One main requirement is to use as less device-internal information as possible, as the aim is to measure what ventilation output actually arrives at the patient. Therefore, an external phase detection is preferred. As an additional advantage, due to its device-independence, the performance measurement can be used for other devices in the future.

Different algorithms to determine the phases of breathing for various applications have been attempted during the last years. Some works use classic zero-crossing or threshold methods [4], [5]. The idea is to recognize the zero crossings of the respiratory flow as it marks the beginning of inspiration as well as expiration. To avoid false detection due to noisy data, the beginning of the respiratory phase can be verified by an additional threshold criterion. Nguyen et al. [3] introduced a method to avoid the typical problems of a zero-crossing algorithm. In order to be unaffected by flow-offsets, not the zero-crossings but inflection points of flow data and epiglottic pressure data are determined.

A similarity of these algorithms is that they are all based on flow curves. The device considered in this paper for the investigation is a pressure-controlled ventilator without an expiratory flow sensor. The data available for phase detection from that device are an inspiratory – only positive – flow and the measured airway pressure.

The main goal of this work was to find an algorithm that can detect inspiration and expiration of different ventilated passive patients in real-time and as accurately as possible without knowing the expiratory flow. This work focuses on the development of the phase detection using model-based simulation with the aim of integrating it into rapid control prototyping in the future.

2 Material and Methods

In this section, the development of the phase detection algorithms is described. The test setup is completely software-based and was implemented and simulated in MATLAB/ Simulink 2019b. A computer simulation of the considered ventilator generates the simulated measured output of airway pressure and inspiratory flow from the ventilator. This simulation consists of the Simulink model of the ventilator, which is identical to the unit's software that controls the ventilation and a simulation model of a patient's lung. The pressure and flow values are used as input data to the performance measurement and thus also for the detection of breathing phases. The emergency ventilator and performance measurement as well as phase detection are examined in more detail below.

2.1 MEDUVENT Standard

The MEDUVENT Standard (Weinmann Emergency Medical Technology GmbH + Co. KG) is a portable emergency ventilator that is capable of invasive and non-invasive ventilation of infants, children and adults [6]. The ventilator provides different ventilation modes. Since the device does not have an expiratory flow sensor, the modes are generated in a pressure-controlled manner. Actual volume-controlled modes can also be generated despite the absence of a continuous flow signal by using pressure regulated volume control (PRVC). The preset tidal volume is delivered with the lowest possible ventilation pressure.

2.2 Performance Measurement

The performance measurement is based on a live data analysis to test whether the ventilator can provide sufficient ventilation for each patient group and ventilation mode. The main structure was taken from [1] and adjusted for the MEDUVENT Standard. The live-data analysis is implemented in MATLAB/ Simulink 2019b. The preprocessing shall be focused in this work. Based on the input data, which are the sensor data from airway pressure and flow provided by the ventilator as well as ventilator settings and patient specific parameters, the phases of breathing are determined.

2.3 Data for the Breath Detection

In this work, three different simulated data sets were used that are representative for the three patient groups adult, child and infant. Table 1 provides representative values of patient-specific parameters like airway resistance (R) and compliance (C). Additionally, it lists ventilation settings for each patient: target values for the respiratory rate (RR), the tidal volume (V_T), the positive endexpiratory pressure (PEEP) and the oxygen flow (O_2 flow).

Table 1: Parameter setting for ventilation simulation of three different patient groups.

	Adult	Child	Infant	
RR	10	20	30	[1/min]
V_T	500	100	100	[mL]
PEEP	5	10	10	[hPa]
R	5	20	50	[hPa/L/s]
C	60	20	10	[mL/hPa]
O_2 flow	3	4	4	[L/min]

Based on the settings given in Table 1 and the Simulink simulation of the MEDUVENT Standard, three data sets were created. In all cases the PRVC mode is chosen. The airway pressure and inspiratory flow for those patients provided by the ventilators simulation are shown in Fig. 1.

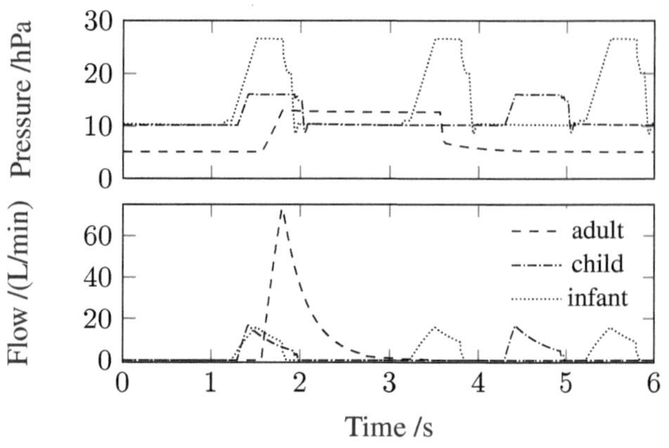

Figure 1: Data sets for three different groups of patients created with the computer simulation of the MEDUVENT Standard ventilator.

To determine the desired detection times for the onset of inspiration and expiration, an assessment by a respiratory expert was performed.

2.4 Breath Phase Detection

All three breath-phase-detection-algorithms presented here share the same basic framework shown in Fig. 2. Besides inspiration and expiration, two phases (possible inspiration and possible expiration) are added to use as a temporary storage for the time of phase transition. The start of inspiration is set retroactively to the start of possible inspiration, when the algorithm goes to the state of inspiration. The transition into expiration works analogously.
The three algorithms, which will be compared in this work, differ in the used criterion (flow or pressure) as well as in the conditions and threshold values that are used to transit between the phases.

2.4.1 Flow based Detection (FBD)

The flow curve for PRVC ventilation provides information about the phases of breathing. The inspiration begins with a strong increase in respiratory flow. After reaching its maximum, the flow decreases exponentially and expiration starts with a strong increase of negative flow [2]. To circumvent that the considered device provides no expiratory flow signal, the zero-crossing is extended by zero-detection and thresholds are adjusted for flow-based detection (FBD), which can be seen in Fig. 2. A positive flow is the criterion for a possible inspiration, while a flow less than or equal to 0 is the indication of a possible expiration. To confirm the respiratory phases, the flow must either exceed a threshold (inspiration) or remain less than or equal to zero (expiration).

2.4.2 Pressure based Detection (PBD)

Unlike the flow signal, the airway pressure curve provides information of both respiratory phases. In PRVC ventilation, starting from the PEEP with the onset of inspiration,

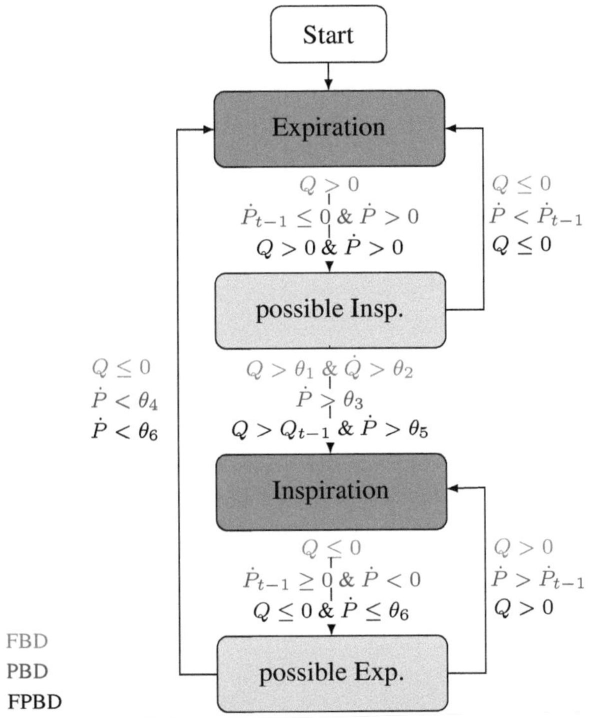

Figure 2: Flowchart of breath phases and possible phase transitions of the three algorithms. The conditions for phase transitions are marked with different colors (flow based detection (FBD) red, pressure based detection (PBD) blue and flow and pressure based detection (FPBD) black), to differ between the algorithms. Q is the flow, $\dot{Q}$ and $\dot{P}$ are the first derivative of flow and pressure provided by the ventilator. θ_i $(i = 1, 2, 3, 4, 5, 6)$ are threshold values, the flow or pressure must exceed for a new phase to be registered.

the airway pressure increases rapidly at first, then more slowly, until it reaches the inspiratory pressure. With the onset of expiration, the pressure decreases fastly back to the PEEP [2]. The pressure-based detection (PBD) algorithm, that is described in Fig. 2, is based on this behavior. It is a combination of the zero-crossing algorithm and threshold criteria using the first derivative of airway pressure instead of flow. A rising or falling zero-crossing of the pressure gradient is the criterion for the transition from expiration to possible inspiration respectively from inspiration to possible expiration. Only when the pressure gradient exceeds or falls below a threshold value the inspiration or expiration is confirmed.

2.4.3 Flow and Pressure based Detection (FPBD)

The flow- and pressure-based detection (FPBD) algorithm is a combination of the previous ones. It uses the physiological information of both, the airway pressure and inspiratory flow and is shown in Fig. 2. For example, to detect the transition from expiration to a possible inspiration both the flow and the pressure gradient have to exceed zero. Only when the pressure gradient exceeds a threshold value and the flow gradient continues to be positive, the inspiration can be confirmed.

3 Results and Discussion

All three detection algorithms were incorporated into the performance measurement and applied in real time for all three patient groups. The deviation in time between the desired onsets of inspiration and expiration and the measured ones were determined and averaged over 60 seconds for the adults and the children and over 30 seconds for the infants. Despite the same simulation, not identical breaths are generated because the controller needs a few breaths to settle. This makes it necessary to average the measured deviation. Each method was able to detect all breaths for all patients apart from one exception. The PBD algorithm missed one onset of inspiration with the child-data. This breath was left out of the calculation of the mean. The results for the detection of the onset of inspiration are shown in Table 2.

Table 2: Results of the three detection algorithms as averaged values of the deviations from the true onset (chosen by an expert) of inspiration for the individual patient groups and as the mean squared error (MSE) of all patients for the respective detection algorithms. Negative deviations mean that detection was too early.

	FBD	PBD	FPBD	
Adult	-1.30	-1.30	-1.30	[ms]
Child	-2.13	-2.00	-2.00	[ms]
Infant	0.22	-95.68	0.22	[ms]
MSE	2.10	3053.3	1.90	[ms^2]

Results of detecting the onset of expiration are given in Table 3. Both tables present the averaged time deviations for all patient groups and all algorithms. Additionally, the mean squared error (MSE) over all patients was determined for each detection method and reported as well.

Table 3: Results of the three detection algorithms as averaged values of the deviations from the true onset (chosen by an expert) of expiration for the individual patient groups and as the mean squared error (MSE) of all patients for the respective detection algorithms. Negative deviations mean that detection was too early.

	FBD	PBD	FPBD	
Adult	-34.27	-1.46	-5.21	[ms]
Child	-2.10	-38.71	24.66	[ms]
Infant	2.05	35.80	6.33	[ms]
MSE	394.26	927.24	225.12	[ms^2]

It is clear that there is not a single method that provides the best results for every patient. There are also differences between inspiration and expiration. While the FBD algorithm produces the best results for detecting the onset of expiration in child- and infant data, it is the method with the largest deviation in adult data. Figure 3 pictures the mean of the detected expiration with all methods on child data set. With PBD the detection accuracy for the adult and the child data set is similar to the other algorithms, while detection

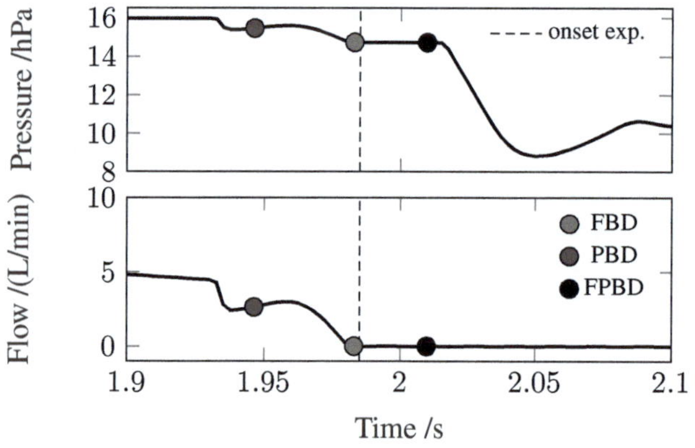

Figure 3: Illustration of the section of a breath from the child data set in which the onset of expiration is located. The dotted line shows the 'true' onset of expiration. The averaged detected time points of all detection algorithms are presented as well.

with this method for the infant data set yields the worst result. It can be seen in Fig. 4. Due to the independence from the flow, the PBD based algorithm detects the onset of inspiration early with increasing pressure.

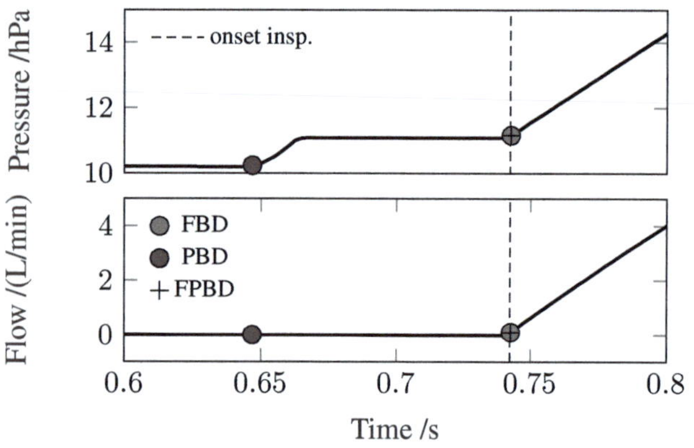

Figure 4: Illustration of the section of a breath from the infant data set in which the onset of inspiration is located. The dotted line shows the 'true' onset of inspiration. The averaged detected time points of all detection algorithms are presented as well.

Although for individual patients the FBD or PBD algorithms achieve more accurate results than the other, the results show that a combination of the advantages of both methods with the FPBD algorithm produces the best results across all patients. Mean squared error across all patient groups is lowest with the FPBD method for both inspiration and expiration.

4 Conclusion

Three algorithms for the detection of breathing phases for the application in performance measurement are introduced. After evaluating the results, we conclude that neither inspiratory flow nor airway pressure is sufficient as a sole criterion to determine respiratory phases sufficiently. Rather a combination of both criteria, as in the FPBD method, is needed to reliably use phase detection in performance measurement. Future studies should include the testing of the algorithms in rapid control prototyping. In addition, the FPBD method can be tested and adjust in order to detect phases of breathing of patients with spontaneous breathing as well.

Acknowledgement

The work has been carried out at Weinmann Emergency Medical Technology GmbH + Co. KG, Hamburg and supervised by Prof. Philipp Rostalski, Institute for Electrical Engineering in Medicine, Universität zu Lübeck.

Author's Statement

Authors state no conflict of interest.

5 References

[1] A. Riebesel, *Design and development of a real-time data analysis to evaluate the performance of emergency ventilators.* (Konzeption und Entwicklung einer Livedatenanalyse zur Bewertung der Performance eines Notfallbeatmungsgeräts. – Masterthesis, Luebeck University of Applied Sciences and Weinmann Emergency Medical Technology GmbH + Co. KG), 2017.

[2] W. Oczenski, H. Andel, A. Werba, *Atmen - Atemhilfen: Atemphysiologie und Beatmungstechnik.* Georg Thieme Verlag, Stuttgart, vol. 7, 2006.

[3] C. D. Nguyen, J. Amatoury, J. C. Carberry, D. J. Eckert, *An automated and reliable method for breath detection during variable mask pressures in awake and sleeping humans.* PLOS ONE, vol. 12, pp. 1–21, 2017.

[4] J. H. T. Bates, G. Schmalisch, D. Filbrun, J. Stocks, *Tidal breath analysis for infant pulmonary function testing.* European Respiratory Journal, vol. 16, pp. 1180-1192, 2000.

[5] D. Khodadad, S. Nordebo, B. Müller, A. Waldmann, R. Yerworth, T. Becher et al., *Optimized breath detection algorithm in electrical impedance tomography.* bioRxiv, pp. 1–15, 2018.

[6] Weinmann Emergency Medical Technology GmbH + Co. KG, *MEDUVENT Standard Beatmungsgerät - Gebrauchsanweisung für Geräte ab Softwareversion 2.1.* Weinmann Emergency Medical Technology GmbH + Co. KG, Hamburg, 2020.

Creating an envelope of an oscillometric signal for the evaluation of blood pressure

Claudius Böhnke [1]
[1] Medical Engineering Science, Universität zu Lübeck, claudius.boehnke@student.uni-luebeck.de

Abstract

The measurement of blood pressure is an important for part the optimal treatment of providing a patient. Fast, effective and patient-friendly performance is facilitated by automated procedures. In order to obtain an accurate blood pressure result, the peaks of the oscillometric signal are analyzed and evaluated to form an envelope curve. Based on this envelope curve, the blood pressure can be calculated. The focus of my work was to develop a general method for creating such envelopes. Therefore, the oscillometric signals were recorded on a healthy person using a laboratory setup. The peak detection and, based on the result, the calculation of the envelope was conducted using the program R. A generally valid method for generating an envelope of an oscillometric signal could be developed. This method is a proof-of-concept and needs further evaluation.

1 Introduction

1.1 Blood pressure

Blood pressure is one of the most frequently recorded vital signs [5], [6]. It is indispensable in perioperative, intensive care and emergency medicine. The heart pumps an average of 60 to 90 times per minute in healthy adults [7]. The force that dilates the elastic arterial blood vessels is induced by blood pressure. It results from the cardiac output, which is distributed throughout the arterial vascular tree. Blood pressure is characterized by systolic blood pressure (SYS) and diastolic blood pressure (DIA). SYS is the maximum pressure within the vessels during systole of the heart whereas DIA is the minimum blood pressure during diastole of the heart [2], [3]. A third specification is the mean arterial blood pressure (MAP). It describes the magnitude of blood pressure as a driving force within the systemic circulation [5]. The typical unit of measurement for blood pressure is millimeters of mercury (mmHg) [4]. In healthy adults, blood pressure is 120/80 mmHg [5].

1.2 Blood pressure measurement

1.2.1 Blood pressure measurement methods

Blood pressure measurement is divided into invasive and non-invasive methods [4]. The most accurate method is invasive blood pressure measurement with an arterial catheter. It is neither a quick option nor comfortable for the patient and is used when permanently accurate results are required [5]. More convenient options are offered by the non-invasive intermittent methods [5]. They are divided into automated and manual methods. Manual methods include palpation and auscultation. In both, an inflatable cuff is used to compress and then decompress the arteries. Palpation involves the pulse and determining the SYS [4], [5]. On auscultation, Korotkoff sounds of the brachial artery are observed and SYS and DIA can be determined [4], [5].

1.2.2 Oscillometric blood pressure measurement

Oscillometric blood pressure measurement is the most commonly used automatic measurement principle [1]. The maximum amplitude of the oscillation of the cuff pressure occurs at a pressure level of MAP [2], [3], [6]. The oscillogram, which represents the amplitude of blood volume oscillation as a function of external pressure, is measured and the blood pressure is evaluated by an empirical algorithm [1], [5]. Blood flow is stopped by automatically inflating a cuff above the SYS. Subsequently, the pressure is continuously lowered (2-3 mmHg per pulse beat) via a valve to below the DIA. There is restricted blood flow between the SYS and the DIA, resulting in periodic expansion and contraction of the brachial artery and thus pulse-synchronous oscillation. An integrated pressure sensor measures the pressure oscillation as an electrical signal. The oscillation starts with very small amplitudes, reaches its maximum at MAP and flattens out [5], [6].

1.3 Oscillation envelope

The algorithms for evaluation of blood pressure require an envelope of the oscillometric signal [1], [3], [4]. One method is called "peak-to-peak". The distance between the maximum and minimum of a peak is measured for each peak. Then these are connected to form an envelope [4], [5]. The "peak-to-base" method works similarly. However, the distance from the maximum of each peak to a selected base is measured and then connected to form an envelope [4]. Once the envelope is determined, an algorithm can evaluate these and calculate results for MAP, SYS, and DIA. One algorithm is the Maximum Amplitude Algorithm (MAA) which determines the maximum amplitude of the envelope as MAP. This is then multiplied by an empirically determined fraction each and SYS and DIA are obtained [1], [4]. The maxima of the slope of the envelope are used in the Derivative Algorithm (DA). For this purpose, the envelope curve is derived and the obtained zero crossings give SYS and DIA. These can be used to calculate the MAP [1], [4]. In the Linear Approximation Algorithm (LAA), the ascending and descending branches of the envelope curve are each represented by an auxiliary line (approximation). These form an intersection point, which is evaluated as MAP. Subsequently, the procedure is the same as for the MAA [1], [4].

2 Material and Methods

2.1 Laboratory setup

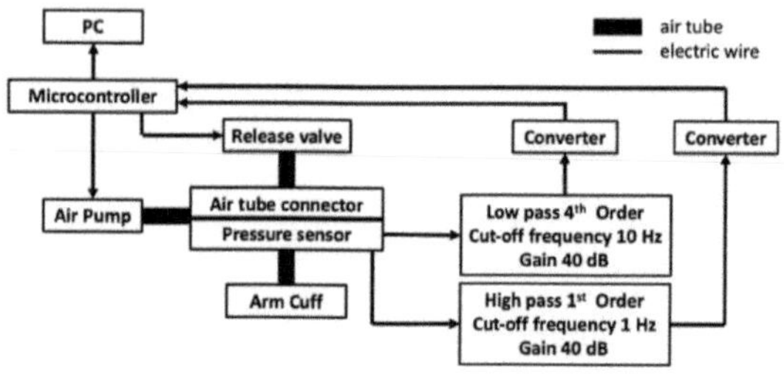

Figure 1: Schematic block diagram of the laboratory setup with electrical connections (thin lines) and pneumatic (air) tubes (thick lines). The transducers are replaced by an oscilloscope.

The block diagram of the setup for evaluation of the oscillometric signal is shown in Fig. 1. The first order high-pass filter is used to obtain the oscillometric signal of the cuff pressure (OSCI). The signal for the static cuff pressure (CP) is obtained through the 4th order low pass filter. The automatic pump enables uniform inflation and deflation of the cuff.

2.2 Oscilloscope

An oscilloscope MDO4104-3 (Tektronix GmbH, Germany, Köln) is connected at the output of both analogue filters and has the possibility to export the acquired data in a comma-separated values file.

2.3 Recording the vital data

The laboratory setup was tested under real conditions and measurements were performed on a test subject (male, 25 years old, no pre-existing conditions present or medication being taken). During the measurement, he sat quietly and did not speak. The inflatable cuff was applied correctly (heart level, 2-3 cm above the crook of the arm, appropriate cuff size with light pressure on the skin) around the upper arm.

2.4 Evaluation of measurement data

Preprocessing of the recorded measurement data was performed with R (version: 1.3.1093; RStudio, PBC). Additional R packages (pracma, 2.2.9; zoo, 1.8 – 8; rPackages) were utilized. These packages are necessary to enable the peak detection.

3 Results and Discussion

3.1 Raw data of the oscilloscope

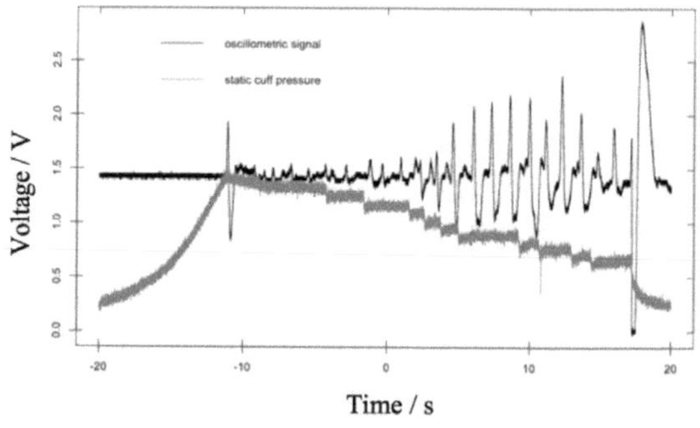

Figure 2: Unfiltered signal for the CP (gray) and OSCI (black) in V versus s.

The oscilloscope recorded data with a data rate of 2.5 kHz. This high temporal resolution with relatively low signal resolution (voltage) results in neighboring values of the same size. The signal can be seen in Fig. 2. In this unfiltered form, peak detection becomes difficult.

3.2 Reduce data rate and filter to a continuous signal

The data rate was reduced by a defined factor. For this purpose, a function was used that determines the bandwidth via the parameter size of the range for the block averaging. Fig. 3a shows the result for any time interval before and after applying the function. The circles represent the individual signal values. The solid line represents the low pass filtered signal. In Fig. 3b, the processed signal is plotted over the entire time interval (for OSZI and CP). The function used summarizes a selected window by an approximation. The process is similar to a high order filter. The window is superimposed over the points of the whole signal and a filtered curve is obtained.

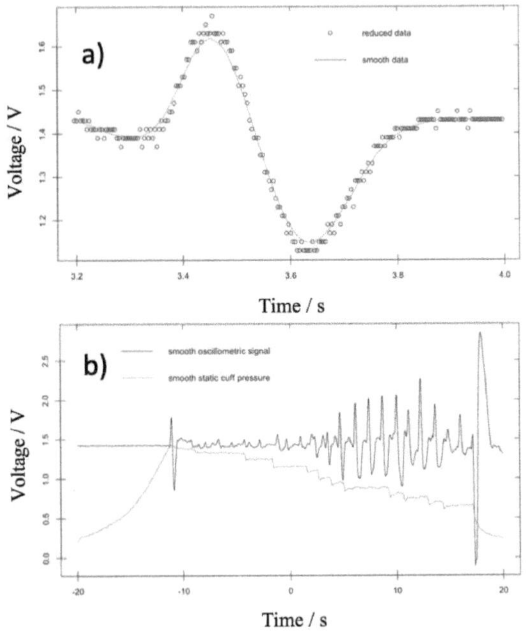

Figure 3: In a) the reduced data of the OSCI are shown as circles. The result filtered using the block averaging function (line) is plotted over a small-time interval. Over the entire time interval and using an approximation, the result for OSCI and CP is shown in b). Both variants give a smooth signal.

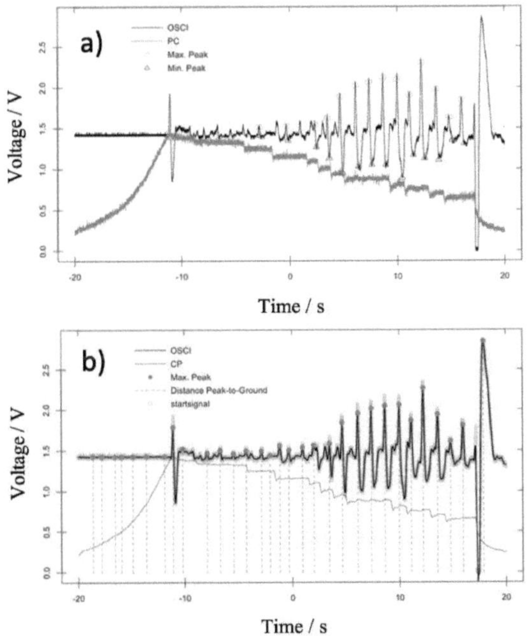

Figure 4: In a) the OSCI and PC traces are shown. The OSCI is marked with circles for the maximum peaks and triangles for the minimum peaks. It can be seen that not all peaks are detected. In b) OSCI and CP are also shown. The circles symbolize the detected peaks. It appears that all peaks are detected. The dashed lines are the peak-to-base distance. The amplitudes of the original signal can be seen by light gray circles.

3.3 Peak Detection

Two different algorithms were evaluated for the peak detection procedure. In Fig. 4a, the peaks are detected by a function that relies on regular patterns to determine. To do this, the entire signal is monitored from start to finish. As soon as a given number of ascending (maximum) or descending (minimum) values are measured, a peak can be detected. The circles represent the maxima and the triangles the minima. Fig. 4b shows the result of an alternative function, which uses an adjustable wide window as well as a ratio of this window to the whole x-axis (in the optimal case a pulse length is set). In this adjusted window all contained points are compared. The highest point is detected as local maximum and is considered as plateau for each point within this window. Both options detect maxima that are real maxima. However, in a) maxima are omitted and in b) maxima are detected which are not of interest (e.g., the first 15 s).

3.3.1 Comparison of peak detection

Table 1: Comparison of peak detection for different Measurements with the number of target peaks

Measurment	Plateau	Patterns	Target
1	29	18	20
2	29	20	21
3	30	14	21
4	28	15	18
5	29	16	17

It can be seen that the method with plateaus detects more peaks overall than the method with regular patterns. However, both do not detect the correct number of target peaks (plateau too many and pattern too few). Overall, it can be seen that the method with plateaus detects all the peaks of the entire signal. Also, the not necessary peaks before the beginning and after the end of the oscillometric signal are detected. The method with regular pattern check, avoids peaks before the beginning and after the end of the oscillometric signal but does not detect all peaks of the signal.

3.4 Envelope Creation

Fig. 5 shows the calculated envelope using the implemented peak-to-peak variant from 1.3. The differences of the detected maxima and minima are calculated. The result is plotted on a graph and the successive points are connected to each other. An envelope of an oscillometric signal is created. It rises to a maximum and then falls. The exception is a clearly visible drop of the envelope curve shortly after the maximum. In Fig. 4a it can already be seen that the oscillometric signal has two peaks behind the avoidable maximum, the first of which lies below and the second above this maximum. The differences to the maximum are accordingly fluctuating. This is the reason for the drop of the envelope curve in Fig. 5.

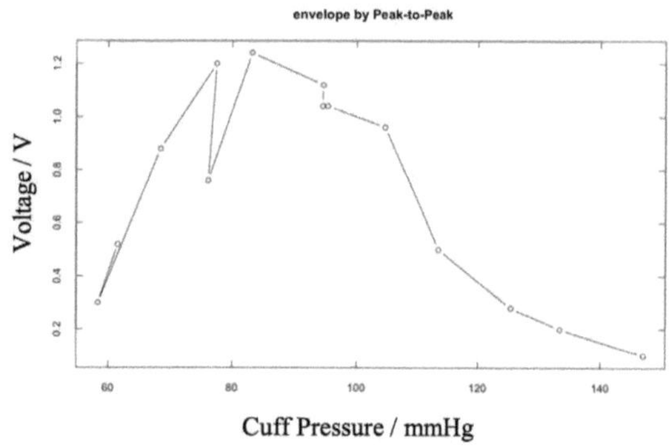

Figure 5: Envelope curve according to the peak-to-peak method. The circles are the obtained values that form the envelope curve. The result shows a clear dip shortly after the supposed maximum. An envelope curve according to the peak-to-base method is ongoing and will be provided later.

3.5 Discussion

The evaluation of the results shows that the detection of the peaks works, and an envelope curve can be generated. The selectivity can be further improved, because in Fig. 4a not all peaks are detected. Fig. 4b shows too many peaks are detected and in particular those before the beginning and after the end of the oscillometric signal. Nevertheless, peaks can be evaluated with both methods. For the peak-to-peak variant, an envelope could be obtained for different oscillometric signals. The dips of the envelope can be explained by the uneven differences of the peak-to-peak. Because of these dips, these envelopes cannot yet be used to evaluate blood pressure by a subsequent algorithm from 1.3. For a direct comparison of the envelopes from peak-to-peak and peak-to-base further evaluation is required. Another problem arises from the reduction of the data rate. In Fig. 3b an approximation is used. The amplitudes of the signal are reduced to an extent that cannot be estimated, which can be seen in Fig. 4b. If the evaluation of these envelopes is used later to infer the blood pressure, errors may result.

4 Conclusion

It could be shown that the laboratory setup records signals for the evaluation of the blood pressure under real conditions. These signals are used to determine the oscillation of blood pressure and static cuff pressure. The oscillometric signal could be evaluated using functions implemented in R. The necessary detection of the peaks for the subsequent creation of an envelope curve worked. However, the resulting envelopes had errors that would make evaluation by an evaluation algorithm from 1.3 difficult. Detection and envelope determination must be improved before further evaluation procedures are possible. It may be necessary to fit the envelopes (e.g., by interpolation) in addition to the general improvement of the detection of the peaks in order to obtain a curve that can be evaluated better. The signal of the oscilloscope can be filtered before reducing the data rate. This can prevent a reduction or distortion of the actual amplitudes. Instead of an oscilloscope, an analogue-to-digital converter can be used. This can better resolve the signal and thus a lower noise output signal can be obtained. The result can be a simpler and better peak detection. The calculation of the envelope curve can also be improved and simplified as a result. The data that is converted from volts to pressure with the envelope and output must be checked for accuracy. In conclusion an arbitrary oscillometric signal could evaluated with this series of measurements. Envelopes based on different peak evaluation methods could be obtained.

Acknowledgement

The work has been carried out at seca GmbH and Co. KG., Hamburg Wandsbek and supervised by Prof. Dr. Philipp Rostalski, Institute for Electrical Engineering in Medicine, Universität zu Lübeck.

Author's Statement

Conflict of interest: Authors state no conflict of interest

5 References

[1] A. Chandraskehar, Y. Mohammad, S. Jin-Oh Hahn, H. Chen-Huan Chen and M. Ramakrishna, *Formulas to Explain Popular Oscillometric Blood Pressure Estimation Algorithms.* Frontiers in Physiology 10, 2019.

[2] P. Csordás, *An improved oscillometric method.* Proc. 14th BME-MIT PhD Mini-Symp.(Budapest, Hungary), pp. 12-5, 2007.

[3] J. Liu, J. O. Hahn and R. Mukkamala, *Error mechanisms of the oscillometric fixed-ratio blood pressure measurement method.* Annals of biomedical engineering 41, no. 3, 2013.

[4] L. Fraccaroli, *Kriterien einer hydraulisch gekoppelten Gewebedruckkurve am Oberarm zur Ermittlung des systolischen Blutdrucks.* PhD diss., lmu, 2018.

[5] P. Elter, *Methoden und Systeme zur nichtinvasiven, kontinuierlichen und belastungsfreien Blutdruckmessung.* Vol. 1013872142. KIT-Bibliothek, 2001.

[6] G. A. van Montfrans, *Oscillometric blood pressure measurement: progress and problems.* Blood pressure monitoring, 6. Jg., Nr. 6, S. 287-290, 2001.

[7] K. Meyer-Waarden, *Einführung in die biologische und medizinische Messtechnik.* Schattauer, 1975.

Acoustic Position Tracking of a Receiver in Reverberant Environments

Svantje Voit [1], Fabrice Katzberg [2], and Alfred Mertins [2]
[1] Robotics and Autonomous Systems, Universität zu Lübeck, svantje.voit@student.uni-luebeck.de
[2] Institute for Signal Processing, Universität zu Lübeck, {f.katzberg, alfred.mertins}@uni-luebeck.de

Abstract

In acoustic applications, it is more simplex to track the position of the receiver using the existing acoustic devices rather than using additional systems, such as optical tracking sensors. In closed room scenarios, audio signals are affected by reverberation which makes this task more complex. In dynamic scenarios, the receiver changes its position continuously leading to time-varying channel characteristics. In common approaches, first the sound field in the volume of interest has to be determined. Thereby, a fast convergence for the dynamic case should be achieved. As a result, information about the position can be generated. In this paper, we present a method for position tracking of a single receiver moving along a random trajectory. For this purpose, the received signal and four excitation signals generated at known positions are used.

1 Introduction

In many cases, it is useful for acoustic applications to determine the unknown position of the receiver in the three-dimensional space. Related to this use, there are methods for source tracking using the receiver's information. Applications can be found in various fields such as teleconferencing systems, smart home, hearing aids or humanoid robots [1], [2]. The localization and tracking is thereby commonly based on the positioning information like directions-of-arrival or source-sensor distances [3].

In both tracking problems, reverberation and a dynamic setup will challenge an accurate localization. Especially in closed room scenarios, reflections from walls and other objects make this difficult, as, in addition to the direct sound, the listener receives also delayed and scaled versions of the signal. This results in the convolution of the excitation signal with the room impulse response (RIR). By reconstructing the RIR from acoustic measurements, the arrival time of the sound from the speaker to the microphone can be estimated from the direct sound peak. In a setup with four speakers at known positions and one moving microphone, four arrival times of the sound can be determined from the respective room impulse responses. From the four arrival times, the four distances between the microphone and the respective speaker are calculated and thus the position in space of the microphone is identified by three-dimensional multilateration [4].

There are several methods for the reconstruction of RIRs. Common static approaches are the use of maximum-length sequences (MLS) or perfect sequences [5]. These sequences have a ideal or nearly ideal auto-correlation function, which is a periodic sequence of Dirac impulses. If the period is at least as long as the length of the RIR, the measurement reduces to a correlation of the received signal with the sequence. RIRs can be obtained by this correlation technique with a low computational demand. In dynamic applications, with time-varying RIRs, fast convergence can be used to minimize the least-mean-square (LMS) error between the measured signal and the output of an adaptive filter with the same excitation sequence as the input signal [6]. In the case of four different excitation signals by four speakers, the measured signal results from the superposition of the convolutions of the respective excitation sequence with the corresponding RIR. Accordingly, the number of unknowns is four times the one compared to the setup with only one input signal.

In this paper, a method is proposed to determine the position of a microphone moving along a random trajectory with varying velocity in a volume of interest. For this purpose, in Section 2.1, a linear system of equations is first set up and in Section 2.2, a stochastic gradient algorithm is presented for tracking the RIRs. In Section 3, an optimization problem is designed to determine the current position for the corresponding measurement of the microphone using the speaker-to-microphone distances obtained from the RIRs. Finally, the localization accuracy is evaluated in Section 4 by testing different simulated room scenarios.

2 Dynamic Measurement Setup

A closed-room scenario with a moving microphone along a randomly chosen trajectory within a volume of interest is considered. Four sources located in the room emit simultaneously predefined signals. Besides, the position of each source is known.

2.1 Linear System Model

The first aim is to determine the four unknown room impulse responses by the dynamic measurements. The sampled RIR of length L from receiver location r on the trajectory to the source k is denoted by $h_{r,k}(n)$ and pooled in the column vector $\mathbf{h}_{r,k}$, where n is the discrete time variable. Since at each position four room impulse responses are to be determined, they are encapsulated in the vector

$$\mathbf{h}_r = [\mathbf{h}_{r,1}^{\mathrm{T}}, \mathbf{h}_{r,2}^{\mathrm{T}}, \mathbf{h}_{r,3}^{\mathrm{T}}, \mathbf{h}_{r,4}^{\mathrm{T}}]^{\mathrm{T}}.$$

Since the length of each RIR is L, $\mathbf{h}_r \in \mathbb{R}^{4L}$ holds. Similarly, the vector of the source signals

$$\mathbf{s}_r = [\mathbf{s}_{r,1}^{\mathrm{T}}, \mathbf{s}_{r,2}^{\mathrm{T}}, \mathbf{s}_{r,3}^{\mathrm{T}}, \mathbf{s}_{r,4}^{\mathrm{T}}]^{\mathrm{T}}$$

is established, where the length of an excitation signal corresponds to the length of a RIR. Assuming a linear time-invariant (LTI) system, each sample b_r recorded by the dynamic microphone at position r arises from the scalar product of the RIRs and the excitation sequences:

$$b_r = \mathbf{s}_r^{\mathrm{T}} \mathbf{h}_r. \quad (1)$$

An odd-length window of W sequential samples

$$\mathbf{b}_r^W = [b_{r-(W-1)/2}, \ldots, b_r, \ldots, b_{r+(W-1)/2}]^{\mathrm{T}}$$

is chosen. Accordingly,

$$\mathbf{h}_r^W = [\mathbf{h}_{r-(W-1)/2}^{\mathrm{T}}, \ldots, \mathbf{h}_r^{\mathrm{T}}, \ldots, \mathbf{h}_{r+(W-1)/2}^{\mathrm{T}}]^{\mathrm{T}} \quad (2)$$

results as a vector containing the sequences of unknown window RIRs with $\mathbf{h}_r^W \in \mathbb{R}^{4LW}$. Using (1) and (2), the system of linear equations

$$\mathbf{b}_r^W = \mathbf{S}_r^W \mathbf{h}_r^W \quad (3)$$

can be set up with the convolution matrix $\mathbf{S}_r^W \in \mathbb{R}^{W \times 4LW}$ of the corresponding source signals within the chosen window.

2.2 Adaptive Filter for System Identification

If the system of equations from (3) is not underdetermined, it can be solved in the least squares sense and a unique estimate for $\mathbf{h}_r^W$ is obtained. However the system is underdetermined by the factor $4L$. Nevertheless, assuming slow variations of the $4LW$ parameters, they can be tracked by using an adaptive filter concept, where a sliding window of hop size one is iteratively chosen from the dynamic samples.

In the following, we show how to reduce the number of window parameters to be tracked. By using a frequency transformation along the positional dimension r, we create Doppler shifts. Assuming that the microphone moves slowly relatively to the sampling frequency of the microphone, these Doppler shifts exclusively live at lower frequencies, i.e., no high spatial frequencies exist along the trajectory window. This structured sparseness is exploited to reduce variables.

Applying a frequency transformation $\mathbf{T}$, such as the discrete cosine transformation (DCT), and eliminating all (spatial) frequencies greater than the R-th frequency, a more compressed representation $\mathbf{c}_r^W \in \mathbb{R}^{4LR}$ with $R \ll W$ of the RIRs can be realized. Using this representation and (3), the measurement process results in

$$\mathbf{b}_r^W = \mathbf{S}_r^W \mathbf{T}^{-1} \mathbf{Z} \mathbf{c}_r^W = \tilde{\mathbf{S}}_r^W \mathbf{c}_r^W \quad (4)$$

with a zero padding matrix $\mathbf{Z} \in \mathbb{R}^{4LW \times 4LR}$.

Accordingly, the underdetermined LMS problem approximated by (4) can be stated as

$$\arg\min_{\mathbf{c}_r^W} \|\mathbf{b}_r^W - \tilde{\mathbf{S}}_r^W \mathbf{c}_r^W\|_2^2.$$

To derive the coefficients of the vector $\mathbf{c}_r^W$, an adaptive filter as shown in Fig. 1 is applied. This involves assigning the filter parameters of $\hat{\mathbf{c}}_r^W$ in such a way that the residuals

$$\mathbf{e}_r^W = \mathbf{b}_r^W - \tilde{\mathbf{S}}_r^W \hat{\mathbf{c}}_r^W$$

are minimized. For this purpose, the parameters are adapted iteratively, according to the respective regressor, by the gradient algorithm

$$\hat{\mathbf{c}}_{r(i+1)}^W = \hat{\mathbf{c}}_{r(i)}^W + \mu \tilde{\mathbf{S}}_r^{W^{\mathrm{T}}} \mathbf{e}_{r(i)}^W$$

with the step size μ and the iteration index i. The influence of the external noise on the adaptation process can be taken into account by adding white noise $\boldsymbol{\eta}$. Since the measurement is dynamic, it is useful to ensure a fast convergence of the filter to the true impulse responses. For this purpose a MLS with a period length of $L_{\mathrm{p}} \geq 4L$ is used as the excitation signals. In addition, the four signals of the individual sound sources must be delayed with respect to each other by the length of one RIR [6]. Consequently, the excitation vectors are orthogonal to each other.

Finally, the relationship

$$\hat{\mathbf{h}}_r^W \approx \mathbf{T}^{-1} \mathbf{Z} \hat{\mathbf{c}}_r^W$$

applies to obtain the estimate of the RIRs from the iteratively identified estimation.

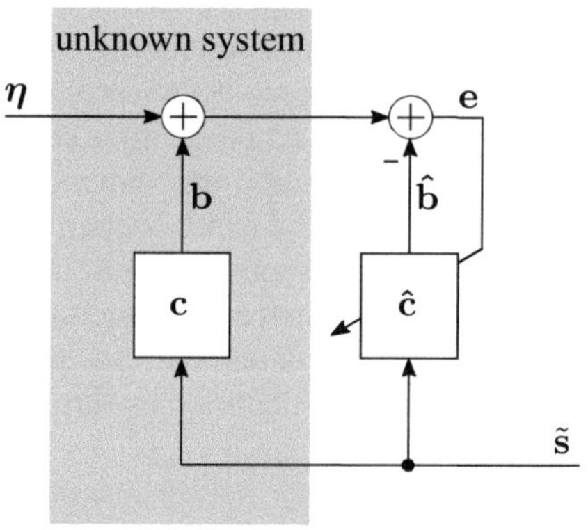

Figure 1: Block diagram of the adaptive filter for system identification.

3 Microphone Localization

For the estimation of the microphone position, the sound sources and their corresponding RIRs are considered separately. First, the distances d_k of the sound sources $k = [1, 2, 3, 4]$ to the measurement position have to be derived. This requires the estimation of the RIR, as well as the knowledge about the sound velocity c_0 and the sampling frequency f_s. From the RIR, the direct sound peak can then be identified by taking the timestep $n_{\max,k}$ from the maximum of $\hat{\mathbf{h}}_r$. The proportional relationship

$$d_k = \frac{n_{\max,k} \cdot c_0}{f_s}. \quad (5)$$

thus yields the four distances.

Knowing the distance from (5), the microphone must be located on the surface of a sphere with the radius equal to this distance. The intersection of the four spheres is the position $\mathbf{x} = [x, y, z]^{\mathrm{T}}$ of the microphone. To be able to uniquely locate the position of the microphone, it must be located within the four spherical surfaces. Moreover, the positions of the sound sources $\mathbf{x}_k = [x_k, y_k, z_k]^{\mathrm{T}}$ have to fulfill certain criteria. For example, they can not be located in one plane. If this is satisfied, the microphone position can be calculated as the solution to the optimization problem

$$\min_{\mathbf{x}} \sum_k \|\mathbf{x} - \mathbf{x}_k\|_2^2 - d_k^2. \quad (6)$$

4 Experiments and Results

For the following experiments, we simulated RIRs and microphone measurements using the image source method [7]. Three different room sizes with different reverberation times as described in Table 1 were considered.

Table 1: Characteristics of the rooms used for the simulations.

Room	x	y	z	reverberation time
(a)	5.8 m	4.9 m	3.2 m	0.125 s
(b)	5.0 m	4.0 m	6.0 m	0.400 s
(c)	3.1 m	7.3 m	4.5 m	0.320 s

The sampling frequency of the RIRs was $f_s = 8\,\text{kHz}$. The positions of the sound sources were placed randomly on a hemisphere surface with a radius of 2 m. An MLS with a period length of $L_p = 2047$ was used for excitation. Measurements were made with a moving microphone following a Lissajous trajectory [8] with an average velocity of $4.28\,\text{km/h}$. The positions listed in Table 2 were chosen as the starting position of the trajectory.

The RIRs were limited to the length $L = 511$. In total, the problem to be solved thus comprises $4LW = 1044484$ sound field variables. Using the method presented in Section 2.2, the variables were restricted to $4LR = 4088$, with $R = 2$. As evaluation criterion for the quality

Table 2: Start positions of the simulated measurement trajectory.

Starting Position	x	y	z
1	2.6 m	3.3 m	1.5 m
2	2.0 m	3.5 m	2.0 m
3	2.2 m	2.3 m	2.5 m

of the position estimation based on the sound field, the mean square error

$$\text{MSE} = \|\mathbf{x} - \hat{\mathbf{x}}\|_2^2$$

is used, where $\mathbf{x}$ contains the true position at the centered location r in each window and $\hat{\mathbf{x}}$ is the corresponding estimated position. The position determination was performed on 23000 samples along the Lissajous trajectory. A step size of $\mu = 0.01$ was chosen for the gradient descent used to iteratively determine the RIRs. For each window position, ten iterations were realized. The zero vector was chosen as the initial estimate. After each window shift, the initial estimate was used again. The external noise was continuously set to $\boldsymbol{\eta} = \mathbf{0}$.

The resulting varying MSEs of the respective rooms and starting positions are shown in Fig. 2 by the corresponding boxplots. Here, Fig. 2(a) represents the deviation with respect to room (a). The three different experiments are related to the three different starting positions of the microphone trajectory. Fig. 2(b) shows the results for the simulated room (b) and Fig. 2(c) for room (c).

Looking at the results, a correlation between the position accuracy and the room scenario is seen. Scenario (a) provides the most accurate position and scenario (b) the least accurate. An improvement can be achieved by a higher sampling frequency f_s and thus an more accurate direct sound peak determination. This can also be achieved by choosing a larger L and therefore more precise estimation of the room impulse responses. To obtain a more robust solution to (6), the number of sound sources can be increased to more than four. However, this involves additional computational cost and increases the number of parameters to be tracked by the adaptive filter.

5 Conclusion

In this paper, a method for determining the position of a receiver during a dynamic measuring process was presented. Knowing the positions of all four sound sources, their respective excitation signals and the measurements of one microphone, a linear system of equations could be established. An adaptive filter was used to solve this by using a reduced representation. From this solution, the position of the microphone could be tracked along the measurement trajectory as the solution of an optimization problem.

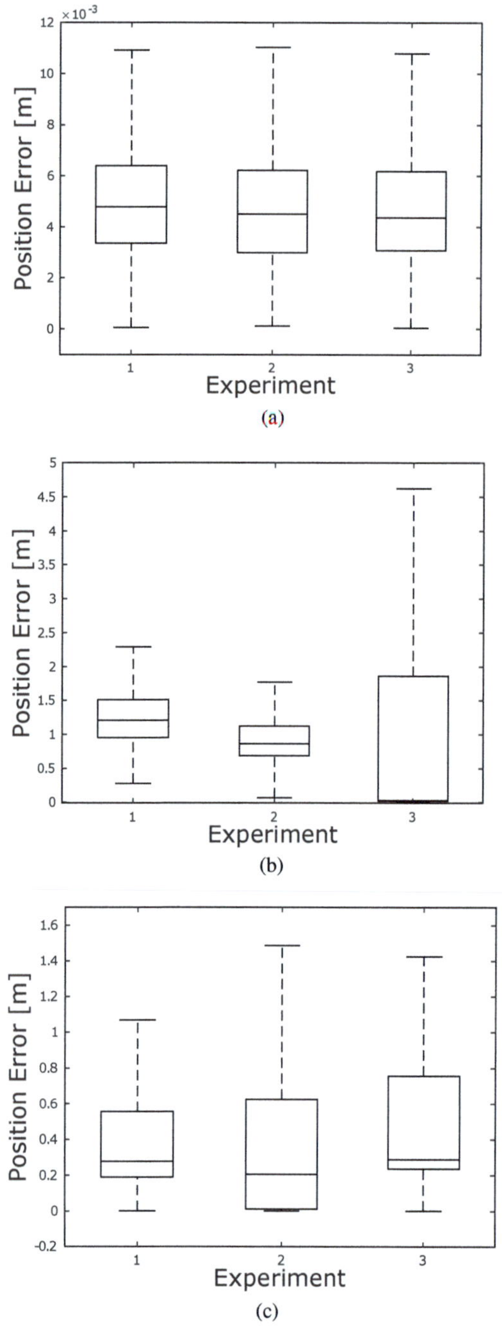

Figure 2: Boxplots of the position deviation for different simulation scenarios.

Acknowledgement

The work has been carried out and supervised by the Institute for Signal Processing, Universität zu Lübeck.

Author's Statement

Conflict of interest: Authors state no conflict of interest.

6 References

[1] V. Tourbabin and B. Rafaely, "Speaker localization by humanoid robots in reverberant environments," pp. 1–5, 2014.

[2] C. Evers and P. Naylor, "Optimized self-localization for slam in dynamic scenes using probability hypothesis density filters," *IEEE Transactions on Signal Processing*, vol. 66, no. 4, pp. 863–878, 2017.

[3] C. Evers, H. Loellmann, H. Mellmann, A. Schmidt, H. Barfuss, P. Naylor, and W. Kellermann, "The locata challenge: Acoustic source localization and tracking," *IEEE/ACM Transactions on Audio, Speech, and Language Processing*, 2020.

[4] W. Torge, *Geodäsie*. Walter de Gruyter, 2008.

[5] C. Antweiler, R. Martin, and U. Heute, "Multi-channel system identification with perfect sequences," *Advances in Digital Speech Transmission*, pp. 171–198, 2008.

[6] C. Antweiler, A. Telle, and P. Vary, "Nlms-type system identification of miso systems with shifted perfect sequences," *Proc. IWAENC*, 2008.

[7] J. Allen and D. Berkley, "Image method for efficiently simulating small-room acoustics," *The Journal of the Acoustical Society of America*, vol. 65, no. 4, pp. 943–950, 1979.

[8] M. Ahlborg, "Bildgebungskonzepte und rekonstruktionsansätze für große bildgebungsvolumen bei magnetic particle imaging," Dissertation, Institut für Medizintechnik, Universität zu Lübeck, 2015.

A Pipeline for Bioelectrical Signal Processing in Cardiac Applications

Jingyu Xie [1], Julia Sauer [2], Jan Grasshoff [2], and Philipp Rostalski [2]

[1] Medical Engineering Science, Universität zu Lübeck, jingyu.xie@student.uni-luebeck.de

[2] Institute for Electrical Engineering in Medicine, Universität zu Lübeck, {j.sauer, j.grasshoff, philipp.rostalski}@uni-luebeck.de

Abstract

Bioelectrical signals can be picked up with electrodes on the skin surface. These signals contain information about the properties of biological systems and can be used to diagnose diseases. Cardiac electrophysiology is one of the most important research fields in medical diagnosis. However, noise and artifacts in the signal processing will negatively affect the signal quality. The electrocardiogram (ECG) signals are subject to various noise sources while passing through different tissues: examples are motion artifacts, crosstalk, electromyography (EMG) artifacts, ambient noise, baseline shifts, and so forth. We present a pipeline in this work to process the measured bioelectrical signals from the chest surface and apply the wavelet denoising method to improve the quality of signals. In addition, the correlation coefficient has been utilized to detect heart diseases and abnormal ECG morphology.

1 Introduction

An electrocardiogram records the electrical activity of the heart using electrodes placed on the body surface. Biomedical engineers aim to use continuous ECG monitoring to investigate the function of heart muscles and heart valves. Electrocardiography has been an established method in diagnosis and treatment of cardiac diseases for decades and is increasingly gaining popularity in other fields. In the intensive care unit, it is typically used to monitor the heartbeat and heart rate [1].

Various noise signals that originate at the electrodes or artifacts in the electronics that amplify the signals and from external sources inevitably affect the ECG measurement. The low-frequency contamination of the ECG frequency spectrum has influence on data quality and causes of low data quality. To maximize the quality of the ECG signal, we need to achieve the signal-to-noise ratio (SNR) with the highest quantity of information from the ECG signal and the minimum quantity of noise contamination. Crosstalk is defined as a form of noise that happens when a bioelectrical signal is detected and produced by a nearby muscle over a non-active muscle. It is mostly due to the volume conduction of electrical activity [2]. Baseline noise comes from the powerline, motion artifact, electronics of the amplification systems, and electrodes. A low-frequency noise (0.5-0.6Hz) is considered as baseline shift. For example, a high-pass filter with a cut-off frequency of 0.5 to 0.6 Hz can be applied to remove it explicitly. Similarly, a notch filter with a cut-off frequency of 50 or 60 Hz can be constructed for the removal of interference in the powerline [3]. Electromyographic noise is also a significant complication in recordings acquired during ambulatory monitoring or exercise. This obscures the low amplitude component and affects the quality of the ECG signal. Generally, the EMG artifact is overlapped with the ECG frequency spectrum and small in amplitude [4]. Wavelet transform (WT) has been utilized for removing noise from the ECG. Previous research has suggested that the wavelet denoising algorithm can be applied to decrease noise in ECG. Low quality of ECG signals causes extracted signals to be inaccurate and leads to misinterpretation and misclassification of the signals. The stationary wavelet transform (SWT) algorithm improves the quality of the denoising.

Template matching with correlation coefficients has been used to detect abnormal ECG in the signal processing when R peaks are detected. The literature survey [5] shows that the related works use cross-correlation. The correlation coefficient will be calculated to determine how similar the two signals are. A correlation coefficient more than an absolute value of 0.9 or greater would represent a strong relationship. Fig. 1 demonstrates the proposed pipeline for bioelectrical signal processing and an approach for anomaly detection using correlation coefficients.

2 Material and Methods

In the following, all processing steps from the pipeline in Fig. 1 will be explained in detail.

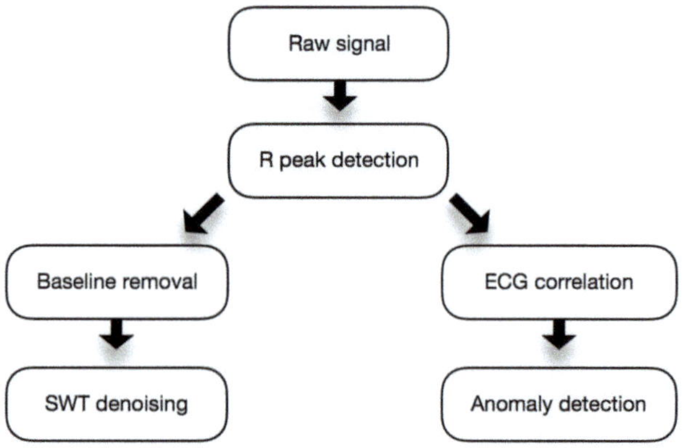

Figure 1: Pipeline flow chart. The flow chart represents the steps in the pipeline and two cases of application. The left part of the figure is mainly used for ECG signal processing. The right part of the figure is mainly applied for anomaly detection.

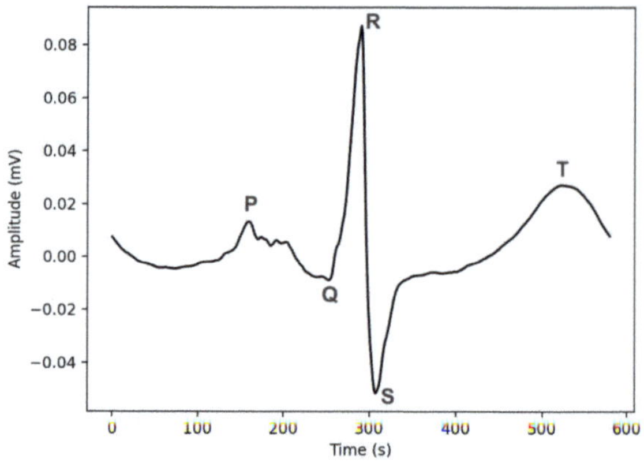

Figure 2: The generated template obtained ECG signal from chest.

2.1 ECG Correlation and Anomaly Detection

This study used multiple datasets from a clinic in Berlin. The fiducial detection of the ECG is fundamental for template generation. To achieve the ECG analysis, it was evident that the R peak is the significant marker that needs to be recognized first. The Pan and Tompkins algorithm [6] was used to detect all the R peaks to calculate the PQRST segment. Signal averaging was used to generate ECG templates for comparing the similarity with sample signals. In order to match the template, the sample segment will be reconstructed by linear interpolation. Correlation coefficients show how similar signals between the template and the sample segment are. Template matching has a relatively limited ability to differentiate between waveforms that are quite similar because it overlooks amplitude information, which is a characteristic of information detection. However, this offers a fast detection method of anomalies. If no ECG template exists, we can compare the current segment with the next segment with the same phase value. A sample of the generated ECG template is presented in Fig. 2.

According to this algorithm, we will first find the ECG R peaks and the phase ϕ_k in frequency domain. Then, each sample of the signal with ϕ_k is compared with the ECG template or its neighboring sample. The neighboring sample is an adaptive template. This method is also named adaptive matching. The neighboring sample is near the current sample in the consecutive ECG beat with the same phase value. If the waveforms of two signals have the same shapes, two samples are correlated with each other. The correlation coefficient is a quantitative standard of the similarity between signals. The amplitude differences between the two signals do not change the correlation coefficient. Accordingly, the correlation coefficient below is purposed as a total *periodicity measure* (PM) [7] for a signal x_k:

$$PM = |\mathrm{corrcoef}\,(x_k, x_{k+\tau_k})| = \frac{|E\left\{x_k x_{k+\tau_k}\right\}|}{\left|E\left\{x_k^2\right\} E\left\{x_{k+\tau_k}^2\right\}\right|^{1/2}} \tag{1}$$

where $E\{\cdot\}$ describes averaging over the time index k. From this definition $0 \leq$ PM ≤ 1, where PM = 0 indicates no linear relationship, and PM = 1 indicates a fully correlation. It is often helpful to use the correlation coefficient to detect abnormity waves. If the samples x_k and $x_{k+\tau_k}$ are uncorrelated, PM value is close to zero [7].

2.2 Baseline Removal and SWT Denoising

Removal of baseline shift is necessary for ECG analysis. The variation of the amplitude might influence the ECG waveform. Therefore, the baseline shift is removed by a traditional highpass filter. In recent years, the wavelet analysis theory has been increasingly investigated in signal denoising. It is essential to remove the wavelet components generated by noise at each scale because the wavelet coefficients have different features at each scale of noise and signal. Furthermore, we can reconstruct the denoised signal with the wavelet inverse transform in the last step. The stationary wavelet transform is proposed based on discrete wavelet transform (DWT), which significantly improves denoising SNR and provides better implementation compared to previous DWT based methods. The first step is to transform the noisy signal into the wavelet domain by decomposing the signal into different levels of approximation and details. Secondly, different threshold values are computed and determined for each coefficient. After this step, the inverse stationary wavelet transforms (ISWT) inverse the thresholded wavelet coefficients in the wavelet domain back to the time domain, which reconstructs the denoised signal. SWT algorithm has no downsampling or decimation process on the approximation and detail of the wavelet coefficients after each level of decomposition through the filter convolution [8]. For denoising, we use a Daubechies wavelet of order two (db2) with a decomposition level of three. Ultimately, the ECG signal is extracted and the result produces a smoother signal. The denoising process can help to improve the measuring precision of ECG signals.

3 Results and Discussion

Section III presents detailed results of the ECG signal processing techniques and discussion about the results.

3.1 ECG Correlation

Cross-correlation can compare the similarity between signals. Signals are correlated with each other if the shapes of the waveforms between two signals are similar. A quantitative measure of the similarity between signals is defined by the correlation coefficient. It is necessary to notice that the amplitude differences between the two signals do not change the correlation coefficient. According to this theory, we match each sample with the generated heartbeat template. Then correlation coefficients will be calculated for one dataset. However, we can also match each sample with the next sample heartbeat if the heartbeat template does not exist. The coefficient PM close to 0 indicates an anomalous signal, which will be considered as an interesting point for ECG analysis. After the iteration of all samples, we get the pictures below.

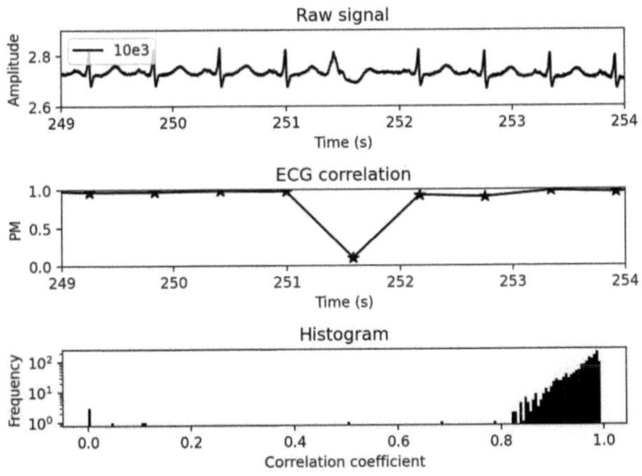

Figure 3: Template matching of a clinical dataset using cross-correlation. Comparison of raw signal from heart muscles (top), correlation coefficient (middle) and frequency (bottom).

Fig. 3 shows the result of the template matching with the generated ECG template. Signal averaging was applied on all heartbeats to create one mean average heartbeats as our ECG template. In our example, nine sequential heartbeats were randomly selected. R peaks were detected and marked with an asterisk. Each R peak corresponds to a correlation coefficient. The correlation coefficient between 251s and 252s is close to 0. This potentially indicates a type of cardiac disease. A small correlation coefficient indicates the anomalous ECG signal. The histogram displays a distribution of all heartbeat samples. For the sample data, a length of 812 seconds includes 1352 R peaks, was completed in a few seconds. Most samples are relatively good for signal processing. Fig. 4 shows another possibility to compare with the neighboring sample, the next heartbeat segment, which has the same effect of anomaly detection. QRS complex by around 251.5s is neither similar to the previous segment nor the next segment. There are two correlation coefficients small than other samples. The determination of outlier by calculating correlation coefficients is performed based on cross-correlation. This method was realized in other datasets. The study's results showed that anomalies could be detected and displayed successfully if R peaks were detected. Nevertheless, we need more data to test this method as a robust detection method thoroughly.

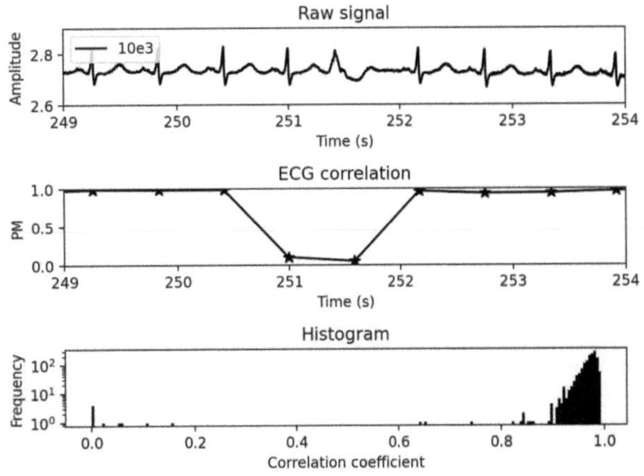

Figure 4: Adaptive matching of a clinical dataset using cross-correlation. Comparison of raw signal from heart muscles (top), correlation coefficient (middle) and frequency (bottom).

3.2 ECG Pipeline

Fig. 5 shows the result of the processing pipeline for ECG signals. The raw ECG signal provides us only the useless numerical signal in a sequence because of the noise in small signal region. Moreover, the baseline shift from ECG signal is effectively removed. The limited interval thresholding with stationary wavelet transform (SWT) enhances the denoising potential of the SWT remarkably and eliminates the EMG artifacts from ECG signals properly. The denoised ECG signal has been successfully produced after denoising.

4 Conclusion

In this work, a pipeline for bioelectrical signal processing was implemented, and anomalies were detected. The implementation and its results show that features of ECG signal with ECG correlation and SWT denoising were effectively extracted. Analysis accuracy can be improved with different coefficients and factors, such as wavelet coefficients. The wavelet method for denoising is extensively applied in comparison with the conventional filtering methods. It

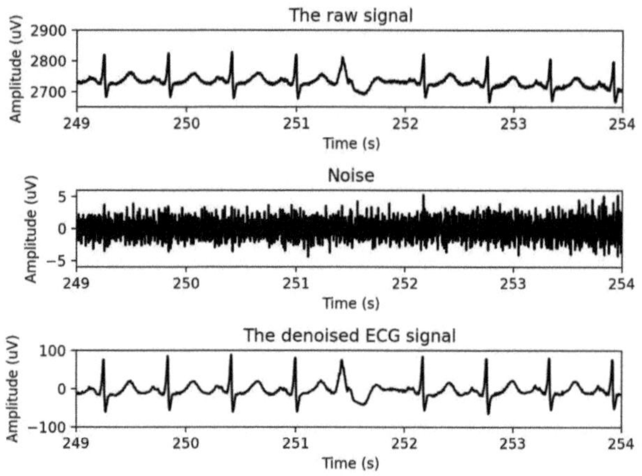

Figure 5: The results of pipeline process for ECG signal and comparison between the original signal (top) and the denoised signal (bottom). It has also shown the removed noise in the measurement (middle).

can maintain some useful local characteristics of the signal. The pipelined processing methods are used in signal processing to increase processing speed. For further research, a more robust system can be implemented, and future works will focus on adapting and testing algorithms with different datasets. More advanced equipment and efficient algorithms will help us determine other important features for future human health.

Acknowledgement

The work has been carried out and supervised by the Institute for Electrical Engineering in Medicine, Universität zu Lübeck. Furthermore, we would like to thank Charite Universitätsmedizin Berlin for the support.

Author's Statement

Conflict of interest: Authors state no conflict of interest.

5 References

[1] L. Sörnmo and P. Laguna, *Bioelectrical Signal Processing in Cardiac and Neurological Applications.* In Biomedical Engineering, pp. 411–452, 2005.

[2] N. Amrutha and V. H. Arul, *A Review on Noises in EMG Signal and its Removal.* International Journal of Scientific and Research Publications, vol. 7, no. 5, pp. 23–27, 2017.

[3] R. Kher, *Signal Processing Techniques for Removing Noise from ECG Signals.* Journal of Biomedical Engineering and Research, vol. 3, no. 101, pp. 1–9, 2019.

[4] S. Abbaspour and A. Fallah, *Removing ECG Artifact from the Surface EMG Signal Using Adaptive Subtraction Technique.* Journal of biomedical physics and engineering, vol. 4, no. 1, pp. 33–38, 2014.

[5] K. Walter, K. Kobayashi, M. Ansermino , G. Dumont, *Removing Cardiac Artifacts From Single-Channel Respiratory Electromyograms.* Physiological measurement, vol. 33, no. 10, pp. 1617–1629, 2012.

[6] J. Pan and W. J. Tompkins, *A Real-Time QRS Detection Algorithm.* in IEEE Transactions on Biomedical Engineering, vol. BME-32, no. 3, pp. 230–236, 1985.

[7] R. Sameni, M. Shamsollahi, C. Jutten, and G. Clifford, *A nonlinear Bayesian filtering framework for ECG denoising.* IEEE Trans. Biomed. Eng., vol. 54, no. 12, pp. 2172–2185, 2007.

[8] N. Osman, H. Shen, F. Ibrahim, W. Abas, H. Rahman, H. Ting, *4th Kuala Lumpur International Conference on Biomedical Engineering 2008.* BIOMED 2008, vol. 21, pp. 99, 2008.

Development of a Software Tool for the Laboratory Management System

Denise Ehlers [1], Sebastian Gerlich [2], Stephan Eisenbrand [3] , and Dennis Kleinewalter [4]

[1] Biomedical Engineering, Luebeck University of Applied Sciences, denise.ehlers@stud.th-luebeck.de
[2] R&D Anesthesia Development, Drägerwerk AG & Co. KGaA, sebastian.gerlich@draeger.com
[3] R&D Anesthesia Development, Drägerwerk AG & Co. KGaA, stephan.eisenbrand@draeger.com
[4] R&D Anesthesia Development, Drägerwerk AG & Co. KGaA, dennis.kleinewalter@draeger.com

Abstract

External regulations and internal processes require a documentation of medical device configurations. The efficiency of searching, planning and structuring device-related information supports the documentation and validation of medical devices. As a method to receive requirements of necessary information, a survey and functional analysis of medical anaesthesia devices, associated software and corporate management programs, is conducted. Creating an overview of automatically generated information using the service interface of the medical device, a software tool is developed. This software tool leads to an efficient and simplified process of laboratory information management with the benefit of preventing errors and providing access for all test engineers via the network.

1 Introduction

A Device Information Exchange Tool, called DIET, is developed to merge different information into a laboratory management system. The process of documentation for medical devices should achieve an increase in efficiency, taking into account the phases of development up to market approval. Thereby the existing synergies between development, market approval, market surveillance till the ending life cycle of a medical device are going to be used. This includes information of the device under test (DUT), which is an important part of the design history file (DHF)[1]. The DHF is a regulatory requirement, demanded by the Food and Drug Administration (FDA) and relates to the requirements of the Medical Device Regulations (MDR)[2].

During the development of the software, existing processes and tools are used as interfaces and their information is implemented. The first to mention is the KANBAN board, which is used to give an overview about processes, projects and tasks [3]. The structure helps to organize the different device information efficiently. The KANBAN is implemented through Atlassian's commercial software Jira. In the following Fig.1 a practical example can be seen. The overview shows three tasks respectively tickets. Usually the tickets, which are titled with numbers, represent working tasks or problems, so called defects. In this case often used information of the medical device can be presented as an overview. The columns are named as laboratories. The tickets, representing medical devices, can be assigned to the laboratories. The single tickets can be assigned to an owner. That means a person is the main responsible for that ticket, the information of the owner can be seen via the image in the right corner of a ticket. Information can be saved into fields like component or label, which helps grouping, searching or filtering special information.

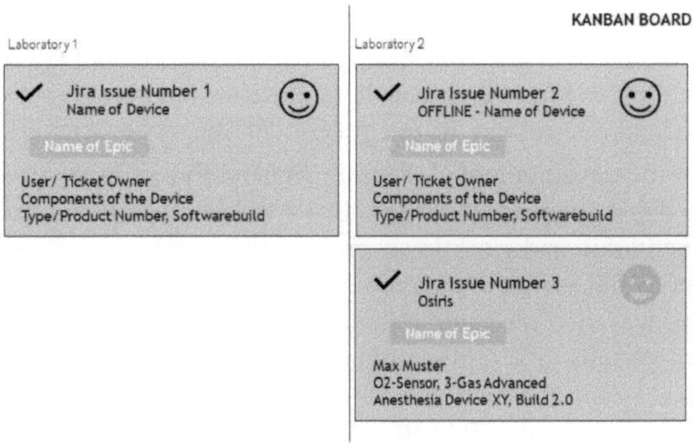

Figure 1: Example for the final design of device tickets with Jira web application as an overview [3].

The aim is to create structures that save time and reduce errors by simplifying and substituting data processing that previously had to be done manually. The issues are known by researchers and mentioned in connection with overcoming the hurdle of manufacturer-dependent models and a lack of standards offering flexible and secure integration of medical devices and IT systems [5]. There are scientific elaborations with equal intentions presenting the diversity of the field [6]. The different kinds of interface processing, which are available [7], demonstrating that often individual solu-

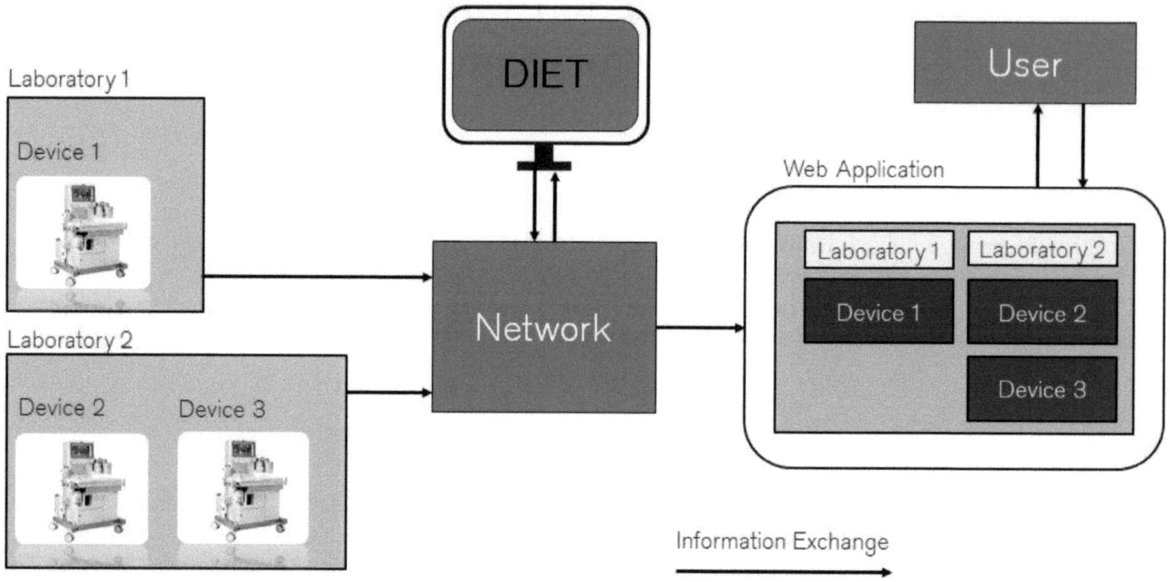

Figure 2: The structure of network communication [8].

tions are necessary to develop, influenced by a lack of standards. Currently, the general medical device information is documented and accessed manually. The DIET should provide a better traceability, thus the creation of a device file and thus also to faster communication paths. That includes the simple and transparent traceability of the configuration of the DUT at any time. Regarding the device connection, the topic is focused on anesthesia devices, but other types of medical devices can be integrated with the same structure.

For the development of the tool, Jira and Python were used. To determine, which information would be useful for documentation and workflows, presentations and surveys were conducted as part of the project. The most relevant information was also read out at the device and transmitted to the Jira system in a semi-automated way. The previous software systems do not provide a connection to the software Jira offering a possible efficient overview about all relevant information.

The medical interface bus browser (MIB browser) is one frequently used application to manually evaluate and manipulate information of the medical devices. It is an established option of the company to extract single information. The DIET can pass information partially automated to the Jira, offering an overview of a continuously updated device history. This assists the requirements of the MDR and FDA to generate information useful for the DUT a part of the DHF. The larger the company structure and the larger the number of medical devices that are integrated and have different configurations, the more complex the management of those devices becomes. The advantage of the DIET as a digital application, which can be used individually configured and being accessible to all users at any place and any time leads to an increase of efficiency for documentation and administration. Receiving advantages for tasks and processes with a complex planning structure using the offered solution of partly automation and creation of digital device file. Therefore the network must be taken into account.

2 Material and Methods

2.1 Medical Device Network

In the Fig. 2 the structure of network communication between DIET and the connected components can be seen. The medical devices, which can be found in Laboratory 1 or Laboratory 2, are connected to the network. The DIET offers the selected information exchange with the usage of the network. Information of the devices can be extracted via the service interface and translated to the web application. The web application, in this case Jira, visualises the content of information in a structured overview. The device tickets are assigned to the Laboratories. The user receives the information and can manipulate or enter additional information to the device tickets.

2.2 Requirement analysis

In order to demonstrate the potential benefits of the tool and to adapt it to the needs of the users, presentations were given and the subsequent feedback processed. The function of the DIET was presented within the team, across the department and specifically in a conference of test engineers. It was analysed, which information have to be provided. Frequently needed information about the hardware components or software components were taken into account, designing the DIET.

2.3 Designing process of the DIET

The designed tool uses the name of the corresponding medical device as well as the IP address and Jira issue ID generated from a configuration file. All devices listed in the configuration file are queried synchronously when the tool is started. The procedure is illustrated in Fig.3. For the testing and implementation 10 anesthesia devices with different configurations were used.

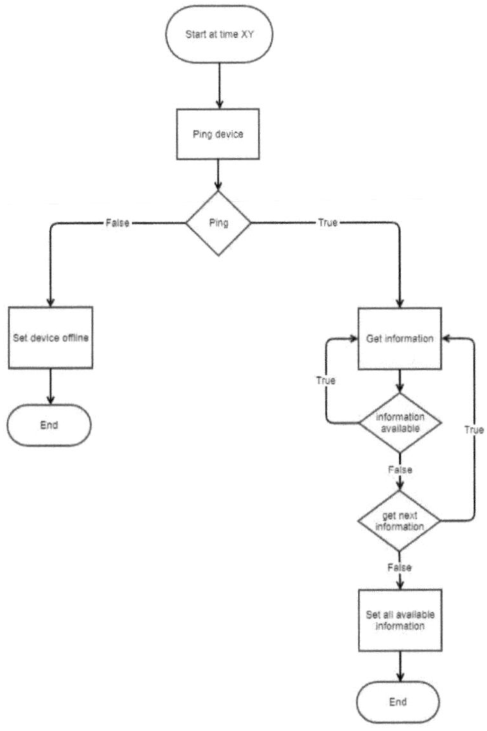

Figure 3: Flow Chart of DIET for interface testing with different anaesthesia devices.

Starting the DIET, the program ping all medical devices, which are listed in the configuration file. To ensure the connectivity of the devices, the ping is executed 5 times after failure of the first trial. If there is no information about the status of the device, the Jira ticket associated with the medical device is set to offline. Gaining access to the device and its data, all necessary information is extracted via the service interface. This query is performed within a loop till all implemented request is accomplished. If some information is not accessible, the next information is requested. If the following information is available, the program jumps back to the previous loop. The program stays running through these loops until all required information steps are collected. Then these information can be transferred to the connected Jira ticket. There are implemented mechanisms in the code to leave the loops via breaks or exceptions.

3 Results and Discussion

The final tool transfers a semi-automated query of device information into a web application. The information is conceptualised so that individual device tickets represent the respective medical devices. The tickets themselves can be manually assigned to the respective laboratories. All devices associated with the department are subordinate to one main ticket. That leads to a better overview and filter option for finding and structuring the anaesthesia devices against ventilation devices.

Using the option of the board as shown in Fig. 1, an optimal visualization can be achieved. Each ticket has an individual Jira Issue Number, which is helpful for traceability and referencing. The information can be referenced directly in confluence, which is used for documentation and transfer of know-how, shared via hyperlink or connected to defect issues. Below that, the device name is listed. If a device is not online, it is shown as offline. This means the device is not connected to the network and thus the information of the device cannot be uptated in the Jira tickets. The last valid information remains displayed. Furthermore, the main ticket, is also listed by name. This is relevant to the extent that devices from other inventories or departments can be integrated into the board for use. The picture of the device owner is displayed in the upper right corner, additionally his name is listed. This information can be helpful in case of queries related to the device. Important frequently used information is stored as components or labels by the DIET. Device components include, for example, information about the installed sensors or mixing units. Information about the device IP address or software build version is stored in the label. Each individual ticket can be opened as a file in order to view further information such as the change history, which is also generated automatically. Manual comments about the device as well as photos can be integrated.

A dynamic file is created, where changes of information stay available. Tickets are created in such a way that they generally cannot be deleted. These facts support in the scheduling of trials or tests. Because information can be found quickly and certain component changes cannot be forgotten to be entered. For compliance with FDA and MDR guidelines, which require device documentation, the DIET serves as a useful tool. In contrast to manually maintained device files, where it is necessary to enter every change to the device, which offers the risk that information is forgotten to be entered, it is not legible or even the device file can be lost during the transport of a device. The DIET can prevent errors in documentation. However, certain aspects must also be taken into account and conditions created for the functionality of the DIET. For example, it is of course necessary that the devices are connected and responsive during the initiated update process. This is because changes from unconnected devices will not be added to the device file. These information can only be updated manually. Unless an accurate solution and establishment has been made for this, approved device files cannot be re-

placed. Other options and further developments of the tool, such as the feedback of occurring failures communicated by the device, can be used as an option and further information. This can potentially facilitate error analyses by the test engineers.
Summarising, the DIET is a facilitation and improvement of the device and documentation related information processing and structuring, Which offers advantages in the detailed information indication and manipulation.

4 Conclusion

The development of the DIET enables partially automated extraction of device information, redirection and presentation with configured device tickets within Jira. For this the device interface is used, which is applied for manipulation and maintenance of the medical devices. Transmission errors can be avoided by directly reading out the device information. Furthermore no changes of information are lost, which is essential for the documentation of medical devices. Thus, the DIET leads to a simplification of approval process for medical devices by offering the documentation partially automated. DIET provides a flexible solution to integrate further information and device types. The device management of the laboratory, which can be used by any computer with access to the internet, leads to a clear and focused overview. DIET supports the guarantee of save devices.

Acknowledgement

The work has been carried out at Drägerwerk AG & Co. KGaA, Lübeck and supervised by Prof. Kallinger, Acoustics and Digital Signal Processing, University of Applied Sciences.

Author's Statement

Conflict of interest: Authors state no conflict of interest. Informed consent: Informed consent has been obtained.

5 References

[1] Johner Institute GmbH Konstanz 2020, *Design History File.* Available: https://johner-institute.com/articles/regulatory-affairs/and-more/technical-file-versus-dhf/ [last accessed on 2021-01-01].

[2] Deutsches Institut für Normung e.V. Berlin 2016, *Medizinprodukte - Qualitätsmanagementsysteme - Anforderungen für regulatorische Zwecke (ISO 13485:2016); Deutsche Fassung EN ISO 13485:2016.* In: Lecture MPRT, SoSe2020, University of Applied Sciences Lübeck].

[3] Atlassian 2020, *Jira Software - How to get started.* Available: https://www.atlassian.com/de/software/jira/guides/getting-started/overview [last accessed on 2020-12-15].

[4] V. Ignat, *Digitalization and the global technology trends.* In: IOP Conf. Ser.: Mater. Sci. Eng. 227 012062, Germany, 2017.

[5] Universität Leipzig 2020, *Transferprojekt ebnet Weg für dynamische Vernetzung von Medizintechnik.* Available: https://www.uni-leipzig.de/newsdetail/artikel/transferprojekt-ebnet-weg-fuer-dynamische-vernetzung-von-medizintechnik-2019-04-09// [last accessed on 2021-01-04].

[6] M. Đordevic, HAW Hamburg, 2016, *Entwicklung eines webbasierten Software- und Informations-Managementsystems für medizinische Geräte.* Available: https://reposit.haw-hamburg.de/bitstream/20.500.12738/8007/1/Bachelorarbeit Milos Dordevic.pdf [last accessed on 2021-01-04].

[7] H. Tanck,M. Heinlein, *Fusion von Medizintechnik und Informationstechnologie.* In: Kramme R. (eds) Medizintechnik. Springer, Berlin, Heidelberg, 2011.

[8] Drägerwerk AG Co. KGaA 2020, *Dräger Atlan® A300/A300 XL Anästhesie-Arbeitsplätze.* Available: https://www.draeger.com/Products/Content/atlan-a300-a300xl-pi-9107092-de-master.pdf [last accessed on 2020-12-15].

10

Image Processing

Automated Camera-Based Laboratory Vessel Detection in a Carbon Dioxide Incubator

Alexandra Jankowski [1] and Philipp Kayser [2]

[1] Medical Engineering Science, Universität zu Lübeck, alexandra.jankowski@student.uni-luebeck.de
[2] Eppendorf Instrumente GmbH, Hamburg, kayser.p@eppendorf.de

Abstract

This paper presents a novel camera-based system for automated laboratory vessel detection in CO_2 incubators. It optimizes the workflow in modern laboratories by automatically creating protocols of incubated samples, pairing them to their user, and facilitating the organization of multi-user laboratories. The presented system improves the cell growth environment of the incubator by reducing the number of necessary door openings and thereby provides an optimized temperature, gas, and humidity control. Moreover, the system provides a method for segmenting partially transparent objects in highly reflecting surroundings. The methods were developed by conceptualizing and constructing a prototype, testing different conventional image processing methods and hardware solutions. The prototype was successfully tested in real-time usage. Several different types of laboratory vessels were used for evaluation. As a result, the prototype sufficiently detects partially transparent generic laboratory vessels in the highly reflecting incubator chamber and creates a protocol optimizing the laboratory workflow and the cell growth environment. The system provides a novel usage of CO_2 incubators contributing to the modernization of contemporary laboratories.

1 Introduction

A Carbon dioxide (CO_2) incubator is a commonly used device in life science laboratories and specifically used when working with cell cultures. By controlling the temperature, humidity, and CO_2 concentration inside its chamber, it provides an optimal environment for cell growth [1]. In many laboratories incubators are jointly used by several scientists. To ensure identification of each specific sample, the users often mark their labware by labeling vessels with individual inscriptions or barcodes. When withdrawing a sample the user has to check the labels. This is time-consuming and leads to undesired multiple incubator openings. Every door opening changes humidity, CO_2 concentration, and temperature in the chamber due to the mixture of the surrounding laboratory air with the chamber. This results in a non-optimal, non-steady cell growth environment. Additionally, every door opening poses a risk for contamination.

This paper presents a novel system based on computer vision, which automatically detects laboratory vessels placed in the incubator, assigns these to their user, and hereby automatically generates a protocol. A display outside the incubator can depict images of the chamber including the vessels and their protocolled information, such as a sample and user identification. The system reduces the number of work steps the scientist needs to complete and therefore increases his or her time efficiency. Checking the display to find a specific sample reduces the number of door openings and results in a more optimal cell growth environment.

2 Material and Methods

2.1 Materials and Setup

The system was developed using Eppendorf's CellXpert® C170i [2]. Regularly, the CellXpert® C170i contains four extractable incubator shelves, each having an approximate size of 52×42 cm^2 and each being placed approximately 15 cm above the other. The developed system is based on foreground segmentation in images of one entire incubator shelf using a bird's-eye-view perspective. A camera is placed centrally above the observed shelf. The distance between two shelves limits the distance between shelf and camera yielding 15 cm. To observe the wide compartment between two shelves an omnidirectional objective is used. Omnidirectional cameras can reach a field of view larger than 180 degrees [3]. Calibration of the omnidirectional camera is done based on the method presented in [4]. A light source is added to the system to lighten the monitored shelf. The camera and the light source are controlled by a computational unit placed outside of the incubator chamber. This ensures that any by the computational unit potentially generated heat has no effect on the cell growth environment within the chamber. An exemplary image of one incubator compartment including a possible setup of labware is shown in Fig. 1, where (a) depicts the raw image captured by the omnidirectional camera and (b) depicts its rectification based on [4].

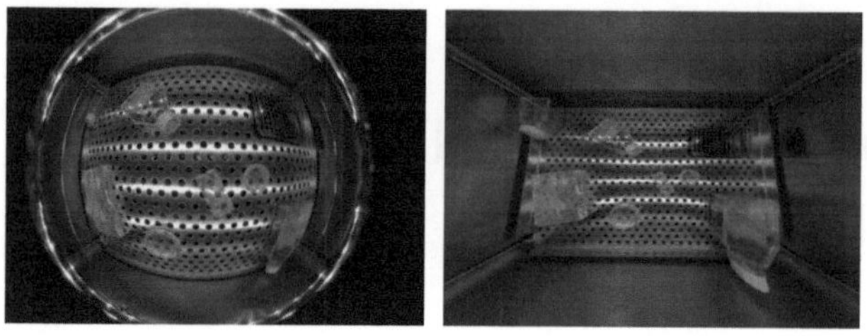

(a) (b)

Figure 1: (a) Raw image of an incubator shelf taken by the omnidirectional camera. (b) Rectification of the raw image.

2.2 Object Segmentation

So long as an incubator door is closed, every object inside is static. Additionally, the chamber is completely dark, meaning there is no light coming in from the outside. Therefore, the newly added system is in full control of the lighting conditions while the door is closed. The presented system detects objects by finding differences in consecutively captured images and is based on conventional image processing methods.

As a first step, an initial background image is captured. As stated above, the setup of objects within the chamber can not change until the door is opened. The system waits for the event of a door opening, received from the incubator's control unit. Consequently, the system waits for the event of a door closing after which it captures an image. This image can now either contain a newly added object, contain a subset of the previously contained objects due to withdrawal or show no difference to the previous state. The following paragraphs describe the image processing methods used to detect the objects by foreground segmentation.

To detect the foreground in an image of the monitored shelf the elementwise absolute difference between the image $I_t(x, y)$ captured at time-step t and the image $I_{t-1}(x, y)$ captured at time-step $t-1$, which denotes the previous door closure event - is computed and defined as

$$F_{\text{diff}}(x, y) = |I_t(x, y) - I_{t-1}(x, y)|, \qquad (1)$$

where $x = 0, 1, 2, \ldots, n-1$ and $y = 0, 1, 2, \ldots, m-1$ with n and m denoting the number of columns and rows, respectively. An elementwise operation is defined as an operation between corresponding pixel pairs in the images [5].

As a second step, a binary image is computed by intensity thresholding, which sets all pixel values with a value smaller than a certain threshold T to zero and all values greater than or equal to T to 255 [5]. It is defined as

$$f_{\text{thresh}}(I(x, y)) = \begin{cases} 255 & \text{if } I(x, y) \geq T \\ 0 & \text{if } I(x, y) < T, \end{cases} \qquad (2)$$

yielding $F_2(x, y) = f_{\text{thresh}}(F_{\text{diff}}(x, y))$ with $T = T_1$.

The task at hand - being the segmentation of labware - faces difficulties specific and unique to the scenario. These are partial transparency of commonly used labware and the environment of the chamber, where both the shelf and the walls are strongly reflecting. Due to its transparency, part of the region inside the vessel boundaries shows very low intensity differences to the background. Contrarily, other image parts show high intensity differences between the background and foreground images in image locations where no object is actually present, formed by reflections of objects on the shelf or walls. Due to these difficulties, the computation of the absolute difference (1) followed by intensity thresholding (2) can be insufficient to segment the objects. As a measure to choose an optimal value for T_1, N. Otsu's method [6] can be used. It is essentially based on examining the image histogram, a detailed discussion would go beyond the constraints of this paper and is here therefore omitted.

To account for the stated problem of transparency, the presented system additionally makes use of the lowpass Gaussian filter kernel, which is defined as

$$M_{\text{gaussian}}(x, y) = \frac{1}{2\pi\sigma^2} \exp(-\frac{x^2 + y^2}{2\sigma^2}), \qquad (3)$$

where σ is the standard deviation. Convolving an image with a Gaussian filter kernel is commonly used for smoothing [5]. The here presented system, however, uses the filter to strongly blur the segmented object parts by choosing a relatively large filter size and σ. When several small but separated segments are in near proximity, the strong filter will blur them into one larger object. These partial segments can originate in the thresholding step from images of transparent labware where weak intensities in $F_{\text{diff}}(x, y)$ were found due to refraction or reflection of light on the vessel surface. Thus, a cluster of small segments is detected instead of the entire object and now blurred into one segment with the Gaussian filtering. Any small segments not near others - meaning not belonging to clusters - will be reduced in intensity. Convolving the image $F_2(x, y)$ with M_{gaussian} yields the image $F_3(x, y)$. In a further step, a second intensity thresholding (2) is used on the blurred image to segment the clusters while removing any stand-alone noisy sections, yielding the binary image $F_4(x, y) = f_{\text{thresh}}(F_3(x, y))$ with $T = T_2$.

As the use of the described twice applied thresholding remains to produce segments with holes and potentially merges near objects during Gaussian blurring, further processing is performed. Erosion denotes a morphological expression used for reducing object sizes and is defined as

$$I \ominus E = \{z | B_z \subseteq I\}, \qquad (4)$$

where I is the binary image, B is the structuring element and z is its referencing point. Dilation is a morphological expression used to enlarge objects. It is defined as

$$I \oplus E = \{z | \hat{B}_z \cap I \neq \emptyset\}, \qquad (5)$$

where $\hat{B}$ is the reflecting mask of B. Opening, defined as

$$I \circ E = (I \ominus E) \oplus E, \qquad (6)$$

denotes a successive application of erosion and dilation and can be used to remove small objects in an image. Closing contrastingly is defined as

$$I \bullet E = (I \oplus E) \ominus E, \qquad (7)$$

and describes the reverse process of first applying dilation and then erosion, which can be used to fill small gaps and holes in objects [5]. The presented system applies closing followed by opening to the image to both fill holes in segmented objects and to remove small objects such as remaining segmentations of reflections or noise, yielding $F_5 = (F_4 \bullet E_1) \circ E_1$. As the Gaussian blurring performed in a previous step also results in enlargement of objects and potentially merges near objects, erosion is applied to reduce the object sizes as a method to reverse the previous enlargement and separate merged objects. The result yields $F_6 = F_5 \ominus E_2$.

Concluding the foreground segmentation, a median filter is applied to F_6 giving the binary image F_7. Applying a median filter M_{med} to an image I is achieved by replacing the value of the center pixel with the median of the values in the region encompassed by M_{med} [5].

Following the described process of foreground segmentation the system removes any segmented objects that are fully outside of a region of interest (ROI). Here, the boundaries of the incubator shelf visible in the image serve as the ROI. The base of any laboratory vessel will always touch the shelf and therefore partially appear inside the denoted region. Any segment appearing fully outside of the ROI can safely be classified as a reflection on one of the sidewalls and therefore be removed. The application of the post-processing steps finally produces the binary image $F(x, y)$.

After computing $F(x, y)$, further processing steps determine whether the changes occurred due to the addition or withdrawal of objects. The sequence of the performed steps is shown in Fig. 2.

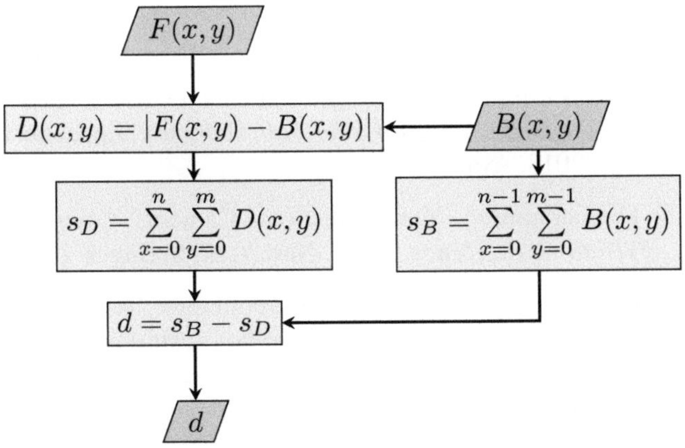

Figure 2: Sequence of steps performed to decide between input or withdrawal. $F(x, y)$ denotes the computed segmentation at the current time-step, $B(x, y)$ denotes the foreground segmentation of the previous time-step and d denotes the resulting value from which can be inferred whether objects have been added or removed.

First, the absolute difference between $F(x, y)$ and the object segmentation of the previous time-step, here denoted as $B(x, y)$, is computed resulting in a binary image $D(x, y)$. Further, the sums of the values over all pixels, defined as

$$s(I(x,y)) = \sum_{x=0}^{n} \sum_{y=0}^{m} I(x,y), \tag{8}$$

is computed of $B(x, y)$ and $D(x, y)$ giving the integers $s_B = s(B(x, y))$ and $s_D = s(D(x, y))$, respectively. Subsequently, the difference $d = s_B - s_D$ is used to decide between withdrawal, input or no change: $d < -d_{min}$ indicates inputted labware, $d > d_{min}$ indicates withdrawn objects, whereas $-d_{min} < d < d_{min}$ indicates no change of labware setup, with d_{min} denoting a minimal change of summed pixel values as even with no change of the setup, d will unlikely equal exactly zero due to noise. Notice, that $D(x, y)$ will serve as $B(x, y)$ in a next time-step $t+1$ as it is the binary image containing segmentations of all currently present objects, whereas $F(x, y)$ merely contains segmentations of the added or withdrawn objects.

The lastly described step concludes the full object segmentation algorithm including a decision about how the scene changed in terms of input or withdrawal of vessels.

3 Results and Discussion

Images with dimensions of 2592 × 1952 pixels were used for evaluation. The described algorithms were used with the following parameters: T_1 was chosen based on N. Otsu's method for optimal thresholding [6], M_{gaussian} was chosen with a filter size of 51 × 51 and $\sigma = 50$, $T_2 = 30$ as a fixed global threshold, the size of the structuring element E_1 was chosen as 25 × 25, the size of the structuring element E_2 was picked as 21 × 21, and finally the size of M_{med} was selected to be 31 × 31.

The presented combined image processing algorithms forming the method for foreground segmentation of partially transparent objects were evaluated using the Jaccard coefficient defined as

$$J = \frac{|G \cap F|}{|G \cup F|}, \tag{9}$$

where F denotes the computed segmentation, here F_7, and G denotes the given ground truth [7]. A number of six different labware setups totaling a number of 40 individual laboratory vessels or vessel stacks were used for evaluation. The computed dice coefficients were averaged giving a result of $\bar{J} \approx 0.83$. Fig. 3 shows the segmentation of laboratory vessels in an exemplary setup, where (a) depicts the segmented foreground F_7 and (b) depicts the contours of the segmentations in the captured and rectified image of the scene. It can be seen that the foreground segmentation detected a reflection on the right side of the image. Additionally, the flask in the top left corner was only partially detected with its parts not merged. The flask on the bottom right corner, on the other hand, shows holes. This serves as an explanation as to why the post-processing steps described in the previous section are useful. After applying them, a result depicted in Fig. 4 (a) is obtained. As a reference to the minimum size a segmentation needs to

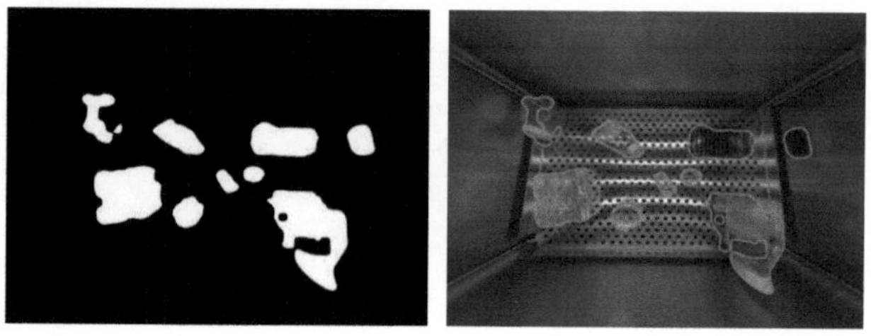

(a) (b)

Figure 3: (a) Binary image with the segmentation of the laboratory vessels depicted in Fig. 1(b). (b) Rectified image of laboratory vessels inside the incubator, where the outlines of the segmentation of (a) are marked in the image.

have to be classified as an object, the size of the smallest commonly used vessel can be taken into account. Here, the post-processing achieves to segment the correct number of objects. Though it is also noticeable that the segmentation was not fully successful as there remain non-segmented *parts* of transparent objects. However, the main goal of the system is object detection to create automated protocols and pair objects to users. Therefore, it suffices to create bounding boxes of the segmentations as depicted in Fig. 4 (b) with the option to display any known information accordingly. In this project, the users were paired with the objects by specifying a user-ID upon input or withdrawal of objects through a user management interface which will here not be further discussed. As noticeable in Fig. 4 (b) some bounding boxes do not encase the entire object due to faults in the segmentation algorithm. While this is undesired it poses little to no difficulty for the user to clearly keep the detected objects apart and correctly find his or her specific sample.

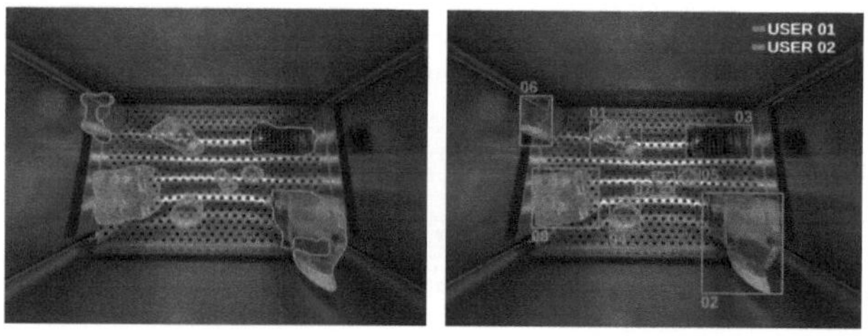

(a) (b)

Figure 4: (a) Depiction of the contours of the foreground segmentation after post-processing. (b) Exemplary resulting object detection depicted with bounding boxes and exemplary user and sample identification numbers.

4 Conclusion

A benefit of the presented system is the ability to detect generic objects. This means the system can detect any laboratory vessels and is not restricted to the tested vessel models. As different laboratories may use different vessel types this is a necessary feature.
The presented system is however unable to separate stacked vessels, as they will always be touching and thereby segmented as one large object by the algorithm. As this is a strict limitation, stacked vessels all belonging to one user can nonetheless be detected adequately.
It can be concluded that the presented system can sufficiently detect laboratory vessels inside the incubator chamber. It can additionally correctly determine whether a vessel has been added or withdrawn or whether there has been no change in the setup of labware. However, the system is unable to track movement when vessels are shifted within the chamber. Instead, it poses a strict limitation to only add or withdraw but not shift the objects. Nonetheless, it serves as a basis for any future developments to track partially transparent objects. The system successfully helps to decrease the number of incubator door openings resulting in a more steady cell growth environment and reducing the number of possible contamination threats. Moreover, the system improves the efficiency of the laboratory workflow.

Acknowledgement

The work has been carried out at Eppendorf Instrumente GmbH, Hamburg and supervised by Prof. Dr. Marcin Grzegorzek, Institute of Medical Informatics, Universität zu Lübeck.

Author's Statement

Conflict of interest: Authors state no conflict of interest.

5 References

[1] R. G. Geraghty et al., "Guidelines for the use of cell lines in biomedical research," *British Journal of Cancer (2014)*, 2014, doi: 10.1038/bjc.2014.166.

[2] I. K. Hartmann and J. Wagener, *CO_2 Incubators - Making the Best Choice for Your Lab*. Hamburg, Eppendorf AG, 2018, Available:

[3] D. Scaramuzza, "Omnidirectional Camera," *Computer Vision: A Reference Guide*, New York, Springer, 2014.

[4] B. Li, L. Heng, K Koser and M. Pollefeys, "A multiple-camera system calibration toolbox using a feature descriptor-based calibration pattern," *2013 IEEE/RSJ International Conference on Intelligent Robots and Systems*, Tokyo, 2013, pp. 1301-1307.

[5] F. C. Gonzalez and R. E. Woods, *Digital Image Processing*. New York, Pearson, 4 ed., 2018.

[6] N. Otsu, "A Threshold Selection Method from Gray-Level Histograms," *IEEE Transactions on Systems, Man, and Cybernetics*, vol. 9, no. 1, pp. 62-66, 1979.

[7] F. Andrade and E. V. Carrera, "Supervised evaluation of Seed-Based Interactive Image Segmentation Algorithms," *2015 20th Symposium on Signal Processing, Images and Computer Vision (STSIVA)*, Bogota, 2015.

Evaluating Interactive Segmentation Methods Across Domains – MVTec ISB: A Novel Benchmark for Evaluating Interactive Segmentation Methods Across Domains –

Matthias Klatt [1,4], Alexander Fertig [2,4], Patrick Follmann [3,4], Niclas Bockelmann [5] and Floris Ernst [5]

[1] Robotics and Autonomous Systems, Universität zu Lübeck, matthias.klatt@student.uni-luebeck.de
[2] Computer Science, University of Applied Sciences Munich, alexander.fertig@hm.edu
[3] Chair of Computer Vision and Artificial Intelligence, Technische Universität München, follmann@mvtec.com
[4] MVTec Software GmbH, Research, {matthias.klatt-ext,follmann, alexander.fertig-ext}@mvtec.com
[5] Institute of Robotics and Cognitive systems, Universität zu Lübeck, {bockelmann, ernst}@rob.uni-luebeck.de

Abstract

With recent developments in Deep Learning (DL), semantic segmentation methods have become very powerful. However, their supervised training requires many and accurate mask labels. In industrial and medical applications, annotations often must be created manually by expert annotators which is expensive and time-consuming. Recent DL-based interactive segmentation methods claim to predict accurate segmentation masks with only a few user interactions. However, the evaluation of such methods was done primarily using simulations on similar images to those of the training set. In this work, we propose a new benchmark for interactive segmentation that consists of a challenging selection of images across various domains and with very different objects. Moreover, our evaluations reveal that an approach without learning component (Watershed) leads to good results in many situations. A modern DL-based method (IOG) needs less interactions, but there is a high variance in accuracy depending on the size and appearance of objects, as well as the exact position of user clicks.

1 Introduction

The segmentation of images is used in a wide field of various applications. Recent deep learning based segmentation networks [1] allow the simultaneous, fast, and robust localization, classification, and measuring of objects within an image. For example, in medical diagnosis image segmentation is applied to locate brain tumor tissues in images on pixel-level [2]. In an industrial context, image segmentation is often used to control processes and ensure quality standards.

Although, a burden to apply this advanced deep learning method is the requirement of highly accurate labelled data. Semantic segmentation demands pixel-level labels, which is mostly done manually with only little assistance. This increases the labelling time and so the expenses to create a labelled dataset.

The existing datasets, that are suitable for semantic segmentation and used in research, often only cover general objects, like in common datasets as COCO [3] or VOC [4], where the objects are mostly without any holes inside. Networks trained with these datasets mostly have a significant drop in performance facing unknown objects. Therefore, these networks only find few applications in the fields of medicine and industry, which deal with highly specialized object types.

Recent developments introduce methods of interactive semantic segmentation, that state to provide accurate labels [5] [6] with the support of manual user clicks. It is claimed the prediction is equivalent to a high-quality label. The advantage in time would decrease the cost of creating suitable labels. However, these methods were evaluated on the large-scale dataset Pascal VOC [4] and evaluated on images of the same domain. This raises the question of their generalization capacities on unseen domains. To examine these generalization capacities, a novel benchmark (c.f. Section 2.1) was set up, which contains a selection of images with various attributes from several domains.

We applied two interactive segmentation methods to this benchmark: the deep learning based *Inside-Outside Guidance* (*IOG*) [6] and the rule-based *Watershed* [7] algorithm. The results were evaluated based on the mean intersection over union (IoU) metric (c.f. Section 2.2).

2 Material and Methods

In Section 2.1, we present our benchmark and in Section 2.2 the evaluation metric IoU. The two methods used in our benchmark are described in Sections 2.3 (*Watershed*) and 2.4 (*IOG*).

Table 1: **Benchmark datasets and image domains.** Some of the MVTec datasets are HALCON (`www.mvtec.com`) example datasets (*) and others are MVTec internal datasets with images from industrial customers (**).

Dataset	Image Domain
Pascal VOC	Everyday photography
COCO	Everyday photography
Cityscapes	Urban street scenes
DAVIS	Everyday photography
MVTec D2S	Supermarket products
MVTec MAD	Defects on objects and within textures
MVTec Pill Bags*	Pills within a bag
MVTec SaC**	High number of small objects in industrial context
MVTec CPOD**	High number of (small) and occluding groceries
MVTec Screws*	Screws on wooden background

2.1 Benchmark

Our novel benchmark, MVTec ISB, consists of 87 images and its purpose is to examine the generalization capacities of the applied methods. The benchmark is kept small in order to be suitable for manual annotation runs by real users. To obtain a meaningful and heterogeneous benchmark, we focused on two main aspects: First, the objects displayed in the images are selected based on following attributes: illumination, contrast, shape, reflection, overlap of objects, number of objects, type of defect, fore- and background texture. Second, the images are selected from a wide range of datasets with various and disparate domains, listed in Table 1. This includes open source datasets (e.g., Cityscapes [8], Pascal VOC [4], COCO [3], and DAVIS [9]), and industrial datasets provided by MVTec for public use (e.g., MVTec D2S [10] or MAD (MVTec Anomaly Detection) [11]). Labels with poor quality were relabeled.
With this, the benchmark stands out with a high variety and informative value on the generalization capacity.

2.2 Mean Intersection-over-Union

The Intersection-over-Union (IoU) is one of the most used metrics in semantic segmentation and is defined as the area of overlap between the predicted segmentation and the ground truth divided by the area of union between the predicted segmentation and the ground truth (GT) [12]:

$$\text{IoU} = \frac{GT \cap prediction}{GT \cup prediction}. \tag{1}$$

The mean IoU (mIoU) of set of objectes inside different images is calculated by taking the IoU of each object and calculate the average.

2.3 Watershed

Watershed transformation is defined on greyscale images. The image is interpreted as a topological map where the segmentation is performed iteratively with markers, set by a user, based on the image intensity.
The annotators can chose between different labels for each marker which are set by them. In our implementation, for clarity, the number of available markers has been set to two, one for the foreground (FG) and one for the background (BG) of the image. The marker size can be adjusted individually, making it easier to label delicate objects.
In our implementation the annotator needs to mark a region of interest first with a bounding box (bbox). In the next step the image is cropped around that region and the annotator can mark an object or the background inside this region. Because of the image cropping it is possible to annotate different objects in an image separately and precisely, while not being confused by several touching or overlapping annotations.

2.4 Inside-Outside Guidance

Inside-Outside Guidance [6] is a DL-based method for interactive semantic segmentation. The authors claim that their method needs three mouse clicks to get high mIOU values even if the image domains are different to the images used for training of the network.
The three needed points are given by two BG mouse clicks to define a bounding box around the object of interest and one FG-click on the object itself. If the predicted annotation is not well enough, it is possible to add more inside (FG) or outside (BG) clicks for further refinement.
To feed the segmentation convolutional neural network with the user interactions around each click, a 2D Gaussian is applied to create two heatmaps. One for the the FG and one for the BG guidance. These two heatmaps are concatenated with the RGB image and are used as five channel input for the model.
To train the interactive segmentation network, the authors adapt a simulation strategy from [5]. The clicks are simulated for training the segmentation network based on the ground truth masks. A bounding box is extracted for each mask, before the box is enlarged by ten pixels to simulate a quickly, but perhaps imprecisely, drawn bounding box of an annotator. The foreground click is generated as the mask center with some random noise applied. We use the same simulation to generate user interactions for *IOG*. We also apply different noise and extension parameters for the drawn bbox during our testing to see how robustly the segmentation network performs if the user interactions are imprecise.
To achieve a realistic user behaviour in the first simulation scenario inaccurate simulations are included as bbox that are smaller than the original GT mask. The simulated bbox is obtained from the GT bbox and extended based on the image size in order to apply different extensions to different image sizes.
In the first scenario the FG click is the GT mask center plus some jitter that depends on the outer radius of the GT mask. The second scenario is similar to the first one with the ex-

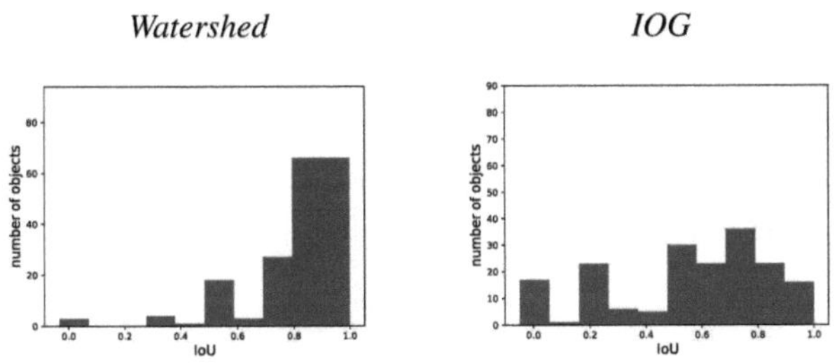

Figure 1: **IoU histograms.** (*Left*) IoUs of all annotations over all runs for *Watershed.* (*Right*) Distribution of IoUs for *IOG* with scenario two and two FG clicks.

Table 2: **Statistics of *Watershed* user benchmark runs.** We show the mean and standard deviation (std) over all annotations made in three different runs.

Data	Mean	Std
IoU	0.80	0.18
Number of Clicks	15.42	11.82
Time per Mask	28.58	24.17
Time per BBox	8.96	4.13

ception that the simulated bbox must enclose the complete GT mask. In the third scenario is the same setting as in [6], like our second scenario but with fixed instead bbox jitter instead of relative to the image size. For this analysis we use the original *IOG* model as in [6] to have a better comparability of the generalization capabilities. The network was trained on Pascal VOC [4] which consists of everyday photography images showing 20 different object categories.

3 Results and Discussion

First, the results for *Watershed* are presented in Section 3.1, followed by an analysis for the simulation with *IOG* in Section 3.2. We discuss the results in Section 3.3.

3.1 Watershed

For *Watershed,* we manually labeled the benchmark dataset three times. Due to the visual feedback of the intermediate result, we refined the annotations with additional FG and BG clicks. If a marker was set, he won't be reset during the annotation process.

Fig. 1 shows a histogram of the IoUs of all annotations with the corresponding ground truth masks for two complete runs. A majority of the annotations have IoU values above 0.8 which indicates a very high accuracy. However, as shown in Table 2, it takes on average more than 37 seconds to annotate an object. The total time required consists of two parts, the required time to draw the bounding box and the actual annotation time to draw *Watershed* markers. The annotation time is compared to the IoU in Fig. 2, where each point is representing one object. Often high IoUs can be achieved in short time, but for some examples even a long annotation time does not lead to high IoU values.

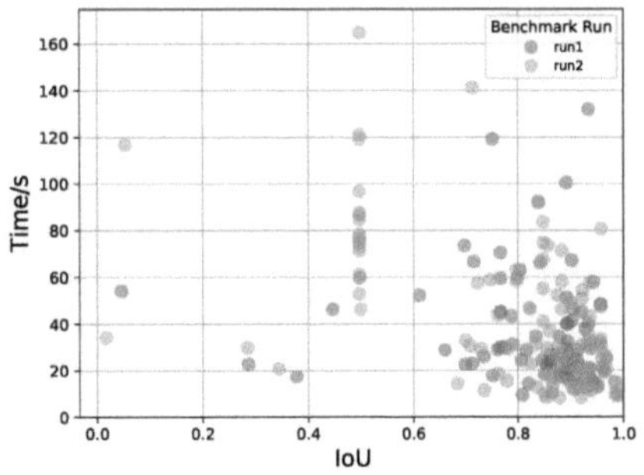

Figure 2: ***Watershed* results: IoU vs. Time.** The annotation time is not correlated to the accuracy. Just two runs are presented for clarity.

Table 3: **Statistics of *IOG* simulated user benchmark runs.** We show the mean and standard deviation (std) for the different simulation settings with two BG clicks for the bbox and one or two FG clicks.

Number of Clicks	Scenario	Mean	Std
3	1	0.35	0.27
3	2	0.51	0.32
3	3	0.50	0.33
4	1	0.39	0.30
4	2	0.56	0.28
4	3	0.53	0.34

3.2 Inside-Outside-Guidance

We evaluate the generalization capability of *IOG* with the help of different simulation settings as described in Section 2.4. The results for the three different simulation scenarios and with one or two FG clicks are shown in Table 3, respectively. Further, an IoU histogram for the second simulation scenario with two FG clicks is depicted in Fig. 1 (*right*).

3.3 Discussion

By evaluating the results manually it can be seen, that *Watershed* gives good results when the object is isolated within the cropped image and the contrast is high. Furthermore, it is advantageous if the object has a homogeneous color. If an object has multiple colors, is transparent or is occluded, the annotation is more challenging. More markers are necessary and increase the annotation time. Furthermore, in difficult situations the markers have to be set more carefully which can be time-consuming. For very low contrast to the background, e.g., due to overexposure, it can happen that an accurate annotation is not possible.

For *IOG*, the simulation works well for objects that are similar to objects shown in PASCAL VOC. Here, an accurate annotation is possible with just three or four clicks. However, for non-convex or very small objects, the simulated click positions are sometimes suboptimal. Also for *IOG*, if many objects overlap or the contrast is very low, it can happen that the method fails. Furthermore, if an object is not

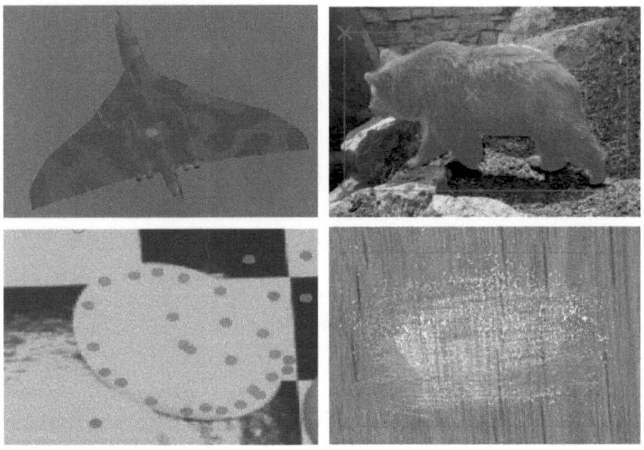

Figure 3: **Qualitative results.** Examples with very accurate results (*top row*) and failure cases (*bottom row*). The result masks are shown as green overlays and the FG and BG clicks by green and red markers.

completely inside the simulated bbox, the IoU drops significantly. If the domain of the dataset to be annotated is very different from Pascal VOC, for *IOG*, accurate annotations cannot be guaranteed with just 3 or 4 clicks.
Good and bad exemplary annotations for *IOG* and *Watershed* are shown in Fig. 3, respectively. We admit that a direct comparison between *Watershed* and *IOG* with user runs should be carried out, but this goes beyond the scope of this work.

4 Conclusion

We introduced a novel benchmark dataset for the evaluation of interactive segmentation methods across domains — MVTec ISB. In particular, the selection of images contains objects with very different characteristics that allows to evaluate the generalizability of methods and find their strengths and weaknesses. We carried out evaluations for two representative methods, *Watershed*, without learning component, and the DL-based *IOG*. Our results show that *Watershed* is versatile enough to obtain good results in most scenarios. In many cases, if there is no domain gap to the training set, *IOG* predicts accurate masks with less user interactions than *Watersheds*. However, if the simulated click-positions do not fit precisely to the underlying object or if the image domain is very different to the training set, the IoU can get very low. In future work, we will include more methods into our benchmark and perform more runs with humans in the loop instead of using simulated click-positions.

Acknowledgement

The work has been carried out at MVTec Software GmbH, Munich and supervised by the Institute of Robotics and Cognitive Systems, Universität zu Lübeck.

Author's Statement

Conflict of interest: Authors state no conflict of interest.

5 References

[1] J. Long, E. Shelhamer, and T. Darrell, "Fully Convolutional Networks for Semantic Segmentation," in *CVPR*, 2015, pp. 3431–3440.

[2] D. Zikic, Y. Ioannou, M. Brown, and A. Criminisi, "Segmentation of Brain Tumor Tissues with Convolutional Neural Networks," *MICCAI-BRATS*, vol. 36, pp. 36–39, 2014.

[3] T.-Y. Lin, M. Maire, S. Belongie, J. Hays, P. Perona, D. Ramanan, P. Dollár, and C. L. Zitnick, "Microsoft COCO: Common Objects in Context," in *ECCV*, 2014, pp. 740–755.

[4] M. Everingham, L. Gool, C. K. Williams, J. Winn, and A. Zisserman, "The Pascal Visual Object Classes (VOC) Challenge," *Int. J. Comput. Vision*, vol. 88, no. 2, pp. 303—338, 2010.

[5] K. Maninis, S. Caelles, J. Pont-Tuset, and L. Van Gool, "Deep Extreme Cut: From Extreme Points to Object Segmentation," in *CVPR*, 2018.

[6] S. Zhang, J. H. Liew, Y. Wei, S. Wei, and Y. Zhao, "Interactive Object Segmentation With Inside-Outside Guidance," in *CVPR*, 2020, pp. 12 234–12 244.

[7] L. Najman and M. Schmitt, "Watershed of a Continuous Function," *Signal Processing*, vol. 38, no. 1, pp. 99–112, 1994.

[8] M. Cordts, M. Omran, S. Ramos, T. Rehfeld, M. Enzweiler, R. Benenson, U. Franke, S. Roth, and B. Schiele, "The Cityscapes Dataset for Semantic Urban Scene Understanding," in *CVPR*, 2016, pp. 3213–3223.

[9] J. Pont-Tuset, F. Perazzi, S. Caelles, P. Arbeláez, A. Sorkine-Hornung, and L. V. Gool, "The 2017 davis challenge on video object segmentation," 2018.

[10] P. Follmann, T. Böttger, P. Härtinger, R. König, and M. Ulrich, "MVTec D2S: Densely Segmented Supermarket Dataset," in *ECCV*, 2018, pp. 581–597.

[11] P. Bergmann, M. Fauser, D. Sattlegger, and C. Steger, "MVTec AD–A Comprehensive Real-World Dataset for Unsupervised Anomaly Detection," in *CVPR*, 2019, pp. 9592–9600.

[12] S. H. Rezatofighi, N. Tsoi, J. Gwak, A. Sadeghian, I. D. Reid, and S. Savarese, "Generalized Intersection over Union: A Metric and A Loss for Bounding Box Regression," *CoRR*, vol. abs/1902.09630, 2019.

Evaluation of the SRM Algorithm of Siemens CERA for CT Half Beam Reconstruction

Clara Thiede [1,2], Maximilian Wattenberg [3,4], Philipp Klein [2], and Mareike Töpperwien [2]
[1] Medical Engineering Science, Universität zu Lübeck, clara.thiede@student.uni-luebeck.de
[2] YXLON International GmbH, Hamburg,{mareike.toepperwien, philipp.klein}@hbg.yxlon.com
[3]Intitute of Medical Engineering, Universität zu Lübeck, wattenberg@imt.uni-luebeck.de
[4] Fraunhofer Research Institution for Individualized and Cell-Based Medical Engineering IMTE, Lübeck

Abstract

Computed tomography (CT) is industrially used for non-destructive testing since the large penetration depth is ideal for visualizing internal structures. The Feldkamp, Davis, and Kress (FDK) algorithm is designed to reconstruct CT-volumes for equidistantly sampled circle trajectories in cone-beam geometry. For trajectories deviating from the classical circle trajectory, Siemens developed a new special reconstruction method (SRM) for their proprietary reconstruction software CERA, which promises better image quality due to an application-specific adapted filtering scheme. In this study, both reconstruction methods were compared for simulated and experimental data obtained in a half beam scan setup, in which the position of the rotation axis is shifted to the edge of the field of view. The experiments show a quality advantage of the SRM compared to the FDK, especially around the rotation axis at the radius corresponding to the half beam overlap, while the reconstruction time is longer. The relative difference, however, decreases with increasing projection data size.

1 Introduction

Computed tomography (CT) is a widely used technique in daily clinical practice to image internal anatomical features in three dimensions. In the last decades, it has become more and more important in the industrial environment for non-destructive testing, e.g. to perform failure analysis or dimensional measurements. Due to its considerable penetration depth, it is ideal for visualizing internal structures.
In contrast to clinical applications, industrial CT allows for rotating the object instead of the X-ray source and the detector, which is mechanically more straightforward. In the classical case, often denoted as circle trajectory, images are acquired in equidistant angular steps during a full 360° rotation of the object. To obtain information about the three-dimensional structure of the object from the recorded projections, a tomographic reconstruction must be performed. Johann Radon provided the mathematical foundations for this in 1917, leading to the widely known filtered back projection (FBP) algorithm, which is valid for parallel beams [1]. In industrial applications, however, most often diverging beams emanating from a quasi point source are used, which requires an adaptation of the FBP algorithm.
The Feldkamp, Davis, and Kress (FDK) algorithm presented in 1984 is the most commonly used reconstruction method for circular CT scans in cone-beam geometry since it is relatively fast [2], [3], [4].
In industrial CT, it is often necessary to scan objects that are larger than the field of view (FOV) provided by the classic circle trajectory. To sample the object sufficiently for reconstruction, only 180°, plus the opening angle of the beam, have to be acquired, leading to redundant information when a 360° scan is performed. This redundancy of information can be used to artificially increase the FOV by moving the rotation axis to the edge of the FOV such that different parts of the object are illuminated during a full 360° scan. In this so-called half beam geometry, the FOV can be extended up to twice its size without increasing the scan time. There are two ways to achieve this:

1. shifting the detector
2. shifting the object (rotation axis).

In this paper, the object shift was analyzed. In Fig. 1 a generic sketch of the setup is shown. Due to the overlap, only the inner part of the sample is illuminated during the entire 360° scan, which, in contrast to the classic circle trajectory, leads to a non-uniform sampling of the volume. Considering that FDK and especially the weighting of the back projection is optimized for circle scans, artifacts are a logical effect of reconstruction of a half beam scan without consideration of the changed geometry. Therefore, an adaptation of the filtering is required. The reconstruction software CERA 6.0 (Siemens Healthcare GmbH, Erlangen, Germany) offers a half beam weighting for the integrated FDK algorithm, but this is considered deprecated and often artifacts, as seen in Fig. 2 occur. Instead, the newly developed special reconstruction method (SRM) algorithm is recommended, which was designed as an alternative to the

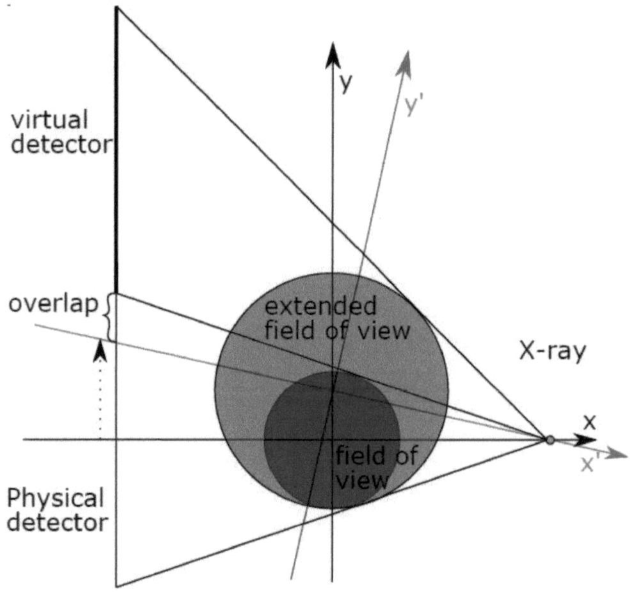

Figure 1: Half beam scan set up with shifted rotation axis configuration allows for a FOV of twice the size (depending on the relative overlap, at least 5% are recommended).

FDK algorithm for trajectories deviating from the circular scan. It is supposed to yield better image quality at the expense of reconstruction time [5].

In this paper, both algorithms were compared for simulated as well as experimental data. The resulting image quality was evaluated using two different visual methods to assess whether the artifacts seen in the FDK reconstruction could be prevented with the SRM algorithm without affecting the image quality in the remaining parts of the volume. Additionally, the difference in reconstruction time for the FDK and the SRM algorithms was evaluated concerning the projection size as well as the number of projections, as cycle time is often a critical factor in industrial applications.

2 Material and Methods

2.1 Data Acquisition

For the investigation of the influence of the reconstruction algorithms on the half beam scan, a mono-material engine head was simulated using aRTist (Analytical Radiographic Testing Inspection Simulation Tool, BAM Federal Institute for Materials Research and Testing, Berlin, Germany). It is a software tool for numerical simulations, which generates realistic radiographs based on virtual part representations and well-defined radiological parameters [6]. For the simulation the following parameters were used: source: tungsten anode, 450 kV acceleration voltage; detector: 768 × 768 pixel with pixel size 0.556 μm; FocusObjectDistance: 450 mm, FocusDetectorDistance: 1200 mm, object shift along y (Fig. 1): 72.06 mm; 1440 projections.

The cross-evaluation for inconsistencies in the real CT-system was executed with a pomegranate on an YXLON FF20 CT, with the settings: microfocus tube, acceleration voltage: 170 kV, tube current: 50 μA; exposure time: 250 ms, 1440 projections; detector: 1792 × 2176 pixel, pixel area: 24.9 × 30.2 cm, 2 × 2 binning, magnification: 6.09. The center of the pomegranate's rotation axis had to be aligned with the edge of the detector with an overlap of 10% to complete the half beam scan.

Due to the deterministic nature of both, the FDK and SRM, the duration of the reconstruction on the same computer does only depend on the size of the data set. Thus, the reconstruction time tests were done on a high-resolution circle trajectory data set, which were sampled to the sizes documented in Table 1 on a reconstruction PC with two Quadro M6000 (RAM: 12 GB) graphics cards. The projections data was scaled with ImageJ (Wayne Rasband, National Institutes of Health, Bethesda, USA) to different sizes, as stated in Table 1. From 307^2 up to 1843^2, all combinations of the number of pixels and projections were tested ten times alternating FDK and SRM. Due to the excessive time required for the reconstruction of data sets with more than 2150^2 pixels, only the tests for the data sets with 4140 projections were performed.

Table 1: Reconstruction time parameters with all tested combinations.

# voxels	# pixels	# projections
3072^3	3072^2	4140
2765^3	2765^2	4140
2458^3	2458^2	4140
2150^3	2150^2	4140
1843^3	1843^2	4140, 2070, 1380, 1035, 828
1536^3	1536^2	4140, 2070, 1380, 1035, 828
1229^3	1229^2	4140, 2070, 1380, 1035, 828
1024^3	1024^2	4140, 2070, 1380, 1035, 828
922^3	922^2	4140, 2070, 1380, 1035, 828
768^3	768^2	4140, 2070, 1380, 1035, 828
614^3	614^2	4140, 2070, 1380, 1035, 828
307^3	307^2	4140, 2070, 1380, 1035, 828

2.2 Image Quality

To evaluate the image quality visually, two different methods were used. The first step was to compare the obtained data. The same slice in the xy-planes, which showcased the centering artifact in the FDK image, was selected for both FDK and SRM. A difference image was calculated from the reconstruction results of SRM and FDK, generated from the same slice, reducing the visual dominance of the object and characterizing the form of the artifacts more clearly.

The second method was a visual comparison of the reconstructed simulated data with the corresponding polygonal surface mesh, which were manually aligned in VGSTUDIO MAX (Volume Graphics GmbH, Heidelberg, Germany), a professional analysis tool for volumetric image data [7]. After defining the surface of the engine head with the method of finding the largest grey value gradient on a

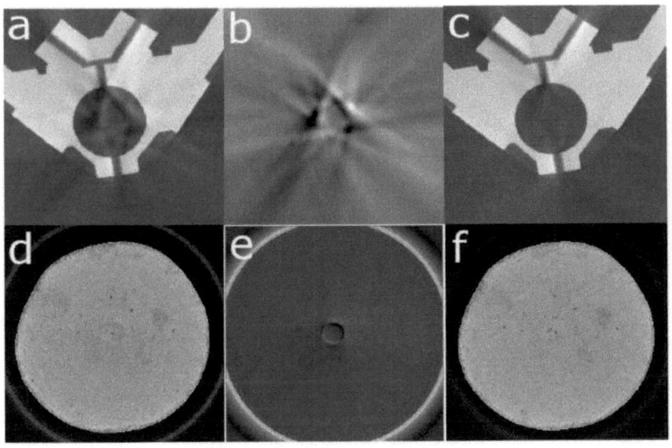

Figure 2: Upper row engine head, lower row pomegranate, (a) and (d) FDK, (c) and (f) SRM, (b) and (e) difference images.

first surface based on the ISO 50 in the histogram, the differences between the surface mesh and the object were visible [8].
The acquired data from the pomegranate was analyzed with the same methods as the simulated data, except that instead of a polygonal surface mesh, the SRM reconstructed volume was utilized as the ground truth. This way the disparity between SRM and FDK was emphasized.

2.3 Reconstruction Time

The median was taken from the ten reconstruction times to prevent influences from outliers. This was necessary because the workstation was used concurrently for other researchers. The reconstruction time was analyzed based on the dependency of projection size, number of projections, and the relative difference of SRM and FDK.

3 Results and Discussion

Visual Image Quality

Fig. 2 shows the generated images with artifacts close to the rotation axis in the FDK image (a). They appear to be round and the radius corresponds to the small overlap that needs to be present in half beam scan. These artifacts in the center are absent in the SRM image (c). The other visible artifacts, which are characterized by dark shadows around the edges of the object, mainly occur because of beam hardening, a well known cause of artifacts due to the polychromatic energy of the X-ray beam. They are similar in SRM and FDK, despite the centering artifacts overlaying the beam hardening artifacts. The difference image (b) only shows the centering artifacts of the FDK, and no structural information remains. Therefore it can be concluded, that SRM provides huge advantages compared to FDK close to the rotation axis, but in the rest of the volume, there is no significant difference. The image of the pomegranate (d) demonstrates the same artifact in the area associated with the overlap. Subtracting the SRM image from the FDK one emphasizes the differences, which in this case is the artifact in the center and the ring around the pomegranate. This ring on the outside is visible in (f) as well, but it is not as prominent as in (d).

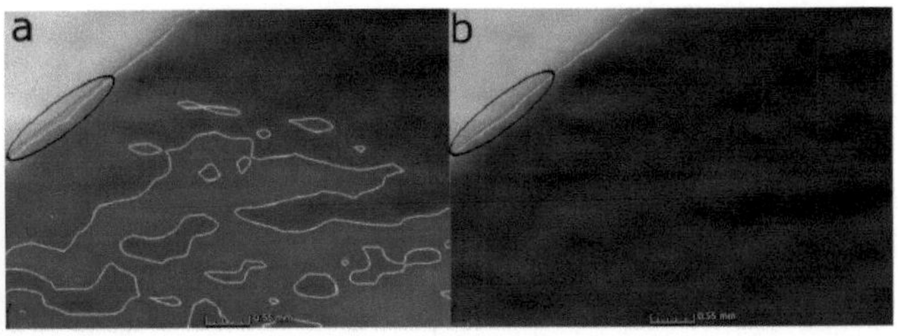

Figure 3: Surface comparison of simulated engine head reconstructed with FDK (a) and SRM (b) with the 3D model.

Detected Surface

Fig. 3 illustrates the comparison of the identified surface of the reconstructed volume with respect to the 3D model (dark grey line). The artifact in (a) in the middle is falsely detected by the algorithm as a surface. No false-positive detection of the surface is present in Fig. 3 (b), due to the smoothness of the background. Other than that, a slight advantage in favor of the SRM algorithm can be seen in the areas circled in black. The white line, which corresponds to the surface based on the SRM volume, matches the ideal object model with high accuracy and can therefore hardly be seen in Fig. 3 (b).

Reconstruction Time

For each projection size considered in this study, the use of the FDK algorithm resulted in a faster reconstruction of the tomographic volume compared to the SRM algorithm. The relative advantage, however, decreases with increasing projection size, leading to almost identical reconstruction times for the largest dataset (Fig. 4 (a)). The slower reconstruction comes from more complex preprocessing, which depends cubically on the size of the projection images. The reconstruction step itself depends quartically on the projection size, meaning at some point the reconstruction is the dominating factor for the total time. This results in a neglectable time difference in preprocessing. At a projection size of 2458^2 pixels in Fig. 4 (a) and (b), the reconstruction time of the FDK algorithm falls below the expected 700 s. This outlier is reproducible and could be a result of handling the storage differently but has not yet been conclusively clarified. Aside from this, the number of pixels follows roughly the expected quartic function (Fig. 4 (b)). The number of projections has a linear impact (Fig. 4 (c)) on the reconstruction time as expected. As the complexity of reconstruction processes at this scale dominates many applications, and due to the small variance within the measurements, the results are assumed to be reliable, despite

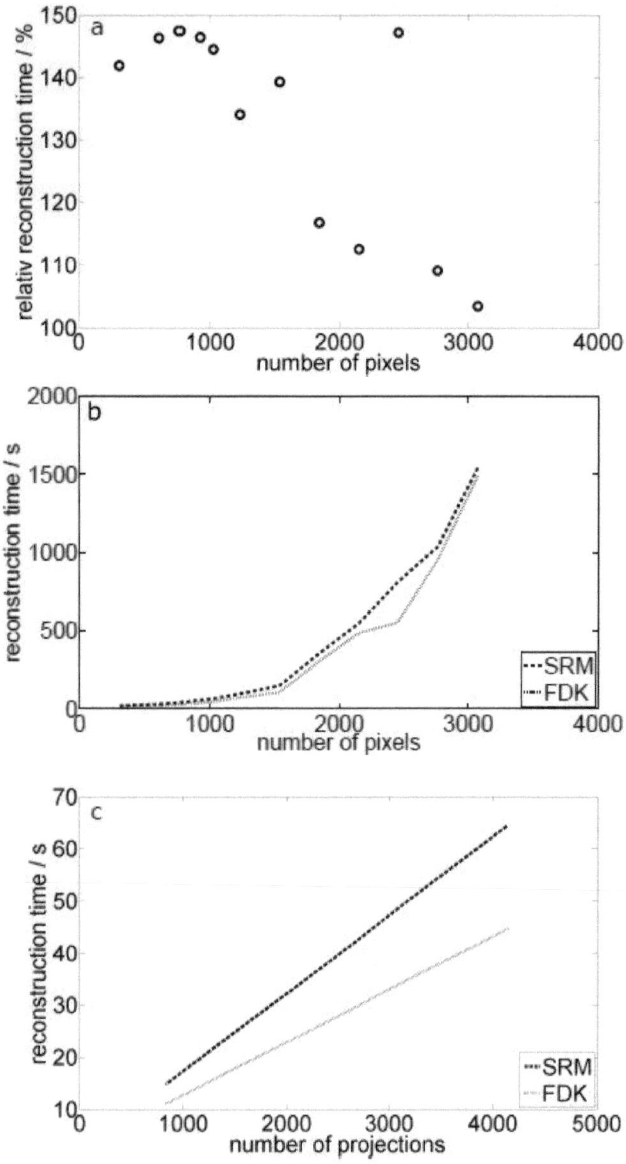

Figure 4: Plots of the reconstruction time (a) relative difference of SRM and FDK, (b) relation pixel size and time (4140 projections), (c) relation number of projections and time (1024^2 pixel).

simultaneous usage of the workstation. However, the results of the current study can be improved by using a PC exclusively for the tests.

4 Conclusion

The present work shows that in the case of CT scans in half beam geometry, the newly developed SRM algorithm has large advantages in terms of image quality compared to the FDK algorithm. The observed artifacts, which in the latter case arise due to unideal filtering in the oversampled region close to the rotation axis, are reduced or have even disappeared completely while the differences in the remaining volume are negligible or even show a small advantage of the SRM algorithm. However, this gain in image quality comes at the price of a longer time needed for reconstruction of the volumes. Especially for small projection sizes, the relative difference is large. It shows a clear advantage of the FDK algorithm, although the absolute time difference is only on the order of a few seconds or even less. With increasing projection size, the relative time difference decreases, resulting in nearly identical reconstruction times for the largest data sets considered in this study.

Acknowledgement

The work has been carried out at YXLON International GmbH, Hamburg, and was supervised by the Institute of Medical Engineering of the Universität zu Lübeck.

Author's Statement

Conflict of interest: Authors state no conflict of interest.

5 References

[1] J. Radon, "Über die Bestimmung von Funktionen durch ihre Integralwerte längs gewisser Mannigfaltigkeiten," *Berichte über die Verhandlungen der königlich sächsischen Gesellschaft der Wissenschaften zu Leipzig. Journal of Mathematical Physics*, no. 69, pp. 262–277, 1917.

[2] L. A. Feldkamp, L. C. Davis, and J. Kress, "Practical cone-beam algorithm," *J. Opt. Soc. Am. A*, vol. 1, no. 6, pp. 612–619, Jun 1984.

[3] T. M. Buzug, *Computed Tomography - From Photon Statistics to Modern Cone Beam CT*. Berlin Heidelberg: Springer Science und Business Media, 2008.

[4] B. Bier, "C-arm Cone-Beam Computed Tomography Reconstruction for Knee Imaging under Weight-Bearing Conditions," Ph.D. dissertation, Friedrich-Alexander-Universität Erlangen-Nürnberg, 2019.

[5] *CERA User manual, English Version 6*, Siemens Healthcare GmbH, 2019.

[6] C. Bellon and G.-R. Jaenisch, "aRTist-analytical RT inspection simulation tool," *International Symposium on Digital industrial Radiology and Computed Tomography*, 2007.

[7] *VGSTUDIO MAX 3.4 Brochure*, Volume Graphics GmbH, 2019.

[8] F. Borges de Oliveira, A. Stolfi, M. Bartscher, L. Chiffre, and U. Neuschaefer-Rube, "Experimental investigation of surface determination process on multi-material components for dimensional computed tomography," *Case Studies in Nondestructive Testing and Evaluation*, vol. 6, 05 2016.

Sparse Normalized Local Binary Patterns – A Structure-Based Depth Measure –

Steffen Hagedorn[1,2] and Jens Dekarz[2]
[1] Robotics and Autonomous Systems, Universität zu Lübeck, steffen.hagedorn@student.uni-luebeck.de
[2] Research and Development: New Technology, Basler AG Ahrensburg

Abstract

We introduce Sparse Normalized Local Binary Patterns (SNLBP), an extension of the structure measure Local Binary Patterns (LBP) for scene depth measurement. LBP cannot be used as a blur measure in a depth from defocus approach since it is not structure-invariant. Our approach proposes a normalization of LBP to achieve structure invariance. Additionally, the depth measure is sparsely restricted to structured image regions. In experiments on a new defocus dataset we investigate if SNLBP qualifies as a depth measure. The results confirm structure invariance and exhibit a correlation of SNLBP and actual scene depth. Determining a mathematical expression for this correlation will be the next step.

1 Introduction

1.1 Problem Statement

Depth measurement is an important part of scene understanding. Conventional stereo vision setups have a broad base width between the two cameras and are susceptible to thermal deformations. Thus, a guaranteed mechanical resilience requires precise and expensive manufacturing. In contrast, small handheld devices are less costly and underly smaller thermal deformations but do not allow for a large base width. When keeping the object at a constant distance, decreasing the base width also decreases the disparity of the stereo images, making the depth measurement less precise. To compensate for this loss in precision, defocus methods can provide additional depth information. Defocus methods leverage the relation of blur and scene depth in 2D projections of 3D scenes.
We propose that defocus method and stereo vision operate on common input images. Both methods have concurring requirements. On one hand, reliable feature points for disparity estimation are mostly described by high frequencies. On the other hand, defocus blur leads to their loss. To resolve the concurring requirements, we use a defocus method that gains depth information from subtle changes in image sharpness.
Local Binary Patterns (LBP) is a method which estimates small changes in image structure. A high amount of image structure implies sharpness. The method is made for focus segmentation and is computationally inexpensive. This work extends the applicability of LBP to scene depth measurement, introducing Sparse Normalized LBP (SNLBP). As the method can work on its own, we disregard the combination with stereo vision for now and focus on fundamental assessment: Does SNLBP qualify as a depth measure?

1.2 Related Work

Defocus methods measure scene depth based on the degree of blur. Extraction of blur information can be performed either in frequency or intensity domain [1], [6].
Frequency domain methods use the fact that sharp regions contain higher frequencies than blurred regions. Generally, they first transform the image from spatial domain into frequency domain and then apply filter banks to extract different frequencies. Backtransformation into spatial domain establishes a relation between frequencies and their location in the image, facilitating blur measurement [1].
Intensity domain methods work either directly on the image intensity or its gradient. Gradient methods are based on the assumption that depth variations correspond to a change in image intensity, i.e. depth information can only be extracted at edges. One example for a gradient method is the Ratio of Gaussians that uses the first spatial derivative and a Gaussian blur model to measure depth [8]. Defocus Magnification also operates on the intensity gradient but uses the second derivative [2].
Image intensity methods mostly rely on local statistical measures and operate directly on pixel values [1]. The underlying assumption is that sharp regions have a higher variance than defocused regions [5]. Local Binary Patterns (LBP) leverages subtle variations of pixel intensity in a local neighborhood to determine blur which is ideal for the combination with stereo vision.

2 Material and Methods

Defocus methods are based on the relation of blur and distance from focal plane, described by the thin lens equation. Our approach uses Local Binary Patterns to measure blur.

2.1 Local Binary Patterns Operator

Local Binary Patterns is a method that is originally applied to segment focused regions of a scene [7]. Therefor, a 3×3 pixels large local neighborhood is masked with different binary patterns. The center pixel of the mask is set as base value. Similarity function $S(x)$ in Eqn. 1 applies a threshold T_{LBP} that determines the largest tolerated deviation $|x|$ from base value. If $|x|$ exceeds T_{LBP}, a pixel is said to deviate from the center pixel, else it is interpreted as similar:

$$S(x) = \begin{cases} 1 & |x| \geq T_{LBP} \\ 0 & \text{else} \end{cases} . \quad (1)$$

$S(x)$ is calculated for eight positions on a circle with radius r_{LBP} (cf. Fig. 1). To determine the values at the positions on the circle, bilinear interpolation is used. This results in nine possible so-called uniform binary patterns (UBP). Uniformity means the property of all neighbor pixels with $S(x) = 1$ to form a connected cluster and all other pixels to form a second connected cluster. Fig. 1 shows the nine UBP. Further, all rotations of a pattern are considered equal. Non-uniform binary patterns are summarized in a 10th category.

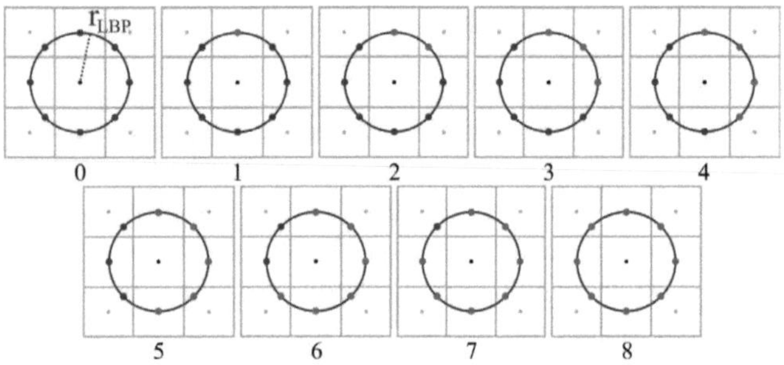

Figure 1: The nine uniform rotationally invariant binary patterns with the center pixel shown as a black dot, interpolated neighboring pixels below T_{LBP} as blue dots, and above T_{LBP} as red dots. All positions on the circle have distance r_{LBP} to the center as shown in pattern 0 [7].

An unambiguous encoding based on $S(x)$ facilitates clear distinction of the patterns and is performed for each pixel. Comparing the histogram of sharp and blurred regions of the LBP-encoded image in Fig. 2 shows that patterns 6 to 9 characterize sharpness. Accordingly, the pixelwise blur

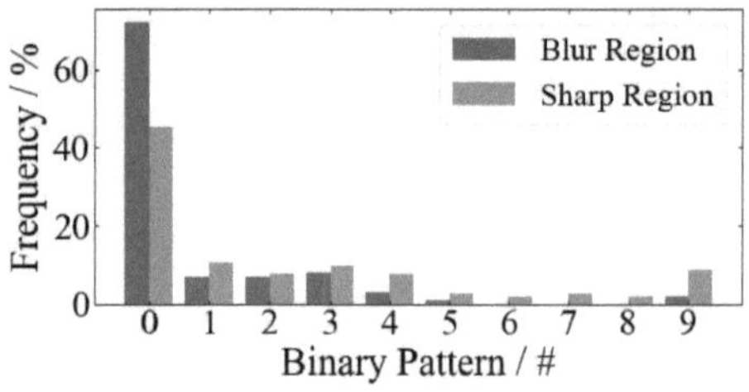

Figure 2: Histogram of LBP in sharp and blurred image regions. Patterns 6 to 9 occur significantly more often in sharp regions [7].

measure m_{LBP} is defined as the mean value over a local window with N pixels, considering only patterns 6 to 9:

$$m_{LBP} = \frac{1}{N} \sum_{i=6}^{9} n(LBP_i) \quad (2)$$

where $n(LBP_i)$ is the number of patterns of type i. In the following, an image where m_{LBP} has been calculated for each pixel is referred to as an LBP map.

2.2 Sparse Normalization

The LBP map represents image structure. Thresholding is sufficient to segment sharp regions [7]. However, we observe that objects at equal distance yield different values for m_{LBP} (cf. Fig 5 (b)). The lack of structure invariance makes the measure unemployable for scene depth measurement. A-priori knowledge on image structure for all image regions resolves this problem. We use a second image that is captured all-in-focus to provide the desired information. In a small base width stereo vision setup, the second image is already available. The general idea of normalization for structure invariance was conceived by [3] but not applied in the context of depth from defocus to our knowledge.
The pixelwise ratio of defocus LBP map (focus on nearest object and shallow depth of focus) and all-in-focus LBP map depends on the degree of blur (m_{LBP}) of a pixel in both images. Close objects are sharp in both images and yield values near one, independent of their structure. Distant objects are blurred in the defocus image and sharp in the all-in-focus image, yielding a ratio directly related to distance. Pixels blurred in both images imply that there simply is no structure and are problematic since they tend to yield a ratio near one, suggesting close distance.
We solve this problem by introducing an additional threshold T_{sparse} (cf. Fig. 3) and consider only pixels that satisfy $m_{LBP} > T_{sparse}$ in the all-in-focus image. This excludes image regions with a low amount of structure. The result is referred to as sparse normalization in the following.

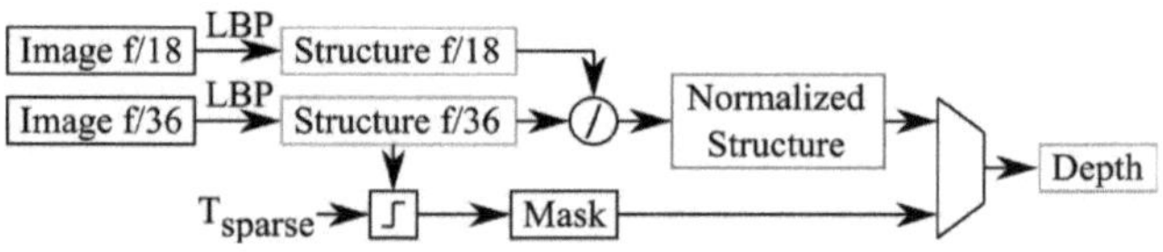

Figure 3: Flow chart of our approach. LBP maps, normalized, and sparse normalized LBP map are outlined in orange, blue, and green, respectively.

2.3 Experimental Setup

Practical experiments were performed on a new defocus dataset. It comprises three targets, shown in Fig. 4, each with the aim of investigating different structures. A target consists of four panels with structures ranging from coarse to fine. Five targets of same type are placed with $\Delta z = 100$ mm between each other along the optical axis, starting at a distance of 1400 mm from the camera's sensor plane. The lateral offset between two consequtive targets is 50 mm.

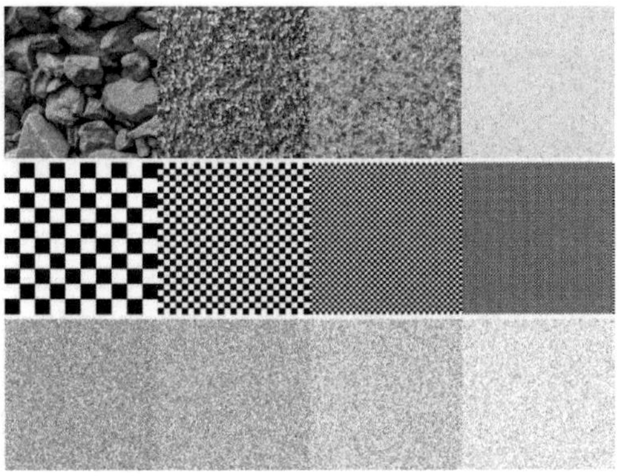

Figure 4: Targets used in the experiments, each ranging from coarse to fine structures. Target (a) exhibits natural structures, (b) repetitive checkerboard structures, (c) noise structures sampled with different black/white-ratios.

Target 0 is the nearest one. For symmetry, the third target is placed on the optical axis.
A Sony Alpha 6500 DSLM with an SEL18200 lens was used to capture the images with constant ISO 1250 and different apertures ranging from f/6.3 to f/36. The resolution was reduced from 24 MP to 1.5 MP. Fig. 5 (a) and (b) show two images of the setup with natural targets shot at f/18 and f/36, respectively, and define the used terminology.

3 Results and Discussion

3.1 Normalization

Fig. 5 (b) and (d) demonstrate how image structure is quantified in the LBP map. Computing the Normalized LBP (NLBP) from these two maps yields the result shown in Fig. 5 (e). Our observations confirm that the main problem are regions with little structure, like the background. Fig. 5 (f) shows that SNLBP improves the result by discarding those regions and introducing structure-invariance. Panels in top and bottom row of the targets are not considered by sparse normalization. In the top row, we assume this happens because the structures are too fine for the camera to resolve and lead to locally homogeneous regions in the image. In the bottom row, structures are too coarse and include nearly homogeneous areas. Both cases lead to patterns 0 to 5 from Fig. 1, consequently not adding to m_{LBP}. Adapting parameters allows to adjust the working range, i.e. the amount of structure the operator is sensitive to. Section 3.2 addresses this topic. The remaining values show a clear progression from bright values at target zero to darker values at target four. Also, the values are nearly constant across all panels of one target. The values on the floor coincide with those of the target at equal distance.
Statistical evaluation confirms these observations. The arithmetic mean is calculated for each panel of each target, not considering zeros in case of the SNLBP map. Fig. 6 (a) and (b) show the averaged values for the LBP map from Fig. 5 (b) and the SNLBP map from Fig. 5 (f), respectively. Our normalization process induces structure invariance. The top row of the natural targets has structures that are too fine for the method with given parameters. Before normalization, the top row panel's graph is between bottom row panels and the second row of panels from the bottom, contrary to our expectation. Sparse normalization eliminated this shortcoming and correctly excluded the top row of the target. Further, the values of target zero are close to one and consistently decrease with the actual target distance. This means that SNLBP correlates with scene depth. Table 1 confirms the visual assessment that all graphs in the sparse normalized plot are closer to each other than without normalization. We compare the relative standard deviations of initial, normalized, and sparse normalized LBP map across all panels of one target. The results show that sparse normalization yields the best result for all structures. It is worth mentioning that the repetetive structures of the checkerboards lead to aliasing effects that impair the results of distant targets.

Table 1: Relative Standard Deviation / %

S	M	T0	T1	T2	T3	T4
NT	LBP	10.4	12.81	16.98	17.94	17.04
NT	N	8.42	5.17	0.76	3.2	5.36
NT	SN	1.88	1.98	1.5	4.57	4.22
CB	LBP	31.12	46.45	54.35	55.54	60.65
CB	N	27.17	5.88	10.13	13.38	11.38
CB	SN	0.6	2.17	7.59	9.56	10.16
NS	LBP	3.71	3.19	4.13	2.39	1.94
NS	N	3.52	3.24	1.83	2.41	3.61
NS	SN	1.11	0.48	1.43	2.54	0.63

S: Structure (NT: Natural, CB: Checkerboard, NS: Noise), **M**: Measure (LBP: Local Binary Pattern Map, N: Normalized LBP Map, SN: SNLBP Map), **T0-T4**: Target Index

3.2 Influence of Parameters

T_{LBP} =0.0001 and $N = 441$ are constant for all results shown in the paper to ensure comparability. T_{sparse} was set to 213 for natural, 170 for checkerboard, and 190 for noise structures. Increasing T_{LBP} or T_{sparse} intensifies the sparseness of the sparse normalized LBP map. Reducing N leads to more noisy LBP maps. r_{LBP} has an important impact on the sparse LBP map. As is demonstrated in Fig. 7, LBP with smaller radius are sensitive to fine structures while a larger radius shifts the sensitivity to coarser structures. The figure also demonstrates that the method is unsuited for very coarse structures with homogeneous regions like the lower panels of the checkerboard targets. When increasing the radius even further, we do not get any meaningful results for our experimental scenes.

4 Conclusion and Future Work

An extension of LBP for depth measurement was introduced. Feasibility of our approach has been proven in prac-

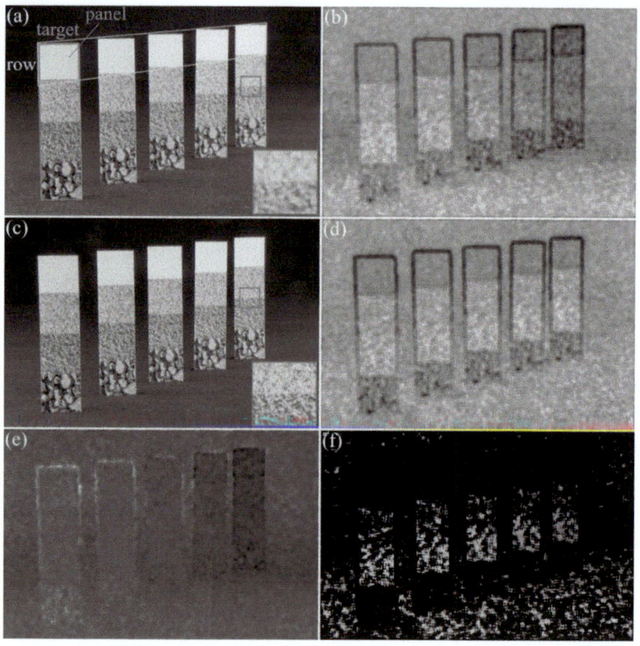

Figure 5: Results of our method. Images with natural structure targets taken at f/18 and f/36 are shown in (a) and (c), respectively. An enlarged cut-out of panels 1 and 2 of the most distant target is shown in the lower right corner, each. Terminology definitions are illustrated in (a). Subfigures (b) and (d) display the LBP maps of the images from (a) and (c), respectively. Here, bright pixels stand for a high amount of structure while dark pixels describe a lack of structure. Division of (b) by (d) yields the normalized LBP map in (e). Bright pixels encode close distance and dark pixels mean large distance. The same applies to our sparse normalized LBP map, displayed in (f). Note that completely black pixels stand for discarded values that do not provide reliable depth information due to lack of structure.

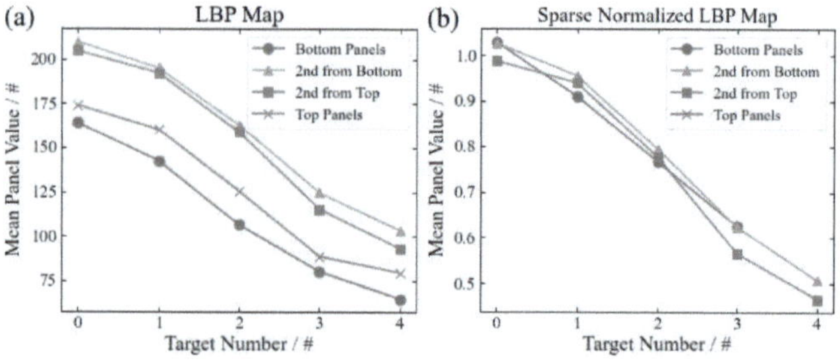

Figure 6: Comparison of LBP map (a) and sparse normalized LBP map (b). Our normalization discards inapplicable values, scales objects in the focal plane to distance 1 and induces structure-invariance.

tical experiments. The results show a correlation of our sparse normalized LBP with actual scene depth, thus qualifying as a depth measure.
Since the method comprises multiple parameters, it is going to be necessary to automize their optimal adaption. Further, it seems advantageous to combine results achived with different r_{LBP} into a single depthmap, hereby extending the sensitivity to a large range of structures. Depending on the application scenario, propagation of sparse to dense depth estimate might be useful. This could be achieved by superpixel-based strategies [4]. For other scenarios it might be benefitial to work on our sparse representation.

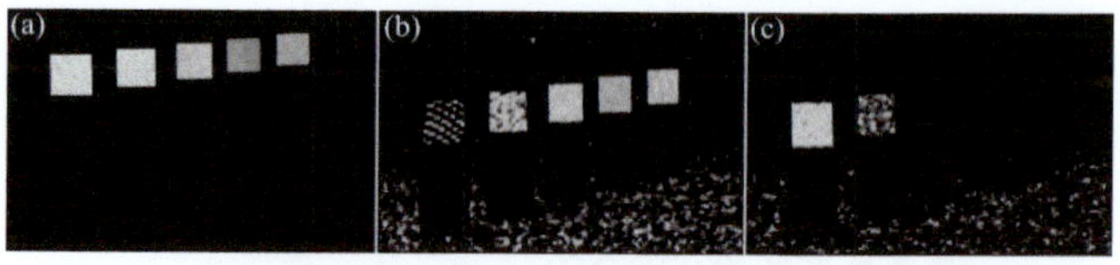

Figure 7: Influence of r_{LBP} on the sparse normalized LBP map demonstrated on checkerboard targets with $r_{LBP} = 1, 3, 4$ in (a), (b), and (c), respectively. A small radius extracts fine structures while large radii are sensitive to coarser structures.

Acknowledgement

The work has been carried out at Basler AG, Ahrensburg and supervised by Prof. Dr. Mattias Heinrich, Institute of Medical Informatics, Universität zu Lübeck. We thank Basler AG for their financial and scientific support.

Author's Statement

Conflict of interest: Authors state no conflict of interest.

References

[1] Usman Ali and Muhammad Tariq Mahmood. "Analysis of blur measure operators for single image blur segmentation". In: *Applied Sciences* 8.5 (2018), p. 807.

[2] Soonmin Bae and Frédo Durand. "Defocus magnification". In: *Computer Graphics Forum*. Vol. 26. 3. Wiley Online Library. 2007, pp. 571–579.

[3] Max Born and E Wolf. *Principles of Optics, 3rd (revised) edition.* 1965.

[4] Ding-Jie Chen, Hwann-Tzong Chen, and Long-Wen Chang. "Fast defocus map estimation". In: *ICIP*. 2016, pp. 3962–3966.

[5] T Vu Cuong, D Phan Thien, and M Chandler Damon. "A spectral and spatial measure of local perceived sharpness in natural images". In: *IEEE Trans. Image Process.* 21 (2012), pp. 934–945.

[6] Jianping Shi, Li Xu, and Jiaya Jia. "Just noticeable defocus blur detection and estimation". In: *Proceedings of the IEEE CCVPR*. 2015, pp. 657–665.

[7] Xin Yi and Mark Eramian. "LBP-based segmentation of defocus blur". In: *IEEE transactions on image processing* 25.4 (2016), pp. 1626–1638.

[8] Shaojie Zhuo and Terence Sim. "Defocus map estimation from a single image". In: *Pattern Recognition* 44.9 (2011), pp. 1852–1858.

Multi-Depth Segmentation on Holographic Data using CNNs

Noah Heldt [1], Philipp Grüning [2] and Falk Nette [3]

[1] Medical Engineering Science, Universität zu Lübeck, noah.heldt@student.uni-luebeck.de
[2] Institute for Neuro- and Bioinformatics, Universität zu Lübeck, Lübeck, Germany, gruening@inb.uni-luebeck.de
[3] Fraunhofer EMB, Lübeck, Germany, falk.hendrik.nette@emb.fraunhofer.de

Abstract

Cell segmentation is a widespread tool to investigate in-vitro cells but still poses a challenge as cells can overlap and therefore occlude each other, when placed in a three-dimensional environment, making it impossible to distinguish them with binary segmentation. We investigate the three-dimensional segmentation capabilities of convolutional neural networks (CNNs) based on raw images captured with Lens-Free Digital Inline Holography, an imaging technique that substantially lowers the cost of microscopes. For this purpose, we simulated challenging training data, featuring overlapping cells, based on real holograms, which we used to train a CNN. In this work, we show that such a network indeed is capable of segmenting the cells while simultaneously extracting their depth information. Therefore, our method could possibly be used to enhance cell tracking capabilities especially for complicated situations featuring crossing cell tracks, by providing the additional depth-information of cells.

1 Introduction

Observing the movement of cells can lead to insights about their function, state and may indicate certain diseases. To yield a sound statistical evaluation, experimental tools need to segment and track cells with high accuracy while also being sufficiently fast for high-throughput analysis. We aim to develop such tools combined with a promising alternative to widefield microscopes: Lens-free digital inline holography (LFDIH) [1]. This low-cost lens-free imaging method can capture a large field of view and yield three-dimensional information. However, a computationally expensive reconstruction is needed to transform the raw input data into informative images for a human observer. For the imaging process, semi-coherent light illuminates the whole sample from above, leading to diffraction artifacts which are captured by a CMOS photochip below the sample. An exemplary image, as well as its algorithmic reconstruction as Phase-Shift Minimum Intensity Projection (PSMIP), can be seen in Fig. 1. A schematic of the microscope is depicted in Fig. 2. Though it has been shown that convolutional neural networks (CNNs) can successfully replace these time consuming algorithms, by being able to learn how to perform the reconstruction of holograms [2], we observed in previous experiments that CNNs could even provide a fast and accurate segmentation of raw data [3]. Therefore, no reconstruction is needed. Although effective, this approach may not sufficiently deal with overlapping or occluded cells. For example, two cells in the same (x, y) position of the image sensor but at different heights, z_0 and z_1, cannot be distinguished by one segmentation map. This can, for example, cause problems for tracking algorithms as the number of cells present in each frame is varying. In this work, we extend CNNs to compute two or more segmentation maps based on their depth, which we call layers. For the above mentioned example, the first cell would appear in a different layer than the second cell. Thus, the cells can be distinguished, which in turn simplifies the tracking.

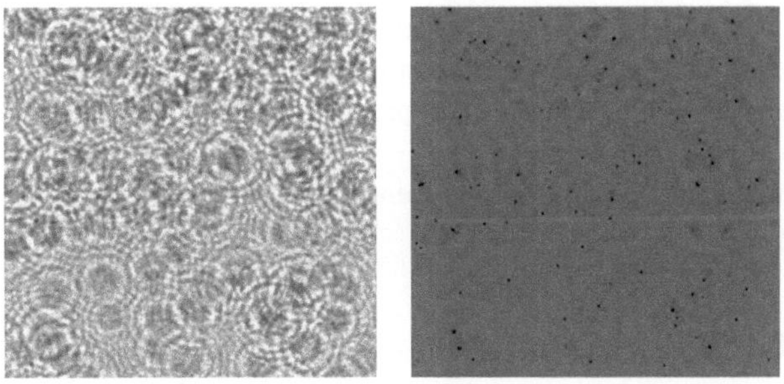

Figure 1: Left: cropped example of the raw holograms. Right: algorithmic reconstruction of the cells.

2 Material and Methods

The reconstruction of holograms is possible because the wave interference and light-matter interaction of the imaging method is known. The light field can be numerically estimated at any distance using e.g. the angular spectrum method, which yields a complex light field, therefore allowing for images depicting the absorption as well as phase-shifting by the sample. However, with this knowledge, the opposite process of generating a hologram from a given reconstruction is also possible. Given a cell in fo-

cus at a distance z, we can propagate this cell to the sensor plane. Apart from imaging artifacts and phase properties of cells, simulated holograms are hard to distinguish from real data, and thus, we can create insightful datasets to evaluate CNN methods. To keep our data as realistic as possible, we used cells from authentic segmentation maps and propagated them to arbitrary depths. We acquired the segmentation maps by thresholding PSMIP reconstructions of LFDIH time-lapse recordings [4] in which cells within a three-dimensional hydrogel were observed.
However, the main drawback of creating data from a single layer segmentation is that no overlapping cells are detected. To overcome this problem, we generated raw data containing overlapping cells by pairing temporally adjacent segmentation maps, and stacking them above each other to form two different layers, which we could use as labels to train our CNN. To create the respective hologram, each cell's depth was chosen randomly, but for the first segmentation map, a fixed threshold was not exceeded. On the other hand, each cell's depth from the second segmentation map had to exceed the threshold. Thus, we obtained data where a set of cells is located nearer, layer 1, and another farther away, layer 2, from the sensor plane. In our case the threshold was chosen to be at half the known height of the hydrogel. An illustration of this can be seen in Fig. 2.
As we used two layers as labels, our CNN needs to provide two output layers as well, having the same height and width as the gray-scale input image, being the corresponding hologram. If a cell exists in the lower half, the corresponding pixels' outputs need to be close to one in the lower layer, indicating that a cell is present. Analog to this, the higher layer predicts the presence of cells existing in the upper half. Zero values are defined as background pixels. Note that the network yields continuous values between zero and one. Thus, a threshold needs to be applied to determine which pixel is assigned the class 'cell' and which pixel 'background'.
Our training- and test-set were each composed of 100 images.

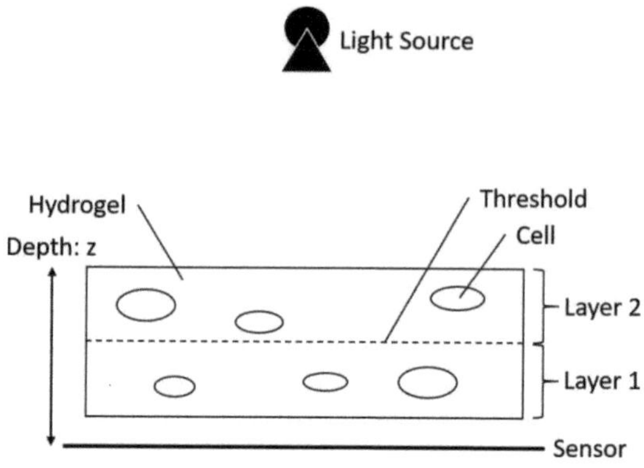

Figure 2: Schematic of LFDIH and how segmentation maps are combined to generate realistic three-dimensional data. Each layer is actually a two-dimensional projection of the cells in its corresponding sub-volume of the hydrogel. Here, Layer 1 is the projection of all the cells in the lower half of the sample while Layer 2 is the one of the cells in the upper half.

3 Experiments

All of our tests were carried out using an u-net [5] with a ResNet-18 [6] encoder, pre-trained on ImageNet [7]. The network was trained on 512 $\times$ 512 pixel crops, using an initial learning rate of 0.1, which was dropped by a factor of ten after one and two thirds of the training process had been completed. Furthermore, we used a batch size of four, a factor of 10^{-4} as weight decay, the Adam optimizer [8], and we trained for 100 epochs. We used binary cross entropy as our loss-function, because we wanted to distinguish two different depths. Therefore, the network would generate two feature maps in which values close to one would indicate that the pixel belonged to a cell. Though in contrast to ordinary multi-class semantic segmentation, where the softmax function enforces that a pixel can only belong to one class, and therefore have a non-zero value only in one feature map, the same pixel could now have a non-zero value in both feature maps, as each of them would represent a volume that could contain a cell at that position. Henceforth, we also substituted the softmax function by a sigmoid function to compute the probability distribution.
For the evaluation we applied a threshold to the probability predictions of the network to create binary predictions. For this, we used the thresholds 0.01, 0.05, 0.25, and 0.5. Based on the used threshold, we first computed the dice score on each layer. Afterwards we computed a bounding box for each cell of the Ground Truth (GT), as well as for each cell of the predictions and computed the Intersection over Union (IOU) between each of the GT and prediction bounding boxes belonging to the same layer. Based on these, we performed a greedy matching to assign to each GT cell the prediction cell with the highest IOU. If the highest IOU was larger then 0.3 the prediction was considered a true positive (TP) and a false positive (FP) otherwise. The number of false negatives (FNs) was then computed by subtracting the number of TPs from the number of GT cells. Based on these values, we then computed the precision, recall and the F1-Score for each layer.
Additionally, we computed the same scores again but only for overlapping and not overlapping cells when using the threshold that yielded the best results. To make this separation possible, we first classified all the GT cells into overlapping and not overlapping ones. For this, a cell was considered to be overlapping if the largest IOU of its estimated bounding box with any other estimated cell bounding box was larger than 0.3. Thereafter, we matched the predictions onto the GT cells by finding the largest positive IOU and assigned the predictions to the same class as their matched GT cells. When there were still unmatched predictions left, we then tried to find matching GT cells in the opposite layer because the chance was high that they originated out of those. Though we could assign nearly all predictions to one of the classes, we still encountered some for which we could not find a match. As those were FPs by definition the recall was

not influenced by their presence or absence in the evaluations. The dice as well as the precision and therefore the F1 score however are. To keep the evaluation fair, we therefore decided to do each of the class evaluations twice. Once only with the cells and predictions that clearly belonged to the respective class, leading to the best case score, as no entire FPs were present, and once with all the cells and predictions that belonged to the class as well as all the unclassifiable predictions, leading to a worst case score, as entire FPs were present. Henceforth, we extended our results to intervals because the scores were dependent on how the unclassifiable predictions were assigned to the classes. Do note that this implies that the results of the two classes are cross-correlated because all the predictions must belong to a class.
Furthermore, we tested how a weighted loss (1) influenced the results by multiplying the loss of every pixel that was above a GT cell pixel by a certain factor, to ensure that predictions in a lower layer would not cause predictions to appear above them, to enforce the desired learning behavior. For this, we used the factors two and three.

$$E_{x\_weighted} = E_x + E_x(Layer_{x-1} > 0) * (w - 1) \quad (1)$$

where w is the weighting factor, E_x is the loss of an arbitrary xth layer and $Layer_{x-1}$ is the label of the layer below layer x.

4 Results and Discussion

The results of our threshold evaluation are shown in Table 1. As expected, lower thresholds tend to create too many FPs, while higher thresholds tend to create too many FNs therefore degrading the results. The recall is also being degraded by the lower threshold because it not only causes FPs but might also cause prediction cells to merge together. The threshold of 0.25 seems to find a good balance for this. Especially the respective F1-Score of nearly 80% indicates that the network's performance is sufficiently high to use its results for cell-tracking. The dice score, which is essentially the F1-Score computed over all pixels, is lower, but shouldn't impact the tracking performance too much, as mainly the position is relevant for the tracking task. Though the lower dice indicates that the CNN seems to struggle with accurately segmenting the cells outline while also predicting the corresponding depth. The performance could possibly be enhanced by the usage of deeper models or by a more sophisticated hyperparameter search.
For the further evaluations we used the threshold of 0.25 and focused on the dice score as it correlates with the other scores, is the most relevant one for the segmentation task and the least dependent on thresholds as it is computed on the segmentation maps itself instead of on the cells which require the matching and classification based on thresholds first.
When comparing the results for the overlapping cells and the not overlapping cells, we found that surprisingly, the network seemed to perform better on overlapping cells than on not overlapping ones even though this is counter intuitive, as one would expect that not overlapping cells would present an easier task. This can be seen in Table 2 and enforces our belief, that the network performs the segmentation task well enough to use it as preprocessing for cell tracking, as it delivers good results even on the difficult, overlapping cells. Additionally one can see that when comparing the results of all cells by layer, we found that the network performed better on the lower layer.

Table 1: Results of the threshold evaluation. One can see that the results are highly influenced by the chosen threshold and that 0.25 yields the best results.

Thres.	Prec.	Rec.	F1	Dice
0.01	0.348	0.324	0.336	0.261
0.05	0.653	0.601	0.626	0.383
0.25	0.862	0.726	0.787	0.534
0.50	0.823	0.568	0.671	0.468

Table 2: Results of the evaluation regarding the different cell types and layer. One can see that the network surprisingly performs better on the overlapping cells and that the lower layer yields better results than the upper layer.

Cell type	Rec.	Dice
Overlapping	0.763	(0.535, 0.536)
Non overlapping	0.597	(0.498, 0.501)
Layer 1	0.742	0.536
Layer 2	0.710	0.531

To better understand the networks performance regarding the different results for the layers, we evaluated it on minimalistic examples featuring all possible cell combinations. I.e. a cell in the lower layer without one above it, a cell in the upper layer without one below it, overlapping cells in both layers, having an IOU of over 0.3, and not overlapping cells in both layers, having an IOU of smaller than 0.3. These, as well as the resulting predictions, can be seen in Fig. 3. Based on these images, we found that a GT cell in the lower layer would not only cause the network to predict a cell at that very position, but that it would also cause the network to predict a cell in the layer above it. This behaviour was the most obvious for GT cells that did not have another cell above them but could be observed for overlapping cells as well. This might indicate that it is advantageous for the network during training to always assume that a detected cell has another cell above it. This could potentially be solved by weighting the Loss or by synthetically creating training data that does feature the same amount of overlapping as non overlapping cells, as there currently are about 1.5 times more overlapping than non overlapping cells in the training set, to break this learning behaviour.
Our evaluation regarding the weighting of the Loss, to prevent this from happening indeed yielded better results when the multiplication factor was chosen to be not too large, as

one can see in Table 3. Though one can also see that the standard deviation of the dice per layer increases with an increasing weighting factor, therefore causing the network to be more inconsistent across images and even different layers, which is a major drawback as consistency is important to make the predictions reliable. Possibly factors which are closer to one may solve this problem.

(a) Lower GT layer.

(b) Upper GT layer.

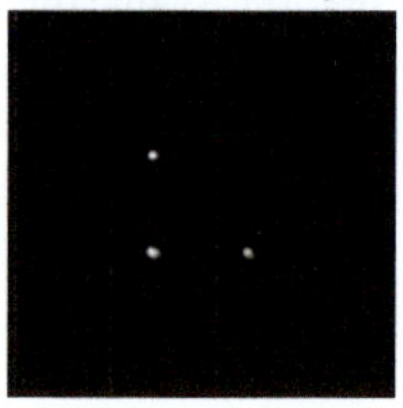

(c) Lower prediction layer.

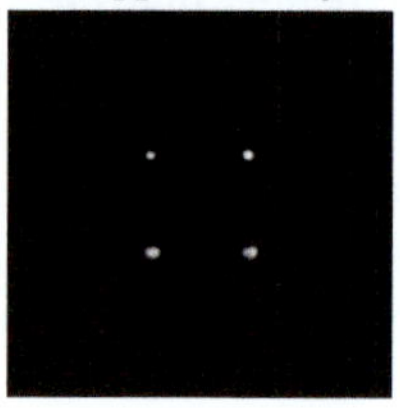

(d) Upper prediction layer.

Figure 3: One can clearly see that there exists an additional prediction in the upper prediction layer without any corresponding GT cell. The GT cells in the lower left of both layers are overlapping due to an IOU of more than 0.3, while the ones on the lower right are not. The colors of the GT layers have been inverted to make them more distinguishable from the predictions.

Table 3: Results of the evaluation regarding the weighting of the loss. The dice was calculated across all cells of all layers. One can see that such a weighting can indeed enhance the performance when the factor is not too large. Though the standard deviation of the dice increases as well.

Factor	Dice	Std.
1.0	0.53	0.030
2.0	0.55	0.116
3.0	0.52	0.133

5 Conclusion

We have presented a method of recognizing cells that are otherwise occluded based on raw holographic images produced by Lens-Free Digital Inline Holography, using the ResNet-18 network. The method therefore poses a promising improvement but still requires further research regarding optimal hyperparameters and especially regarding additional layers to enhance the longitudinal resolution of the images. The latter is particularly important to make it feasible for practical usage such as allowing for more accurate cell tracking using lens-less devices. Situations with crossing cell tracks or generally many cells could benefit the most from our method, as these would likely lead to overlapping ones, which otherwise could not be distinguished.

Acknowledgement

The work has been carried out at the Institute for Neuro- and Bioinformatics, Universität zu Lübeck in cooperation with the Pattern Recognition GmbH, Lübeck, Germany and the Fraunhofer Research Institution for Marine Biotechnology and Cell Technology, Lübeck, Germany and supervised by Prof. Dr.-Ing. Erhardt Barth.
The authors thank Ms. Dr. Ana Cristina Guerra de Souza for data acquisition and Mr. Prof. Dr. Tamás Laskay, Ms. Mareike Ohms and Mr. Daniel Dömer for provision of primary human neutrophils. This work was partly funded by the European Regional Development Fund (ERDF).

Author's Statement

Conflict of interest: Authors state no conflict of interest.

6 References

[1] L. Repetto, E. Piano, and C. Pontiggia, "Lensless digital holographic microscope with light-emitting diode illumination," *Optics letters*, vol. 29, no. 10, pp. 1132–1134, 2004.

[2] Y. Rivenson, Y. Wu, and A. Ozcan, "Deep learning in holography and coherent imaging," *Light: Science & Applications*, vol. 8, no. 1, pp. 1–8, 2019.

[3] P. Gruening, F. Nette, A. C. Guerra de Souza, N. Heldt, and E. Barth, "Direct inference of cell positions using lens-free microscopy and deep learning," in submission.

[4] M. K. Kim, "Principles and techniques of digital holographic microscopy," *SPIE reviews*, vol. 1, no. 1, p. 018005, 2010.

[5] O. Ronneberger, P. Fischer, and T. Brox, "U-net: Convolutional networks for biomedical image segmentation," in *International Conference on Medical image computing and computer-assisted intervention.* Springer, 2015, pp. 234–241.

[6] K. He, X. Zhang, S. Ren, and J. Sun, "Deep residual learning for image recognition," in *Proceedings of the IEEE conference on computer vision and pattern recognition*, 2016, pp. 770–778.

[7] J. Deng *et al.*, "Imagenet: A large-scale hierarchical image database," in *2009 IEEE Conference on Computer Vision and Pattern Recognition*, 2009, pp. 248–255.

[8] D. P. Kingma and J. Ba, "Adam: A method for stochastic optimization," 2017.

DPHelmet: Pre-training on Public Data to Boost Differentially Private Machine Learning

Moritz Kirschte [1] and Esfandiar Mohammadi [2]
[1] Medical Informatics, Universität zu Lübeck, moritz.kirschte@student.uni-luebeck.de
[2] Institute for IT Security, Universität zu Lübeck, esfandiar.mohammadi@uni-luebeck.de

Abstract

Recent work shows that Machine Learning (ML) models can leak information about training data, which in medical applications translates to sensitive patient data. Prior work proposes privacy-preserving ML methods that protect patient data. Yet, existing methods have either a high learning capacity but are unsuited for privacy-protecting modifications (e.g., neural networks) or limited learning capacity (e.g., SVMs) but are suited for privacy-protecting modifications. This work aims to achieve the best of these two approaches: pre-training on related public data sets and privacy-preserving post-training on sensitive data. We base pre-training on a contrastive learning task, called SimCLR and post-training on differentially private SVMs, which we ported to ScikitLearn. We evaluate our method on a $4\,k$ points large, high-dimensional image data set (tf_flowers), achieving an accuracy of $> 80\,\%$ with acceptable privacy guarantees. We show that our method achieved on CIFAR-10 almost comparable performance to prior work on privacy-preserving ML.

1 Introduction

Recent work has shown privacy attacks on machine learning (ML) models that extract information about the training data. In medical applications the training data constitute sensitive patient data, leading to severe privacy concerns. Whenever such models are used in an unprotected environment, strong privacy guarantees are indispensable. There is a growing body of literature on privacy-preserving ML [1], [2], [5], [9] that is based on a well-understood privacy notion: differential privacy (DP) [3].

For simple learning tasks, such as so-called convex optimization (including support vector machine classification, SVC for short), there are effective DP ML techniques [1]. Yet, for some applications, SVCs perform far worse than neural networks. While there are methods [2] for DP training of neural networks (e.g., DP-SGD), these methods lead to a stark deterioration of their accuracy.

There is a way of combining these two advantages if useful unlabelled public data sets are available. In a pre-training phase on a related public data set, a low-dimensional embedding can be trained via a neural network that enables the effectively utilizing DP convex ML methods (e.g., SVCs), trained on sensitive data. Recent advances [6], [7] on unsupervised pre-training methods enable the effective utilization of such public data sets. Public data sets exist for a variety of important applications such as image classification like lesion detection in medical applications [12].

Prior work has shown that pre-training a neural network on public data and using DP-SGD to fine-tune the neural network with sensitive data can lead to promising results. As mentioned above, neural networks have, however, inherently far more leakage than convex optimization problems. As convex ML methods can successfully learn on small data sets, these methods are suited and widely used for medical applications. In this work we illustrate how non-convex pre-training methods can be utilized on public data to learn simplifying representations such that even simple DP convex ML methods can be successfully applied, resulting in effective and privacy-preserving ML methods.

Summary of contribution. First, we present a novel DP ML method by combining self-supervised pre-training methods with DP convex ML.
Second, using an image classification benchmark data set (ImageNet), we illustrate the generalization potential of this kind of DP ML method. The experiments show (using tf_flowers) a competitive accuracy of $> 80\,\%$ for acceptable privacy guarantees.
Third, to compare our approach to prior work on DP ML with pre-training (DP-SGD), we evaluate the performance on benchmark data (CIFAR-10). While our simple DP convex ML methods result in slightly less accurate models than DP-SGD with pre-training, we achieve an accuracy of $> 60\,\%$ on CIFAR-10 for acceptable privacy guarantees.

2 Material and Methods

2.1 Preliminaries: Differential Privacy

The privacy notion that we consider in this work is called differential privacy (DP) [3]. In the context of ML, differential privacy requires that a given ML method does not leak more information about the training data set than can be denied by the training party.

Definition 1 (Differential Privacy) *Let Obs be the set of observations, and $RV(Obs)$ be the set of random variables over Obs, and $\mathcal{D}$ be the set of all databases. A randomized algorithm $M : \mathcal{D} \to RV(Obs)$ for all pairs of databases $\mathcal{D}, \mathcal{D}'$ that differ in at most 1 element is a (ε, δ)-DP mechanism if for all tests $S \subseteq Obs$ we have*

$$\Pr[M(D) \in S] \leq \exp(\varepsilon) \Pr[M(D') \in S] + \delta. \quad (1)$$

The ε-value characterizes the degree of deniability that an algorithm achieves. The δ-value quantifies the probability that the deniability guarantee fails. Typically, the parameter in the range $\varepsilon \leq 1$ are considered to provide high deniability and $1 < \varepsilon \leq 8$ might be acceptable in some applications. The parameter δ is typically $\delta \leq 10^{-4}$. In line with prior work on DP ML [2], we discuss the accuracy in the low-privacy regime i.e. $1 < \varepsilon \leq 8$.

2.2 Preliminaries: Contrastive Learning

Self-supervised pre-training methods on unlabelled data recently made tremendous advances, e.g., the contrastive learning technique SimCLR [6], [7]. Its goal is to learn an efficient and linearly separable representation. Most notably, it only slightly underperforms supervised training.

Given an image, SimCLR transforms this image into two different images by applying two data augmentation transformations (e.g., rotation, cropping, color jitter) randomly. SimCLR can be seen as attracting similar images while repelling dissimilar images. The similarity notion that SimCLR uses is binary: if two images are the result of transformations from the same image, they are similar; otherwise they are dissimilar. The contrastive loss rewards the closeness of those similar images (positive pair) while simultaneously punishing the closeness of dissimilar images (negative pair).

Definition 2 (Contrastive Loss) *Let $\mathcal{T}$ be a set of image transformations, be $f(\cdot)$ a base encoder, and $g(\cdot)$ a projection head (both neural networks). Let $\mathcal{D}$ be a distribution over images. For a temperature τ, and the cosine similarity $sim(u, v) = \frac{u^T v}{\|u\|\|v\|}$, the following term is minimized ($h_{i,b} := f(t_b(x_i))$ and $z_{i,b} := g(h_{i,b})$) and h is output:*

$$\mathop{\mathbb{E}}_{\substack{(x_i)_{i=1}^N \sim \mathcal{D} \\ t_0, t_1 \sim \mathcal{T}}} \left[-\, log \frac{\exp\left(sim(z_{i,0}, z_{i,1})/\tau\right)}{\sum\limits_{\substack{b \in \{0,1\} \\ 1 \leq k \leq N \\ k \neq i}} \exp\left(sim(z_{i,0}, z_{k,b})/\tau\right)} \right]. \quad (2)$$

Wang et al. [11] visually illustrated that the contrastive loss leads to a unit hypersphere where every data point is distributed in such a way that similar images lay close together (i.e. have a large cosine distance). Former is called the uniformity assumption (the loss's nominator), the latter alignment assumption (denominator). With neither of which successfully training could be performed, thus they have to be balanced out carefully for maximum performance.

2.3 DP-SVC

In this work, we consider convex optimization problems, which are optimization problems where every local minimum is a global minimum. More specifically, we focus on a risk minimization problem: $\arg\min_f \sum_{i=1}^n \ell(f^T x_i, y_i)$, for a model f, a data set $(x_i, y_i)_{i=1}^n$ and a convex loss function ℓ. This problem is a variant of Chaudhuri et al.'s work on regularized empirical risk minimization for DP convex ML methods, such as training a DP linear SVC [1]. In that work, the resulting model is slightly perturbed, using carefully calibrated noise, to achieve DP convex ML.

Chaudhuri et al. require that the influence of every training data point x_i be bounded. So, we clip their norm to a given bound c as follows:

$$clipped(x_i, c) = \begin{cases} c \cdot x_i / \|x_i\|, & \text{if } \|x_i\| > c \\ x_i, & \text{otherwise} \end{cases}. \quad (3)$$

Definition 3 (DP-SVC) *For a given loss function ℓ, a predictor $f \in \mathbb{R}^p$ (i.e. coefficients plus intercept) on a data set $D := (x_i, y_i)_{i=1}^n$, and a function $R(\cdot)$ that controls the margin span, SVC considers the following R-regularized objective $J(f, \mathcal{D}) = C \sum_{i=1}^n \ell(f^T \cdot clipped(x_i, c), y_i) + \frac{1}{2} R(f)$. DP-SVC with parameters (C, c, σ) computes on input D $f^*_{priv} = b + \arg\min_f\ J(f, \mathcal{D})$ with $b \sim \mathcal{N}(0, \sigma^2 I_p)$ chosen from a multivariate normal distribution, where I_p is the identity matrix for a feature dimension p.*

Chaudhuri et al. prove differential privacy bounds for output perturbation for different perturbation distributions [1, Theorem 6 & Corollary 8]. Bun et al. show precise privacy bounds for the output-perturbation with multivariate Gaussian noise [5, Lemma 2.5]. Mironov shows how these bounds can be translated to (ε, δ)-DP bound using [9, Proposition 3]. We combining these results in Theorem 3.1.

Theorem 3.1 (DP-SVC) *If in DP-SVC, ℓ is convex and differentiable with $|\ell'(z)| \leq 1$ for all z, $N(\cdot)$ is 1-strongly convex and differentiable, then for all $\alpha \geq 2$, $0 < \delta \leq 1$, and $\varepsilon' > 0$, DP-SVC with parameters (C, c, σ) is*

$$(\varepsilon, \delta) := \left(\frac{\alpha (2C \cdot c\varepsilon')^2}{2\sigma^2} + \frac{\log(1/\delta)}{\alpha - 1}, \delta \right) -\text{DP}. \quad (4)$$

In our experimental evaluation, we compute α that minimizes the (ε, δ)-DP parameters from (4).

We would like to apply the method from Theorem 3.1 to ScikitLearn's highly optimized SVC implementation. However, Theorem 3.1 formally requires a differentiable loss function, and ScikitLearn's SVC implementation implicitly uses the non-differentiable hinge-loss. We nevertheless do use the hinge loss with the following argumentation. We use a differentiable approximation of the hinge loss: the family of Huber losses. Huber losses can approximate the hinge loss with arbitrary precision while satisfying the prerequisites of Theorem 3.1 (bounded first derivative). We can let the Huber loss approximate the hinge loss beyond machine precision, resulting in a situation where on the respective machine the hinge loss and a sufficiently precise Huber loss would output the same result.

Multi-class DP-SVC. For the extension to multi-class classification (*multi-class DP-SVC*), we use the one-vs-one (OVO) scheme. In the OVO scheme, training takes place on every combination of classes, thus for m classes $\frac{m(m-1)}{2}$ classifiers in total. Afterwards, all classifiers voted to which class a data point belongs.
Mironov proves that these privacy bounds are only slightly worse when using n classifiers [9, Proposition 1].

Corollary 3.1.1 (Multi-class DP-SVC) *If n DP-SVC classifiers are applied together on the same dataset $\mathcal{D}$ in an OVO scheme, then for all $\alpha \geq 2$, $0 < \delta \leq 1$, and $\varepsilon' > 0$ the so-called multi-class DP-SVC with parameters (C, c, σ) is*

$$(\varepsilon, \delta) := \left(n \frac{\alpha(2C \cdot c\varepsilon')^2}{2\sigma^2} + \frac{\log(1/\delta)}{\alpha - 1}, \delta \right) - \mathrm{DP}. \quad (5)$$

Optimizing for α shows that the noise parameter σ has to be scaled by a factor of $\mathcal{O}(\sqrt{n})$.

2.4 Our Method: DPHelmet

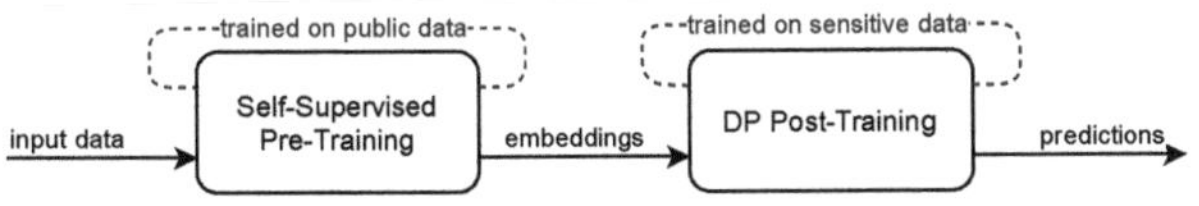

Figure 1: Differentially private machine learning, utilizing pre-training on public data.

Our method illustrates how the advantages of self-supervised learning on public data sets can be combined with DP convex ML methods on sensitive data sets as depicted in Fig. 1. The self-supervised ML model maps the inputs to a low-dimensional embedding space that is designed to be linearly separable. It is furthermore trained on public data with the contrastive loss. We apply DP convex ML on this reduced space for post-training using private data.
The efficiency of DP-convex optimization is further accelerated by the uniformity assumption of the contrastive loss essentially restricting the feasible embedding space. In detail, knowing the approximate embedding space distribution beforehand allows finding tighter sensitivity bounds for DP-SVC by clipping towards the expected mean which is data-independent. Here a clipping bound c of $\log_2(p)$ has been selected, for a feature dimension p.

3 Results and Discussion

3.1 Generalization ability

We illustrate the proposed method's generalizability by applying it to the high-dimensional ImageNet2012 data set [8] for pre-training. The post-training experiments have been taken on the tf_flowers [10] data set, originating from TensorFlow's transfer learning tutorial. It contains $3,670$ high-resolution images of flowers of the classes *daisy*, *dandelion*, *roses*, *sunflowers*, and *tulips* with only *daisy* overlapping with an ImageNet class. These have been scaled down to $224 \times 224 \times 3$ to be fed into an ImageNet pre-trained SimCLR-v2 on a ResNet-152 (3x, with selective kernels) backbone (795 M parameters).

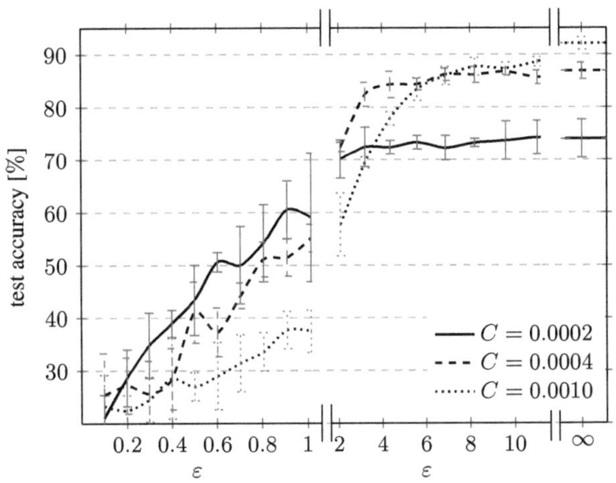

Figure 2: On tf_flowers trained DP-SVC ($\delta = 10^{-4}$) using 5-fold cross-validation ($n\_train\_samples = 2,936$). Pre-trained has been with SimCLR-v2 on ImageNet2012 using a ResNet-152 (3x, SK) resulting in an $6,144$ d code space.

The pre-training evaluation took place on a linear classifier reaching 79.8 % top-1 accuracy and 94.9 % top-5 accuracy respectively. Post-training performance is depicted in Fig. 2. Despite having significantly less training data than features it still reaches a decent performance emphasizing the importance of a strong pre-training technique.

3.2 Comparison to non-convex DP ML

A DP version of Stochastic Gradient Descent called DP-SGD has been introduced by [2]. It is to be considered as the baseline of highly non-convex optimization by being applicable to arbitrary neural networks. Abadi et al. evaluated the DP-SGD algorithm by pre-training (using SGD without privacy protection) on public data and fine-tuning on sensitive data. As a public data set, they use the CIFAR-100 data set, and, as a sensitive one, they use CIFAR-10. To achieve a meaningful comparison, we utilize exactly the same data sets as examples for public and private data sets.
Introduced by [4] both CIFAR-100 and CIFAR-10 are a $50,000$-strong collection of thumbnail-sized colored images of size 32×32 having 100 and 10 classes respectively. Both datasets are having disjoint classes thus being perfectly suited to be treated as a public-private dataset combination.
For pre-training, SimCLR-v1 has been trained on CIFAR-100 with the default settingsfor CIFAR-10. Most notably, a modified ResNet-18 has been chosen as a backbone and training has been performed for $1,000$ epochs on a 512 batch size with a temperature parameter of $\tau = 0.5$ and using a learning rate of 1.0. Transformations included random color jitter with a strength of 0.5 as well as random flipping and cropping.

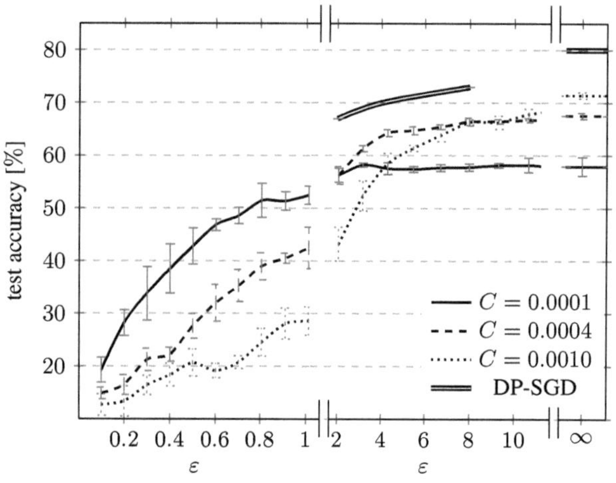

Figure 3: On CIFAR-10 trained DP-SVC ($\delta = 10^{-5}$) using 5-fold cross-validation ($n\_train\_samples = 50\,k$). Pre-trained has been with SimCLR-v1 on CIFAR-100 using a modified ResNet-18 resulting in an 512 d code space.

Evaluation of SimCLR took place on a linear classifier using CIFAR-100 test data with 65.4 % top-1 accuracy and 89.6 % top-5 accuracy respectively. Post-training performance is depicted in Fig. 3. It shows that our simple approach of using output perturbation is not able to beat DP-SGD on CIFAR-10 but already achieves reasonable classification accuracy. As applying objective perturbation is expected to yield stronger DP convex ML methods, our results support the conjecture that DP convex ML methods applied on pre-trained models can lead to effective privacy-preserving ML methods.

4 Conclusion & Future Work

We have presented a method for pre-training with contrastive learning large neural networks on unlabelled public data and post-training on sensitive training data DP convex ML methods. We show that we achieve comparable performance to prior work (DP-SGD), where pre-training was done with labelled data.
We see a high potential for utilizing DP ML methods that are amenable to privacy-preserving modifications. This work concentrates on output perturbation and achieves promising results. More sophisticated approaches, such as objective perturbation [1] for SVCs or gradient boosted decision trees, have the potential to achieve even higher accuracy results while providing strong DP guarantees, in particular when combined with tighter DP guarantees. Additionally, pre-training can be further improved by using debiasing techniques or hard negative sampling.

Acknowledgement

The work has been carried out and supervised at the Institute for IT Security, Universität zu Lübeck. Furthermore, we would like to thank Marven Kummerfeldt, Saman Ardalan, Niclas Kath, Théo Giovanna, David Sommer, and Alexander Viand for fruitful discussions about the topic.

Author's Statement

Conflict of interest: Authors state no conflict of interest.

5 References

[1] K. Chaudhuri, C. Monteleoni and A. D. Sarwate, *Differentially private empirical risk minimization.* JMLR, vol.12, no. 3, pp. 1069–1109, 2011.

[2] M. Abadi, A. Chu, I. J. Goodfellow, H. B. McMahan, I. Mironov, K. Talwar and L. Zhang, *Deep learning with differential privacy.* In: ACM CCS, ACM, pp. 308–318, 2016.

[3] C. Dwork, F. McSherry, K. Nissim and A. Smith, *Calibrating noise to sensitivity in private data analysis.* In: TCC, Springer, Berlin, Heidelberg, pp. 265–284, 2006.

[4] A. Krizhevsky and G. Hinton, *Learning multiple layers of features from tiny images.* 2009.

[5] M. Bun and T. Steinke, *Concentrated differential privacy: simplifications, extensions, and lower bounds.* In: TCC, Springer, Berlin, Heidelberg, pp. 635–658, 2016.

[6] T. Chen, S. Kornblith, M. Norouzi and G. E. Hinton, *A Simple Framework for Contrastive Learning of Visual Representations.* In: ICML, PMLR, pp. 1597–1607, 2020.

[7] T. Chen, S. Kornblith, K. Swersky, M. Norouzi and G. E. Hinton, *Big self-supervised models are strong semi-supervised learners.* arXiv preprint arXiv:2006.10029, 2020.

[8] O. Russakovsky et al. *Imagenet large scale visual recognition challenge.* IJCV, vol. 115, no. 3, pp. 211–252, 2015.

[9] I. Mironov, *Rényi differential privacy.* In: IEEE CSF, IEEE Computer Society, pp. 263–275, 2017.

[10] The TensorFlow Team, *Flowers.* 2019.

[11] T. Wang and P. Isola, *Understanding Contrastive Representation Learning through Alignment and Uniformity on the Hypersphere.* In: ICML, PMLR, pp. 9929–9939, 2020.

[12] K. Yan, X. Wang, L. Lu and R. M. Summers, *DeepLesion: automated mining of large-scale lesion annotations and universal lesion detection with deep learning.* JMI, vol. 5, no. 3, p. 036501, 2018.

11

Medical Imaging

Dynamic Positioning of an OCT-Scanbeam using 3D Object-Tracking in Stereo Microscope Images

Felix Müller [1], Richard Neffin [2], Marc Krug [2], and Heinz Handels [3]
[1] Medical Informatics, Universität zu Lübeck, felix.mueller@student.uni-luebeck.de
[2] HAAG-STREIT SURGICAL GmbH & Co. KG , R&D - Zweigstelle Lübeck,
{richard.neffin, marc.krug}@haag-streit.com
[3] Institute of Medical Informatics, Universität zu Lübeck, handels@imi.uni-luebeck.de

Abstract

This paper describes the development of an algorithm to detect the position of an object in 3D space using images captured by a surgical microscope (Haag-Streit Hi-R 1000). Afterwards the detected 3D position is used to dynamically project the scan beam of an Optical Coherence Tomography Device (OCT) to enable adaptive OCT imaging. Both devices, microscope and OCT, are developed by the Haag-Streit-Surgical GmbH & Co. KG and are essential components of the research and development of the Haag-Streit-Group. The images which the microscope delivers are obtained by a prototype stereo camera. The paper presents how classical computer vision approaches, in an experimental setup, can be used to solve the problem of finding the 3D position of an object based on 2D image information. Furthermore, problems that occur by transferring the experimental approach to the actual surgical microscope are discussed.

1 Introduction

The surgical microscope and the OCT-Device work together in an intraoperative scenario to provide additional OCT image information beside the regular microscope image information. To obtain good image information several steps and interactions with both devices are involved. The microscope has to be focused onto the surface of the tissue to be examined, to obtain satisfactory sharpness in the microscope images. The OCT-Device has to adjust the optical path length so an actuator motor can move the OCT-scanbeam to the object plane to obtain an OCT image. The user needs to interact with many devices at the same time adjusting many settings to get sufficient image results in terms of microscope and OCT imaging. Therefore, it is advantageous to develop a method to automatically adjust the OCT-scanbeam position based on the image information provided by the microscope.

2 Material and Methods

Recently a functional sample has been developed at Haag-Streit-Surgical that enables a stereo imaging approach to capture the microscope image data. This prototype consists of two simple RaspberryPi model V1 pinhole cameras. The classical approach to detect the 3D position of an object based on 2D stereo imaging is the triangulation method. Triangulation computes a 3D position that corresponds to two additional, corresponding points of the same scene captured in the 2D images of the two stereo cameras [1], [2].
The experimental setup consists of the same model V1 stereo cameras that are build in the functional sample. The cameras are connect to a standard raspberry pi computing module, in this case the StereoPi v.09. This RaspberryPi-Stereo-Camera-Module serves as an experimental device to develop and test the algorithms for stereo imaging and 3D position computing. After successful development and testing on this experimental device, the algorithm is tested and evaluated in relation to the actual prototype camera connected to the surgical microscope.
The experimental approach, based on traditional stereo imaging, delivers sufficient results for detecting the 3D position of an object. However, although the experimental approach gets good results, there arise several problems regarding the actual prototype camera connected to the surgical microscope. The presented results show that regular triangulation is not sufficient to compute the 3D position correctly. Instead this paper introduces another approach to determine a 3D position of an object based on 2D image data in form of ArUco Markers [4]. ArUco is an open source library embedded into the OpenCV library. It consists of squared fiducial Markers that are easy to detect and more stable in terms of determining their 3D position. They deliver better results for the 3D position computation than regular triangulation and get sufficient results in context with the functional sample and the surgical microscope. This more accurate determination of the 3D position leads to a better adjustment of the OCT-scanbeam to automatically provide a good OCT image.

2.1 Camera Calibration

To use the two stereo cameras for stereo imaging, triangulation and ArUco marker detection the two cameras need to be calibrated. This calibration provides their intrinsic camera parameters, camera matrix $\mathbf{K}$ and distortion coefficients $\mathrm{p1}, \mathrm{p2}, \mathrm{k1}, \mathrm{k2}, \mathrm{k3}$, and their extrinsic camera parameters, rotation matrix $\mathbf{R}$ and translation matrix $\mathbf{t}$ [1], [3]. To compute these parameters, typically several images of a chessboard are taken from different perspectives, which serve as references for the calibration. Those calibration images are necessary because the calibration process requires some correspondences between environment points and their projection in the camera images from different viewpoints. In general, these correspondences are obtained from the corners of the chessboard patterns.
The resulting intrinsic and extrinsic camera parameters allow to describe a transformation from the 2D images to the 3D world. Two corresponding 2D image points $\mathbf{x}$ and $\mathbf{x}'$ within the 2D camera coordinate systems are transformed to a corresponding 3D object point $\mathbf{X}$ in the 3D world coordinate system.

$$\mathbf{x} = \mathbf{K}[\mathbf{R}|\mathbf{t}]\mathbf{X} \tag{1}$$

To use triangulation and compute the 3D point $\mathbf{X}$, the 3×4 projection matrix $\mathbf{P}$ needs to be derived from $\mathbf{K}$, $\mathbf{R}$ and $\mathbf{t}$. The projection matrices $\mathbf{P}$ and $\mathbf{P}'$ of the first and second camera can be used to calculate the 3D object point $\mathbf{X}$ that corresponds to the two 2D image points $\mathbf{x}$ and $\mathbf{x}'$.

$$\begin{gathered}\mathbf{PX} = \mathbf{x} \quad \text{and} \quad \mathbf{P}'\mathbf{X} = \mathbf{x}' \\ \text{with } \mathbf{P} = \mathbf{K}[\mathbf{R}|\mathbf{t}] \text{ and } \mathbf{P}' = \mathbf{K}[\mathbf{I}|\mathbf{0}]\end{gathered} \tag{2}$$

Note that in order to use triangulation and determine the 3D object point, one of the cameras needs to be chosen as the origin. This applies that one of the projection matrices will be a concatenation of a 3×3 identity matrix $\mathbf{I}$ and a 1×3 null vector $\mathbf{0}$.
The intrinsic and extrinsic camera parameter are also needed to detect ArUco markers and determine their 3D position. Using ArUco markers the calibration process can even be improved by mixing ArUco markers into the chessboard creating a so called ChArUco board. This kind of calibration is superior since the provided corners are much more accurate and occlusions and partial views are allowed, so that not all the corners need to be visible in all the viewpoints. In the end, it is a more stable and less error-prone approach for calibration, but in general, the classic chessboard approach achieves sufficient results as well.

2.2 Triangulation

To determine a 3D object point $\mathbf{X}$ from two corresponding 2D image points $\mathbf{x}$ and $\mathbf{x}'$ a transformation $\mathcal{T}$ needs to be formulated so that

$$\mathbf{X} = \mathcal{T}(\mathbf{x}, \mathbf{x}', \mathbf{P}, \mathbf{P}'). \tag{3}$$

The projection matrix $\mathbf{P}$ can be used to estimate the pose of a 3D object point $\mathbf{X} = (X, Y, Z)$ that projects to two 2D image points $\mathbf{x} = (x, y)$ and $\mathbf{x}' = (x', y')$ by perspective projection. Therefore, the equations $\mathbf{PX} = \mathbf{x}$ and $\mathbf{P}'\mathbf{X} = \mathbf{x}'$ in (2) can be combined to a linear equation of the form $A\mathbf{X} = 0$ where A is

$$A = \begin{bmatrix} x\mathbf{p}^{3\mathrm{T}} - \mathbf{p}^{1\mathrm{T}} \\ y\mathbf{p}^{3\mathrm{T}} - \mathbf{p}^{2\mathrm{T}} \\ x'\mathbf{p}'^{3\mathrm{T}} - \mathbf{p}'^{1\mathrm{T}} \\ y'\mathbf{p}'^{3\mathrm{T}} - \mathbf{p}'^{2\mathrm{T}} \end{bmatrix}. \tag{4}$$

The projection matrix coefficients $\mathbf{p}^{i\mathrm{T}}$ are determined from the intrinsic and extrinsic camera parameters, such as the focal length, and the motion parameters $\mathbf{R}$ and $\mathbf{t}$. In the OpenCV Library the homogeneous Direct Linear Transform method (DLT, see [1]) is used to solve this linear equation $A\mathbf{X} = 0$ and determine the 3D position $\mathbf{X}$.

2.3 ArUco Marker

2.3.1 Marker Detection

To determine the 3D position of an ArUco marker relative to the stereo cameras the pose of the marker has to be estimated. The first step is to detect the marker within the images provided by the cameras. This automatic detection consists of several steps to detect the marker rectangle and extract the markers internal binary code that identifies each marker individually [4], [5].
First, an image segmentation is applied to allow the extraction of prominent contours in the gray-scaled images. Therefore, the ArUco implementation uses a local adaptive thresholding approach because it proved to be very robust to different lighting conditions.
The threshold image is used to extract a set of image contours. Some of those contours are not important because the goal is to only extract the contour of the ArUco markers. So the unnecessary contours are filtered out and only the marker contours are kept.
The inner region of a marker's extracted contour will be analyzed to determine the marker's id. To do so the marker's contour first is freed from its perspective distortion. Afterwards the resulting image needs to be binarized to extract it's id by dividing it into a regular grid and assigning the values 0 or 1 to each grid element, depending on the values of the majority of pixels within each element.
The id obtained from the binarized image identifies each marker individually. It evaluates if the marker is the type of marker that actually belongs to the marker dictionary that the algorithm tries to detect or if it is just part of the environment. Finally the pose of the marker in respect to the camera can be computed.

2.3.2 Marker Pose Estimation

If a camera is calibrated and a marker is detected in the camera's images, then it is possible to estimate its pose related to the center of the marker. The detection of the four corners of the marker allows to use planar pose estimators to estimate the relative pose of the camera center regarding to the center of the detected marker. The ArUco pose estimation method is based on the robust plane pose algorithm (Robust Planar Pose, RPP) that solves the perspective n point problem (see solvePnP in OpenCV [3]). So the pose estimation method gives the extrinsic rotation and translation parameters $\mathbf{R}$ and $\mathbf{t}$. Those parameters describe the projective transformation of a 3D object point $\mathbf{X} = [\mathrm{X_w}, \mathrm{Y_w}, \mathrm{Z_w}, 1]$, that represents the center of the marker, from the 3D world coordinate system to the 2D camera coordinate system, where the marker center is represented by a corresponding 2D image point $\mathbf{x} = [\mathrm{x}, \mathrm{y}, 1]$. This projective transformation is given by:

$$\mathbf{x} = \mathbf{K}[\mathbf{R}|\mathbf{t}]\mathbf{X}$$

$$\Leftrightarrow \begin{bmatrix} \mathrm{x} \\ \mathrm{y} \\ 1 \end{bmatrix} = \begin{bmatrix} \mathrm{f_x} & 0 & \mathrm{c_x} \\ 0 & \mathrm{f_y} & \mathrm{c_y} \\ 0 & 0 & 1 \end{bmatrix} \begin{bmatrix} \mathrm{r_{11}} & \mathrm{r_{12}} & \mathrm{r_{13}} & \mathrm{t_1} \\ \mathrm{r_{21}} & \mathrm{r_{22}} & \mathrm{r_{23}} & \mathrm{t_2} \\ \mathrm{r_{31}} & \mathrm{r_{32}} & \mathrm{r_{33}} & \mathrm{t_3} \end{bmatrix} \begin{bmatrix} \mathrm{X_w} \\ \mathrm{Y_w} \\ \mathrm{Z_w} \\ 1 \end{bmatrix} \quad (5)$$

Using the joint rotation-translation matrix $[\mathbf{R}|\mathbf{t}]$ in homogeneous form, the coordinates X_c, Y_c, Z_c of the 2D image point (x, y) in the camera coordinate system c can be obtained by

$$\begin{bmatrix} \mathrm{X}_c \\ \mathrm{Y}_c \\ \mathrm{Z}_c \\ 1 \end{bmatrix} = \begin{bmatrix} \mathrm{r_{11}} & \mathrm{r_{12}} & \mathrm{r_{13}} & \mathrm{t_1} \\ \mathrm{r_{21}} & \mathrm{r_{22}} & \mathrm{r_{23}} & \mathrm{t_2} \\ \mathrm{r_{31}} & \mathrm{r_{32}} & \mathrm{r_{33}} & \mathrm{t_3} \\ 0 & 0 & 0 & 1 \end{bmatrix} \begin{bmatrix} \mathrm{X_w} \\ \mathrm{Y_w} \\ \mathrm{Z_w} \\ 1 \end{bmatrix}. \quad (6)$$

With the intrinsic camera matrix $\mathbf{K}$, those coordinates can then be projected to the 2D image point (x, y). In case of a pinhole camera the 2D image points can be derived from

$$\mathrm{x} = \frac{\mathrm{X}_c \cdot \mathrm{f}_x}{\mathrm{Z}_c} + \mathrm{c_x} \text{ and } \mathrm{y} = \frac{\mathrm{Y}_c \cdot \mathrm{f}_y}{\mathrm{Z}_c} + \mathrm{c_y}, \quad (7)$$

with intrinsic parameters f_x and f_y which are the focal length of the camera and $(\mathrm{c}_x, \mathrm{c}_y)$ the principle point which is usually close to the image center.

However the projection will not result in the correct coordinates (x, y) if the images are distorted. Of course the used cameras are not free from radial or tangential lens distortion. Their images must be freed from the distortion to get sufficient projections. The distortion coefficients $\mathrm{p1}, \mathrm{p2}, \mathrm{k1}, \mathrm{k2}, \mathrm{k3}$, provided as part of the intrinsic camera parameters by the camera calibration, can be used to free the images from the distortion effects.

2.4 OCT-scanbeam Positioning based on Aruco Marker Position

To position the OCT-scanbeam the actuator motor that is build in the OCT device needs to be moved. This motor adjusts the optical path length so that the light of the object plane can interfere with the reference light and produce an OCT image of the targeted tissue. This means the actuator value, that controls this actuator motor, needs to be adjusted to meet the distance measured by the ArUco marker detection and 3D position determination. The problem is that in the surgical microscope environment the measured distance between marker and camera is also affected by the zoom Z and focus F value of the microscope. Considering this, the distance measurement based on the ArUco markers needs to include those two parameters into the distance calculation as well. There exists a zoom and focus state that can be considered "neutral". In this "neutral" state the marker appears uninfluenced by zoom or focus. This can be used to set every measurement D in relation to the "neutral" state to free the measurements from the zooming and focusing effects and simultaneously prevent the real measured distance. Afterwards the distance can be converted in actuator values AC by setting it into relation with the actuator value in "neutral" state $\mathrm{AC_{neutral}}$. By default, one actuator step equals 0.004 centimeters (1 AC $=$ 0.004 cm) and the following relation applies to compute the required actuator value:

$$\mathrm{AC} = \mathrm{AC_{neutral}} - \frac{\left(\left(\frac{\mathrm{Z}}{\mathrm{Z_{neutral}}} \cdot \mathrm{D}\right) - (\mathrm{F_{neutral}} - \mathrm{F})\right)}{0.004} \quad (8)$$

3 Results and Discussion

The first thing to evaluate is how accurate the approach to calculate the 3D position of an object, compared to the manual measured, real distance to the cameras, actually is.

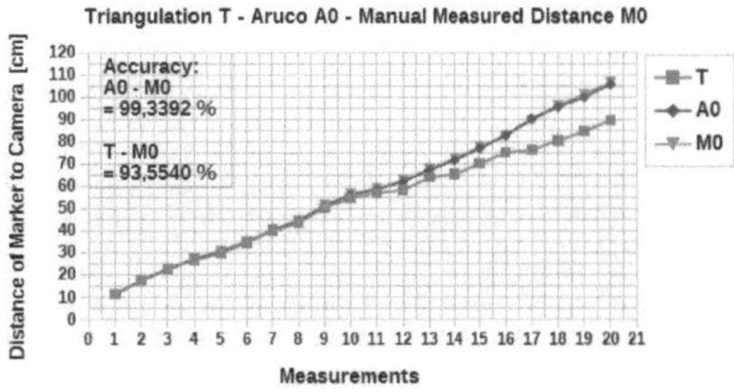

Figure 1: Comparison of the distance measurements between the center of one of the stereo cameras to the center of an ArUco Marker using the experimental RaspberryPi-Stereo-Camera-Module.

Fig. 1 shows how accurate various distances, computed with the triangulation $\mathbf{T}$ and ArUco method $\mathbf{A0}$, match the manual measured distances $\mathbf{M0}$ between the center of a marker and the center of one of the two cameras. The triangulation approach loses accuracy with increasing distance of the marker to the camera. The ArUco approach however maintains very good accuracy comparing the measured and computed distances ($99,3392$ % on a distance interval of 10 to 110 cm).

Secondly the positioning of the OCT-scanbeam, based on

the distance measurements between the functional sample combined with the surgical microscope and the detected ArUco markers, is evaluated. The actuator value margin, in which the OCT-scanbeam is positioned correctly and results in a good OCT image, is only a few millimeters (typically 3,8 - 4,0 mm = 95 - 100 actuator values (AC)). Therefore, the resulting measurement are divided into three classes as shown in Fig. 2.

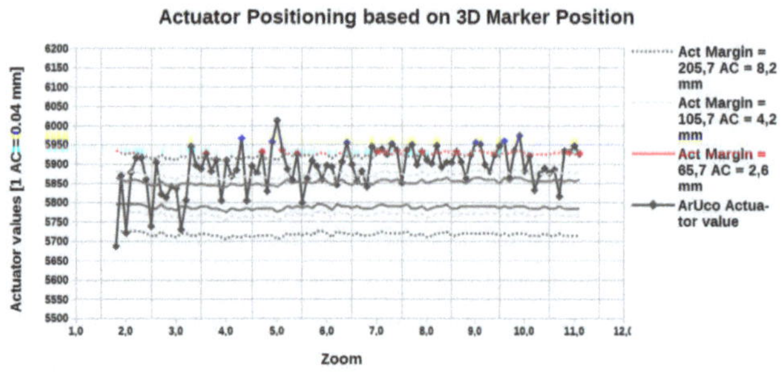

Figure 2: Classification of actuator values to evaluate the OCT-scanbeam positioning. The resulting actuator values are classified based on the quality of the OCT images received by positioning the scan beam using the respective actuator values.

Actuator values that lie in the inner margin (2.6 mm) are nearly perfect and deliver an optimal OCT image. Values that lie between the inner and the middle margin (4.2 mm) are not perfect but still pretty good in showing the tissue structure as an OCT image, so all values that fall in this two margins are considered "good". Values that lie between the middle and the outer margin do not really result in a good OCT image but are still considered "acceptable". Those resulting images still show a shadow of the examined tissue structure and a slight manual adjustment of the actuator motor again results in good images. All values that lie outside the outer margin (8.2 mm) result in images which do not show any structures of the target anymore. Those are classified as "bad" results.
Table 1 shows the overall classification result of all measured actuator values.

Table 1: Classification of overall 282 measured actuator values with varying distances between surgical microscope and ArUco marker. Note that Fig. 2 only shows an exemplary fraction of the overall measurements.

Class	Num Points	Percentage %
Good	69	24.70
Acceptable	118	41.84
Bad	95	33.69

4 Conclusion

As shown in Fig. 1, the ArUco approach to detect an 3D object works exceptionally well and precisely determines the 3D position of the object. Triangulation works also fine but only in a limited area and yet is not as accurate as the ArUco approach and therefore unsatisfactory. After all the resulting distance measurements strongly depend on the camera calibration. The real challenge is to achieve sufficient accuracy using the surgical microscope. As seen in Fig. 2 the computation of the actuator values, based on the measured distances between marker and cameras, leads to resulting values that are often not as accurate as desired. Still, some values imply accuracy that is sufficient to position the OCT-scanbeam to automatically provide a good OCT image of the detected target. Note that the reason why ArUco markers are used in the first place is that triangulation led to inaccurate distance measurement results. The triangulation method was not applicable to the microscope environment because the internal structure of the microscope lenses led to extremely inaccurate distance results. To get better results the process needs to be optimized in terms of the surgical microscopes inner structures. Understanding how exactly its lenses, zoom and focus influence each other, it may be possible to achieve an even more accurate determination of the distance between an ArUco marker and the cameras and a more accurate positioning of the OCT-scanbeam.

Acknowledgement

The work has been carried out at the research and development department of Haag-Streit-Surgical GmbH & Co. KG, Lübeck and supervised by the Institute of Medical Informatics, Universität zu Lübeck.

Author's Statement

Conflict of interest: Authors state no conflict of interest.

5 References

[1] R. Hartley and A. Zissermann, *Multiple View Geometry in Computer Vision*. Computer Vision and Image Understanding, Vol. 68, No. 2, November, 1997.

[2] K. Kanatani, Y. Kanazawa and Y. Sugaya, *Advances in Computer Vision and Pattern Recognition*. Springer International Publishing AG 2016.

[3] G. Bradski, *The OpenCV Library*. Dr. Dobb's Journal of Software Tools, version 4.5.1-dev, Camera Calibration and 3D Reconstruction.

[4] S. Garrido-Jurado, R. Munoz-Salinas, F. J. Madrid-Cuevas and R. Marin-Jimenez, *Automatic generation and detection of highly reliable fiducial markers under occlusion*. University of Cordoba, Pattern Recogn. 47, 6 (June 2014).

[5] G. Bradski, *The OpenCV Library*. Dr. Dobb's Journal of Software Tools, version 4.5.1-dev, ArUco Markers Detection.

Intertemporal Slice-to-Volume matching in Cardiac CT Perfusion Imaging

Danil Zamnius [1], Mattias Heinrich [2], Steffen Lukas [3], Hanna Siebert [2]
[1] Biomedical Engineering, Universität zu Lübeck, danil.zamnius@student.uni-luebeck.de
[2] Institute for Medical Informatics, Universität zu Lübeck, {heinrich, siebert}@imi.uni-luebeck.de
[3] Charité University Hospital Berlin, steffen.lukas@charite.de

Abstract

We present an automated affine image registration method based on Modality Independent Neighbourhood Descriptor (MIND), which identifies the location of a 2D slice within a 3D volume at different acquisition time points in a 4D cardiac perfusion sequence. The method was found to be robust to intertemporal contrast change, noise and reconstruction artefacts. The accuracy of registration parameters was evaluated on a dynamic myocardial CT perfusion dataset (Charité University Hospital Berlin) by simulating transformation parameters of the known truth, ranging between ± 5.71° for rotation and ± 4mm for translation. The validation demonstrates the average errors of 0.69° for rotation and 0.60 mm for translation. These results are comparable with best achievable parameter estimation, given the image resolution of 0.5 mm.

1 Introduction

Image registration is the method of image data alignment from two or more sources into a single coordinate system. Source images may have various dimensionality and not in all cases does the dimensionality match. In our case, as an alternative to image registration of the same dimensionality, we aim to find a 2D plane, within a given 3D image volume which corresponds to a match to the given 2D image input. Additionally, as we use a 4D CT perfusion sequence, we choose our 2D plane and 3D volume to be at different acquisition time points.

There is a number of clinical applications, where slice-to-volume image registration can be employed. It can be particularly useful in image fusion during guided interventions, real-time motion correction and 3D reconstruction, as slice-to-volume methods have superior runtime performance in comparison with volume-to-volume registration methods [1]. Our particular choice in slice-to-volume matching is also due to its possible application in multimodal image registration, where its high runtime performance can be useful to register contrast enhanced MRI and CT.

However in this work, we would like to explore an image registration method of CT perfusion, which in its turn can be of great importance in clinical use. There are two main components which add the challenge for intertemporal registration methods, as they simultaneously have to overcome contrast variations over time and account for chest motion as well as cardiac deformation.

At present, slice-to-volume image registration has received a lot of attention from the research community globally. The existing slice-to-volume registration methods have not yet reached universal robustness and runtime performance in image registration tasks for clinical applications. The extensive literature review [2, 3], demonstrates an absence of an algorithm solving the slice-to-volume registration problem for a large number of circumstances. Moreover, cardiac CT Perfusion (CTP) registration is accompanied with additional challenges, such as time-dependent variations of iodinated contrast tracer concentration resulting in non-linear intertemporal intensity changes.

We present a slice-to-volume image registration algorithm, which jointly addresses challenges of speed performance, robustness to noise, aforementioned contrast changes, dimensionality mismatch, and intertemporal motion.

2 Material and Methods

Given a fixed image slice $I_f \in R^{H \times W}$ and moving image volume $I_m \in R^{H \times W \times D}$, we intend to find an optimal affine transformation $\Theta \in R^{3 \times 4}$ that would align a pair of images of two different time points. We aim at robustness in a setting of contrast variability, motion artefacts and noise. The example of two CT perfusion images is shown in Fig. 1. The images demonstrate the iodinated contrast bolus, which passes through the heart and attenuates X-rays proportionally to the iodine content in tissue. This creates a non-linear intensity relation between two images.

Feature extraction. Instead of registering an image pair in image space I, we choose to perform registration in feature space F, by using the modality-independent neighbourhood descriptor (MIND) with self-similarity context (SSC)

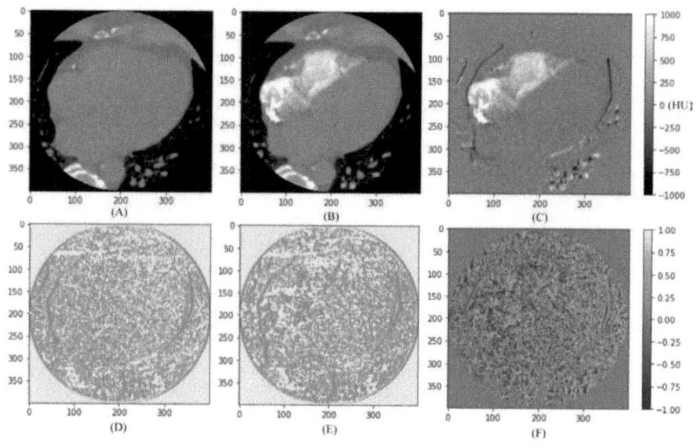

Figure 1: The comparison of two images of a sequence of t1 = 0s (no presence of contrast tracer) and t2 = 5.2s (maximal presence of contrast tracer in the Right Ventricle (RV)) (a, b) – a pair of images of time t1 and t2; (c) – difference between images (d, e) – a pair of MIND-descriptors (only first channel is shown) of time t1 and t2; (f) – difference between corresponding MIND descriptors, showing that contrast differences are substantially reduced by the descriptor.

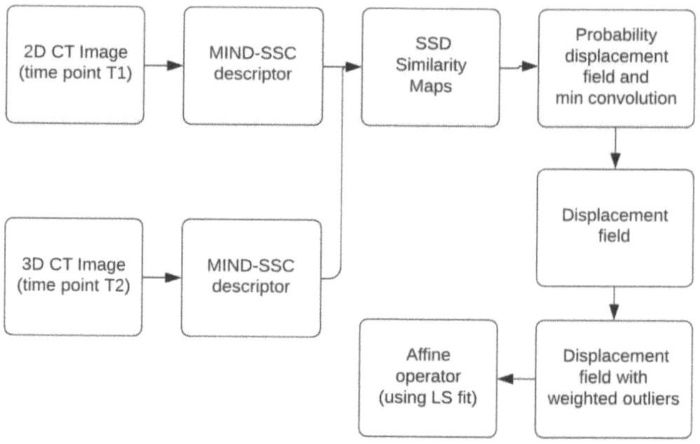

Figure 2: A graphical outline of the presented method. The feature maps computed based on MIND descriptor are resulting in SSD similarity map. This allows computing the displacement vectors for each of the control points of the defined grid. Accuracy of transformation parameter estimation is improved by employing outlier weighting before final LS fitting.

[4, 5]. As it can be seen from the Fig. 1 (d, e, f), the use of MIND descriptor demonstrates a substantial decrease in intertemporal contrast change between corresponding images of cardiac perfusion sequence.

By means of MIND descriptor, a number of features, which describe image structures is extracted. The feature extraction using MIND descriptor results in features $F_f \in R^{C \times H \times W}$ and $F_m, \in R^{C \times H \times W \times D}$. The features are down-scaled to the size of 64 x 64 for H x W (corresponds to 2 x 2 mm), using trilinear interpolation to sample images from the defined discrete grid [6].

Instead of estimating the parameters of affine transformation globally, we estimate the local displacement for each point of 64 x 64 control grid. This allows us to explore the influence of local intensity variation on deformation and identify outliers across each point of the grid. Optimised deformation field with a reduced weight of outliers may result in a more accurate estimation of global affine transformation [7]. The overall graphical outline of the set-up is shown in Fig. 2.

Dissimilarity computation. The sum of squared differences (SSD) is computed between each control point of feature F_f and the corresponding search region of the feature F_m . This results in 6D dissimilarity cost map. $D \in R^{C \times H \times W \times r \times r \times r}$, where r is a search range along each dimension. Afterwards, the dissimilarity cost map is summed along the channel dimension, which results in 5D dissimilarity cost map $D \in R^{H \times W \times r \times r \times r}$ as shown in Fig. 2.

The resulted 5D dissimilarity cost tensor is smoothed in a spatial dimension using an average-pooling layer with stride 1 and the kernel size 7. Next, based on smoothened dissimilarity cost map, the probability for every displacement can be computed with min convolutions [6], which is calculated in displacement dimensions using max-pooling and average-pooling with a stride size of 1 and a kernel size of 3.

Afterwards, we compute the contribution of every discrete displacement pair for all positions along with $15 \times 15 \times 15$ possible displacements. In order to have the lowest SSD value as the maximum value, we negate it and apply the Softmax along the displacement dimension. For more technical insights, see [6]. Finally, we obtain the weighted contributions of all displacement values by broadcasting and multiplying with coordinates of displacement points. This results in 2D displacement field $D \in R^{H \times W}$.

Affine transformation estimation. The estimation of an affine transformation based on the displacement field is performed in two steps, by firstly estimating the initial approximate plane position and secondly perform more accurate post-fitting using outlier rejection. Initially, we estimate a preliminary affine transformation $\Theta \in R^{3 \times 4}$, which corresponds to fitting a plane, which slices the given volume. To achieve it, we warp the points of the centrally placed (reference) plane using the estimated displacement vector field. Then, using two sets of points of central and estimated planes, we approximate the affine transformation which matches two sets of points using Least-Squares (LS) fitting.

During the LS fitting step, we represent each point of the plane $P(x, y, z)$ as a vector $p = (x, y, z, 1)$. Since we know the coordinates of each vector of the plane p (or point P), we can estimate the affine transformation matrix A so that $p = Ap$, where the matrix A is 4×4 elements with 9 unknowns. In this way, we aim to find a minimum of a function with respect to Θ as shown in Equation 1.

$$f(\Theta) = argmin^{\Theta} \sum_{n=1}^{N} ||(Ap^i - p^i - W)||^2 \qquad (1)$$

The initial displacement field, however, may contain outliers which lead to the less optimal estimation of the affine operator. One of the challenges associated with the LS regression method is a lack of robustness to the outliers, which may stem from the noise or CT reconstruction artefacts. Particularly, a point situated far away from the plane will have a strong impact on the LS solution. One of the logical remedies is an iterative discarding (or using low weights) for the points situated further away from the plane and recomputing LS fitting to the data remained. Therefore, after the initial LS fit, we form the matrix $W \in R^{H \times W}$ with the error weights in its corresponding entries and solve regression including outlier weighting map W [7], as shown in Equation 1. We decrease the weights of outliers by subtracting a weighting map, which is based on the weighted distances of outliers to the plane. This results in a smoother displacement field, as shown in Fig. 3 (a) and (b).

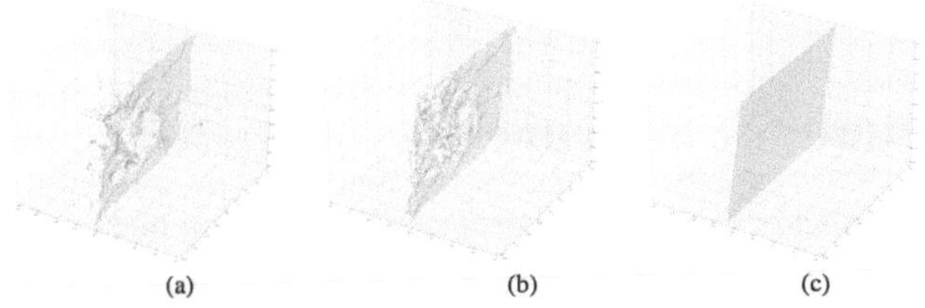

Figure 3: (a) – warped points of the centrally placed plane by estimated deformation field (b) – a warped plane with decreased weight of the points situated further away from the plane (outliers) (c) – final LS fit of the estimated plane.

2.1 Validation

The accuracy of the method is validated based on the distance between estimated and simulated transformation parameters. Given a single slice and a volume, if the affine transformation Θ_{GT} mapping two images is known, we can compute the distance between Θ_{GT} and estimated transformation Θ_{EST}, where each distance per parameter is $|\Theta^i_{GT} - \Theta^i_{EST}|$. In other words, we sample an arbitrary slice and evaluate the accuracy of the defined position in a volume.

For simulating an affine transformation, we create a pseudo-random set of affine parameters, added to the linear operator (± 0.1 with uniform distribution), which corresponds to a range of ± 5.71° for rotation, ± 4mm for translation (capturing more than 10% of the image volume) as well as shear and scaling. In the results section, we present the corresponding evaluation by registering 100 random slices from 30 dynamic CT perfusion images with the time-points t1 = 0s (no presence of contrast tracer) and its corresponding 10 volumes with t2 = 5.2s (maximal presence of contrast tracer in the RV).

3 Results and Discussion

For the validation of our method, we first compare the robustness between several distance metrics for the intertemporal contrast changes and artefacts in Cardiac CT perfusion dataset. We present the comparison of Mean of Absolute Differences (MAD), MAD of corresponding MIND-descriptors, and Mutual Information (MI) as shown in Fig. 4.

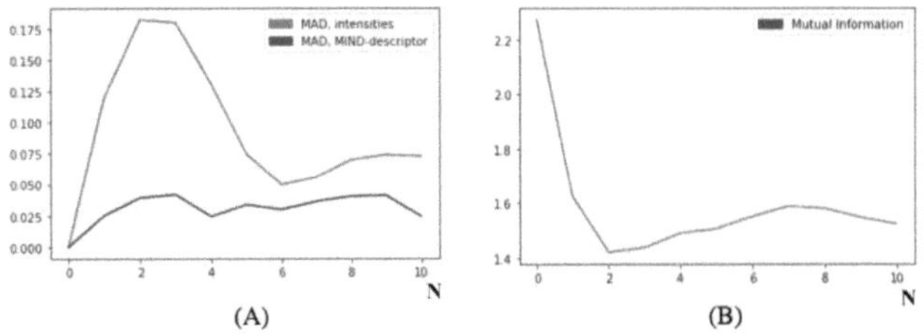

Figure 4: Comparison of distances of images of a sequence and image of its first time-point t=0 using various metrics, where N along x-axes is a number of time points. (a) The Mean of Absolute Distance (MAD) of images and MAD of its corresponding MIND-descriptors. (b) The Mutual Information (MI).

As it is seen from the graph, while the intertemporal MAD and MI of images show the change corresponding to the passage of a contrast bolus, the MAD of MIND-descriptors remains flat, which demonstrates the robustness for its use in image registration.

The further accuracy of the algorithm is validated by registering different temporal sequences of Charité 4D Dynamic CT Perfusion Pilot Study (Charité Universitätsmedizin, Berlin). We use a clinical study dataset featuring 30 temporal cardiac CT perfusion sequences, which were preprocessed and scaled to have an isotropic voxel size of 0.5 mm. The dataset has been also temporally registered, which allows us to validate the accuracy between estimated and synthetic ground truth transformations.

The accuracy is analysed based on error mean and a standard error of difference (SEM) from the synthetic ground truth transformation. The mean error values were calculated for a rotation and a translation, based on results of registering 30 CT Perfusion images as shown in Table 1. As the ablation strategy, we exclude the MIND descriptor and outlier rejection components from the algorithm.

As shown in Table 1, the use of MIND-descriptor and outlier rejection results in improvement of accuracy. The average registration error using both methods for rotation is 0.69° and for translation is 0.60 mm, and without outlier rejection is 0.85° and 0.69 mm respectively. This demonstrates the effectiveness of the outlier rejection method. These results are comparable with best achievable parameter estimation, given the image resolution of 0.5 mm. The high accuracy results when including MIND-descriptor demonstrates its robustness to the local intertemporal contrast changes, which increases the accuracy of estimating individual SSD displacements. The approximate runtime of the presented algorithm is about 3-4 sec, which has a capacity for further improvement for real-time registration, where the volumetric image does not necessarily have to be processed every iteration of registration.

Among comparable works, which also provide the valida-

Table 1: The assessment of registration accuracy based on the mean error and standard error of the difference between estimated and simulated transformation parameters for CTP images. We represent the table using the following coding: **Unregistered** – unregistered simulated dataset; **SSD w OR** – use of SSD metric with outlier rejection; **MIND w/o OR** – MIND-descriptor without outlier rejection; **MIND w OR** both outlier rejection and MIND-descriptor.

Unregistered			SSD w OR			MIND w/o OR			**MIND w OR**		
Rotation (°) – Mean Error/SEM											
$\Delta\theta x$	$\Delta\theta y$	$\Delta\theta z$	$\Delta\theta x$	$\Delta\theta y$	$\Delta\theta z$	$\Delta\theta x$	$\Delta\theta y$	$\Delta\theta z$	**$\Delta\theta x$**	**$\Delta\theta y$**	**$\Delta\theta z$**
2.86	2.86	2.86	3.86	2.41	3.51	0.91	0.89	0.75	**0.72**	**0.86**	**0.51**
0.97	0.97	0.97	0.72	0.47	0.58	0.48	0.34	0.14	**0.46**	**0.26**	**0.19**
Translation (mm) – Mean Error/SEM											
Δx	Δy	Δz	Δx	Δy	Δz	Δx	Δy	Δz	**Δx**	**Δy**	**Δz**
2.00	2.00	2.00	1.28	1.01	2.12	0.68	0.89	0.52	**0.52**	**0.82**	**0.46**
1.35	1.35	1.35	0.36	0.31	0.41	0.25	0.54	0.45	**0.25**	**0.34**	**0.35**

tion metrics in the context of slice-to-volume registration is [8], where they formulate the registration problem as a graph optimization problem using discrete labelling. The work uses a discrete estimation of a linear transformation by means of Markov Random Field (MRF), where the pairwise MRF is modelled. The nodes are linked to rigid parameters, and edges represent a connection of variables. The accuracy evaluated using an MRI cardiac dataset resulting in the average registration error of 4.77° for rotation and 5.32mm for translation, which has a considerably higher error than one of the presented algorithm. However, the accuracy results might not be directly compared due to differently defined search ranges and a larger voxel size of MR images. Nevertheless, the runtime of the MRF discrete method is about 9 min, which is considerably longer than the runtime of our proposed method (4-5 s).

However, despite our method proved to be accurate and has a low registration mean error, the question of stability shall be further addressed. The standard error of difference (SEM) is 0.46° for rotation and 1.88 mm for translation. In about 5% of the cases, the error can reach more than 1.50° for rotation and 1.20 mm for translation. Depending on the clinical application, the problem of increasing robustness needs to be considered. Additionally, the search range of our method is 30% of the full image volume, which may result in low robustness at estimating larger deformations.

4 Conclusion

In this work, we present a slice-to-volume image registration algorithm for motion correction cardiac images using MIND descriptor. The accuracy validation demonstrates robustness against the intertemporal alteration of contrast agent as well as the presence of motion. In our accuracy validation, we register 30 pairs of CT perfusion image slices into a reference CT volume in different timepoints. The average registration error of algorithm with the outlier rejection for rotation is 0.69° and for translation is 0.60 mm. The accuracy of registration results is superior in comparison to another slice-to-volume registration method. In the work of Porchetto et al. [8] both registration error and runtime are considerably higher. The presented method of slice-to-volume registration has potential for effective application in the medical image analysis tasks such as motion correction, volume reconstruction and image fusion during image-guided surgeries. In the future work, we intend to explore the possibility of full 4D CT perfusion temporal volume matching as well as modality independent MRI-CT slice-to-volume registration.

Acknowledgement

The work has been carried out at Charité University Hospital Berlin and supervised by the Institute of Medical Informatics, Universität zu Lübeck.

Author's Statement

Conflict of interest: Authors state no conflict of interest.

5 References

[1] E. Ferrante and N. Paragios, Slice-to-volume medical image registration: A survey," Med. Image Anal., vol. 39, pp. 101–123, 2017.

[2] V. Mani and S. Arivazhagan, Survey of medical image registration," J. Biomed. EngTech., vol. 1, no. 2, 2013.

[3] A. Sotiras, C. Davatzikos, and N. Paragios, Deformable medical image registration: A survey," IEEE Trans. Med. Imaging, vol. 32, no. 7, pp. 1153–1190, 2013.

[4] M. P. Heinrich, M. Jenkinson, M. Brady, and J. A. Schnabel, Globally optimal deformable registration on a minimum spanning tree using dense displacement sampling," in MICCAI , 2012, pp. 115–122.

[5] M. P. Heinrich, M. Jenkinson, B. W. Papież, M. Brady, and J. A. Schnabel, Towards realtime multimodal fusion for image-guided interventions using self-similarities," in MICCAI, 2013, pp. 187–194.

[6] M. P. Heinrich, Closing the gap between deep and conventional image registration using probabilistic dense displacement networks," in MICCAI, 2019, pp. 50–58.

[7] I. Y. Ha and M. P. Heinrich, Modality-agnostic self-supervised deep feature learning and fast instance optimisation for multimodal fusion in ultrasound-guided interventions," Comput. Methods Biomed., 2021.

[8] R. Porchetto, F. Stramana, N. Paragios, and E. Ferrante, Rigid slice-to-volume medical image registration through Markov random fields," in MICCAI, Springer, 2016, pp. 172–185.

Ultrasound Medical Imaging: Comparison of Methods for Adjusting Speed of Sound of Human Tissue in Water

Timir Barua [1], Felix von Haxthausen [2], Verónica García-Vázquez [2]
[1] Biomedical Engineering, Luebeck University of Applied Sciences, timir.barua@stud.th-luebeck.de
[2] Institute for Robotics and Cognitive Systems, Universität zu Lübeck, {vonhaxthausen, garciavazquez}@rob.uni-luebeck.de

Abstract

In ultrasound, image distortion is produced if speed of sound in a medium differs from 1540 m/s (speed assumed in ultrasound machines). Our study compared several methods reported in previous literature to adjust the speed of sound in tap water using a wire phantom immersed in different water baths. Distances between wires from ultrasound volumes were compared to ground truth distances from a computed tomography scan. Water at room temperature resulted in large errors (mean error 3.25 mm) as expected. Increasing water temperature to 50 °C is not a feasible approach since the ultrasound probe did not work and the phantom was deformed. Dissolving a specific amount of salt in water depending on water temperature is a better approach than mixing 7% glycerol with water at room temperature since the former provides more accurate results (mean error 0.89 mm) and is less expensive than the latter (mean error 1.36 mm).

1 Introduction

Ultrasound imaging is a relatively low-cost, harmless, non-invasive and mobile technique [1]. Real-time acquisition also makes ultrasound a widely used imaging modality for intra-operative procedures in comparison with magnetic resonance imaging (MRI) and computed tomography (CT) [2]. In CT, ionizing radiation can cause cancer. However, a disadvantage of ultrasound imaging is its operator dependency.

Two-dimensional (2D) ultrasound acquires 2D images and requires that sonographers mentally reconstruct these images into three-dimensional (3D) structures [3]. Furthermore, transducer movements and patient breathing cause out-of plane motion that changes the anatomical plane acquired. In addition, reproducing an ultrasound image in follow-up studies is cumbersome [3]. These problems are solved by means of 3D ultrasound, which acquires ultrasound volumes of the region of interest. Moreover, distances and volumes of body organs may be more accurate compared to measurements obtained with 2D ultrasound [1].

An ultrasound transducer (also known as ultrasound probe) transmits sound waves into the human body and captures echoes (specifically, reflected and scattered sound waves), which are processed to generate ultrasound images. Most ultrasound machines assume that sound waves travel at 1540 m/s to calculate distances to the transducer [1]. Distortion is produced if the speed of sound in a medium differs from this average speed of sound through human tissue [1]. This is the case when immersing a wire phantom in water at room temperature to acquire ultrasound images of the wires since the speed of sound of this medium is approximately 1485 m/s [1]. In order to achieve the average speed of sound of human tissue in water, previous literature presented different solutions. Boctor et al. [2] and Treece et al. [4] increased the temperature of water close to 50 °C. Tap water was specified in [4]. By mixing 9.5% $\pm$ 0.25% ethanol with distilled water (temperature of the mixture 20 °C $\pm$ 0.75 °C), the speed of sound was 1540 $\pm$ 1.5 m/s, reported by Martin and Spinks [5]. Pace et al. [6] used a solution of 7% glycerol in water. Kleis and Sanchez [7] described the dependence of the speed of sound in sodium chloride (NaCl) solutions with temperature. To our knowledge there is no previous literature comparing these methods to match the assumed speed of sound.

The aim of our study was to compare several methods to adjust the speed of sound of 1540 m/s in water in terms of feasibility, distortion reduction and cost. A wire phantom was immersed in different water baths and acquired with a 3D ultrasound probe. The distances between wires from those ultrasound volumes were compared to ground truth distances from a CT scan to evaluate image distortion.

2 Material and Methods

2.1 Wire Phantom

The 3D model of the fCal-3.1 calibration phantom was downloaded from Plus 3D model catalog of Plus toolkit (https://plustoolkit.github.io/). This phantom was designed for freehand spatial ultrasound calibration for structures of up to 30-cm depth. All pieces (specifically, one front piece, one back piece, five spacers and one sensor block) were 3D-printed with an Anycubic i3 Mega 3D printer and polylactic acid (PLA) filament. These eight pieces were joined with six bolts (DIN933 - M6x80 PA6.6) and six nuts (DIN555/934 M6 - PA 6.6). Ten wires of nylon (thickness 0.35 mm) were placed in parallel between the front piece and the back piece (distance between both pieces 40 mm) at different depths using the phantom holes. Fig. 1 shows the phantom built and Fig. 2 (left) illustrates the wire configuration.

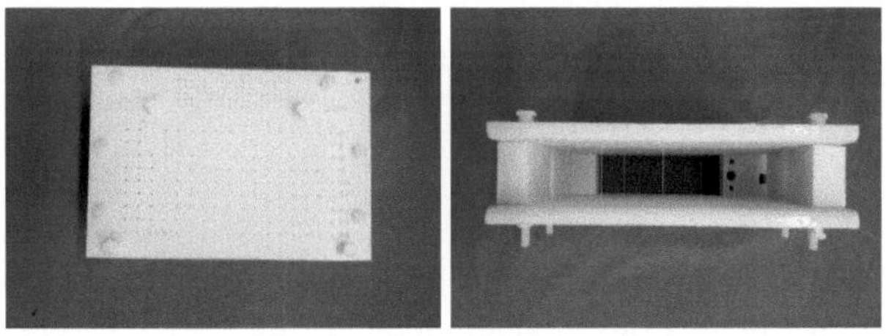

Figure 1: Wire phantom. Lateral view (left) and bottom view (right).

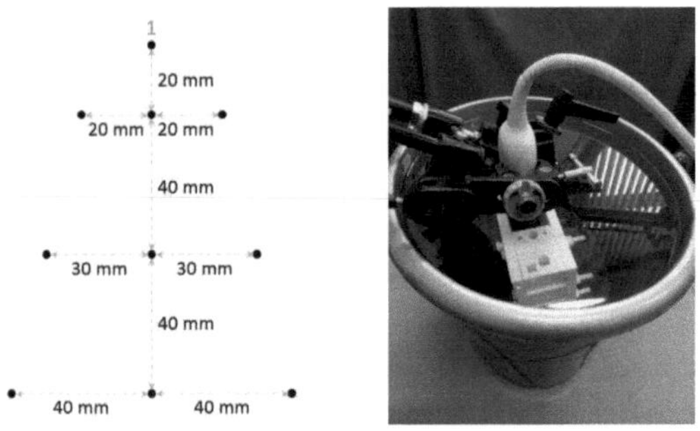

Figure 2: Wire configuration (left) and experimental setup (right).

2.2 Study Protocol

In this study, four different setups were conducted where the wire phantom was placed inside a bucket that contained warm water, water at room temperature, water with glycerol or water with salt. Acoustic foam was attached to the bottom (inner side) of the bucket with silicone hot melt glue to avoid sound echoes from the bottom of the bucket. Each setup (changing the foam each time) with its ultrasound acquisition and temperature measurement was repeated three times. Specifications of each setup are presented as follows:

- Warm water: The bucket was filled with 12 liters of tap water after heating up the water to approximately 50 °C.
- Water: The bucket was filled with 12 liters of tap water at room temperature. This setup was included to assess the image distortion when the speed of sound of the medium does not match 1540 m/s.
- Glycerol solution: The bucket was filled with 1 liter of glycerol 85% (cost 15.94 €) mixed with 11 liters of tap water at room temperature. Therefore, the percentage of glycerol of this solution was 7.08.
- Salt solution: A specific amount of table salt (which is usually 97% to 99% NaCl) was dissolved in 12 liters of tap water at room temperature. This amount was calculated considering that salinity in NaCl solutions depends on the speed of sound and temperature of the solution as follows [7]:

$$S(c,T) = a_2(T) + a_3(T)c \quad (1)$$

where

$$a_2(T) = -101.682 - 0.857118\,T - 0.0237298\,T^2 + 0.000453213\,T^3 - 2.17401E-6\,T^4 \quad (2)$$

$$a_3(T) = 0.0722597 + 0.000412596\,T + 1.46562E-5\,T^2 - 2.65803E-7\,T^3 + 1.27778E-9\,T^4 \quad (3)$$

where S is salinity in percentage, c is speed of sound in m/s (1540 m/s in our case) and T is temperature in degrees Celsius (the initial temperature of the tap water in our case). Assuming 100% NaCl in table salt, the amount of salt s (in grams) was calculated as follows:

$$s = V * S/100 \quad (4)$$

where V is the volume of water in milliliters. Table 1 shows the initial temperature of the tap water for each repetition of this setup, its corresponding salinity to obtain a speed of sound of 1540 m/s in the NaCl solution using (1)-(3) and the corresponding amount of salt dissolved in the 12 liters of water using (4). The cost of 500 grams of table salt was 0.17 €.

Table 1: Settings of the salt solutions

Repetition	Initial temperature	Salinity	Salt amount
1	21.1 °C	4.77%	572.4 g
2	21.0 °C	4.79%	574.8 g
3	21.2 °C	4.75%	570.0 g

For each setup and repetition, ultrasound volumes of the ten wires of the wire phantom were acquired with a 3D ultrasound probe (X6-1, Philips healthcare) (Fig. 2, right) and the EPIQ 7 ultrasound system (Philips Healthcare) with the following settings: intensity gain 37%, angle 30°, depth 16 cm and frequency (volume acquisition) 3 Hz. Ultrasound data were transferred from the ultrasound station to the medical image processing software 3D Slicer (https://www.slicer.org/) (specifically, *Plus Remote* module) by means of a proprietary network protocol (provided by Philips) and Plus toolkit. For each volume, its matrix size was 416 x 291 x 98 voxels and its voxel size was 0.58 x 0.57 x 0.95 mm^3.

A CT scan of the wire phantom was acquired with a Siemens SOMATOM Definition AS+ CT scanner to obtain the ground truth distances between the wires. The acquisition parameters were as follows: voltage 120 kVp, exposure 166 ± 4 mAs (mean ± standard deviation), slice thickness 0.40 mm and pixel size 0.25 x 0.25 mm^2.

2.3 Image Processing

The following process was applied to an ultrasound volume of each setup and repetition, and to the CT volume. After loading the volume in 3D Slicer, each wire was segmented using *Threshold*, *Scissors* and *Islands* tools to remove regions that did not belong to that specific wire. A 3D model was created from each segmented wire and this, in turn, was adjusted to a straight line with *Marksup to Model* module and the following settings: (Curve type) global least squares polynomial; (Fitting) point sorting indices and polynomial order 1; (Tube properties) radius 0.17 mm, number of sides 20 and segments per point 1. The distance from each point of the wire line at the top of the phantom (wire number 1, Fig. 2) to the closest point of each of the other nine wire lines was computed with *Model to Model Distance* module (absolute closest point option). For each pair of lines (nine in total), the distances (more than 4000 values) were saved in VTK file format and loaded in MATLAB to calculate the mean and the standard deviation.

For each pair of lines (nine in total) of each setup and repetition, the error was calculated subtracting the CT mean distance (ground truth) from the ultrasound mean distance.

3 Results and Discussion

Table 2 shows the temperatures of the medium for each setup and repetition when acquiring the ultrasound volumes. In the case of the warm water, ultrasound volumes were not recorded since, in the first repetition, there was an error message of ultrasound probe getting hot when immersing the probe. In addition, the wire phantom was deformed by the warm water (Fig. 3) so the phantom was built again to continue with our study. For the second and third setups, the temperatures were slightly different among repetitions. For the salt solution and for each repetition, the temperature when scanning was close to the initial temperature (Table 1).

Table 2: Temperatures of the medium for each setup and repetition (rep) when acquiring the ultrasound volumes

Setup	1st rep	2nd rep	3rd rep
Warm water	50.0 °C	-	-
Water	23.2 °C	21.8 °C	21.3 °C
Glycerol solution	23.0 °C	20.9 °C	22.0 °C
Salt solution	21.1 °C	20.7 °C	20.9 °C

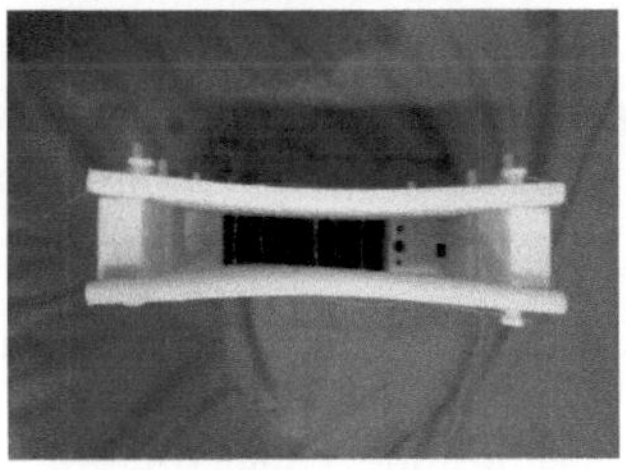

Figure 3: Deformed wire phantom (bottom view).

Standard deviation of the distances for each pair of wires should ideally be zero since the wires were placed in parallel. The process of computing these distances is more reliable in the case of the CT scan compared to the ultrasound setups since its median and range of the standard deviations (0.12 mm and 0.01 mm respectively) are lower (Fig. 4). This is because the wire segmentation was less accurate in the case of the ultrasound volumes due to ultrasound artifacts and noise. Nevertheless, the standard deviations of the distances are less than 0.3 mm for the ultrasound setups, which are acceptable considering the voxel size.

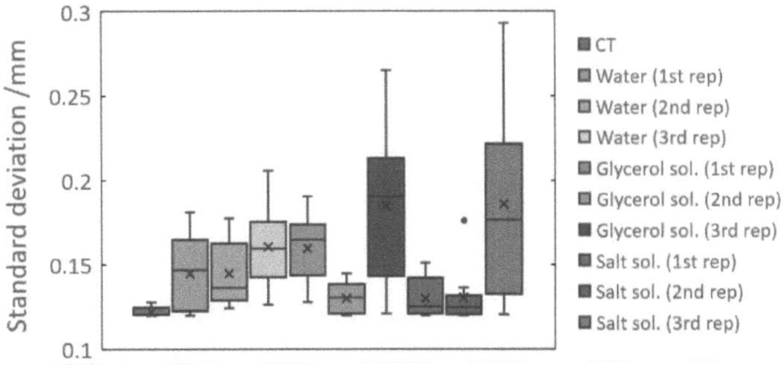

Figure 4: Box plot of the standard deviations of distances for the nine pairs of wires. Crosses and dots represent means and outliers respectively. Solution (sol.) and repetition (rep).

Table 3 shows the errors for each setup combining all repetitions, where the largest values (mean error 3.25 mm) correspond to water at room temperature (as expected) and the smallest values (mean error 0.89 mm) correspond to salt solutions. Glycerol solutions provided a mean error of 1.36 mm with repetitions at slightly different room temperatures. Increasing glycerol percentage may reduce errors but this method is more expensive than salt solutions. All minimum errors are positive. Therefore, the speed of sound in these mediums was smaller than 1540 m/s since the wires appeared further in the ultrasound images than in reality [1].

Table 3: Errors for each setup combining all repetitions

Error (mm)	Water	Glycerol solution	Salt solution
Mean	3.25	1.36	0.89
Standard deviation	1.37	0.50	0.35
Minimum	1.26	0.59	0.37
Maximum	5.60	2.39	1.67

Fig. 5, Fig. 6 and Fig. 7 illustrate the linear relationship between error and ground truth distance (positive regression slope, R-squared values mostly larger than 0.7) for water, glycerol solutions and salt solutions respectively. Assuming that the ultrasound probe was parallel to the wires, those figures show that wires at the same depth (Fig. 2) did not provide similar errors (as is the case of linear probes [1]). Our 3D ultrasound probe is a sector probe so the radius (image in polar coordinates) is scaled by the ratio between assumed speed of sound and real speed [1]. The dispersion of the errors (Table 3) is partly explained by this systematic error.

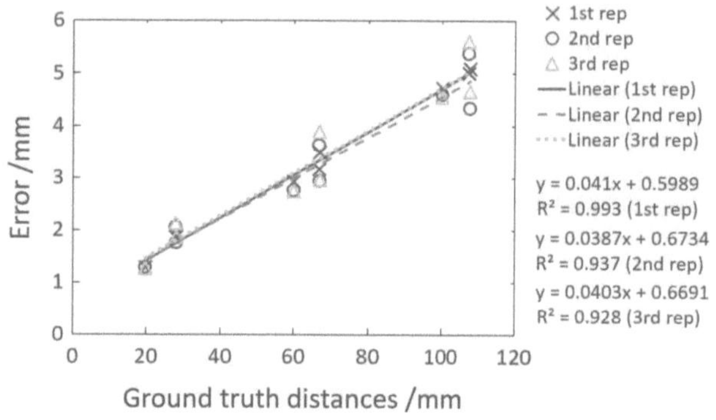

Figure 5: Error versus ground truth distance for the water. A scatter plot per each repetition (rep) that includes its trend line, its equation and its R-squared value.

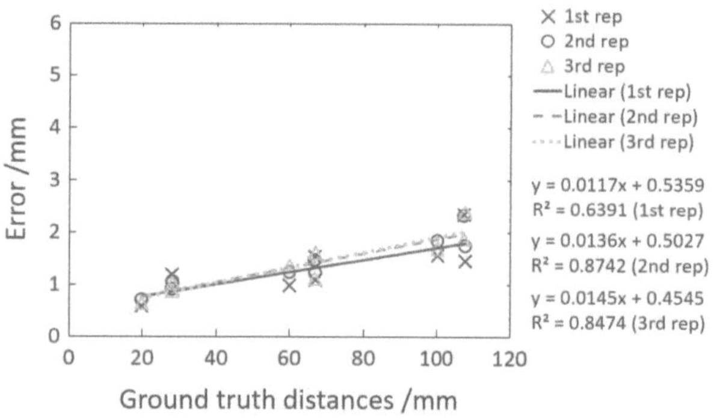

Figure 6: Error versus ground truth distance for the glycerol solution. Same figure explanation as in Fig. 5.

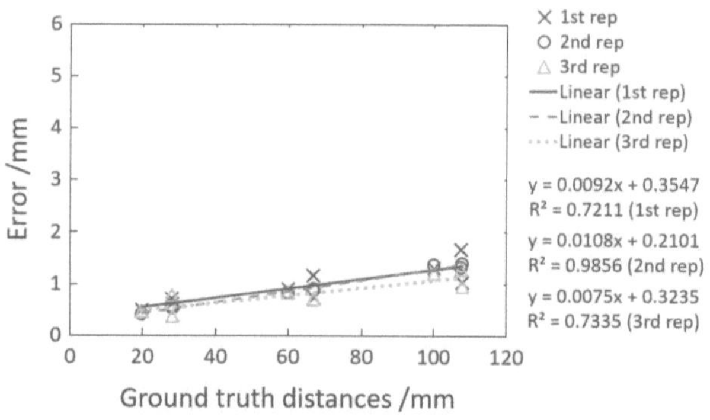

Figure 7: Error versus ground truth distance for the salt solution. Same figure explanation as in Fig. 5.

4 Conclusion

This study compared several methods to adjust the speed of sound in tap water to the average speed of sound through human tissue. Increasing the temperature to 50 °C is not a feasible approach since ultrasound probes may not work and phantoms may be deformed. Dissolving a specific amount of salt in water depending on the water temperature is a better approach than mixing 7% glycerol with water at room temperature since the former provides more accurate results and is less expensive than the latter. In both setups, the error increases with the distance to the sector probe. Further experiments (for example, freehand spatial ultrasound calibration) will be done immersing phantoms in salt solutions.

Acknowledgement

The work has been carried out and supervised by the Institute for Robotics and Cognitive Systems, Universität zu Lübeck. This study was supported by the German Federal Ministry of Education and Research (grant number 13GW0228).

Author's Statement

Conflict of interest: Authors state no conflict of interest. Informed consent: Not applicable.

5 References

[1] L. Mercier, T. Langø, F. Lindseth and L. D. Collins, *A review of calibration techniques for freehand 3-D ultrasound systems.* Ultrasound in Medicine & Biology, vol. 31, no. 4, pp. 449–471, 2005.

[2] E. M. Boctor, A. Jain, M. A. Choti, R. H. Taylor and G. Fichtinger, *A rapid calibration method for registration and 3D tracking of ultrasound images using spatial localizer.* Proceedings of SPIE, Medical Imaging 2003: Ultrasonic Imaging and Signal Processing, vol. 5035, pp. 521-532, 2003.

[3] E. Boctor, A. Saad, D-J Chang, K. Kamel and A. M. Youssef, *PC-based system for calibration, reconstruction, processing, and visualization of 3D ultrasound data based on a magnetic-field position and orientation sensing system.* Computational Science - ICCS 2001, Lecture Notes in Computer Science, vol. 2074, pp. 13–22, 2001.

[4] G. M. Treece, A. H. Gee, R. W. Prager, C. J. C. Cash and L. H. Berman, *High-definition freehand 3-D ultrasound.* Ultrasound in Medicine & Biology, vol. 29, no. 4, pp. 529-546, 2003.

[5] K. Martin and D. Spinks, *Measurement of the speed of sound in ethanol/water mixtures.* Ultrasound in Medicine & Biology, vol. 27, no. 2, pp. 289-291, 2001.

[6] D. F. Pace, A. D. Wiles, J. Moore, C. Wedlake, D. G. Gobbi and T. M. Peters, *Validation of four-dimensional ultrasound for targeting in minimally-invasive beating-heart surgery.* Proceedings of SPIE, Medical Imaging 2009: Visualization, Image-Guided Procedures, and Modeling, vol. 7261, 726115, pp. 1-12, 2009.

[7] S. J. Kleis and L. A. Sanchez, *Dependence of speed of sound on salinity and temperature in concentrated NaCl solutions.* Solar Energy, vol. 45, no. 4, pp. 201-206, 1990.

Deep learning-based image registration for voxel-based morphometry

Zhibin Xin [1], Mattias Heinrich[2], for the Alzheimer's Disease Neuroimaging Initiative[3]

[1] Roboitics and Autonomous Systems, Universität zu Lübeck, zhibin.xin@student.uni-luebeck.de

[2] Institute for Medical Informatics, Universität zu Lübeck, heinrich@imi.uni-luebeck.de

[3] Data used in preparation of this article were obtained from the Alzheimer's Disease Neuroimaging Initiative (ADNI) database. The investigators within the ADNI contributed to the design and implementation of ADNI but did not participate in analysis or writing of this report.

Abstract

This paper describes a sub-project of Alzheimer's disease progression. Voxel-based morphometry (VBM) will be used in this project for the analysis of the brain. To speed up the registration of brain MRI scans, the process involved in VBM, this sub-project aims at building a learnable registration model by applying deep learning techniques. Currently, the sub-project has trained a fast registration model by ADNI data, which is able to predict registered images within half a minute. In the future, brain segmentation may be applied to this sub-project to further improve the quality of registration.

1 Introduction

VBM is a technique involving the voxel-wise gray matter comparison between two groups of subjects [1], such as normal control (NC) and Alzheimer's disease (AD), or AD and mild cognitive impairment (MCI). This technique is widely used for the analysis of neuroanatomical images.

Image registration, as one of the steps involved in VBM technique, is a process of aligning a moving image to the space of fixed image so that their corresponding features can be easily compared [2], which improves the accuracy of gray matter comparison work. However, traditional method of image registration align moving images to fixed ones by optimizing an objective function for each pair of images, which is computationally and time expensive when processing large sets of high-resolution 3D medical images. Normally, it takes hours to register a single 3D image by traditional method. Therefore, many image registration methods based on deep learning techniques have emerged in recent years. In deep learning-based approaches, the iterative alignment process can be replaced by a learnable convolutional neural network model to extract features of input images and predict spatial deformation for registration. Although the training process of the network could be also time-consuming, once the training is finished, the model can predict spatial transformation fast. This sub-project applies the deep learning-based method to the registration of brain MRI scans to prepare for the future VBM analysis.

Since VBM analysis requires mapping all subjects into the same anatomical space for gray matter comparison, all subjects need to be registered to the same fixed image. The fixed image can be chosen from a random subject but this would result in bias, so an atlas needs to be constructed. Atlas represents an average volume and is usually constructed by jointly and repeatedly aligning a dataset of brain MR volumes and averaging them together [3].

Therefore, in order to build a deep learning-based image registration model, two steps are needed, constructing atlas and training model by taking constructed atlas as fixed image.

2 Material and Methods

2.1 Dataset

The used dataset is ADNI T1-weighted brain image [4], which includes 1700 subjects. 500 subjects in this dataset belong to the NC group and the rest are AD or MCI.

2.2 Atlas Construction

A common approach of atlas construction is choosing an initial atlas or simply averaging all images, then align all images to it and a better atlas can be estimated by averaging the aligned images. The process will be iterated until convergence [5]. Since the process requires many iterations and involve many pairwise registrations in each iteration, it is very time and computation consuming. In order to speed up the process of atlas construction, a deep learning-based one provided by VoxelMorph [6] was used]. The structure of the network for generating atlas is shown in Fig.1.

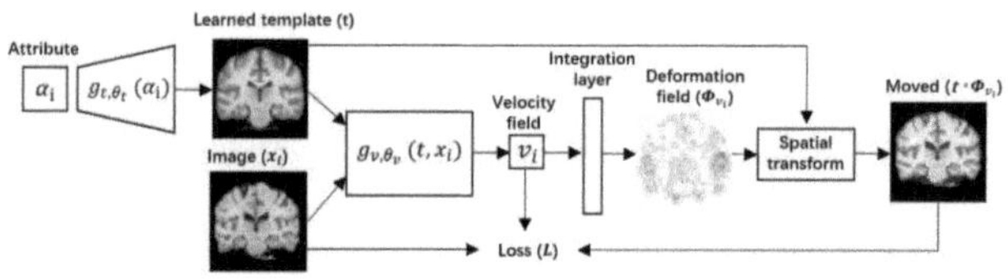

Figure 1: Structure of atlas generation network [5]

In this model, θ denotes the pixel intensity value to be estimated and α, latent variables (e.g. age and gender). The $g_{t,\theta_t}(\cdot)$ is a generative network that outputs atlas, and $g_{v,\theta_v}(\cdot)$ is a U-Net network with ReLU activation function for image registration. There are two versions of atlas can be generated by this model. The first one, conditional atlas, requires latent variables for generating an atlas with respect to a certain group (e.g. the atlas for a certain age group). The second one, unconditional atlas, does not need the input of latent variables and generates a global atlas for all groups. Since an atlas for registration of all subjects is required in this sub-project, the unconditional atlas was used. At the beginning of the learning process, a rough atlas is generated by simply averaging all input images. During the training process, the generative network yields an atlas in each iteration, and the atlas is registered with the other input image to output velocity field (i.e. deformation). After that, the generated atlas is warped to the space of the input image by applying the deformation field. While optimizing the global network, the generative network can produce a better atlas.

2.3 Learnable Image Registration Model

In terms of model training, VoxelMorph provides an unsupervised learning-based model. The general structural can be seen in Fig.2. $g_\theta(f, m)$ is a U-Net taking fixed and moving image as input, and generating a deformation field. By applying the generated deformation field to the moving image, the image will be warped to the anatomical space of the fixed one. The transformation process is optimized by minimizing 2 loss terms, similarity, and smoothness. For measuring similarity, there are 3 common metrics, mean squared, mutual information [7] and cross-correlation [8]. The optimization problem can be written as:

$$\widehat{\phi} = \arg\min_{\phi} L(f, m, \phi) \tag{1}$$

$$= \arg\min_{\phi} L_{sim}(f, m \circ \phi) + \lambda L_{smooth}(\phi) \tag{2}$$

where f, m and ϕ respectively denotes fixed image input, moving image input and deformation field. $m \circ \phi$ represents wrapping of m by ϕ and λ, the weight of smoothness loss.

In addition, if the data is labeled with segmentation, this method can be supervised by applying a deformation field to moving image segmentation, and an additional dice loss will be taken into consideration for measuring the overlap between warped segmentation and fixed image segmentation. This auxiliary function can be used for improving the performance of image registration.

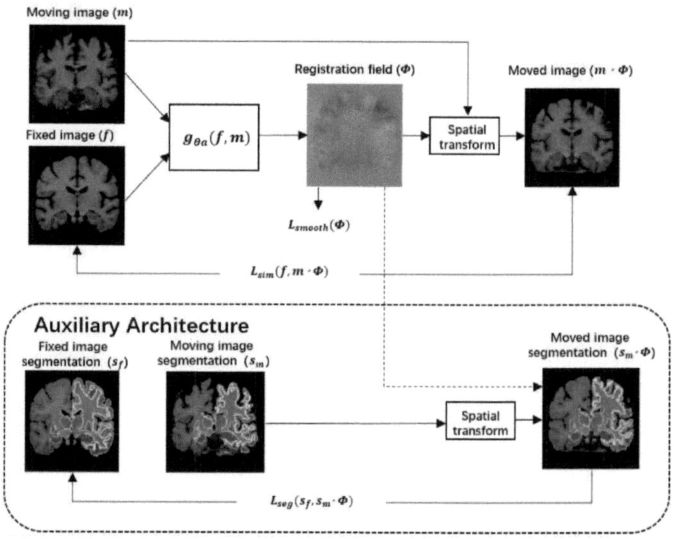

Figure 2: Structure of VoxelMorph network [6]

3 Experiment

As mentioned above, the goal of this sub-project is training a deep learning-based model for fast registration and preparing for the following analysis. Before working on the final analysis, the function of classifying different groups (i.e. AD, MCI, and NC) should be reached. The approach of classification that will be used in this project is exploring the deformation field of 3 different subjects. Therefore, in order to better distinguish the deformation field of data of different groups when aligned with the atlas, only data of NC group was used in the atlas construction and model training phase.

Firstly, in order to improve the performance of VoxelMorph model, all scans have to be preprocessed. Standard steps of data preprocessing, including motion correction and conform, Talairach transform computation, intensity normalization, and skull stripping were applied by using FreeSurfer [9].

Before decided to use FreeSurfer for data preprocessing, this sub-project also tried to apply several currently available deep learning-based approaches to reduce the time consumption because the standard processing by FreeSurfer takes around 20 minutes for each sample. However, many samples processed by these approaches have significant non-brain tissues left.

In addition, given the computational expense and architecture of U-Net used in the training phase, all scans were cropped into an appropriate size, 160x194x224. As shown in Fig.3, the input scan will undergo four downsamplings in the encoder part, so the size of scans should be multiple of 16 to ensure size consistency of feature maps in the encoder and decoder parts while concatenation.

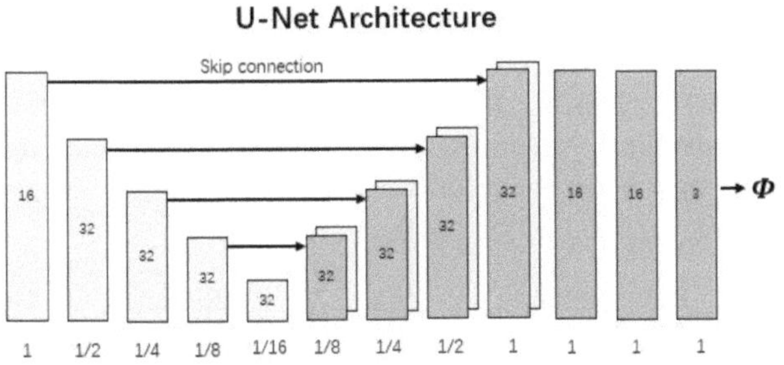

Figure 3: Architecture of U-Net used in deep learning-based image registration model [6]. The number in each layer denotes the number of feature maps. The U-Net uses ReLU as the activation function.

After data preprocessing, all NC data was used for generating the atlas. The generated atlas is taken as a fixed image through the whole deep learning model training phase. 500 NC subjects were divided into 400 training data, 50 evaluation data, and 50 test data. Different hyperparameters setup, learning rate, batch size, and optimizer, was applied for trying to investigate the best one. In addition, visual inspection was used for quality control of registration. During the training phase, the model state in each 10 epoch is saved for tracking the performance of the trained model in different periods.

In the beginning, the trained model did not perform well. The significant difference can be easily noticed by visual inspection. The example of bad registration is shown in Fig. 4. The right-side scale denotes the image intensity.

After investigation, the problem was discovered on the constructed atlas. The atlas cannot be used directly after being constructed, but the Talairach transformation and intensity normalization need to be applied to the atlas to ensure that both fixed images and moving images are in the Talairach space. All moving images are mapped to Talairach space and normalized after data preprocessing.

4 Results and Discussion

A complete training phase for one model with 400 training samples and 1000 epochs took about 4 days but in the test phase, the average time to predict warped image is only 21.04 seconds. Currently, the best hyperparameter setup is learning rate = 1e-4, adam optimizer and batch size = 1 with the average test loss = 0.0327. Because of a large number of parameters, only a small batch size (e.g. 1 or 2) is allowed to be used. Otherwise, the allocation of parameters will exceed max system memory. The example of brain image registration by the currently trained model can be seen in Fig.5.

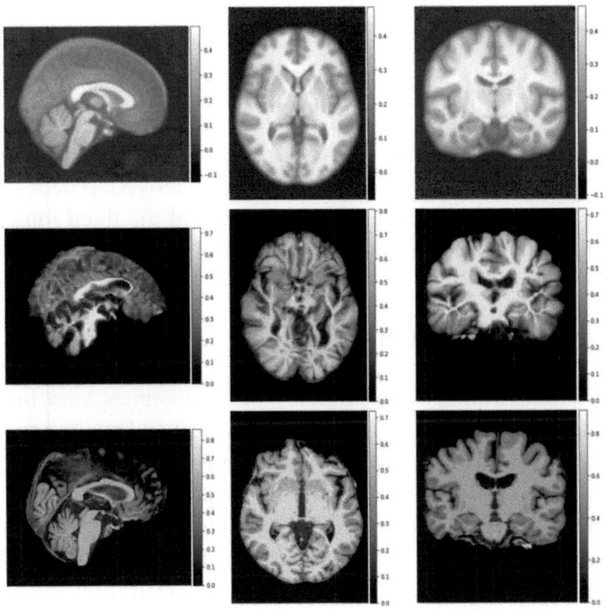

Figure 4: Example of bad registration. Each row from top to bottom is mid slices of fixed image, warped image and moving image in 3 different plane.

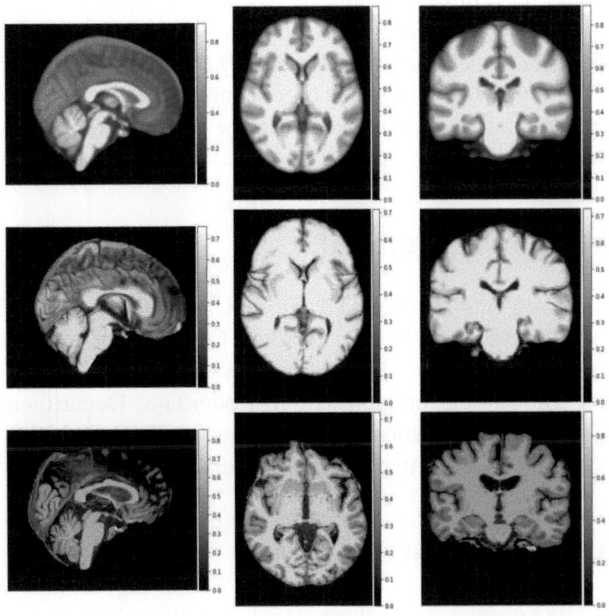

Figure 5: Example of registration predicted by current model. Each row from top to bottom is mid slices of fixed image, warped image and moving image in 3 different plane.

Although the alignment of brain outlines is good, there are still significant differences between the internal structure (especially the sagittal plane) of the fixed image and the moving image. By checking the registration performance of the models in the last 200 periods, even if the training loss is not significantly reduced, the internal structure of the registered image is still improving. Therefore, training with more epochs may help improve the registration performance of the model.

Moreover, a weakly supervised manner can be introduced for further improvement of internal structure by applying the spatial transformation to the segmentation of moving images. In this way, another loss term, the overlap between warped segmentation and segmentation of the fixed image, can be included in the optimization problem.

5 Conclusion

The trained image registration model consumes very little time when predicting new moving images. This is a very prominent advantage of the deep learning-based approach, and it is also the desired result of this sub-project. However, since this sub-project is still trying to build a deep learning model with better registration performance, it is hard to make a conclusion in terms of image registration quality of the deep learning-based approach. Moreover, the time spent on atlas construction in this sub-project has not been compared with the traditional pairwise registration approach.

Hence, in future work, training with more epochs will be carried out and weak supervision will be introduced to improve the registration performance of the internal structure of the brain. In addition, the time spent on atlas construction between pairwise registration and the deep learning-based approach will be compared.

Acknowledgement

The work has been carried out at Universität zu Lübeck and supervised by both of Institute for Medical Informatics, Universität zu Lübeck, and Dr.Vikram Venkatraghavan, Biomedical Imaging Group Rotterdam, Departments of Medical InformaticsRadiology, Erasmus MC, University Medical Center Rotterdam, the Netherlands.

Author's Statement

Conflict of interest: Authors state no conflict of interest.

6 References

[1] J. Ashburner and K. J. Friston, "Voxel-based morphometry—the methods," *Neuroimage*, vol. 11, no. 6, pp. 805–821, 2000.

[2] J. V. Hajnal and D. L. Hill, *Medical image registration.* CRC press, 2001.

[3] M. De Craene, A. du Bois d'Aische, B. Macq, and S. K. Warfield, "Multi-subject registration for unbiased statistical atlas construction," in *International Conference on Medical Image Computing and Computer-Assisted Intervention*, pp. 655–662, Springer, 2004.

[4] S. G. Mueller, M. W. Weiner, L. J. Thal, R. C. Petersen, C. R. Jack, W. Jagust, J. Q. Trojanowski, A. W. Toga, and L. Beckett, "Ways toward an early diagnosis in alzheimer's disease: the alzheimer's disease neuroimaging initiative (adni)," *Alzheimer's & Dementia*, vol. 1, no. 1, pp. 55–66, 2005.

[5] A. V. Dalca, M. Rakic, J. Guttag, and M. R. Sabuncu, "Learning conditional deformable templates with convolutional networks," *arXiv preprint arXiv:1908.02738*, 2019.

[6] G. Balakrishnan, A. Zhao, M. R. Sabuncu, J. Guttag, and A. V. Dalca, "Voxelmorph: a learning framework for deformable medical image registration," *IEEE transactions on medical imaging*, vol. 38, no. 8, pp. 1788–1800, 2019.

[7] P. Viola and W. M. Wells III, "Alignment by maximization of mutual information," *International journal of computer vision*, vol. 24, no. 2, pp. 137–154, 1997.

[8] B. B. Avants, C. L. Epstein, M. Grossman, and J. C. Gee, "Symmetric diffeomorphic image registration with cross-correlation: evaluating automated labeling of elderly and neurodegenerative brain," *Medical image analysis*, vol. 12, no. 1, pp. 26–41, 2008.

[9] B. Fischl, "Freesurfer," *Neuroimage*, vol. 62, no. 2, pp. 774–781, 2012.

Automatic Segmentation of the Femoral Artery from 2D Ultrasound Images

Ana V. Estrada Lugo [1], Felix von Haxthausen [2], Niclas Bockelmann [2] and Floris Ernst [2]
[1] Biomedical Engineering, Luebeck University of Applied Sciences, ana.veronica.lugo@stud.th-luebeck.de
[2] Institute for Robotics and Cognitive Systems, Universität zu Lübeck, {vonhaxthausen, bockelmann, ernst}@rob.uni-luebeck.de

Abstract

Ultrasound (US) is one of the most popular imaging modalities, but one of its disadvantages is the high sensitivity to noise and artifacts. In order to facilitate the identification of structures during surgical interventions, the easy interpretation of the images is a challenging task to address. This work compares three different approaches of the U-Net: Conventional U-Net, U-Net with one encoder of two channels and a U-Net with two encoders to automatically segment the femoral artery from 2D ultrasound images. The latter two architectures followed a sequential structure, where each Ultrasound image is considered a slice of the whole volume and its segmentation will affect directly the prediction of the next image. Ultrasound scans from five different volunteers were collected to produce a dataset of 10,557 US images and their respectively manual segmentation. The evaluation Dice scores were 0.8191, 0.6331 and 0.7250 for the Conventional U-Net, U-Net with one encoder of two channels and a U-Net with two encoders respectively. Those metrics show a better performance on the Conventional U-Net compared to the Sequential U-Net approaches for the femoral artery segmentation. This could be attributed to the misalignment of the slices being used in those networks. A possible improvement could be assumed in the implementation of a spatial calibration for the ultrasound probe. Overall these results indicate promising approaches for an automatic segmentation using 2D ultrasound data.

1 Introduction

Ultrasound (US) is one of the most used imaging modality due to its low cost, non-invasive nature, real time display and relative safety [1]. Nevertheless, US also presents drawbacks such as high sensitivity to artifacts and noise during acquisition and a complex interpretation of the images which requires years of training and experience. These challenges could be addressed through deep learning, a machine learning subset that extract pieces of information needed to inform future predictions or make a decision [2]. This allows us to develop automatic US analysis, which could improve not only the diagnostic of a pathology but also enhance medical interventions by reason of a more accurate image-guided tool. The main applications of deep learning for US include: computed aided diagnostics, regression, classification and tissue segmentation [3]. The scope of this project was the segmentation of the femoral artery since cardiovascular diseases are one of the most frequent causes of death in western nations [4]. The procedures to treat these cardiovascular diseases are minimally invasive, but require the use of contrast agent which could lead to kidney damage for the patient. They also require continuous radiation caused by X-Rays during the operation, which with a prolonged exposure could be harmful for both, patients and physicians. For this reason ultrasound is an excellent option to guide through these endovascular procedures, due to its real time display and its low risk associated with radiation. The combination of US and deep learning allows us to go further in terms of non-invasive intra-operative procedures, with the first step in this work being the segmentation of the artery. This serves as a basis for later developments regarding vessel reconstruction and other applications.

2 Material and methods

2.1 Data acquisition

Data acquisition was performed with a 2D linear US probe (L12-3, Philips Healthcare) along with a US station (EPIQ7, Philips Healthcare) and images were transferred in real time to the computer using a network protocol provided by the manufacturer. The complete dataset consisted of US images of the femoral artery from five healthy volunteers. The scan for each one of the subjects started below the inguinal ligament following a superior-to-inferior movement and ending at the adductor hiatus. This protocol was repeated three times for each proband, for a total of 10,557 2D US images (Table 1). Binary ground truth masks for the femoral artery were created via manual segmentation using *Slicer* [5] and the guidance of an experienced physician in

US imaging. Once every image had its corresponding mask, training, validation and testing datasets were defined with a split of 60%, 20% and 20% respectively. The validation dataset was used to evaluate the performance of the network during training while the testing dataset was used to evaluate the accuracy on images that were never seen before by the network.

Table 1: Summary of images per proband

	Run 1	Run 2	Run 3	Total
Proband 1	733	767	669	2,169
Proband 2	1098	938	917	2,953
Proband 3	522	530	548	1,600
Proband 4	704	756	683	2,143
Proband 5	566	551	575	1,692
Total				*10,557*

The image size of US images and masks were 512x323 pixels. The intensities of our US images were in the range of (0,255). For our ground truth masks we have two classes, the femoral artery and the background (0,1).

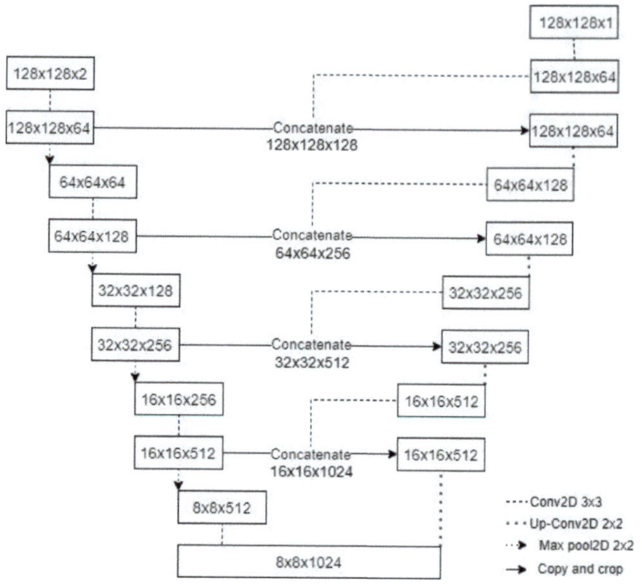

Figure 1: Schematic of *U-Net with single encoder of two channels*. US image and previous prediction concatenate before going through the U-Net.

2.2 Deep learning segmentation approaches

Conventional U-Net

The first segmentation approach is based on the well-known 2D U-Net architecture [6]. Each block in the encoder path has a two 3x3 convolution, each followed by an activation function; in this case, a rectified linear unit (ReLU) and a 2x2 max pooling with a downsampling stride of 2. In the decoder path each block consists of a 2x2 upconvolution, a concatenation with the output block having the same shape in the encoder path and a double 3x3 convolution, each followed by a ReLU. This network produces an output with the same shape as the input.

U-Net with single encoder of two channels

For this approach 2D US images were stacked forming a continuous volume that represent the femoral artery. This network follows a sequence where each US image is considered a slice of the whole volume and will be segmented, this segmentation will affect directly the prediction of the next slice since it will be concatenated with the next slice and will conform the input image of our network. A schematic overview of the network is given in Fig. 1, this concatenation will offer a more detailed extraction of features, such as location. In consequence improve the accuracy of our segmentation.

U-Net with double encoder

Similar to the previous approach, this is a sequential architecture that takes each US 2D image as a slice of a continuous volume. For this case, the obtained prediction and the next US image to segment are the inputs of our network. In this architecture, each one of the input images is processed by its own encoder. The concatenation occurs at the bottleneck of the U-Net as shown in Fig. 2. Afterwards the resultant image is processed by a single decoder, which concatenates with the original US input, and follows the same expansive path as the original U-Net.

The proposed double encoder network was presented so we could extract the spatial information from the previous volume slice independently, without compromising the extraction of the most characteristics features of the US image.

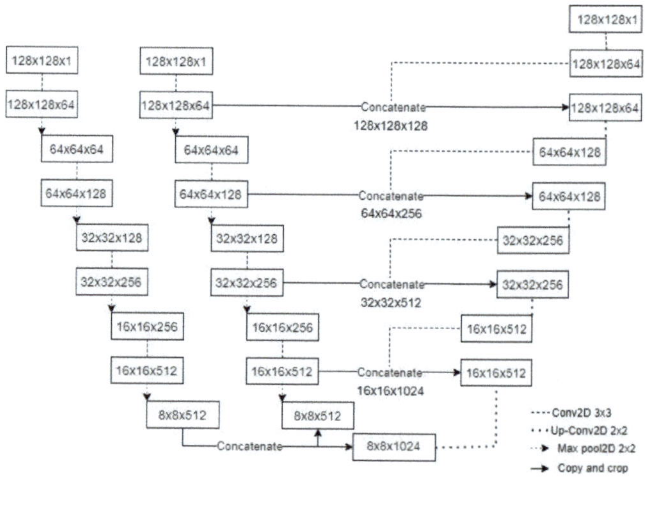

Figure 2: Schematic of the *U-Net with double encoder*, in this approach the US image and previous prediction go through their own encoder and merge in the bottleneck of the U-Net.

2.3 Training specifications

The networks were coded in Python with PyTorch as the preference deep learning framework and trained on NVIDIA DGX A100. Images from our datasets were downsampled from 512x323 to 128x128, in order to decrease memory and computational requirements. The networks were trained using a Binary cross entropy loss with a starting learning rate (LR) of 0.0001. If after four epochs our validation loss did not decrease, the LR was multiplied by a factor of 0.1. Each network training consisted of 30 epochs with a batch size of 25.

3 Results and Discussion

The segmentations of our different approaches were assessed and compared to our manual segmented ground truth by calculating the Dice score. This evaluation was performed for our training, validation and testing data as shown in Table 2.

Table 2: Comparision of dice scores and losses for femoral artery segmentation

Modality	Dice Score
Training	
Conventional U-Net	0.9624
U-Net single encoder of two channels	0.8130
U-Net two encoders	0.8047
Validation	
Conventional U-Net	0.8322
U-Net single encoder of two channels	0.7917
U-Net two encoders	0.7646
Test	
Conventional U-Net	0.8191
U-Net single encoder of two channels	0.6331
U-Net two encoders	0.7250

Comparing the results between our approaches (Figure 3), we found some differences in their performance and accuracy. Overall, the *Conventional U-Net* approach achieved the highest Dice score in validation and testing with a 0.8322 and 0.8191 respectively. On the other hand, the Dice score for the remaining approaches was not as high compared to the conventional network. The stacked images that represent the artery 3D volume are not aligned, causing some discrepancies on the location of the vessel from one slice to another, making it harder to our network to reach good metrics and learn the vessel features. Since we consider the stacked slices as a volume, it is expected that one image is the continuation of the other, so this misalignment affects differently depending the chosen approach. In the *U-Net with single encoder with two channels* our network output has the distance deviation between slices and the overall prediction loss, since we form a loop where this output concatenates with the next US image to predict, the error is carried on since is considered part of the input. On the *U-Net with double encoder* approach this misalignment error does not impact so drastically due to the separate feature extraction. Here, the vessel segmentation is not compromised because the US image has a greater impact in the prediction and is not merged into one with the previous slice and its segmentation and spatial information.

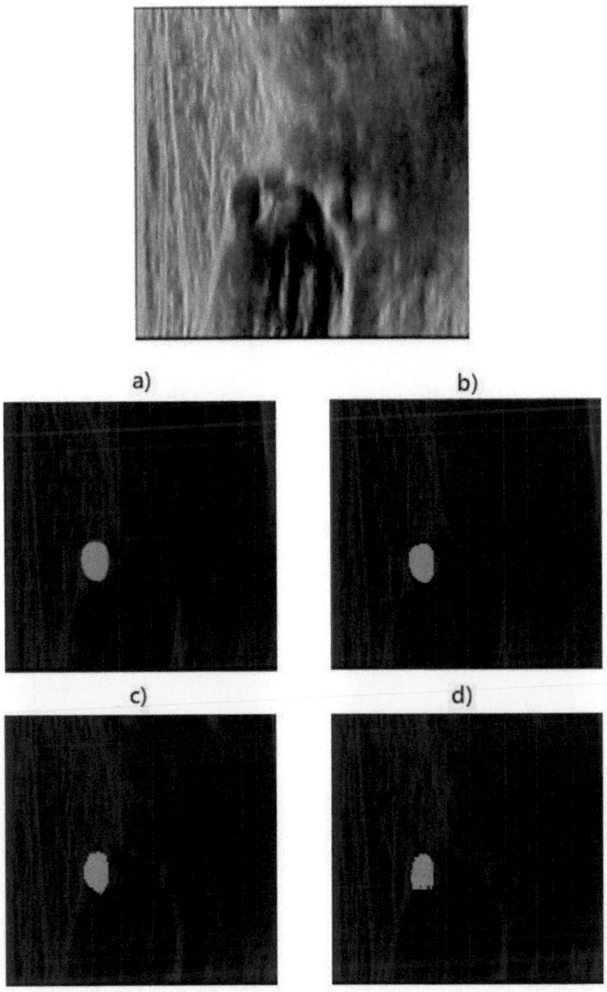

Figure 3: Comparision of one US image with its respective mask and the predicted segmentations. a) Ground truth, b) *Conventional U-Net*, c) *U-Net with single encoder of two channels*, d) *U-Net with double encoder*

4 Conclusion

For our purposes the *Conventional U-Net* was the best approach to segment the femoral artery due to its highest Dice score through all the modalities: training, validation and testing. Although our *U-Net with single encoder of two channels* and our *U-Net with double encoder* ideas are promising, the evaluation results can be improved. In order to do this, a spatial calibration of the US probe must be implemented prior to the US scan so we can have a better definition of the vessel, its distance limits, and with this avoid the spatial position misalignment. In addition, a post processing could refine and improve our final segmentation. In the future, this work could branch out and include the segmentation of the femoral vein so physicians could so have a more complete overview of the surgical space and improve the endovascular intra-operative procedure. Overall, we have implemented an accurate algorithm for segmentation of the femoral artery for 2D ultrasound images.

Acknowledgement

Parts of this work were supported by the German Federal Ministry of Education and Research (BMBF, project KI-LAB-Lübeck, grant number: 01IS19069)

This work has been carried out at the Institute for Robotics and Cognitive Systems, Universität zu Lübeck.

Author's Statement

Conflict of interest
The authors declare that there were no conflicts of interest.

Ethical approval
The research related to human use complies with all the relevant national regulations, institutional policies and was performed in accordance with the tenets of the Helsinki Declaration, and has been approved by the authors' institutional review board or equivalent committee.

Informed consent
Informed consent has been obtained from all individuals included in the presented study.

5 References

[1] S. Liu, Y. Wang, X. Yang, B. Lei, L. Liu, S. Xiang Li, D.Ni and T.Wang *Deep learning in medical ultrasound analysis: A review*. Engineering, vol. 5, Issue. 2, pp. 261–275, 2019. Available: http://www.sciencedirect.com/science/article/pii /S2095809918301887

[2] H. Saleh *Applied deep learning with pytorch*. Packt publishing, 2019.

[3] L.J. Brattain, B.A. Telfer, M. Dhyani, J.R. Grajo, A.E. Samir *Machine learning for medical ultrasound: status, methods, and future opportunities*. Abdom Radiol 43, 786–799 (2018). Available: https://doi.org/10.1007/s00261-018-1517-0

[4] S. Mendis, P. Puska, B. Norrving *Global Atlas on Cardiovascular Disease Prevention and Control*. World Health Organization, Geneva 2011.

[5] A. Fedorov, R. Beichel, J. Kalpathy-Cramer, J. Finet, J.C. Fillion-Robin J, S. Pujol, et. al *3D Slicer as an Image Computing Platform for the Quantitative Imaging Network*. Magnetic Resonance Imaging. (2012).

[6] O. Ronneberger, P. Fischer and T. Brox, *U-Net: Convolutional networks for biomedical image segmentation*. In: Medical Image Computing and Computer-Assisted Intervention (MICCAI). Springer, LNCS, Vol.9351: pp 234–241, 2015. Avaliable: http://lmb.informatik.uni-freiburg.de/Publications/2015/RFB15a

[7] B.R. Thomson, J. Nijkamp, O. Ivashchenko, F. van der Heijden, P. Fischer, J.N. Smit, N.F.M. Kok, K.F.D. Kuhlmann, T.J.M. Ruers and M. Fusaglia, *Hepatic vessel segmentation using a reduced filter 3D U-Net in ultrasound imaging*. In: International Conference on Medical Imaging with Deep Learning, arXiv:1907.12109v1, 2019.

[8] L.A. Groves, B. VanBerlo, N. Veinberg , A. Alboog, T.M. Peters, and E.C.S. Chen, *Automatic segmentation of the carotid artery and internal jugular vein from 2D ultrasound images for 3D vascular reconstruction*. In: International Journal of Computer Assisted Radiology and Surgery, 2020. Available: https://doi.org/10.1007/s11548-020-02248-2

[9] T. Nemoto, N. Futakami, M. Yagi, A. Kumabe, A. Takeda, E. Kunieda and N. Shigematsu *Efficacy evaluation of 2D, 3D U-Net semantic segmentation and atlas-based segmentation of normal lungs excluding the trachea and main bronchi*. Journal of Radiation Research, Vol. 61, No. 2, pp. 257–264, 2020. Available: https://doi.org/10.1093/jrr/rrz086

[10] R.J.G. van Sloun, R. Cohen and Y.C. Eldar *Deep learning in ultrasound imaging*. arXiv:1907.02994v2, 2019.

Neural networks for Compton camera imaging: Estimating initial and transferred energies of prompt gamma radiation

Julius J. Friedemann Werner [1,2], Nadja Kohlhase [2], Andreas Bolke [2] and Magdalena Rafecas [2]
[1] Medical Engineering Science, Universität zu Lübeck, julius.werner@student.uni-luebeck.de
[2] Institute of Medical Engineering, Universität zu Lübeck, {werner,kohlhase,bolke,rafecas}@imt.uni-luebeck.de

Abstract

Compton cameras have been proposed for proton therapy dose monitoring using secondary prompt gamma radiation. The quasi-continuous spectrum of the prompt gamma radiation demands event by event estimation of the initial photon energy for Compton camera image reconstruction. We propose to use neural networks for estimating the initial photon energy and the energy transferred in the first interaction between photon and detector. Monte-Carlo simulations produced the training and evaluation data sets for this study. The estimated energies and corresponding scattering angles were compared to the ground truth and current estimation techniques. A rise in angular uncertainty was observed. The number of potentially usable events increased by 13 % compared to current estimation techniques. This increase is relevant for image reconstruction in clinical application settings with limited numbers of prompt gamma photons. Further improvements of network architecture and training are needed to reduce the enlarged angular uncertainty.

1 Introduction

Compton cameras are imaging devices for mid to high energy photons based on Compton kinematics. They rely on coincidence detection. Two or more signals are assumed to be caused by the same photon if detected within a predefined time window (~ ns). Such a collection of signals is called a *coincidence*. The line connecting the first two interactions is part of the scattered photon's path. Assuming the first interaction is Compton scattering, the scattering angle θ can be calculated using the formula

$$\cos\theta = 1 - \frac{m_e c^2 \Delta E_1}{E_0(E_0 - \Delta E_1)} \tag{1}$$

with electron mass m_e and speed of light c. This calculation relies on an accurate estimation of the initial photon energy E_0 and the energy transferred from the photon to an electron in the Compton scattering process, ΔE_1. The calculated scattering angle and the known segment of the photon's path constrain the photon's origin to the surface of a cone as illustrated in Fig. 1. An image reconstruction algorithm estimates the photon source distribution based on a set of such cones from several *coincidences*.

The correct estimation of energies E_0 and ΔE_1 is especially challenging in applications like prompt gamma imaging for proton therapy dose monitoring. The prompt gamma radiation produced by the interaction of the proton beam with the patient's tissue covers an energy range from a few keV up to 14 MeV and higher [1]. An estimation of the initial photon energy E_0 is needed for each detected event to calculate the scattering angle θ.

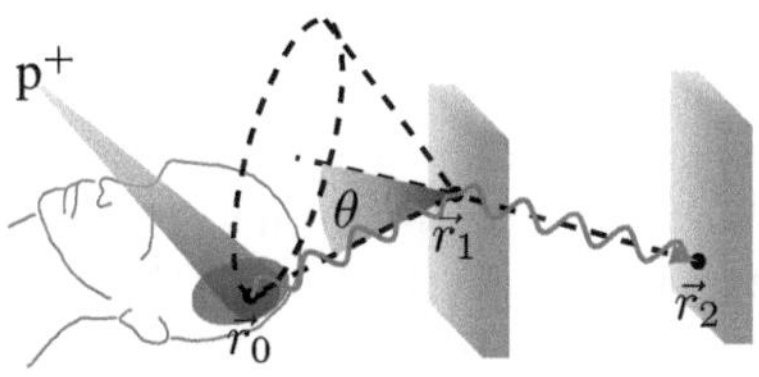

Figure 1: Proton beam, patient and Compton camera.

The simplest method to estimate E_0 is to assume that the second interaction was a photoelectric absorption. Therefore the initial photon energy is entirely absorbed by the detector and can be calculated as

$$E_{0,C} = \Delta E_{1,C} + \Delta E_{2,C}. \tag{2}$$

$\Delta E_{1,C}$ and $\Delta E_{2,C}$ are the energies recorded in the first two interactions and $E_{0,C}$ denotes this current estimation of initial energy. However, the probability of photoelectric absorption decreases for higher photon energies. For instance, if the photon undergoes pair production or Compton scattering in the second interaction, the initial photon energy E_0 is underestimated. Such photons still carry some of their energy, thus $E_0 \geq \Delta E_{1,C} + \Delta E_{2,C}$.

For events with three or more interactions (*multiples*), the second interaction is assumed to be Compton scattering. Then the initial photon energy can be estimated from the interaction positions and the first two measured energies [2]. In both cases, the correct estimation of the scattering angle and the reconstruction rely on measuring the scattered electron's kinetic energy. The measured energies tend to underestimate the true kinetic energies due to so-called *es-*

Table 1: Estimations and their respective symbols.

symbol	description
E_0	initial photon energy
ΔE_1	transferred photon energy
θ_{geom}	scattering angle using (3)
$\theta_{E_0,\Delta E_1}$	scattering angle using E_0 and ΔE_1
$E_{0,\text{C}}$	estimation E_0 using (2)
$\Delta E_{1,\text{C}}$	detected energy, first interaction
θ_{C}	scattering angle using $E_{0,\text{C}}$ and $\Delta E_{1,\text{C}}$
$E_{0,\text{NN}}$	neural network estimation of E_0
$\Delta E_{1,\text{NN}}$	neural network estimation of ΔE_1
θ_{NN}	scattering angle using $E_{0,\text{NN}}$ and $\Delta E_{1,\text{NN}}$

caping electrons. After the interaction, the recoiling electron transfers its kinetic energy in multiple Coulomb scattering interactions with atoms in the detector. High kinetic energies, thin detectors, and low-density detector materials increase the electron's likelihood to leave the detector. In such cases, the electron's residual kinetic energy decreases the measured energy $\Delta\tilde{E}_i$ [3]. In [4] the number of *escaping electrons* in Monte Carlo simulations of a Compton camera prototype was reported to be 20 % and 40 % at an initial photon energy of 3 MeV and 6 MeV, respectively.
Alternatively, the energy can be included as a further unknown into the tomographic reconstruction process [5]. However, this approach requires highly complex models able to describe all relevant physical effects. We propose to estimate the initial photon energy and correct the measured energy of the first interaction using a neural network to improve the estimated scattering angle. This study is limited to two interaction events (*doubles*), constraining the problem posed to the neural network.

2 Material and Methods

2.1 Simulation and data extraction

Symbols and names are defined for the different estimations and ground truth variables in Table 1. This study is based on Monte Carlo simulations with the toolkit GATE 9.0, dedicated to emission tomography simulations [6]. Within the simulation, proton beams impinge on a cuboid water phantom. The proton beam energy was sampled from a discrete spectrum from 120 MeV to 123 MeV in steps of 1 MeV convoluted with a Gaussian distribution with a standard deviation of 1 MeV. For each discrete proton energy numE9 protons were simulated. The simulated Compton camera is based on a prototype developed by the CLaRyS collaboration [4]. It consists of seven $9 \times 9 \times 0.2\,\text{cm}^3$ silicon detectors (*scatterers*) and one $21 \times 28 \times 3\,\text{cm}^3$ bismuth germanate (BGO) scintillation detector (*absorber*). The camera was placed perpendicular to the proton beam with a distance of 10 cm to the first scatterer. All detectors were simulated as continuous blocks without substructure. Detector uncertainties were not considered at this point.
The simulation was executed in two steps. First, the proton beam interacting with the water phantom was simulated. The resulting photons were recorded. Based on this data, the interactions of photons and Compton camera were simulated. The resulting data is a list of *coincidences*.

Table 2: Evaluation and training data sets.

set	# *doubles*	proton energy
train	360 000	120 MeV to 123 MeV
evaluate	10 000	120 MeV

In the Monte Carlo simulation, each nonelastic photon interaction with the detector produces secondary particles. These deposit at least some of their energy in interactions like Coulomb scattering. Each of these interactions is saved separately by GATE as a *hit*. The proposed Compton camera cannot differentiate these *hits*. Thus all *hits* belonging to the same photon interaction are combined to so-called *singles* using the ideal adder module for Compton cameras provided by GATE [7]. This module allows recovering the true initial and deposited energies of the photon interaction. Secondary particles with a mean range below 1 mm in the detector material were not simulated to avoid infrared divergence. Their energy was counted back to the *hit* producing the particle (*range cut*). If two or more *singles* are observed within 2 ns, they were stored as a *coincidence* and assumed to originate from the same photon.
Further post-processing was implemented using C++. When two photons interact within the same detector element in a narrow sequence, they produce two distinct *singles* which would not be resolved in a real detector. Therefore all *singles* in the same detector layer and *coincidence time window* were combined, using an energy weighted centroid. The initial photon energies E_{ini} and final photon energies E_{final} were summed. The transferred energy from photon to secondary particles ΔE_1 was calculated as $E_{\text{ini}} - E_{\text{final}}$. E_0 was set to the source energy of the first *single* in the layer. This leads to the sum of transferred energies potentially being higher than E_0 if two or more uncorrelated photons are involved. *Coincidences* with more than two *singles* were not further considered. The number of *doubles* used in this study is listed in Table 2.
The most important figure of merit for using any energy estimation in image reconstruction is the angular error. The reference angle θ_{geom} was calculated geometrically

$$\theta_{\text{geom}} = \arccos\left(\frac{(\vec{r}_1 - \vec{r}_0)\cdot(\vec{r}_2 - \vec{r}_1)}{||\vec{r}_1 - \vec{r}_0||_2\,||\vec{r}_2 - \vec{r}_1||_2}\right) \qquad (3)$$

using the two interaction positions $\vec{r}_1$ and $\vec{r}_2$ and the source position $\vec{r}_0$, compare Fig. 1. Thus, the source position lies on the cone surface defined by the interaction positions and the angle θ_{geom}, which makes this the desired angle for the reconstruction.

2.2 Neural Network

The proposed neural network consists of five fully connected hidden layers of fifty perceptrons each. The posi-

tions and deposited energies of the first and second detector interactions $\vec{r}_1$, $\vec{r}_2$, $\Delta E_{1,\mathrm{C}}$ and $\Delta E_{2,\mathrm{C}}$ are the network's input data. They were varied in each iteration of the neural network training process, using the proposed detectors' uncertainties given in [3, 4]. The output values are the estimated initial energy $E_{0,\mathrm{NN}}$ and corrected deposited energy of the first interaction $\Delta E_{1,\mathrm{NN}}$. These are used for the scattering angle estimation θ_{NN} following (1). The network was implemented in Python using *PyTorch*.
The activation function leaky rectified linear unit (lReLU)

$$\mathrm{lReLU}(x) = \begin{cases} x, & x \geq 0 \\ 0.01x, & x < 0 \end{cases} \tag{4}$$

was used for all neurons of the network. This choice favors positive output values. They are required, as the output values represent energies. Constraining the output values to positive values using the rectified linear unit as an activation function led to output value 0 for almost all input values. Skip connections have been included to speed up and stabilize the learning process using the knowledge that $E_0 \geq \Delta E_{1,\mathrm{C}} + \Delta E_{2,\mathrm{C}}$ and $\Delta E_1 \geq \Delta E_{1,\mathrm{C}}$ are lower bounds for the output values. They were added to the respective network output before the last activation function. The network only learns the correction of the energies.
The network training followed the stochastic gradient descent algorithm with learning rate 0.01 and momentum 0.1. The L_1 norm of the differences between the network output and desired output was used as the loss function. Optimization steps were taken after averaging the gradient calculated from processing 900 *doubles*. For each iteration, the event order was randomized. 1000 iterations over the complete training data set were performed. These parameters were chosen after a preliminary parameter study.

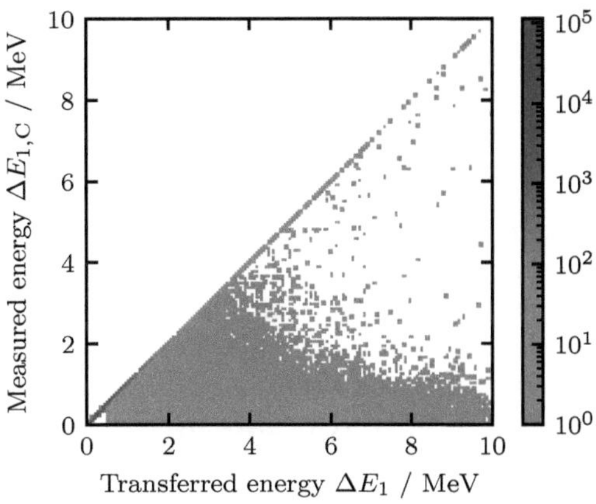

Figure 2: Histogram of the measured energy $\Delta E_{1,\mathrm{C}}$ (first interaction) and the energy transferred from the photon to secondary particles ΔE_1.

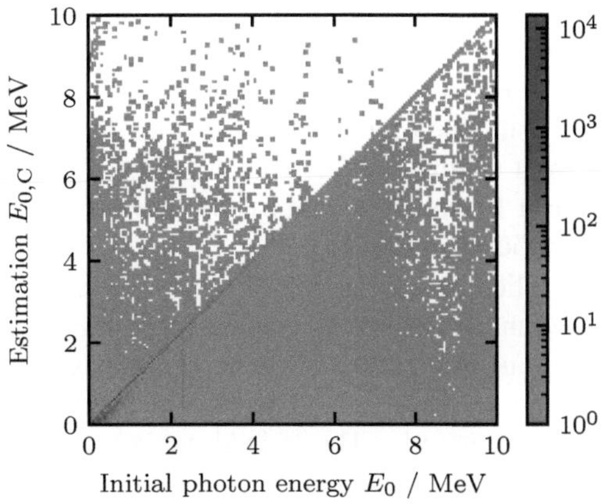

Figure 3: Histogram of the current estimation of the initial energy $E_{0,\mathrm{C}}$ and photon source energy E_0.

3 Results and Discussion

3.1 Simulation analysis

The training data was analyzed to better understand the inverse problem posed to the neural network. In Fig. 2 a 2D-histogram of the measured energy $\Delta E_{1,\mathrm{C}}$ and the energy transferred from the corresponding photon to secondary particles ΔE_1 is shown for the training data set. A significant number of events have measured energies considerably lower than the transferred energy (values below the angle bisector). Remarkably, for transferred energies ΔE_1 above 3 MeV, 87 % of measured energies $\Delta E_{1,\mathrm{C}}$ are below 1 MeV. This effect may result from the *escaping electrons* large mean path length within the *scatterer* compared to the detector's thickness of 2 mm. The limited path length of ~2 mm translates to a deposited energy of ~1 MeV. *Range cuts* in the simulation lead to the perfect measurement of transferred energies ΔE_1 below 0.5 MeV visible in Fig. 2.
Fig. 3 shows the potential to improve the current estimation of the initial photon energy $E_{0,\mathrm{C}}$. Any deviation from the angle bisector results in wrong cone angles. The vertical lines correspond to discrete lines in the prompt gamma spectrum, i.e., specific de-excitation energies of specific elements within the water phantom, like 4.4 MeV for ^{12}C. The excited ^{12}C atoms result from the reaction of ^{16}O with a high energy proton [1]. Values above the angle bisector are likely artefacts from the combination of multiple *singles* in the same layer described in Section 2.1. Both 2D-histograms indicate, that even with a perfect detector resolution, no direct relationship between measured energy and the desired energy is present for many *doubles*. This has to be taken into account when designing and evaluating energy reconstruction methods.

3.2 Neural network

The evaluation data set with mean proton energy 120 MeV was used for assessing the neural network performance compared to the current estimations. The cumulative histograms of the absolute difference of the estimated energies $E_{0,\mathrm{C}}$ and $E_{0,\mathrm{NN}}$ to E_0 as well as $\Delta E_{1,\mathrm{C}}$ and $\Delta E_{1,\mathrm{NN}}$ to ΔE_1 are shown in Fig. 4. The large error rate is similar for the current estimations $E_{0,\mathrm{C}}$ and $\Delta E_{1,\mathrm{C}}$ and the neural network estimations $E_{0,\mathrm{NN}}$ and $\Delta E_{1,\mathrm{NN}}$ (horizontal sections). The small error rate increases significantly for the neural network estimation of the transferred energy $\Delta E_{1,\mathrm{NN}}$ compared to $\Delta E_{1,\mathrm{C}}$. This is equivalent to an increased energy uncertainty.

Three scattering angle estimations $\theta_{E_0,\Delta E_1}$, θ_{C} and θ_{NN} are compared to the geometric angle θ_{geom}. The first angle $\theta_{E_0,\Delta E_1}$ was calculated using the true initial photon energy E_0 and true transferred photon energy ΔE_1 in (1), demonstrating the effect of an ideal estimation of initial and transferred energies. The second angle θ_{C} was calculated using the measured energy $E_{1,\mathrm{C}}$ and $E_{0,\mathrm{C}}$. This is the angle estimation currently used for reconstruction in our group. For the third angle θ_{NN} the energies given by the neural network $E_{0,\mathrm{NN}}$ and $\Delta E_{1,\mathrm{NN}}$ were used. The cumulative histogram in Fig. 4b shows a reduction of large absolute angular errors by the neural networks estimation θ_{NN} compared to $\theta_{E_0,\Delta E_1}$ and θ_{C}. The increased energetic uncertainty observed in Fig. 4a translates to a rise of angular uncertainty visible in Fig. 4b. Not all combinations of initial photon energy E_0 and transferred energy ΔE_1 are physically meaningful, as the right side of (1) must be inside $[-1, 1]$. The histograms in Fig. 4b show an increase in valid energy combinations of 13 % by using the neural network estimation θ_{NN} instead of the current estimation θ_{C}. This potential rise in usable *doubles* must be weighed against the increase of angular uncertainty shown in Fig. 4b.

This study relied entirely on simulations. An actual Compton camera can not provide the required measurement of the initial and transferred energies on an event by event basis. A verified simulation is needed to produce the training data for the neural network. The trained network can then be deployed to correct the usual Compton camera data output.

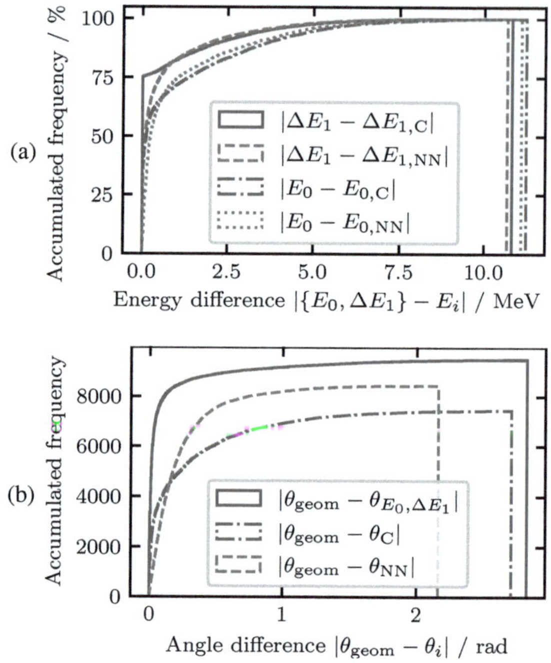

Figure 4: Cumulative histograms of the absolute difference between the ground truth and its estimations.

4 Conclusion

A neural network was developed to improve the estimation of initial photon energy and energy transferred to secondary particles in a Compton camera. The observed increase of usable *doubles* might improve the statistics within image reconstruction procedures towards low count clinical applications. Future studies will address the decreased angular resolution by adapting the network architecture and training. Also the effects of the new estimations on the image reconstruction and proton therapy dose monitoring need to be investigated.

Acknowledgement

The work has been carried out and supervised by the Institute of Medical Engineering, Universität zu Lübeck. Computing resources were provided by the North German Supercomputing Alliance (HLRN). We would like to thank Mattias Heinrich (IMI, Lübeck, Germany) for providing helpful information.

Author's Statement

Conflict of interest: Authors state no conflict of interest.

5 References

[1] J. M. Verburg, H. A. Shih, and J. Seco, "Simulation of prompt gamma-ray emission during proton radiotherapy," *Physics in Medicine & Biology*, vol. 57, no. 17, p. 5459, 2012.

[2] R. Kroeger, W. Johnson, J. Kurfess, B. Phlips, and E. Wulf, "Three-compton telescope: theory, simulations, and performance," *IEEE Transactions on Nuclear Science*, vol. 49, no. 4, pp. 1887–1892, 2002.

[3] M. Fontana *et al.*, "Monitoring ion beam therapy with a Compton camera: simulation studies of the clinical feasibility," *IEEE Transactions on Radiation and Plasma Medical Sciences*, vol. 4, no. 2, pp. 218–232, 2020.

[4] M. Fontana, D. Dauvergne, J. M. Létang, J.-L. Ley, and E. Testa, "Compton camera study for high efficiency spect and benchmark with anger system," *Physics in Medicine & Biology*, vol. 62, no. 23, p. 8794, 2017.

[5] E. Muñoz *et al.*, "A spectral reconstruction algorithm for two-plane Compton cameras," *Physics in Medicine & Biology*, vol. 65, no. 2, p. 025011, 2020.

[6] D. Sarrut *et al.*, "A review of the use and potential of the GATE Monte Carlo simulation code for radiation therapy and dosimetry applications," *Medical Physics*, vol. 41, no. 6 Part1, p. 064301, 2014.

[7] A. Etxebeste *et al.*, "CCMod: a GATE module for Compton camera imaging simulation," *Physics in Medicine & Biology*, vol. 65, no. 5, p. 055004, 2020.

Towards Effective Contrastive Pretraining for Medical Image Segmentation

Finja A. Ottink [1], Gregor Koehler [2], and Mattias P. Heinrich [3]

[1] Medical Informatics, Universität zu Lübeck, finja.ottink@student.uni-luebeck.de

[2] Division of Medical Image Computing, German Cancer Research Center (DKFZ), Heidelberg, g.koehler@dkfz-heidelberg.de

[3] Institute of Medical Informatics, Universität zu Lübeck, heinrich@imi.uni-luebeck.de

Abstract

The application of many supervised machine learning models in the medical domain fails due to a lack of sufficient annotated data. To reduce the costly and time-consuming annotation effort, we aim to train models requiring fewer labels, thus achieving increased data efficiency. Recent advances in self-supervised learning enable learning accurate models for 2D image classification and object recognition despite restricted access to annotated data. Self-supervised learning methods allow pretraining neural networks in an unsupervised way, followed by fine-tuning for a downstream task with limited annotations. We developed a contrastive self-supervised learning approach, CSSL-Seg, based on the contrastive method SimCLR, extended for the task of medical image segmentation in three-dimensional space. CSSL-Seg achieves Dice scores approaching those of the supervised baseline, nnU-Net, however not meeting the aspiration of surpassing it in the low-data regime which strongly recommends conducting further research.

1 Introduction

Medical image data is of major importance for diagnostics and therapy as it conveys important information about a patient's state of health. As an enormous amount of medical image data are generated daily and need to be analyzed, machine learning-based models are being increasingly employed in the medical field for assistance. However, the application of many supervised machine-learning models in the medical domain fails due to a lack of annotated data. Despite the availability of large amounts of data, only a small fraction possesses annotations because they need to be manually created by physicians in a costly and time-consuming process [1].

Advances in self-supervised learning have shown to enable learning accurate models for 2D image classification and object recognition despite limited availability of annotations [2]. Transferring this idea to problems of medical image processing, mainly working in the three-dimensional image space, and integrating it into approaches that work in the low-data-regime could help overcome this issue.

In this work, we pursue the goal of fewer required annotations in the context of biomedical image segmentation, a predominant problem in medical image processing which is essential for analyzing the acquired data and making quantitative statements about it [3], [4]. We propose a self-supervised learning approach based on the contrastive method SimCLR [5], extended for the task of medical image segmentation in three-dimensional space. The aim is to enable segmentation models to be trained with less annotation effort and thus achieve increased data efficiency. Self-supervised learning pretrains a network in an unsupervised way, followed by fine-tuning for a downstream task with limited annotations [6]. In detail, our main contributions are:

- We enable using contrastive learning approaches in the context of encoder-decoder neural network architectures.
- We explore the usefulness of contrastive pretraining in the context of medical image segmentation of images containing pathologies.
- We propose new data augmentation strategies tailored to contrastive pretraining in the context of 3D images.

2 Material and Methods

2.1 Data

To evaluate the proposed approach, we use the 2019 MICCAI Kidney and Kidney Tumor Segmentation Challenge (KiTS19) dataset [7]. The dataset comprises 300 abdominal 3D CT scans of kidney cancer patients split into 210 training and 90 test cases. The structures of interest to be segmented include kidneys and kidney tumors. Since reference annotations are not publicly available for the test set, we exclusively consider the public training set in our approach, further splitting the training set into training and validation and using the challenge's validation set as a hold-out test set to report the final performance. Data preprocessing is performed equivalently to nnU-Net [3] to facilitate the comparison during evaluation.

2.2 Semantic Segmentation

Semantic segmentation of biomedical images is a predominant problem in medical image processing. In the context of computer-aided diagnosis and therapy, it represents an essential mean for analyzing the acquired data and making quantitative statements about it. Its scope is diverse, including diagnostics, therapy planning, intra-operative systems, radiotherapy, and tumor growth monitoring [3], [4].
In general, semantic segmentation is considered as classification on pixel-level because it assigns each pixel to a class prevalent in the image without distinction between multiple instances of the same class. Opposed to standard classification tasks, it incorporates localization information, resulting in more informative outputs while requiring a more expensive annotation [4].
A very successful neural network architecture for biomedical image segmentation is the U-Net with its encoder-decoder architecture, proposed in [8]. A depiction of a modified version of this architecture is shown in Fig. 2. First, the encoder captures a large spatial context by reducing the input resolution, which results in small feature maps that contain high-level semantic information. From this representation, the decoder is tasked with reconstructing low-level details. For network optimization during training, stochastic gradient descent with pixel-wise cross-entropy loss is employed.
Due to the diversity of biomedical tasks, the design of segmentation methods that achieve strong performance usually involves considerable manual interaction with expert knowledge and experience needed, as even small errors can lead to significant degradation of the results. Despite the success of many proposed U-Net-based architectures, most of them are tailored to specific datasets and tasks [3].
In [3], nnU-Net, an automatic U-Net configuration was proposed to alleviate the need for expert knowledge when confronted with new tasks, covering preprocessing, network architecture, training, and postprocessing. It is based on the U-Net architecture [8] and outperforms most existing segmentation approaches without manual intervention, setting a new state-of-the-art for biomedical image segmentation.

2.3 Self-Supervised Pretraining

Self-supervised learning, a subset of unsupervised learning, aims to learn meaningful representations of the given data without human supervision, but by constructing and employing pseudo-labels, defined by the structure of the input data itself, in tasks referred to as *pretext tasks*. To learn meaningful representations and prevent the model to collapse to trivial representations, the pretext task must not be overly simple to solve. Such representations can subsequently be exploited for different types of *downstream tasks*, potentially requiring fewer labeled data. Different downstream tasks can therefore serve as an instrument to assess the quality of the representations obtained in the pretext task by using the resulting neural networks as a pre-initialization of the model which then simply needs to be fine-tuned for solving the downstream task. In this paper, we evaluate the learned representations of the proposed method by fine-tuning the model on the KiTS19 segmentation dataset as a downstream task and restricting the model's access to labeled data in order to test the label-efficiency when pretraining the model.
Contrastive learning is a specific self-supervised learning variant. During pretext training, the network is tasked with solving a discrimination task and differentiate between positive and negative samples. It seeks to maximize the similarity between similar data samples ("positive pairs") by driving their representations in the latent space closer together while pushing apart the representations of diverse data samples ("negative pairs"). To learn meaningful visual representations, this concept relies on extensive data augmentation [5], [6].

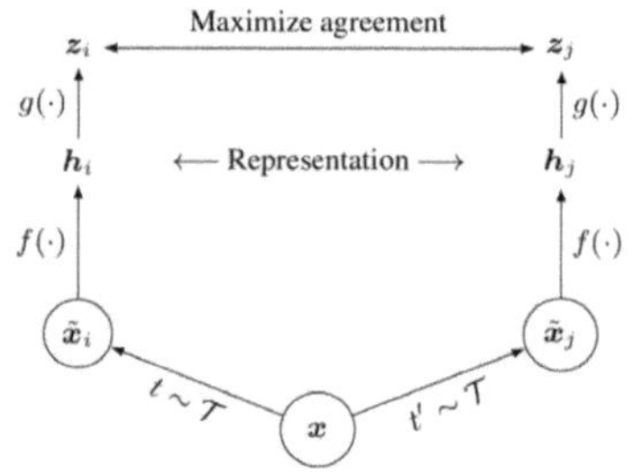

Figure 1: Concept of the SimCLR [5] pretext task including data augmentation $\mathcal{T}$, extraction of representations with an encoder f and mapping them into another space, where the contrastive loss is applied, using a projection head g.

A successful contrastive learning approach, called "a simple framework for contrastive learning of visual representations", referred to as SimCLR, was proposed in [5]. Fig. 1 illustrates the concept of the SimCLR pretext task. First, the input data x is transformed using data augmentation $\mathcal{T}$ which results in two differently augmented, corresponding views $\tilde{x}_i$ and $\tilde{x}_j$, representing the positive pair. The views are fed through an encoder f to extract representations $h_{i,j}$. These representations are subsequently fed through a non-linear projection head g, which maps the representations to a space where the contrastive loss is applied. In [5], the authors show that applying the contrastive loss after mapping the representations using g is beneficial for the downstream task. Aside from extensive data augmentation, which renders the pretext task more difficult due to strongly varying positive pairs, large batch sizes proved to be advantageous for designing a demanding pretext task. Large batch sizes are associated with more negative samples available during training, making the discrimination task more challenging [5].

2.4 CSSL-Seg

In this work, we propose *CSSL-Seg*, a contrastive self-supervised learning approach for segmentation which can operate directly in the three-dimensional image space usually present in medical images. The aim is to enable segmentation models to be trained with less annotation effort and thus achieve an increased data efficiency which is particularly relevant in the medical context due to the scarcity of expert-annotated data. The developed approach consists of a pretext task training based on SimCLR and adapted to the challenges of medical imaging, as well as a downstream training strategy to make efficient use of the learned representations for segmentation tasks.

Pretext Training

For pretext training, we extend the general SimCLR framework proposed in [5], depicted in Fig. 1, to allow exploiting contrastive pretraining for medical images. As we are interested in performing 3D segmentation based on nnU-Net in the downstream task, we realize the necessary transfer of the pretrained model to the downstream task in a simple way by imposing architecture consistency. To this end, we split the typical 3D U-Net network architecture used in [3], illustrated in Fig. 2, in two parts, the encoder and decoder. During pretext training, we use the 3D CNN encoder to extract representations for the contrastive loss. However, due to memory limitations, this 3D CNN encoder operates on patches sampled from the original 3D volume, leading to a patch-based contrastive task rather than an instance contrastive task as in [5].

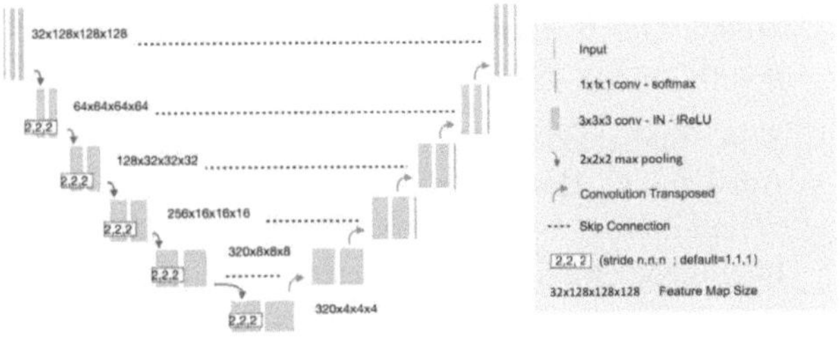

Figure 2: 3D U-Net network architecture for the KiTS19 dataset adapted from [3]. The left half represent the encoder, the right half shows the decoder.

Another important adaption for the medical imaging domain concerns data augmentation, which represents a major aspect of the contrastive approach. Compared to standard SimCRL, we apply 3D transformations and use different transformation modules tailored to the intricacies of medical images. To obtain a sufficiently strong data augmentation, for which an example is illustrated in Fig. 3, we compose various types of transformations, including spatial transformations (rotations, scaling, different deformations and mirroring), color transformations (changing contrast and brightness as well as gamma transforms), noise augmentations (Gaussian noise and Gaussian blur), cropping, and masking a region in the data to model occlusions.

Downstream Training

The enforced architecture consistency proposed in this paper allows for easy downstream training on segmentation

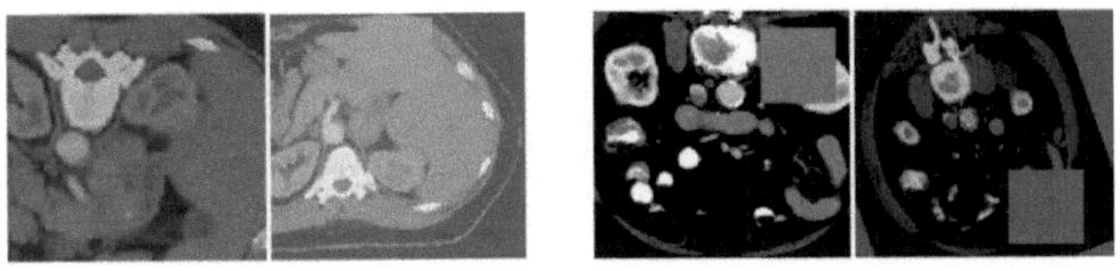

Figure 3: Example of data augmentation applied in pretext training. The 2D image slices, extracted from the 3D data, depicted closely side by side represent correlated views.

tasks. In order to fine-tune the representations learned during pretext training, we propose to make use of the pretrained U-Net encoder without the projection head, in conjunction with a randomly initialized U-Net decoder. In order to allow the decoder to adapt to the representations given by the encoder, we employ a *warm-up* training strategy for fine-tuning, where the encoder is not trained until a certain number of warm-up epochs is reached.

3 Results and Discussion

In this section, we demonstrate experiments to evaluate the potential performance gains of the proposed contrastive learning method in the context of downstream segmentation tasks. To assess the performance and test the label-efficiency achieved by pretraining a U-Net encoder, we use the encoder obtained by the self-supervised pretext training as a starting point for fine-tuning the model on the KiTS19 segmentation dataset. To this end, we use various fractions of labeled data, including 10%, 25%, 50% and 100% of the complete labeled dataset. For robustness reasons, we randomly select several subsets for each respective fraction of labeled data to fine-tune the model, and for evaluation, we compute the mean value over all subset trainings belonging to one fraction of labeled data. The metric applied to evaluate the quality of the predicted segmentation maps relative to their ground truths is the widely used Dice score [4]. To evaluate whether self-supervised pretraining provides a performance gain over supervised training, especially in the low-data regime, a comparison to the supervised nnU-Net, as well trained on the same fractions of labeled data, is drawn.

The results achieved, depicted in Fig. 4, show that up to now, the proposed approach is not able to achieve the desired results. Although they are very close to those of the supervised baseline, they do not surpass it, which was an aspired aim, especially for the low-data regime. Based on the standard deviation, it can be stated that the performance of the downstream training for various labeled data fractions using different subsets for fine-tuning vary more the less annotated data are used during training. This suggests that the choice of data when training with a small amount of annotated data is relevant and has an impact on the performance, as the network learns the representations based on the data available during the training process. In particular, data with pathologies, which applies to the KiTS19 dataset, are very diverse, further supporting the need for a meaningful choice of samples for the labeled data fractions.

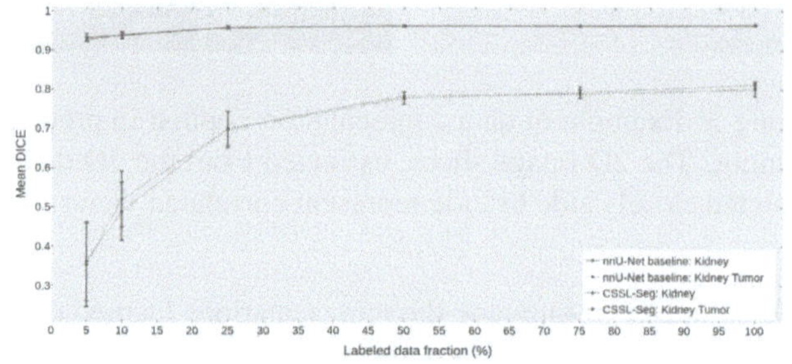

Figure 4: Results achieved with CSSL-Seg in terms of Dice scores and comparison to the supervised baseline.

Despite the current results, it is desirable to use self-supervised learning for medical image segmentation in the presence of limited annotations. If successful, this would be a relevant achievement and a step forward in terms of reliable training of neural networks in the medical domain despite a lack of annotated data.
In [9], the same idea of constructing a contrastive learning approach for medical image segmentation was pursued, which yields promising results. Therefore, we assume that the approach of using contrastive learning for medical image segmentation is useful in principle, but our approach requires further development, for which there are still many options.

4 Conclusion

A lack of sufficient annotated data poses the problem of training reliable and robust machine learning models, which are essential for a successful application, especially in the medical domain. In this context, we proposed an approach for contrastive self-supervised pretraining of CNN encoders for label-efficient semantic segmentation. The results show, that the aspiration of surpassing the performance of the supervised baseline in the low-data regime is not yet met. Nonetheless, there are plenty of opportunities to further develop and enhance the approach. A major challenge, owing to memory limitations of current hardware accelerators, is negative sample mining, which represents an important basis for the success of contrastive learning approaches. Here, further research is required to alleviate the need for large numbers of negative samples. Moreover, distinct fine-tuning options can be explored that may have a substantial impact on performance, as common segmentation network architectures have to balance both the encoder and decoder during optimization. Another interesting aspect concerns the influence of different data augmentation variants on the quality of the learned representations. In future work, another important aspect is to investigate the generalization ability of the approach on further datasets.
To summarize, it can be stated that the proposed CSSL-Seg approach is a first and promising step towards effective contrastive pretraining for medical image segmentation and leaves room for improvement. For this reason, we believe it is worth pursuing further research on this topic.

Acknowledgement

The work has been carried out at the Division of Medical Image Computing, German Cancer Research Center (DKFZ), Heidelberg and supervised by the Institute of Medical Informatics, Universität zu Lübeck.

Author's Statement

Conflict of interest: Authors state no conflict of interest.

5 References

[1] S. P. Singh et al., *3D Deep Learning on medical Images: a Review*. In: Sensors, MDPI, vol. 20, no. 5097, 2020

[2] O. J. Hénaff et al., *Data-efficient Image Recognition with Contrastive Predictive Coding*. In: International Conference on Machine Learning, PMLR, pp. 4182–4192, 2020

[3] F. Isensee, P. F. Jaeger, S. A. A. Kohl, J. Petersen and K. H. Maier-Hein, *Automated Design of Deep Learning Methods for biomedical Image Segmentation*. In: arXiv preprint arXiv:1904.08128, 2019

[4] S. A. Taghanaki, K. Abhishek, J. P. Cohen, J. Cohen-Adad and G. Hamarneh, *Deep Semantic Segmentation of natural and medical Images: a Review*. In: Artificial Intelligence Review, Springer, pp. 1–42, 2020

[5] T. Chen, S. Kornblith, N. Norouzi and G. Hinton, *A simple Framework for Contrastive Learning of visual Representations*. In: arXiv preprint arXiv:2002.05709, 2020

[6] A. Jaiswal, A. R. Babu, M. Z. Zadeh, D. Banerjee and F. Makedon, *A Survey on Contrastive Self-Supervised Learning*. In: Technologies, Multidisciplinary Digital Publishing Institute, vol. 9, no. 2, 2021

[7] N. Heller et al., *The State of the Art in Kidney and Kidney Tumor Segmentation in contrast-enhanced CT Imaging: Results of the KiTS19 Challenge*. In: Medical Image Analysis, vol. 67, 2021

[8] O. Ronneberger, P. Fischer and T. Brox, *U-Net: Convolutional Networks for biomedical Image Segmentation*. In: Medical Image Computing and Computer-Assisted Intervention – MICCAI 2015, Springer International Publishing, pp. 234–241, 2015

[9] K. Chaitanya, E. Erdil, N. Karani and E. Konukoglu, *Contrastive Learning of global and local Features for medical Image Segmentation with limited Annotations*. In: arXiv preprint arXiv:2006.10511, 2020

FlowNet application for 3D image registration

Chenzhang Li [1], Mattias Heinrich [2]
[1] Robotics and Autonomous Systems, Universität zu Lübeck, chenzhang.li@student.uni-luebeck.de
[2] Institut für Medizinische Informatik, Universität zu Lübeck, heinrich@imi.uni-luebeck.de

Abstract

Deep learning has made many significant improvements in medical image processing. FlowNet estimates the optical flow of the input image by a supervised method. However, this is only applicable to the estimation of optical flow for 2D images. We propose a 3D image registration method using FlowNet to abdominal CT images for alignment. Our experiments first fine-tune the FlowNet network using the segmentation loss of the image, three sets of orthogonal 2D images are obtained by slicing the 3D images, and the optical flow field is obtained by FlowNet, which is then reconstructed into a 3D optical flow field that is used as the deformation field of the images for alignment. To enhance the alignment effect, inverse consistency constraints are also added. The Dice coefficients are used as an evaluation of the experimental results. As a result of our method, the dice score improved from 36.4% to 54.6%.

1 Introduction

Image registration refers to searching for a correspondence that makes one image align to another image, where the unchanging image is the fixed image. The image that changes is the moving image. In the medical field, registration is often used to compare CT or MRI images of the same patient at different times for the same location, or to see an organ more specifically using different imaging equipment for the same location at the same time. It can help the physician to get a better understanding of the patient's condition from multiple perspectives.

The traditional registration method can be divided into traditional registration methods and learning-based registration methods. The traditional registration method requires iterative optimization of the image based on similarity criterion to make the highest similarity between the moved image and the fixed image. This method is time-consuming, but it is more effective and stable. Learning-based methods usually refer to registration methods using neural network training, using a large amount of data to train a registration model, and using the trained model to directly register the new image. The training process of this method is slower, but the prediction process is much faster than the traditional method. Due to the lack of sufficient ground truth training data with deformation fields and the huge cost of manual labeling, learning-based training methods are divided into supervised methods[1] and unsupervised learning methods[2].

Optical flow is the 2D instantaneous velocity field of a pixel point in an image. The optical flow field is the amount of movement of the same pixel point in frame t to frame $t+1$ and reflects the movement information of an object in two adjacent frames. This movement may be caused by a camera movement or by the objects' movement. FlowNet[3] uses an end-to-end convolutional neural network for optical flow estimation. The input to the model is two frames and the output is the optical flow from the first frame to the second frame. We can use the obtained optical flow field as the deformation field for the registration problem to align the two images, but this is only applicable to the registration between 2D images and cannot be used for common medical images such as CT.

To train a model for medical image alignment applications requires the use of large datasets of medical images, but these are often not easily available, due to privacy protection and supervision issues. However, using pre-trained 2D optical flow models does not depend on access to large medical datasets. Due to the high optimization of the software hardware for 2D convolution the 2D model can be processed very quickly (although it needs to be processed on multiple planes) So we achieved predictions in three orthogonal two-dimensional views by using a pre-trained FlowNet and fine-tuning it to fit the new data, and combining them into a three-dimensional deformation field.

2 Material and Methods

In this section, we briefly describe the FlowNet network structure and how to fine-tune the pre-training models to improve the results.

2.1 Optical flow prediction

The input to the FlowNet network is a pair of images and the output is a dense optical flow field. As shown in Fig. 1 The network consists of an encoding module with 9 layers of convolution and ReLU activation function layers and a

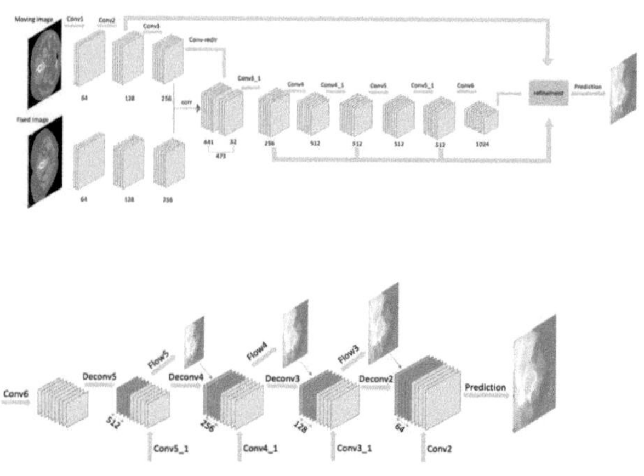

Figure 1: FlowNet-C network structure, the top figure is the encoding module, corr represents for correlation operation. The bottom figure is the decoding module. The final predicted optical flow field is one-fourth of the original size[3].

decoding module with 4 layers of deconvolution and ReLU activation function layers. There are no fully connected layers, so there is no limit to the size of the input image.The authors designed two network structures, FlowNet Simple and FlowNet Corr, which differ mainly in the coding module. FlowNet Simple directly combines the input pair of images by channel as input, while FlowNet Corr processes the pair of images separately and applies the convolution layer separately to extract features, and then the features of the two images are matched which is equivalent to a convolution of the features of the two images and there are no weights to be trained. This step is called correlation. The decoding module consists of multiple upconvolutions and unpooling, while the optical flow can be predicted directly on low-resolution feature maps at different scales, which not only extracts deep information but also obtains low-level information. The final output is the optical flow field. However, the final result is still a quarter of the input image size, and since refinement at higher resolutions does not help to improve the training results, the result is directly reverted to the original input size using bilinear upsampling. We use this optical flow field as a correspondence between the two images to guide the image alignment. Because this is a supervised learning problem, a large number of optical flow ground turth are needed for training, but the existing dataset is too small to satisfy the training requirements and the manual labelling is very expensive, so the authors created the Flying Chairs dataset[3], simulated the motion by adding some virtual chairs to the background image and artificially synthesised a large number of datasets with optical flow ground turth by affine transformation.

2.2 Fine-tune FlowNet-C model

We fine-tune the FlowNet-C pre-trained model, using 3D CT images with manually annotated segmentation information as input data for improved applicability to medical image data. Since FlowNet-C network can only predict the optical flow field of 2D images, in order to adapt it to 3D medical images, we sliced the 3D medical images in 3 dimensions: sagittal, coronal and axial. The 2D slices were fed as training data into the FlowNet-C network. Due to the lack of ground truth, we use an end-to-end weakly supervised learning approach to fine-tune the network, using label supervision as auxiliary information to help train the network and segmentation information is only used in training[4].

The Spatial Transformation Networks[5] approach helps us to perform unsupervised end-to-end training. The moving and fixed images are processed through a convolutional neural network to generate an optical flow field (which can be used as a deformation field), a sampling grid generator to generate a regular network of the same size as the image, and add it to the deformation field to obtain a sampling network, and then resample the moving image through the sampler to obtain a moved image, which is a process that can compute gradients backwards.

Calculating the loss of similarity between the fixed and moved images. The similarity loss is used to measure the similarity between images, and when two images have the same grey value, MSE Loss is usually used:

$$L_{sim} = \frac{1}{N}\sum_{i=1}^{N}(y_i - \hat{y}_i)^2 \tag{1}$$

MSE loss is used to predict the mean of the sum of squared errors at the corresponding points of the data and the corresponding points of the original data, and N is the number of samples.

When using label-supervised training, the deformation field is also applied to the moving segmentation to generate the moved segmentation and to calculate the segmentation loss between the fixed and moving segmentation:

$$L_{Dice} = \frac{2|X \cap Y|}{|X| + |Y|} \tag{2}$$

$|X \cap Y|$ represents the intersection between element X and element X, $|X| + |Y|$ represents the total number of elements, and the coefficient 2 indicates that the denominator was double-counted for the common elements between the numerators. Dice coefficient is a similarity measure function that is used to calculate the similarity between samples and takes values in the range $[0, 1]$, where 0 means no overlap at all and 1 means complete match. It is used to evaluate the results of the registration in this experiment.

This dice loss is derived from the dice coefficient, it is used as the loss function for the segmentation loss.:

$$L_{Diceloss} = 1 - \frac{2|X \cap Y|}{|X| + |Y|} \tag{3}$$

It is also necessary to impose a spatial smoothness constraint on the deformation field ϕ that penalizes the gradient of the deformation field, because maximizing the similarity of the images may cause the network to produce discontinuous deformation fields[6].

$$L_{smooth}(\phi) = \sum_{p} \|\nabla\phi(p)\|^2 \quad (4)$$

Finally the total loss is calculated using the deformed image with the fixed image, which is back-propagated and continuously optimized to minimize the value of the loss function.

2.3 Inverse consistency transformation

The inverse consistency approach[7][8] indicates that we cannot just consider the forward optical flow field from the moving image to the fixed image without considering the inverse transformation from the fixed image to the moving image. The transformation from the moving image to the fixed image should be equal to the inverse transformation from the fixed image to the moving image, and this inconsistency may cause the results obtained from the alignment to not actually reflect the correspondence between the two images. The inverse consistency loss is defined as[7]:

$$L_{inv} = \left\|\mathbf{F}_{AB} - \widetilde{\mathbf{F}}_{AB}\right\|_2 + \left\|\mathbf{F}_{BA} - \widetilde{\mathbf{F}}_{BA}\right\|_2 \quad (5)$$

$\mathbf{F}_{AB}$ represents the forward transformation of A and B. $\widetilde{\mathbf{F}}_{AB}$ represents the forward deformation field of B and A as a moving, using the inverse deformation field of B and A for its transformation. $\mathbf{F}_{BA}$ and $\widetilde{\mathbf{F}}_{BA}$ in the same way We reduce the inverse consistency error between the forward and backward deformation by optimizing multiple iterations.
The process of FlowNet alignment on 3d images is as follows: the fixed image and moving image are sliced by sagittal, coronal and axial to obtain three sets of 2D orthogonal images, which are fed into the FlowNet to obtain the forward and backward optical flow fields respectively, then the inverse consistency error between them is reduced by iterating the inverse consistency function, the three optical flow fields with the smaller inverse consistency error are trilinear unsampled to obtain a 3D optical flow field, a spatial transformation is performed on the moving image to obtain the aligned moved image, and then iterative optimization is performed (the moved image is repeated as the moving image again).

3 Results and Discussion

3.1 Data Pre-processing

We performed experiments on the abdominal organ dataset provided by Learn2Reg Task3, which contains 30 3D ct images of the abdomen and 13 abdominal organ segmentations manually labelled by two experienced physicians. The size of the images is 192x160x256 and the dataset has been provided with the same voxel resolution and general preprocessing of the spatial dimension, and also with affine preregistration. The dataset also provides a registration guide file that specifies the correspondence between the fixed and moving images in the dataset. From this we can obtain 45 pairs of trainable images (one image can be used as a fixed image for multiple moving images). In the pre-processing phase we first normalise the images to the range [0,1] and then resample them to a size of 256x256x256.

3.2 Experimental results

The FlowNet-C pre-trained on flying chairs was fine-tuned by segmentation loss, and 15360 2D images were sliced from 20 3D images for training, leaving 10 images for testing. From these, 2160 images with clear markings and low noise were selected as the training set. We used PyTorch for training, K80 GPU and CUDA 10.1 for acceleration, Adam as the optimization method, batch size = 4, epoch=100, learning rate is 1e-5, and the regularization term coefficient is chosen as 10. The segmentation information was evaluated using the dice coefficient.

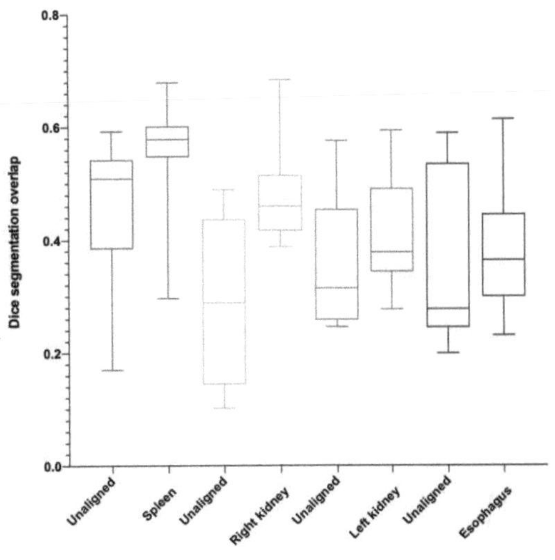

Figure 2: We present the dice coefficients for 4 of the 13 labels, with unaligned indicating that they did not go through the FlowNet network.

We applied pre-trained FlowNet-C on all three dimensions of the images and we tested the images in the dataset. Using the fine-tuned frontal model, we tested the remaining images. As shown in Fig. 2 we improved the image alignment of the spleen, left kidney, right kidney and oesophagus markers from 36.4% to 54.6%. our method successfully applied FlowNet-C to the alignment of 3D images, and the registration results were computed in only 0.63s.

3.3 Discussion

By using ITK-SNAP software to view the 3d ct images, it was found that the slices in the outer layers of the images were without segmentation labels and contained unidentifiable tissue organs. This was difficult for us to perform semantic supervision, and we carefully examined the dataset to find the range of slices that contained clear semantic information as well as tissue organs. And because of using 2D slices, some of the spatial information of the images may be lost, which does not help us to get better alignment results. Also, FlowNet-C is sometimes not ideal in the face of large tissue deformations. Fig.3 shows the three planes in which we obtained the slices and shows the aligned images. It can be seen that the registration has some effect.

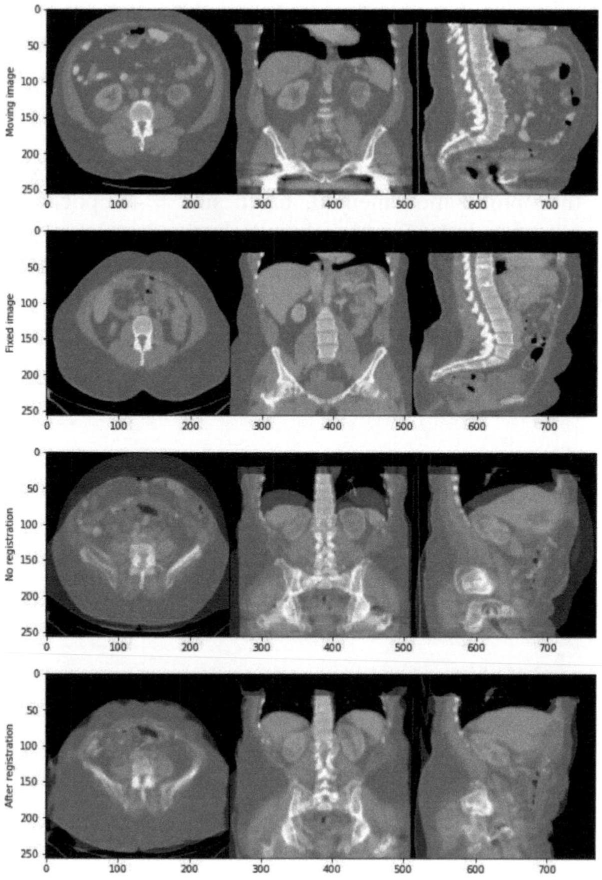

Figure 3: From left to right, axial plane, coronal plane, sagittal plane, 3D image slicing is also implemented in this way.

4 Conclusion

We successfully applied the FlowNet network to 3D image registration, for which we sliced the 3D images and fine-tuned the network using segmentation losses. An inverse consistency constraint was used to adjust the predicted optical flow field for better performance, and our experimental results also show that the alignment does improve. In future work, we will use additional datasets to fine tune our model for improved accuracy in 3d registration.

Acknowledgement

The work has been carried out at Institut für Medizinische Informatik and supervised by Prof. Dr. Mattias Heinrich,Universität zu Lübeck.

Author's Statement

Conflict of interest: Authors state no conflict of interest.

5 References

[1] S. Miao, Z. J. Wang, and R. Liao, "A cnn regression approach for real-time 2d/3d registration," *IEEE transactions on medical imaging*, vol. 35, no. 5, pp. 1352–1363, 2016.

[2] B. D. de Vos, F. F. Berendsen, M. A. Viergever, M. Staring, and I. Išgum, "End-to-end unsupervised deformable image registration with a convolutional neural network," in *Deep learning in medical image analysis and multimodal learning for clinical decision support*, pp. 204–212, Springer, 2017.

[3] P. Fischer, A. Dosovitskiy, E. Ilg, P. Häusser, C. Hazirbas, V. Golkov, P. van der Smagt, D. Cremers, and T. Brox, "Flownet: Learning optical flow with convolutional networks," *CoRR*, vol. abs/1504.06852, 2015.

[4] A. Hering, S. Kuckertz, S. Heldmann, and M. P. Heinrich, "Enhancing label-driven deep deformable image registration with local distance metrics for state-of-the-art cardiac motion tracking," in *Bildverarbeitung für die Medizin 2019*, pp. 309–314, Springer, 2019.

[5] M. Jaderberg, K. Simonyan, A. Zisserman, and K. Kavukcuoglu, "Spatial transformer networks," *arXiv preprint arXiv:1506.02025*, 2015.

[6] G. Balakrishnan, A. Zhao, M. R. Sabuncu, J. V. Guttag, and A. V. Dalca, "Voxelmorph: A learning framework for deformable medical image registration," *CoRR*, vol. abs/1809.05231, 2018.

[7] J. Zhang, "Inverse-consistent deep networks for unsupervised deformable image registration," *arXiv preprint arXiv:1809.03443*, 2018.

[8] G. E. Christensen, *Inverse Consistent Image Registration*, pp. 219–250. Boston, MA: Springer US, 2005.

Dynamic Mode Decomposition applied to Positron Emission Tomography Data - Investigation of Dopamine Processing in Parkinson's Disease

Tilman Wegener [1], Jessie Fanglu Fu [2], Ivan Klyuzhin [3], Martin McKeown [4], A. Jon Stoessl [5] and Vesna Sossi [2]
[1] Medical Engineering Science, Universität zu Lübeck, tilman.wegener@student.uni-luebeck.de
[2] University of British Columbia, Physics and Astronomy, Vancouver, Canada, {jfu, vesna}@phas.ubc.ca
[3] University of British Columbia, Physics and Astronomy, Vancouver, Canada, ivansk@physics.ubc.ca
[4] University of British Columbia, Division of Neurology, Vancouver, Canada, martin.mckeown@ubc.ca
[5] Djavad Mowafaghian Centre for Brain Health, Vancouver, Canada, jon.stoessl@ubc.ca

Abstract

Parkinson's Disease (PD) is characterised by the loss of dopaminergic function in the striatum, a part of the basal ganglia. Using multi-tracer *Positron Emission Tomography* (PET) and a previously published data-driven approach - *Dynamic Mode Decomposition* (DMD) - we investigated whether distinct spatio-temporal patterns exist in different aspects of presynaptic dopaminergic processing in PD patients. Differences in these patterns may reflect unique contributions from each aspect of dopaminergic dysfunction to disease initiation, disease progression and potential compensatory mechanisms. Our results are as follows: 1.) *[^{11}C]-dihydrotetrabenazine* (DTBZ) tracer results replicated previous findings of DMD applied to a different cohort on a higher resolution PET scanner. This demonstrates the robustness of the DMD approach, while 2.) *[^{11}C]-d-threo-methylphenidate* (MP) and *[^{18}F]-fluoro-L-DOPA* (FDOPA) tracer analysis results are novel and related to compensatory and regulatory effects at different disease stages.

1 Introduction

Parkinson's Disease (PD) is the second most common progressive neurodegenerative disease [1]. There is currently no cure available and the mechanisms of this disease are still largely unknown. PD is characterized by the loss of dopaminergic neurons in the brain, more specifically in the substantia nigra and their projections into the striatum, in the form of specific spatio-temporal patterns. This nigrostriatal dopaminergic pathway is crucial for the production of movement. In PD patients, the posterior striatum contralateral to the body side more affected by movement symptoms is affected first by loss of dopaminergic function, followed by degeneration in the anterior striatum [1].
Functional neuroimaging techniques such as *Positron Emission Tomography* (PET) can be used to track disease progression and to better understand disease mechanisms [2], [3]. Different PET tracers allow us to investigate different parts of dopaminergic processing which are affected differently over the course of the disease, manifesting in different spatio-temporal patterns. Differences in these patterns may reflect contributions from each aspect of dopaminergic processing to disease initiation, disease progression and potential compensatory mechanisms [4].
Dynamic Mode Decomposition (DMD) can be used to extract these patterns. DMD is a data-driven multivariate analysis tool that allows to simultaneously extract coherent spatio-temporal patterns [5]. The applicability of DMD to study progressive changes of PET tracer binding values in PD has previously been shown in [1].
In this work, we applied DMD to three PET tracers, which label different aspects of presynaptic dopaminergic processing (see Fig. 1):

- *[^{11}C]-dihydrotetrabenazine* (DTBZ): Labels the *Vesicular Monoamine Transporter Type 2* (VMAT2). Estimates dopaminergic terminal density and is the most direct estimate for the loss of dopaminergic function in the striatum [2].
- *[^{11}C]-d-threo-methylphenidate* (MP): Labels the membrane-bound *Dopamine Transporter* (DAT) and estimates the reuptake from the synaptic cleft into the cytoplasm [3].
- *[^{18}F]-fluoro-L-DOPA* (FDOPA): Assesses dopamine synthesis and storage [2].

To extract and compare the spatio-temporal patterns obtained with different tracers, we applied DMD to the tracer data sets in a large PD cohort. After preprocessing of the data, we applied DMD to each tracer on a voxel level to extract spatio-temporal patterns in the putamen (a part of the striatum that is largely involved in motor control). We then compared these patterns to find information about disease

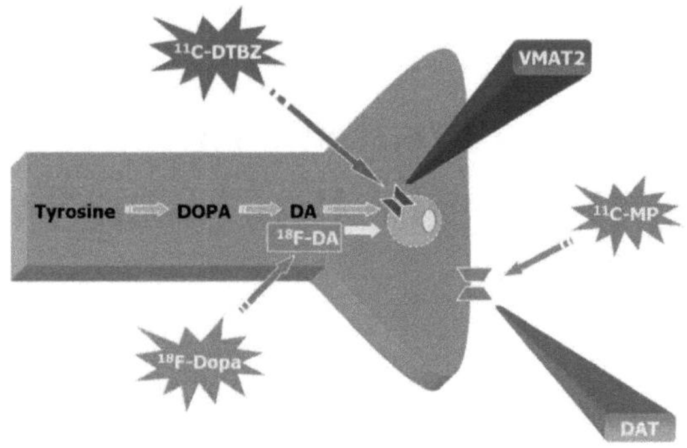

Figure 1: Presynaptic dopaminergic neuron and the binding points of the PET tracers DTBZ, MP and FDOPA [6] (*DA* = Dopamine).

and compensatory mechanisms in PD. We also compared our results to previously published univariate analysis results of the same data set [4] and with results of DMD applied to DTBZ scans performed with a higher resolution PET scanner in a different PD cohort [1].

2 Material and Methods

2.1 Study Participants and multi-tracer Positron Emission Tomography Imaging

Sixty-nine PD patients were scanned using DTBZ (disease duration 1-22 years), seventy-three patients using MP (disease duration 1-26 years) and fifty patients using FDOPA (disease duration 1-22 years). Scans were performed on the ECAT 953B tomograph (CTI/Siemens, Knoxville, TN) in three-dimensional mode. More details on study participants and the imaging protocol can be found in [4].

2.2 Image Processing

PET images were frame-to-frame realigned to correct for motion using *Statistical Parametric Mapping* (SPM) [7]. The PET images for all subjects were then brought into a common space. For this, a template for each tracer was created by rigidly registering and averaging scans of a cohort of healthy subjects performed on the same scanner. Images were rigidly and non-linearly registered to the tracer specific template. *Parametric non-displaceable Binding Potential* (BP_{ND}) images were calculated for DTBZ and MP using the *Simplified Reference Tissue Model 2* (SRTM2) [8] and parametric uptake rate constant (KOCC, min^{-1}) images were generated for FDOPA using the Patlak graphical method [9]. The transformation from each template to the *Montreal Neurological Institute* (MNI) space was calculated based on [10] by using rigid and non-linear registration. This transformation was then applied to the individual scans bringing them into MNI space. Left and right putamen of each PET scan was masked using the MNI segmentation and separated into more and less affected putamen based on the mean DTBZ putaminal BP_{ND}. The segmentation of the putamen was checked for each scan to ensure a high segmentation quality.

2.3 Dynamic Mode Decomposition

DMD is a data-driven analysis technique. It combines the ability to extract coherent spatial modes and their associated temporal dynamics with the dimensionality reduction capability of *Principal Component Analysis* (PCA) [5]. Our goal was to model the temporal progression of PET tracer values in the putamen of PD subjects over disease duration. The following description of the DMD algorithm follows the description in [1]:
Each PET scan was treated as a snapshot at disease duration $k\Delta t$ and stretched into a column vector x_k. A constant time difference Δt of one year between measurements is assumed. Images of different patients with the same disease duration were averaged to reduce noise. To make results between different tracers comparable, each vector x_k was demeaned. The vectors were then concatenated to form the matrices

$$X_{t-1} = [x_1, ..., x_{t-1}] \tag{1}$$

and

$$X_t = [x_2, ..., x_t] \tag{2}$$

where X_t is the by Δt into the future advanced version of X_{t-1}. The progression from X_{t-1} to X_t can be modeled as

$$X_t = A\, X_{t-1} + \epsilon \tag{3}$$

using the unknown linear operator A and the residual ϵ. DMD models a linear regression of the non-linear dynamics relating X_{t-1} and X_t by eigendecomposition of A. By applying singular value decomposition to $X_{t-1} (= U \Sigma V^*)$ and using its pseudo inverse $X^{\dagger}_{t-1}$, A can be approximated as

$$A \approx X_t\, X^{\dagger}_{t-1} = X_t\, V\, \Sigma^{-1}\, U^*. \tag{4}$$

However, direct eigenvalue analysis of A is computationally too expensive. Instead, we project A into a reduced dimensional space, similar to PCA-based dimensionality reduction. We truncate the previously computed matrices U, S and Σ (to U', S' and Σ') so that they only contain the components which describe the highest variance in X_{t-1}. We then use U', V' and Σ' to project A into a reduced dimensional space:

$$\hat{A} = U'^*\, A\, U' = U'^*\, X_t\, V'\, \Sigma'^{-1} \tag{5}$$

We now calculate the eigendecomposition of $\hat{A}$ ($\hat{A} W = \Lambda W$). The first eigenvalues of A and $\hat{A}$ are identical and their eigenvectors Φ are related by a linear transformation. The DMD modes (eigenvectors of A) are therefore defined as

$$\Phi = X_t\, V'\, \Sigma'^{-1}\, W \tag{6}$$

and their associated temporal curve as

$$T(t) = \frac{x_1}{\Phi}\, exp\left(\frac{log(\Lambda)\, t}{\Delta t}\right). \tag{7}$$

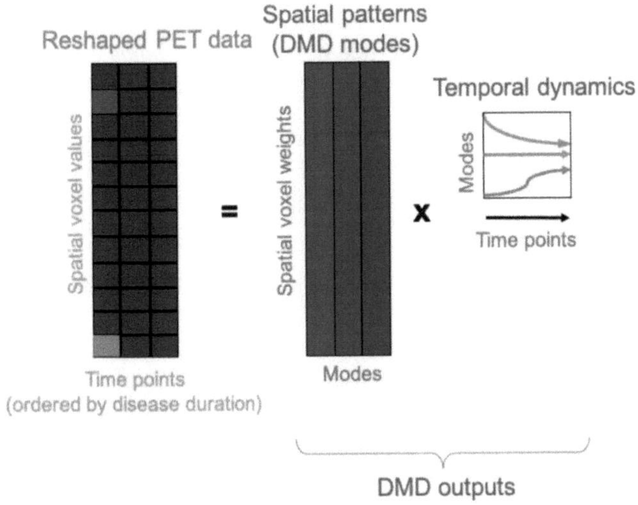

Figure 2: DMD decomposes the spatio-temporal progression of the PET tracer data into spatial patterns and their associated temporal progression curves [1].

In summary, DMD decomposes the input data into two parts: The spatial patterns or DMD modes Φ and their associated temporal dynamics curve $T(t)$ (see Fig. 2).

3 Results and Discussion

For each tracer individually, DMD was applied to the binding values of the less and more affected putamen together. DMD extracted one spatio-temporal pattern accounting for at least 80% of the total variance for each PET tracer.
For all three tracers, the spatial maps of the first DMD component showed an anterior-posterior gradient on both sides, with all three gradients looking very similar (see Fig. 3). This anterior-posterior gradient was previously observed when applying DMD to a PD cohort scanned with DTBZ on a PET scanner with higher spatial resolution [1]. The gradient for DTBZ and MP was more prominent in the less affected putamen compared to the more affected side (see Fig. 3) as also shown in [1].
The temporal curves of all gradients decreased gradually with disease progression (see Fig. 4). However, slope and intercept of the temporal curves were different. DTBZ, which is a direct measure of dopaminergic terminal loss and least sensitive to regulatory changes [11], had the slowest decay rate of all tracers. MP and FDOPA reflect a combination of both dopaminergic terminal degeneration and regulatory changes. The expression of the anterior-posterior gradient in MP and FDOPA is very high in early disease (<10 years) and then decreases. Univariate analysis of the same data set indicated that this gradient might be due to downregulation of DAT density (MP) in the posterior putamen in early disease and upregulation of dopamine synthesis (FDOPA) in the anterior putamen [12]. Downregulation of DAT (MP) in early disease may serve a functional role to maintain constant synaptic dopamine level in presence of dopaminergic terminal loss. Upregulation of dopamine synthesis (FDOPA) in the anterior putamen might be to keep dopamine concentration in the remaining synapses high. The breakdown of these compensatory mechanisms might lead to progression of motor symptoms.

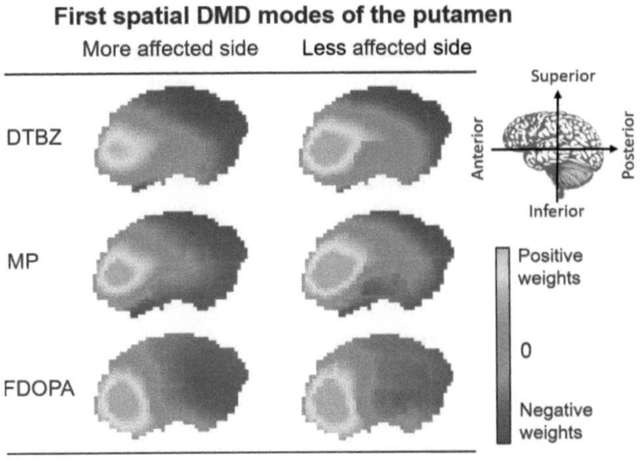

Figure 3: Extracted spatial patterns for DMD applied to the tracer binding values of the more and less affected putamen. All three tracers showed an anterior-posterior gradient of dopaminergic degeneration in both the less and more affected sides.

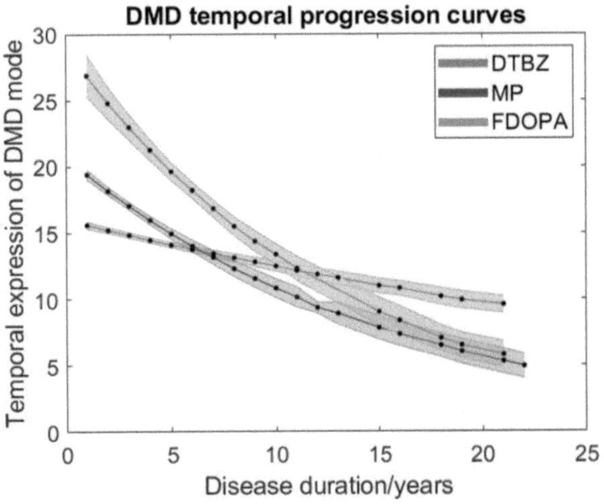

Figure 4: DMD temporal progression curves (with standard deviation calculated using leave-one-out cross-validation) for the tracers DTBZ, MP and FDOPA, associated with the spatial patterns in Fig. 3.

4 Conclusion

DMD is designed to extract spatial features that are most sensitive to disease progression, whereas previous univariate analysis correlates progression with fixed predefined features ([6] and [4]). By comparing our findings with previously obtained results from a different PD cohort scanned on a PET tomograph with higher spatial resolution, we demonstrated the robustness of the DMD approach.

Our results showed that the expression of the anterior-posterior gradient is more sensitive to disease progression than mean putaminal binding. This suggests that PD has a different impact on anterior and posterior putamen. While DTBZ mainly reflects direct disease-induced dopamine denervation, distinct temporal progression curves obtained with MP and FDOPA may suggest upregulation of dopamine synthesis in the anterior putamen and downregulation of dopamine reuptake in the posterior putamen in early PD, which may be of compensatory nature. These compensatory mechanisms may breakdown as the disease progresses, which could lead to progression of motor symptoms in advanced disease.

Acknowledgement

The work has been carried out at the PET/MRI Imaging Group at the University of British Columbia, Canada and was supervised by Prof. Magdalena Rafecas, Institute of Medical Engineering, Universität zu Lübeck.
The authors thank the UBC PET scanning and the TRIUMF radio-chemistry production staff. The volunteer subjects who generously donated their time to this research are also most gratefully acknowledged. The study was financially supported by the *Natural Sciences and Engineering Research Council of Canada* (NSERC), Brain Canada, and *Canadian Institutes of Health Research* (CIHR) and Michael Smith Foundation of Health Research. AJS is supported by the Canada Research Chairs program. JF receives scholarship funding from the Isotopes for Science and Medicine program (NSERC-CREATE). TW is supported by ENEN+ project that has received funding from the EURATOM research and training Work Programme 2016-2017 (1755576) and the PROMOS Study or Internship Abroad Scholarships which has received funding from the *German Academic Exchange Service* (DAAD).

Author's Statement

Conflict of interest: Authors state no conflict of interest.
Informed consent: Informed consent has been obtained from all individuals included in this study.
Ethical approval: The research related to human use complies with all the relevant national regulations, institutional policies and was performed in accordance with the tenets of the Helsinki Declaration, and has been approved by the UBC Ethics Committee.

5 References

[1] J. F. Fu, I. S. Klyuzhin, M. J. McKeown, A. J. Stoessl, and V. Sossi, "Novel data-driven, equation-free method captures spatio-temporal patterns of neurodegeneration in Parkinson's disease: Application of dynamic mode decomposition to PET," *NeuroImage: Clinical*, vol. 25, p. 102150, 2020.

[2] A. J. Stoessl, "Neuroimaging in Parkinson's disease: from pathology to diagnosis," *Parkinsonism & related disorders*, vol. 18, pp. S55–S59, 2012.

[3] A. J. Stoessl, W. W. Martin, M. J. McKeown, and V. Sossi, "Advances in imaging in Parkinson's disease," *The Lancet Neurology*, vol. 10, no. 11, pp. 987–1001, 2011.

[4] R. Nandhagopal, L. Kuramoto, M. Schulzer, E. Mak, J. Cragg, C. S. Lee, J. McKenzie, S. McCormick, A. Samii, A. Troiano *et al.*, "Longitudinal progression of sporadic Parkinson's disease: a multi-tracer positron emission tomography study," *Brain*, vol. 132, no. 11, pp. 2970–2979, 2009.

[5] P. J. Schmid, "Dynamic mode decomposition of numerical and experimental data," *Journal of fluid mechanics*, vol. 656, pp. 5–28, 2010.

[6] R. Nandhagopal, M. J. McKeown, and A. J. Stoessl, "Invited article: functional imaging in Parkinson disease," *Neurology*, vol. 70, no. 16 Part 2, pp. 1478–1488, 2008.

[7] W. D. Penny, K. J. Friston, J. T. Ashburner, S. J. Kiebel, and T. E. Nichols, *Statistical parametric mapping: the analysis of functional brain images*. Elsevier, 2011.

[8] Y. Wu and R. E. Carson, "Noise reduction in the simplified reference tissue model for neuroreceptor functional imaging," *Journal of Cerebral Blood Flow & Metabolism*, vol. 22, no. 12, pp. 1440–1452, 2002.

[9] C. S. Patlak and R. G. Blasberg, "Graphical evaluation of blood-to-brain transfer constants from multiple-time uptake data. generalizations," *Journal of Cerebral Blood Flow & Metabolism*, vol. 5, no. 4, pp. 584–590, 1985.

[10] I. S. Klyuzhin, J. F. Fu, A. Hong, M. Sacheli, N. Shenkov, M. Matarazzo, A. Rahmim, A. J. Stoessl, and V. Sossi, "Data-driven, voxel-based analysis of brain PET images: Application of PCA and LASSO methods to visualize and quantify patterns of neurodegeneration," *PloS one*, vol. 13, no. 11, 2018.

[11] T. Vander Borght, M. Kilbourn, T. Desmond, D. Kuhl, and K. Frey, "The vesicular monoamine transporter is not regulated by dopaminergic drug treatments," *European journal of pharmacology*, vol. 294, no. 2-3, pp. 577–583, 1995.

[12] C. S. Lee, M. Schulzer, R. de la Fuente-Fernández, E. Mak, L. Kuramoto, V. Sossi, T. J. Ruth, D. B. Calne, and A. J. Stoessl, "Lack of regional selectivity during the progression of Parkinson disease: implications for pathogenesis," *Archives of neurology*, vol. 61, no. 12, pp. 1920–1925, 2004.

Adding DICOM Support for an Industrial X-Ray Inspection Software

Pia-Sophie Lampert [1], Frederik Kaiser [2] and Maik Stille [3, 4]
[1] Medical Engineering Science, Universität zu Lübeck, piasophie.lampert@student.uni-luebeck.de
[2] VisiConsult X-ray Systems & Solutions GmbH, info@visiconsult.de
[3] Institute of Medical Engineering, Universität zu Lübeck, stille@imt.uni-luebeck.de
[4] Fraunhofer Research Institution for Individualized and Cell-Based Medical Engineering, Lübeck, Germany

Abstract

DICONDE (Digital Imaging and Communication in Non-Destructive Evaluation) is a standard that builds on DICOM and offers manufacturers and users of non-destructive evaluation (NDE) a way to store and exchange image data. With the development of a software application that enables the use of DICONDE, it should be possible to read, generate and process DICONDE images. This will allow many advantages, such as better interoperability, as proprietary data will no longer be created.

1 Introduction

Companies involved in the design and testing of engineering equipment and systems often need to generate and store non-destructive examination (NDE) test data. Such NDE data can be useful in cases where a defect is discovered in a part or in the event of a failure of the part during operation. Such NDE test data can include digital images, such as X-ray images.

However, proprietary data formats are often used in the process, creating numerous, incompatible 'island archives' of NDE data from different sources [1]. As a result, there are often conflicts with cross-system data integration, and data cannot be readily shared between providers and customers or between suppliers and government agencies [2]. One solution for inefficient data sharing is DICONDE.

With this, not only the problem of missing interoperability is solved, but one also gains more certainty regarding quality and process. Organizations have more confidence when their departments and suppliers apply recognized standards, as processes and results become more transparent and easier to compare with those of other market players. Further benefits include fewer transaction costs, because internal and external transaction costs are lower when the same definitions and data models are used within the company and between business partners. Furthermore, another advantage of using a standard is the promotion of synergetic partnerships.

After all, standards are essentially codified knowledge. Before a standard can be developed, however, best practices must first be widely accepted by experts. Organizations can take advantage of this synergy because the resulting reliable source of knowledge can help them raise their level of development and connect more easily with partners [3].

2 Material and Methods

For the development of a software application that provides the use of DICONDE, a basic understanding of the DICOM and DICONDE standard is first essential.

2.1 DICOM

Digital Imaging and Communications in Medicine (DICOM) is a standard for exchanging and storing medical imaging information and related data. It became a central standard in radiology and is increasingly used in other medical fields [4]. The objective of the DICOM standard is to enable communication of diagnostic and therapeutic information, images, and associated data of any kind. Connectivity, compatibility, and work-flow optimization are the main intentions. Cooperating with the users themselves, manufacturers define the main characteristics of this standard [4].

One part of the DICOM standard describes the data structure, the components, and construction of a DICOM file. The first section of a DICOM file is the header (Fig. 1) and contains only metadata. Every DICOM file covers much other information beyond the image pixel data in a very organizational and standardized way. All information is grouped into datasets. These datasets contain multiple so-called data elements. After the initial header, of which each DICOM file has at least one but often several, the primary data set is following.

A data element is the smallest unit of a DICOM file, it is the coded information of a specific attribute. The attributes' data structure consists of a Tag, Value Representation, Value Length and Value Field.

The Tag of each attribute is an 8-digit hexadecimal number composed of a 4-digit group number and a 4-digit element number (gggg,eeee). Attributes that are related to each other are often grouped in the same group. The element number refers to the specific attribute within the group. Furthermore, no two attributes have the same tag. The Value Representation is a two-place string code and defines the data type of the value. It is predefined for every attribute and can be referred to in the DICOM dictionary. The next section, Value Field, indicates the length of the entry. Each entry has an odd length and will be padded with space (ASCII 0x20) to have an even length. This even Value Length is due to the fact that the final encoding type of DICOM files is binary. Finally, the Value Field contains the actual information of a given attribute. Fig. 1 illustrates the just described DICOM data structure.

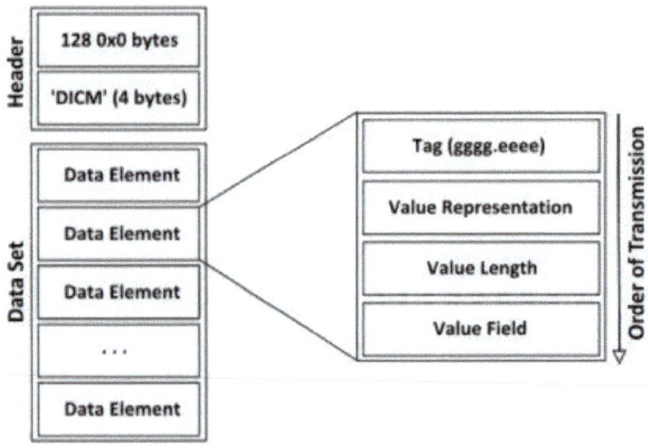

Figure 1: data structure in a DICOM file, including the data structure of a DICOM data element

In addition, each attribute has a name that indicates the information of the attribute. This name is actually not part of the DICOM file itself and has to be looked up in the DICOM dictionary. Furthermore, the Value Multiplicity provides information about the number of values. A data element does not have to have only one value, but can also have a list of values. The Requirement Type is part of the DICOM data structure. An attribute, encoded as a Data Element, may or may not be required in a Data Set, depending on that Attribute's Data Element Type. This information is kept in the Requirement Type.
Besides the defined DICOM tags, there are also Private Data Elements. Implementations may require communication of information that cannot be contained in Standard Data Elements. Private Data Elements are intended to be used to contain such information. They have the same structure, but the group number used in the Element Tag of Private Data Elements shall be an odd number (Standard Data Element always have an even group number).
Table 1 summarizes the DICOM data structure of a data element based on an example.
The actual pixel data can also be found in a data element. The individual pixel values are stored as a data stream in the value of the DICOM tag with the name 'Pixel Data'. It can contain either a single slice or multiple slices of the acquired image information.
Moreover, another major component of the DICOM standard covers the communication and exchange of information in medical image data management.

2.2 DICONDE

DICONDE stands for „Digital Imaging and Communication in Non-Destructive Evaluation“ and provides the industry a standard data format and a uniform communication protocol. DICONDE builds on the DICOM standard and extends it with elements of the non-destructive evaluation [5]. The most crucial difference between the two standards is the naming of the tags. For this purpose, DICOM tag names that are not usable in the non-destructive examination are replaced by other names and extended by additional tags. ASTM International (American Society for Testing and Materials) develops the DICONDE standard, and for this, ASTM produces sets of tags for non-destructive material testing (see Fig. 2). ASTM International is an international standards organization based in the USA. It publishes technical standards for products and services. So DICONDE overrides and extends DICOM in order to make it applicable in industrial inspection [6].

Attribute Name	Tag	VR	VM	Type	Description
Component					
Component Name	(0010,0010)	PN	1	2	Component Name or Part name
Component ID Number	(0010,0020)	LO	1-N	2	Component ID or Part ID
Other Component IDs	(0010,1000)	LO	1-N	3	Additional Component IDs when multiple parts in one image
Other Component Names	(0010,1001)	PN	1	3	Additional Component IDs when multiple parts in one image
Component Manufacturing Date	(0010,0030)	DA	1	2	
Patient Sex	(0010,0040)	CS	1	2	Required for DICOM compliance. Should either contain zero value or the enumerated value of "O" for OTHER.
Component Notes	(0010,4000)	LT	1	3	
Component Manufacturing Procedure	(0014,0025)	ST	1	3	
Component Manufacturer	(0014,0028)	ST	1	3	
Component Welder IDs	(0014,0100)	LO	1-N	3	A text string identifying the individual or machine performing welding operations on the component.
Material					
Material Name	(0010,2160)	SH	1	2	Steel, copper, etc. (16 char. max.)
Material Grade	(0014,0042)	ST	1	3	
Material Properties Description	(0014,0044)	ST	1	3	
Material Notes	(0014,0046)	LT	1	3	
Geometry					
Material Thickness	(0014,0030)	DS	1-N	3	Wall/material thickness in mm
Material Pipe Diameter	(0014,0032)	DS	1-N	3	Retired
Material Isolation Diameter	(0014,0034)	DS	1-N	3	Retired
Component Shape	(0014,0050)	CS	1	3	General description of the shape of the test piece. See 7.4.1.1for additional information.

Figure 2: Snippet of the ASTM DICONDE Component Module [7]

Like the DICOM standard, DICONDE generates data in a hierarchical and systematic structure. Following the DICOM standard, the data is organized in the hierarchy of study, series and instance (Fig. 3). This allows for the inspections to be grouped and categorized within a system.

2.3 DCMTK

The DICOM Toolkit (DCMTK) from OFFIS is a collection of libraries and applications that together implement large parts of the DICOM standard. DCMTK contains applications for examining, creating, and converting DICOM image files, editing storage media, sending and receiving DICOM images in a network, and sample servers for the DICOM Image Archive Services and "Modality Worklist". DCMTK is implemented in a mixture of ANSI C and C++ and is provided as an open source software in source code [8]. The OFFIS-Institute is a non-profit association at the University of Oldenburg.

Table 1: example data structure of a DICOM data element

Tag ID	Tag Name	Value Representation	Value Length	Value Multiplicity	Mandatory	Value
(0008,0060)	Modality	CS	2	1	1	CT
(0010,0010)	Patient Name	PN	8	1	2	John Doe

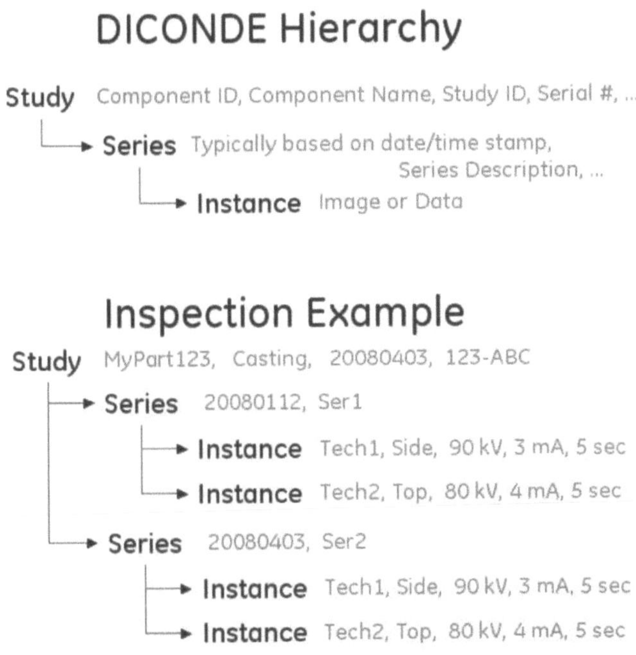

Figure 3: Hierarchy of a DICONDE file

2.4 Implementation

The development of the software application can be divided into three basic steps: being able to read and process a DICONDE file, being able to display DICONDE tags and being able to generate a DICONDE file.

2.4.1 Step 1: Read a DICONDE file

In order to read and display a DICONDE file, a few steps must be followed. If one wants to read the image data itself, which means the individual gray values for each pixel, one has to read the value of the 'Pixel Data' tag. This tag has the Value Representation 'OW' and thus contains binary data. In order to interpret this data correctly, the number of pixels (in x- and y-direction) and the data length (8- or 16-bit) must first be read out.
In addition, a DICOM file contains much more information in the attributes that can be read and processed. This information can be accessed with a sequential readout of the dataset. It is important to distinguish between the different Value Representations so that the values can be interpreted correctly. After reading out the tags using the DCMTK library, the data is converted into internal tag classes that take the different data types into account.
Another point to keep in mind is that the DCMTK library will reflect the DICOM names and descriptions when reading the tags. However, as mentioned above, there are differences in the tag names between DICOM and DICONDE. To take this into account, a dictionary has been created that contains all tags that are named differently in DICONDE or that only exist in DICONDE. Thus, when reading a tag, it must also be checked whether the tag is contained in the dictionary, and if so, the name must be adjusted.

2.4.2 Step 2: Display DICONDE Tags

The different internal tag classes are implemented according to the Model-View-Viewmodel pattern, so that a customized display of the different data types in the user interface is easy to implement. The use of data binding creates the possibility to easily exchange the view without making changes to the code. This enables an easier way to display an attribute with a text differently than an attribute with data as a value.

2.4.3 Step 3: Create a DICONDE file

In the third step, it should be possible to generate DICONDE images with the DICONDE software application. To this, some more information is needed than just the pixel values generated by the X-ray device. It is not enough to convert only the pixel values into a DICONDE file.
For a start, a DICONDE tag must be created that contains the pixel values as value. This can be done with the DCMTK library. It is important that the individual values are passed in byte format since the 'Pixel Data' tag has a given Value Representation. Furthermore, there are some required tags, that must be specified in order to create a valid DICONDE file. These include, for example, component name and study date. For all required tags, a value must be specified, otherwise, it is not possible to create the DICONDE file.
When creating the tags, different cases can be considered. On the one hand, some values can be specified directly in the code, for example date and time. In this case, the current time or date will be taken as value. Then there are values that can be taken from the X-ray device, such as the device properties. And finally, there is information that has to be entered manually by the user. It should also be possible for the user to specify additional information by manually creating new tags.

3 Results and Discussion

3.1 Step 1: Read a DICONDE file

Step 1, reading a DIOCNDE file, has been implemented. It is now possible to read a file with the extension ".dcm". In doing so, the image pixel data can be read out and displayed in the image display program of the internal software. Furthermore, a list of all defined tags can be generated and saved in internal data structures.

3.2 Step 2: Display DICONDE Tags

The implementation of step 2 could be achieved, too. The saved attributes can be displayed in a list (see Fig. 4). As shown in Fig. 4, the tags have been sorted according to the DICONDE modules for a better overview.

3.3 Step 3: Create a DICONDE file

Finally, a short prospect shows the expected results for step 3, creating a DICONDE file. When this step is implemented, all DICONDE tags that are automatically filled in should be displayed in a list. In addition, all required tags that have not yet been assigned to a value should also be included in this list. These tags should be color-coded so that they can be easily identified. Additionally, it should be possible to add further tags with an add button.
Since DICOM not only provides the data structures for storing and exchanging image data but also offers many other possibilities, such as network communication, etc., there are now many more ways to expand and optimize the product.

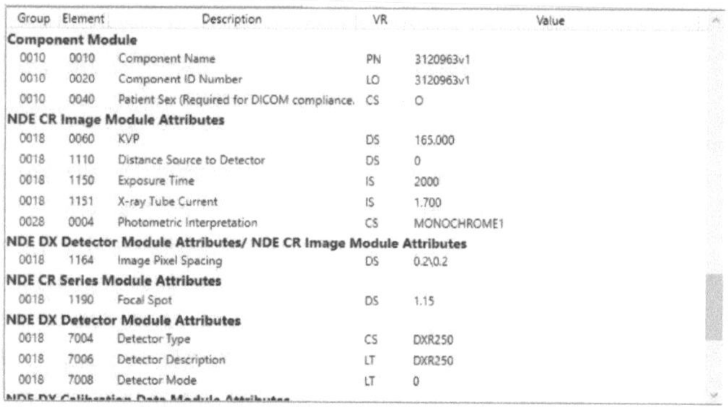

Group	Element	Description	VR	Value
Component Module				
0010	0010	Component Name	PN	3120963v1
0010	0020	Component ID Number	LO	3120963v1
0010	0040	Patient Sex (Required for DICOM compliance.	CS	O
NDE CR Image Module Attributes				
0018	0060	KVP	DS	165.000
0018	1110	Distance Source to Detector	DS	0
0018	1150	Exposure Time	IS	2000
0018	1151	X-ray Tube Current	IS	1.700
0028	0004	Photometric Interpretation	CS	MONOCHROME1
NDE DX Detector Module Attributes/ NDE CR Image Module Attributes				
0018	1164	Image Pixel Spacing	DS	0.2\0.2
NDE CR Series Module Attributes				
0018	1190	Focal Spot	DS	1.15
NDE DX Detector Module Attributes				
0018	7004	Detector Type	CS	DXR250
0018	7006	Detector Description	LT	DXR250
0018	7008	Detector Mode	LT	0

Figure 4: list of DICONDE tags, sorted by DICONDE modules

4 Conclusion

Proprietary data formats can cause many disadvantages in NDE, such as poor interoperability. The introduction and use of a standard would solve these problems.
Therefore, the DICONDE standard was developed from the DICOM standard. DICOM can be used to store and exchange medical image information and furthermore provides a way for nondestructive evaluation manufacturers and users to share image data with some extensions to this standard.
With the help of the DCMTK toolkit from OFFIS, a software application will be developed that enables the use of DICONDE. The implementation can be divided into three steps, reading a DICONDE file, displaying the tags, and creating a DICONDE file.
Looking ahead, it can be said that with the integration of the DIOCNDE standard, many more DICOM services can be used and implemented.

Acknowledgement

The work has been carried out at VisiConsult X-ray Systems & Solutions GmbH and supervised by the Institute of Medical Engineering, Universität zu Lübeck.

Author's Statement

Conflict of interest: The author Pia-Sophie Lampert receives an expense allowance from VisiConsult X-ray Systems & Solutions GmbH for her work in association with this article. All other authors state no conflict of interest.

5 References

[1] E. Neuser and S. Montagna, *ASTM und DICONDE konformes Management von NDT Daten.* DGZfP (DACH) Jahrestagung 2015, 10-13 May, Salzburg, Austria (DGZfP 2015), 2015.

[2] T. W. Birdwell, J. B. Ross, R. C McFarland and C. R. Hammond, *Method of processing test information.* US patent US20040210586A1, 2007.

[3] P. Brunnengraeber and A. Pasupuleti *The Role of Integration in NDT Quality Assurance Chain.* The NDT Technician, Volume 16, Issue 2, pp. 1-3, 2017.

[4] P. Mildenberger, M. Eichelberg and E. Martin, *Introduction to the DICOM standard.* Eur Radiol 12, pp. 920–927, 2001.

[5] M. Jobst, A. Koetz and S. Clendening *The Value of DICONDE in Multi-Modal NDT Environments.* 10th European Conference on Non-Destructive Testing, Moscow 2010, June 7-11 (ECNDT 2010), 2010.

[6] C. Voelker *If a Picture Is Worth 1,000 Words, then Pervasive, Ubiquitous Imaging Is Priceless.* Available: https://www.astm.org/SNEWS/OCTOBER2003/voelkeroct03.html [last accessed on 2021-01-18].

[7] ASTM International, *E2339-15 Standard Practice for Digital Imaging and Communication in Nondestructive Evaluation (DICONDE).* West Conshohocken, PA, downloaded 2018. www.astm.org

[8] OFFIS e.V., *DCMTK - DICOM Toolkit.* Available: https://dicom.offis.de/dcmtk.php.en [last accessed on 2021-01-11].

Studying the response of magnetic particles to rectangular excitation fields in the context of Magnetic Particle Imaging

Tobias Klemme [1], Alexander Neumann [2],
[1] Medical Engineering Science, Universität zu Lübeck, tobias.klemme@student.uni-luebeck.de
[2] Institute of Medical Engineering, Universität zu Lübeck, neumann@imt.uni-luebeck.de

Abstract

Magnetic particle imaging (MPI) is a new promising imaging modality introduced by B. Gleich and J. Weizenecker in 2005 [1]. The basic imaging process uses excitation of magnetic nanoparticles with magnetic fields. By measureing a spatial unique particle response, the spatial distribution of magnetic nanoparticles can be obtained using algebraic reconstruction methods. Since the particle response depends on the applied excitation field, different types of excitation fields can be advantageous for different types of applications or reconstruction methods [2]. This work studies the effect of rectangular excitation fields in comparison to typically chosen sinusoidal excitation in order to gain knowledge that can help finding improved excitation fields for applications like MPI or magnetic particle hyperthermia (MPH). The simulations show that the use of rectangular excitation fields increases the amplitude of higher order harmonics depending on the rise time of the excitation field. Additionally it is shown that the usage of rectangular excitation fields may be advantageous for MPH.

1 Introduction

MPI uses the spatial unique response of magnetic nanoparticles in order to obtain their spatial distribution. The basic imaging approach uses static magnetic fields to create a field free point (FFP). Outside the FFP the magnetic particles are aligned with the static magnetic field (saturated). The application of an additional dynamic magnetic field causes that only particles within the FFP are excited by the dynamic field, since the amplitude of the excitation field is considerably smaller than the static magnetic field. By moving the FFP, the object can be sampled and a spatial unique particle response is measured. The particle response of the excited particles is usually described using Langevin's theory of paramagnetism, which models the magnetization with the non-linear Langevin function. This non linearity of the particle response introduces higher order harmonics in the detected particle signal. The spatial particle response is obtained using receiver coils, measuring the induced signal, which is proportional to the derivative of the magnetization. The usage of a simple receiver coil yields the problem that the induced signal of the excitation field will overlay the particle signal at the excitation frequency in the receiver coil, making it technically challenging to obtain the particle signal at this frequency. Therefore the received signal is usually high or bandpass filtered, leaving only higher order harmonics in the signal. Based on an algebraic reconstruction method, the desired spatial particle distribution can be obtained using a system matrix (SM) containing the spatial frequency response of the magnetic particles. Using this SM based approach the image quality and resolution is in particular dependent on the amplitude and number of harmonic frequencies within the measured particle response, making a particle response containing many high amplitude harmonics advantageous. The excitation field greatly influences the particle response and the corresponding spectrum, studying the influence of different excitation fields on the particle response can hence help to find optimized excitation fields for different applications such as imaging or MPH [3]. This paper focuses on the application of rectangular excitation fields using different rise times τ and alternating rectangular excitation. Therefore especially the influence on the particle signal and spectrum is studied. The results are obtained using a simulation model considering both, Néel and Brown relaxation by solving the coupled equations of motion. Due to the presence of thermal white noise these equations are stochastic differential equations, which are solved using the Euler-Maryuama scheme.

2 Material and Methods

2.1 Simulation

The simulations performed in this paper are based on the simulation intruduced by A. Neumann et al. [4]. In order to fully describe the particle dynamics of magnetic particles, coupled equations of motion are required, considering the dynamic of the particle magnetic moment (Néel rotation) as well as the mechanical (Brownian) rotation, which are coupled due to the magnetic anisotropy. The calculation of the particle dynamics are performed using spherical and Euler coordinates. The appropriate description of the coupling is achieved by a combination of the Landau-Lifschitz-Gilbert equation (LLG) [5] describing the dynamics of a magnetic moment $\vec{m}$ in a magnetic field $\vec{H}$ and adapted Euler equations that are used to describe rotational dynamics within fluids [4]-[6]. The LLG is given by

$$\begin{aligned}\frac{\partial\vec{m}}{\partial t} &= \underbrace{-\frac{\gamma}{1+\alpha^2}\vec{H}_{\text{eff}}}_{\vec{\omega}_{\text{L}}}\times\vec{m} \\ &+ \underbrace{\frac{|\gamma|\alpha}{(1+\alpha^2)M_{\text{S}}V_{\text{M}}}\left(\vec{m}\times\vec{H}_{\text{eff}}\right)}_{\vec{\omega}_{\text{D}}}\times\vec{m} \\ &= (\vec{\omega}_{\text{L}}+\vec{\omega}_{\text{D}})\times\vec{m} = \vec{\omega}_m\times\vec{m}\end{aligned} \tag{1}$$

where the first term describes the Larmor precession and the second term the damping or relaxation of the magnetic moment. Here γ is the gyromagnetic ratio, α the damping constant, V_{M} the magnetic (core) radius and M_{S} the saturation magnetisation, where the modulus of the magnetic moment can be written as $|\vec{m}|= M_{\text{S}}V_{\text{M}}$. Furthermore the Euler equation for particles in viscose media can be written as

$$\mathbf{I}\frac{\partial\vec{\omega}_n}{\partial t} + \vec{\omega}_n\times(\mathbf{I}\vec{\omega}_n) + 6\eta V_{\text{H}}(\vec{\omega}_n - \Omega) = \vec{\tau} \tag{2}$$

$\vec{\omega}_n$ is the angular velocity, $\mathbf{I}$ the inertia tensor, η the viscosity, V_{H} the hydrodynamic volume of a particle and Ω the vorticity. Assuming the inertia of the particle and the vorticity can be neglected (2) is simplified to

$$6\eta V_{\text{H}}\vec{\omega}_n = \vec{\tau}. \tag{3}$$

The damping term in (1) can be rewritten to

$$6\eta_{\text{M}}V_{\text{M}}\vec{\omega}_D = \vec{m}\times\vec{H}_{\text{eff}}, \tag{4}$$

where $\eta_{\text{M}} = M_{\text{S}}(1+\alpha^2)/6\gamma\alpha$ is the magnetic viscosity. Since the particle magnetization can also relax due to particle rotation (4) has to be rewritten to

$$6\eta_{\text{M}}V_{\text{M}}(\vec{\omega}_{\text{D}} - \vec{\omega}_n) = \vec{m}\times\vec{H}_{\text{eff}}. \tag{5}$$

Analogue (3) is rewritten to

$$6\eta V_{\text{H}}\vec{\omega}_n + 6\eta_{\text{M}}V_{\text{M}}(\vec{\omega}_n - \vec{\omega}_{\text{D}}) = \vec{\tau}_{\text{eff}} \tag{6}$$

because the rotation of the magnetic moment causes a torque in the opposite direction of the mechanical friction. Combining those equations results in the following angular velocities

$$\vec{\omega}_n = \frac{1}{6\eta V_{\text{H}}}(\vec{m}\times\vec{H}_{\text{eff}} + \vec{\tau}_{\text{eff}}) \tag{7}$$

and

$$\begin{aligned}\vec{\omega}_m = &-\frac{\gamma}{1+\alpha^2}\vec{H}_{\text{eff}} + \left(\frac{|\gamma|\alpha}{(1+\alpha^2)M_{\text{S}}V_{\text{M}}}(\vec{m}\times\vec{H}_{\text{eff}})\right. \\ &\left.+\frac{1}{6\eta V_{\text{H}}}((\vec{m}\times\vec{H}_{\text{eff}}) + \vec{\tau}_{\text{eff}})\right),\end{aligned} \tag{8}$$

where $\vec{\omega}_n$ and $\vec{\omega}_m$ are the angular velocities of the particle/magnetic moment. The vector $\vec{n}$ describes the particle orientation. The effectice magnetic field and torque are given by

$$\vec{H}_{\text{eff}} = -\frac{\partial U}{\partial\vec{m}} + \vec{H}_{\text{noise}} \tag{9}$$

and

$$\vec{\tau}_{\text{eff}} = -\vec{n}\times\frac{\partial U}{\partial\vec{n}} + \vec{\tau}_{\text{noise}}. \tag{10}$$

Equation (9) and (10) include white noise terms due to thermal fluctuations. These can be described by the following correlations

$$\langle H_{\text{noise,i}}(t)H_{\text{noise,j}}(t')\rangle = 2\frac{k_{\text{B}}T\alpha}{\mu_0|\vec{m}|\gamma}\delta_{\text{i,j}}\delta(t-t') \tag{11}$$

$$\langle F_{\text{noise,i}}(t)F_{\text{noise,j}}(t')\rangle = 12\eta V_{\text{H}}k_{\text{B}}T\delta_{\text{i,j}}\delta(t-t'). \tag{12}$$

Using the assumption that the particles exhibit an uniaxial anisotropy the energy is given by $U = -\vec{m}\cdot\vec{H} - KV_{\text{M}}(\vec{e}\cdot\vec{n})^2$ with $\vec{e} = \vec{m}/(M_{\text{S}}V_{\text{M}})$ being the normalized magnetic moment. In Euler or spherical coordinates the corresponding Langevin equations can be written as

$$\frac{\partial\vec{\Phi}_n}{\partial t} = E_{313}\left(\vec{\Phi}_n\right)\cdot\vec{\omega}_n \tag{13}$$

and

$$\frac{\partial\vec{\Phi}_m}{\partial t} = E_{\text{spherical}}\left(\vec{\Phi}_m\right)\cdot\vec{\omega}_m, \tag{14}$$

where E_{313} and $E_{\text{spherical}}$ are projection matrices and $\vec{\Phi}_n = (\phi_n, \theta_n, \psi_n)$ and $\Phi_m = (\theta_m, \phi_m)$ the given Euler angles /spherical coordinates. The vectors $\vec{m}$ and $\vec{n}$ can be transformed from the spherical or Euler coordinates with

$$\vec{m} = M_S V_M\begin{pmatrix}\sin(\theta_m)\cos(\phi_m)\\ \sin(\theta_m)\sin(\phi_m)\\ \cos(\theta_m)\end{pmatrix} \tag{15}$$

and

$$\vec{n} = \begin{pmatrix}\sin(\theta_n)\sin(\psi_n)\\ -\sin(\theta_n)\cos(\psi_m)\\ \cos(\theta_n)\end{pmatrix}. \tag{16}$$

Equation (13) and (14) are stochastic differential equation solved by application of the Euler-Maryuama scheme [7].

2.2 Rectangular excitation field

The implementation of the used rectangular excitation field is done using charging and discharging curves with a given rise time τ.

The mathematical description of the implemented field can be written as

$$H_{\sqcap}(t) = \begin{cases} H_0\left(1-\exp^{-\frac{t}{\tau}}\right) + H_{\text{offset}} & t \le \frac{T}{2} \\ H_0\exp^{-\frac{t}{\tau}} - \left(H_0 - H_{\sqcap}\left(\frac{T}{2}\right)\right) + H_{\text{offset}} & t > \frac{T}{2}\end{cases} \tag{17}$$

where H_0 is the Field amplitude and T the period duration. Equation (17) gives an expression for rectangular excitation without sign change. A rectangular excitation with alternating sign can be simply achieved by introducing a phase and field offset in (17) resulting in

$$H_{\sqcap\sqcup}(t) = H_{\sqcap}(t + \phi) + H_o. \tag{18}$$

Fig. 1 shows the implemented rectangular excitation field, where the rectangular excitation with alternating sign is plotted in blue and the pulsed rectangular excitation in orange.

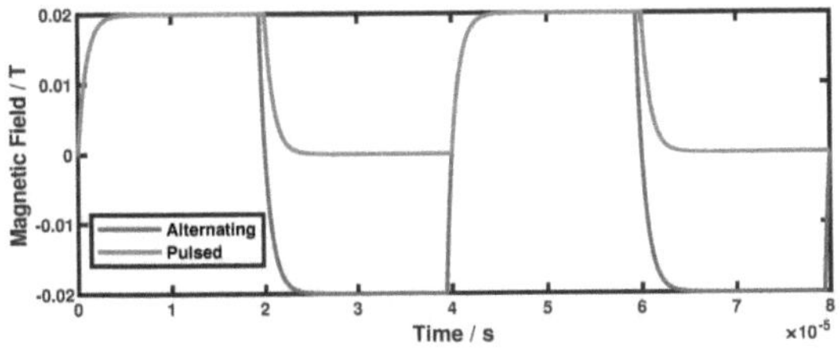

Figure 1: Alternating rectangular excitation Field (blue) and pulsed rectangular excitation (orange), $\tau = 0.3\ \mu s$.

2.3 Simulation parameters

The simulations within this work are carried out using the magnetic field strength of 20 mT and a excitation frequency of 25 kHz. Simulated particles have a core diameter of 24 nm and a hydrodynamic diameter of 50 nm. M_S is set to 477464 A/m being the saturation magnetization of iron and the anisotropy constant K is given by 4000 $\mathrm{kJ/m^3}$. The surrounding of the particle is water, having a viscosity of 1 mPa s and a temperature of 295 K. The damping constant α is set to 0.1. Within the simulation the time step used to solve the equations of motion is set to 5 ps, where the overall simulation time is set to 240 μs which corresponds to six periods of the excitation frequency. The actual output of the simulation is re-sampled to a time step of 0.02 μs. The simulations are performed on a ensemble of 2000 particles. In the following evaluation the first period of the particle response is neglected in order to avoid initialisation artefacts due to non periodicity, since the initial particle orientation and initial magnetic moment orientation is random.

3 Results and Discussion

Fig. 2 shows the used excitation fields, were the rise time τ is set to 0.3, 0.6, 0.9, 2, 3 and 8 μs. Additionally a sinusoidal excitation field is included. The associated particle response is plotted in Fig. 3, where (a) shows the normalized magnetic moment and (b) the derivative of the curves in (a), representing the induced signal in a receiver coil. In Fig. 3 (a) it can be clearly seen, that the rectangular excitation has faster switching times. The induced signal shown in Fig. 3 (b) increases significant with faster rise times due to obvious reasons.

Fig. 4 shows the amplitude of the harmonic frequencies in the spectra of the induced signals shown in Fig. 3 (b). The amplitude and amount of higher order harmonics increases significant with a rectangular excitation and shortening of

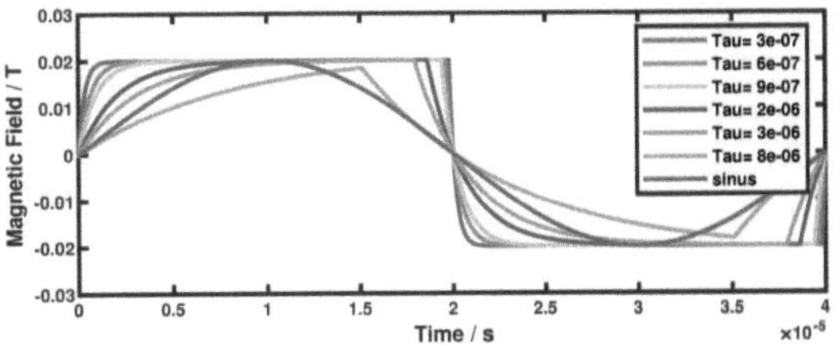

Figure 2: Excitation fields with the used rise times $\tau = 0.3$, 0.6, 0.9, 2, 3 and 8 μs.

(a)

(b)

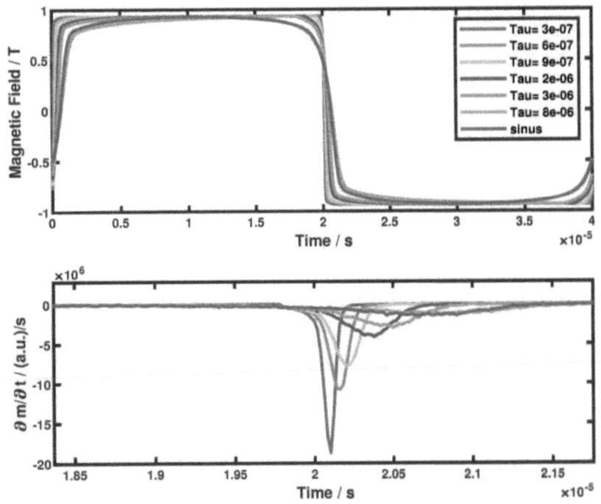

Figure 3: (a) Normalized magnetic moment of the given excitation field with the used rise times $\tau = 0.3, 0.6, 0.9, 2, 3$ and 8 μs and the particle response to sinusoidal excitation as a reference. (b) Derivative of the normalized magnetic moment representing the induced signal (for better visualization only the time interval when the magnetization switches is shown).

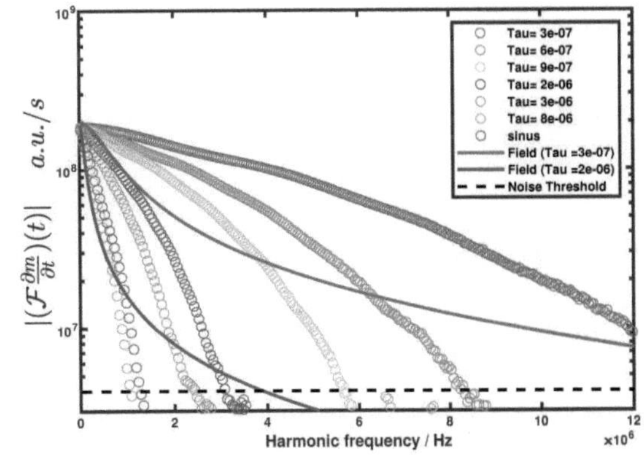

Figure 4: Amplitude of the harmonic frequencies in the spectra of the signal shown in Fig 3 (b). As a comparison the harmonics of the signal induced by the normalized rectangular excitation field is shown as a line plot ($\tau = 0.3, 2\mu$s).

the rise time τ when compared to the sinusoidal excitation. Nevertheless it has to be considered that the particle signal and the associated spectra are strongly dependent on the used particle parameters and surrounding e.g. viscosity and temperature as shown in previous works [8],[9]. Consequently differently chosen parameters such as the viscosity, temperature or particle diameter may lead to different results. Considering the increased amplitude of high frequency harmonics the use of rectangular excitation might appear beneficial. However it has to be taken into account, that the rectangular excitation field will overlay the particle signal at multiple frequencies depending on the shape of the rectangular field. Therefore Fig. 4 includes the harmonic frequencies occurring in the spectrum of the signal which is induced by direct throughput of the excitation field for the excitation fields with τ = 0.3 and 2 μs. These additional frequency components of the excitation field will make the filtering of the particle response more difficult and requires techniques such as the usage of gradiometer receiver coils. Another use case of rectangular excitation might be in applications such as MPH, where the excitation fields are used to heat the nanoparticles for example to destroy tumour tissue. Fig. 5 shows the hysteresis of particles excited with a rectangular field in comparison of particles that are sinusoidal excited. The area of the hysteresis loop using rectangular excitation is noticeably larger and increases with decreased rise times τ, meaning heat generation is more efficient since the generated heat is proportional to the area of the hysteresis loop. The opening of the hysteresis is caused by a increasing phase lag of the particle response relative to the excitation field.

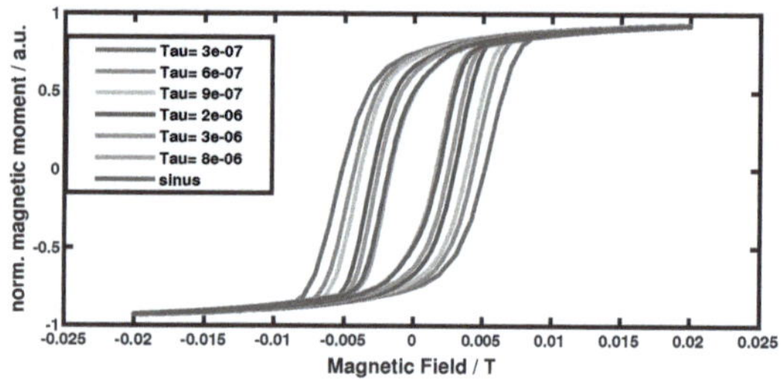

Figure 5: Hysteresis loops for rectangular and sinusoidal excitation.

4 Conclusion

Within this work it has been shown how excitation fields e.g. alternating rectangular excitation affects the particle signal and its spectrum. Additionally the rise time of the excitation fields have been varied in order to examine the effects of different rise times. The shortening of the rise time results in an expected increase of amplitude for higher order harmonics. This increase of amplitude for higher order harmonics might be beneficial for MPI imaging, although the throughput of the rectangular excitation field complicates the filtering process in order to only get the desired particle signal. Furthermore the impact of rectangular excitation on the particle hysteresis has been studied, indicating that rectangular excitation might favour heat generation in applications like MPH [3]. In [2] it is shown how the application of pulsed excitation field can help to improve image quality in MPI in connection with the X-space reconstruction method [10]. Further study of particle behaviour using rectangular or pulsed excitation in combination with different particle parameters e.g. viscosity, particle diameter, anisotropy will help finding improved excitation fields for MPI or MPH.

Acknowledgement

This work has been carried out at the Institute of Medical Engineering, Universität zu Lübeck.

Author's Statement

The author's state no conflict of interest.

5 References

[1] B. Gleich and J. Weizenecker, "Tomographic imaging using the nonlinear response of magnetic particles," *Nature*, vol. 435, no. 7046, pp. 1214–1217, 2005.

[2] Z. W. Tay, D. Hensley, J. Ma, P. Chandrasekharan, B. Zheng, P. Goodwill, and S. Conolly, "Pulsed excitation in magnetic particle imaging," *IEEE transactions on medical imaging*, vol. 38, no. 10, pp. 2389–2399, 2019.

[3] S. Dutz and R. Hergt, "Magnetic particle hyperthermia—a promising tumour therapy?" *Nanotechnology*, vol. 25, no. 45, p. 452001, 2014.

[4] A. Neumann and T. M. Buzug, "Stochastic simulations of magnetic particles: Comparison of different methods," *International Workshop on Magnetic Particle Imaging*, p. 213, 2018.

[5] Y. P. Kalmykov and W. T. Coffey, *The Langevin Equation*. World Scientific Publishing Company, 2017.

[6] M. Shliomis and V. Stepanov, "Theory of the dynamic susceptibility of magnetic fluids," *Advances in Chemical Physics: Relaxation Phenomena in Condensed Matter*, vol. 87, pp. 1–30, 1994.

[7] P. E. Kloeden and E. Platen, *Numerical solution of stochastic differential equations*. Springer Science & Business Media, 2013, vol. 23.

[8] T. Klemme, T. M. Buzug, and A. Neumann, "Exploring parameters of magnetic particles in 1d field excitation," *International Journal on Magnetic Particle Imaging*, vol. 6, no. 1, 2020.

[9] C. Shasha, E. Teeman, and K. M. Krishnan, "Harmonic simulation study of simultaneous nanoparticle size and viscosity differentiation," *IEEE Magnetics Letters*, vol. 8, pp. 1–5, 2017.

[10] P. W. Goodwill and S. M. Conolly, "Multidimensional x-space magnetic particle imaging," *IEEE transactions on medical imaging*, vol. 30, no. 9, pp. 1581–1590, 2011.

Implementation of a medical Android application for measuring EEG data and storing them onto a remote server

Ricardo Stolze [1], Ralf Hauffe [2], Jacob Kanev [3] and Frédéric Li [4]

[1] Medical Informatics, Universität zu Lübeck, ricardo.stolze@student.uni-luebeck.de
[2] COO at eemagine Medical Imaging Solutions GmbH, rhauffe@ant-neuro.com
[3] Senior software developer at eemagine Medical Imaging Solutions GmbH, jacob.kanev@eemagine.com
[4] PhD student at Institute of Medical Informatics, Universität zu Lübeck, li@imi.uni-luebeck.de

Abstract

Electroencephalography (EEG) is used to measure currents produced by the brain, and can be used for many different applications, like sleep analysis, emotion detection or as a part of brain computer interfaces. Many EEG recording setups have been developed to investigate such applications. Hence most of them are unwieldy and allow only local data recording, a setup using an Android device, an *eego* signal amplifier (ANT Neuro GmbH) and a *waveguard* dry electrode cap (ANT Neuro GmbH) for EEG recording is proposed in this paper. To ensures light hardware, which can stream the measured data directly onto a remote server. Basic tests have been carried out to guarantee that the proposed application is indeed capable of recording satisfactory EEG data. Further tests to compare the measured data to state of the art technology should be done in the future.

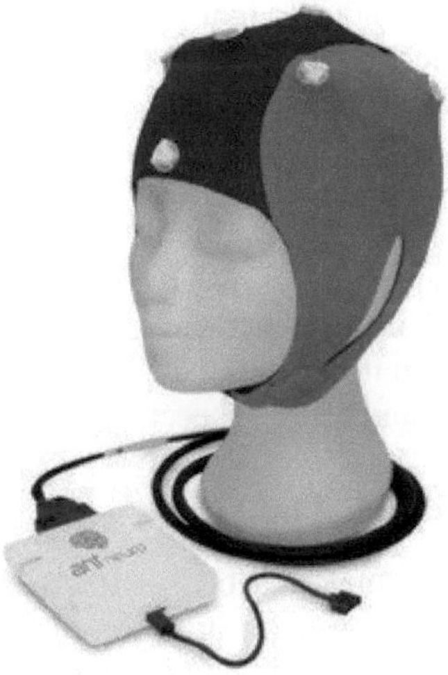

Figure 1: 8-channel *waveguard* [1] touch sensor cap combined with a *eego* [2] signal amplifier

1 Introduction

For millennia understanding the human brain has been of high interest for humankind. Starting in ancient Egypt [3], countless operations on head and brain have been performed. Back then mostly for healing purpose, but in modern times many more additional applications have been developed. A big step in understanding the brain functionality was the development of the electroencephalography (EEG) which is still used in modern medicin and neuroscience. The EEG first was used in 1942 by Hans Berger [4]. He was the first to measure the electrical currents produced by the brain without opening the skull. Instead he used ordinary radio equipment to record and amplify the signals and thereby laid the foundation for modern EEG measurement. Nowadays, many different applications are build on data, measured using EEG, like emotion recognition [5] or sleep state detection [6]. For sleep analysis in particular, an immediate feedback of the measured signals is of high interest for the society. By detecting sleeping states, one could be prevented from falling asleep in monotonous but dangerous situations, for example while driving.

For such applications a mobile EEG setup is needed. Since many clinical EEG setups rely on non-mobile computers or wet electrodes, which are difficult to set up [7], they cannot be used. Other setups are using long term EEG [8] or Android devices [9] to acquire data, but can not share them via the internet . This feature would be of advantage for data heavy analysis methods, like modern deep neural networks, since the data could be processed on a remote server.

The proposed EEG setup aims at combining a light, small and mobile EEG setup with the benefits of heavy high performance data analysis devices and global storage. Therefore it uses an Android device as an interface between the EEG measuring hardware shown in Fig. 1 and a remote sever to which the measured data is send.

A benefit of using Android devices is their broad accep-

tance in nowadays society. The most used technical device for people under 53 is the smartphone [10]. At the same time, smartphones contain all needed technology for simple data processing tasks. This makes smartphones ideal tools for EEG applications. Together with a set of electrodes and a signal amplifier (Fig. 1), nothing more is needed to measure brain waves, and send them to a server for immediate processing, analysis and storage.
Information regarding the hardware setup and an introduction to the developed software is provided in Section 2. Section 3 shows the results of the proposed design and highlights additional features Android provides, that will be of use for future medical products. The conclusion is drawn in Section 4.

2 Material and Methods

This chapter will give a short overview over the hardware and software developed to obtain a lightweight EEG recording system. The hardware setup includes the signal amplifier, the sensor cap and the Android device. Afterwards the developed Android application is described.

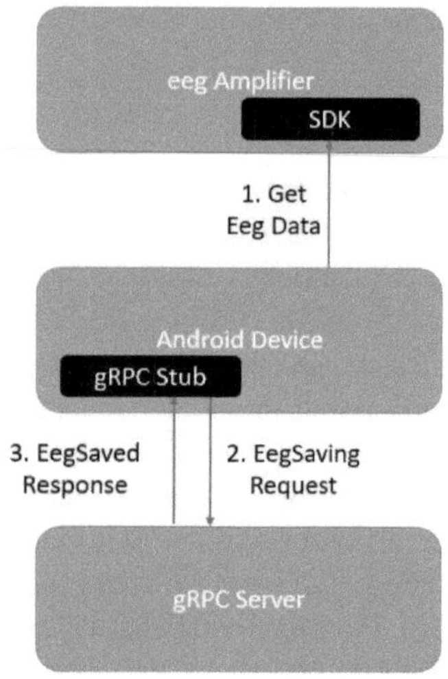

Figure 2: The Android Device is the central part in the presented approach as it connects the EEG amplifier and the storage on the server

2.1 Hardware

The hardware setup used in this approach consist of three different devices. First one is the *8-channel waveguard touch cap* (ANT Neuro GmbH) [1], which uses Ag/AgCl coated soft polymer electrodes to measure the brain functionality. By using dry electrodes, no conductive paste needs to be applied to the skin, which makes the cap easy to use and safe against signal losses. Using usual wet electrodes would also work together with the proposed amplifier and an Android device. They are often the first choice for measuring EEG in a clinical or laboratory environment, but are less practical for everyday usage. Attaching single electrodes onto the right spots, while using the perfect amount of conductive paste, could be too hard for novice users [7]. That is why recording EEG in everyday life situations benefits highly from using a *waveguard* cap.
Because the currents on a scalp skin are very low, they must be massively amplified before being displayed. Therefore the signals measured by the cap are passed to an *eego rt 8* signal amplifier (ANT Neuro GmbH) [2], which is characterized by its low weight and small design,and can supply high quality EEG signals from up to 8 channels and sampling rates ranging from 500 up to 2048 Hz. It comes without a power supply, so it needs to be powered by the Android device. Using an Universal Serial Bus (USB) the signals are then transferred to a *Google Pixel 3* Android Smartphone running with a clean version of *Android 11*, the latest version of Android.

2.2 Software

The application presented in this paper consists of three different software components, which are compiled into one Android package file. This file is used by Android powered devices to install an application. The main component of this app is written in Java and implements the applications main logic, which is described in Section 2.2.1. It integrates the following software elements to ensure a proper functionality of the application. First, an *intent filter* is used to listen for information send by the operating system. In the proposed application it is used to start the application when the amplifier gets attached to the phone via USB. The second component is a *Software Development Kit* (SDK), which provides all necessary functionality to interact with the *eego* amplifier and record data. The recorded data are then send to a remote server using *gRPC*, the third software component, which is an open source remote procedure call (RPC) framework developed at Google in 2015. Further information are given in sections 2.2.2, 2.2.3 and 2.2.4 for the intent filter, SDK and gRPC respectively.

2.2.1 The Application Life Cycle

In Android development, each User Interface is called an *activity*. It presents all the information, that are important for the user, handles user input and implements the logic behind the application. The application presented in this paper only needs one single activity to handle all the logic needed for measuring and storing EEG signals.
One activity always has a life cycle, which defines how the activity should behave in its different states. It must build the user interface when first created, handle the input as long as it is active and free resources when closed.
The proposed application is created when the Android device opens it due to an intent request, or when the user starts it manually. When first created, the activity sets up the user interface. It includes buttons used to initiate an EEG recording or a data stream to the server. Information regarding the attached amplifier is displayed in text fields and a graph is implemented to plot the measured data. Furthermore the

permission to use the USB device is gathered, and a connection to the server is established.
While the activity is displayed on the device, the user can start an EEG recording. For storing measured data, some additional data are needed and gathered from a database positioned on the server. This includes information regarding the patient and the way the EEG is recorded. The actual EEG scan happens multiple times per second, depending on the sampling rate. Each time, the recorded data are read by the Android device and temporarily stored. Another thread sends a request every second to the server via gRPC to store all recorded data. This kind of multi threading ensures a better usability of the app by preventing it from a freezing screen due to long lasting processes.
When all the EEG is recorded and the app gets shut down by the user, all resources are freed, to ensure a constant level of good performance from the Android device.

2.2.2 Intent filter

The first important component implemented is an *intent filter*. It is listening for attached devices on the USB-port of the Smartphone. If an *eego rt 8* gets attached to the port, an intent is send by the Android device to all applications installed. If an application has a matching intent filter implemented, the application receives the order to handle the intent event. The application presented in this paper, when receiving a USB permission intent specified with the *eego* amplifier id, awakes and asks the user for permission to interact with the amplifier. If the permission is granted, the app can start a data stream and connect data provided by the amplifier.

2.2.3 eego Amplifier Software Development Kit

The proposed *eego* amplifier was developed to be used with many different hardware setups. Therefore a SDK is provided by its manufacturers. The SDK provides a C++ interface, which includes all the necessary functionality to create an amplifier object, open a stream and poll for any data that has been acquired. This data can then be send back to the main application for further processing and storing. Since the SDK is written in C++, a Java Native Interface (JNI) is used to integrate it properly into the Java application.

2.2.4 gRPC and Protocol Buffers

To store measured data sets on the server, *gRPC* is included in the application. Using gRPC, a client can call a method implemented on another machine as if it were local. Therefore the client needs a *stub* providing the methods implemented by the server. A stub in terms of software development is a piece of code, working as a placeholder code distributed over the system. Using the stub, it is possible to send messages, including the called method and its associated parameters, and return types. When the server receives such a call, it executes the method and sends an answer back to the client. gRPC supports different languages, so the client and server don't have to be written in the same languages.
To serialize data, gRPC uses *Protocol Buffers*, which use a *proto file* to define the data structure. In this file, each gRPC service is defined as a RPC method with its parameters, and return types. Those are specified as protocol buffer messages, small components containing name-value pairs called *fields*. By using *protoc*, which is a compiler for proto files, the necessary data access classes are generated to integrate gRPC into the application.

3 Results

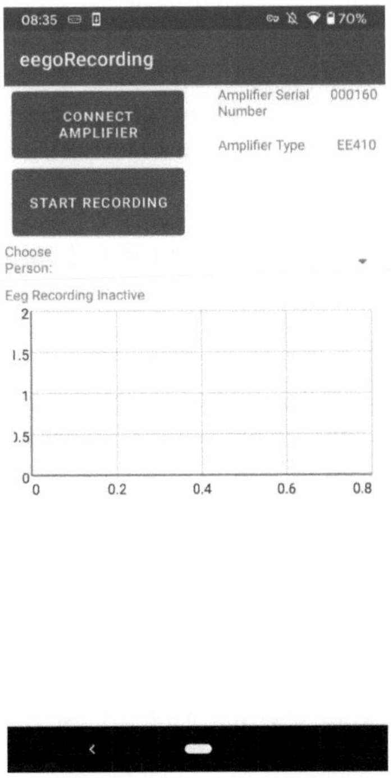

Figure 3: The graphical user interface of the presented application. There are buttons to initiate an amplifier connection and start the data acquisition, as well as a dropdown menu to choose the patient file from the patient database stored on the remote server. After connection to the amplifier, its serial number and type are being displayed. When recording, the gathered data is plotted in a figure

The GUI of the proposed application is shown in Fig. 3. It includes buttons to connect to the amplifier and start the data collection. After the Android device connected to the amplifier, some characteristic amplifier data, its serial number and type are displayed in the upper right corner of the GUI. To assign the gathered data to a patient on the remote server, a drop down menu was included from which to choose an available patient. While the main purpose is to store the data on the remote server, it can also be plotted directly as a graph in the application. For a wireless communication between the Android device and the remote server, gRPC calls were used. They provide an easy, but at the same time efficient and extensive opportunity to share data between remote devices, even for application written

in many different languages, which provides an extensive interface to all kind of different storage setups.
To verify the correct functionality, EEG was measured once and stored into a database on a remote server. No more comparison to other state of the art approaches has been done due to a lack of time during the internship.

4 Conclusion

In this paper a lightweight EEG-recording solution relying on Android smartphones was presented. Therefore an application was programmed with the purpose to interact with an EEG signal amplifier to gather an EEG signal and send it to a remote server using gRPC. The application is designed to work together with an *eego* system amplifying gathered currents from a *waveguard* cap. Furthermore it can store the data on a remote server using remote procedure calls and the gRPC framework.
The goal of minimizing the hardware setup in terms of weight and size has been successfully achieved. The amplifier and the Android device can be carried around easily inside of a backpack or even a pocket. The used *waveguard* cap guarantees a stable, research-grade EEG signal recording even in non laboratory environments [1]. Due to the used gRPC messaging, the EEG data can now be accessed at each time during recording for proper analysis or additional processing.
The application has been verified by a successful recording and storing of EEG data. How good the recorded signals are in comparison to other EEG recording setups has not been tested yet due to a lack of time and will be done in the future. Furthermore, proper bug fixing has to be done to make sure, that the Android application works at any time. Also, signal processing, like blinking artefact removal, could be implemented to be done by the Android application directly on the device. This could prevent the application to send unnecessary data to the server to save data volume and storage space.

Acknowledgement

The work has been carried out at eemagine Medical Imaging Solutions GmbH in the department of software development and supervised by Dr.-Ing. R. Hauffe, COO at eemagine Medical Imaging Solutions GmbH, J. Kanev, senior software developer and project manager at eemagine Medical Imaging Solutions GmbH and Dr.-Ing. habil M. Grzegorzek, Institute of Medical Informatics, Universität zu Lübeck.

Author's Statement

Conflict of interest: Authors state no conflict of interest.

5 References

[1] ANT Neuro (2018), *waveguard™touch.* Available: https://www.ant-neuro.com/sites/default/files/2018-01-08_wt_brochure_A4_HR.pdf

[2] ANT Neuro (2018), *eego™mini-series product range.* Available: https://www.ant-neuro.com/sites/default/files/SLS-SM-0040rev01%20eego_mini_brochure_A4%202018-01-08.pdf

[3] S. Finger, *Origins of Neuroscience: A History of Explorations into Brain Function.* In: Oxford University Press, 2001.

[4] M. Teplan, *Fundamentals Of Eeg Measurement.* In: Measurement Science Review, Volume 2, Section 2, 2002.

[5] Y. Liu, O. Sourina, M. k. Nguyen, *Real-Time EEG-Based Emotion Recognition and Its Applications.* In: Transactions on Computational Science XII, 2011. https://doi.org/10.1007/978-3-642-22336-5_13

[6] R. D. Bickfort, *Electroencephalography.* In: Adelman G. ed. Encyclopedia of Neuroscience, Birkhauserm, Cambridge, 371-373, 1987.

[7] G. Di Flumeri et al., *The Dry Revolution: Evaluation of Three DifferentEEG Dry Electrode Types in Terms of Signal SpectralFeatures, Mental States Classification and Usability.* In: Sensors 19, no 6, 2019. https://doi.org/10.3390/s19061365

[8] C. Lin et al., *Wireless and Wearable EEG System for Evaluating Driver Vigilance.* In: IEEE Transactions on Biomadical Circuits and Systems, vol.8, no.2, 2014. doi: 10.1109/TBCAS.2014.2316224.

[9] M. Pineyro Salvidegoitia et al., *Out and about: Subsequent memory effect captured in a natural outdoor environment with smartphone EEG.* In: Psychophysiology, 56:e13331, 2019. https://doi.org/10.1111/psyp.13331

[10] C. Bröhl et al., *Desktop PC, Tablet PC, or Smartphone? An Analysis of Use Preferences in Daily Activities for Different Technology Generations of a Worldwide Sample.* In: Zhou J., Salvendy G. (eds) Human Aspects of IT for the Aged Population. Acceptance, Communication and Participation. ITAP 2018. Lecture Notes in Computer Science, vol 10926. Springer, Cham. https://doi.org/10.1007/978-3-319-92034-4_1

12

Machine Learning / AI

Comparison of deep reinforcement learning algorithms for Catheter-based interventions

Jacqueline Ritter [1], Maximilian Dietrich Schwarzmann [2], Lennart Karstensen [3] and Marcin Grzegorzek [4]

[1] Medical Informatics, Universität zu Lübeck, jacqueline.ritter@student.uni-luebeck.de
[2] Informatics, Karlsruhe Institute of Technology, maximilian.dietrich.schwarzmann@ipa-extern.fraunhofer.de
[3] Fraunhofer IPA, Mannheim, lennart.karstensen@ipa.fraunhofer.de
[4] Institute of Medical Informatics, Universität zu Lübeck, grzegorzek@imi.uni-luebeck.de

Abstract

Smart Assistance for Catheter-Based Interventions, in short STACIE, is a project by Fraunhofer IPA. It focuses on the autonomous control of endovascular catheters and guidewires within the human body with the help of deep reinforcement learning [1]. The currently used method is Deep Deterministic Policy Gradient with Hindsight Experience. In this paper more suitable algorithms are investigated and experimentally compared. The methods are chosen from a pool of various deep reinforcement learning algorithms. They meet the requirements of STACIE. In order to compare the chosen algorithms Twin Delayed Deep Deterministic Policy Gradient (TD3) and Soft Actor-Critic (SAC) we implemented a tilt maze environment. The results show that both algorithms are capable of learning to tilt the maze plane such that the ball reaches an arbitrary goal.

1 Introduction

The project on which this paper is based is called Smart Assistance for Catheter-Based Interventions, in short STACIE. It is carried out by the Fraunhofer Institute for Manufacturing Engineering and Automation (IPA). The long-term aim is to support physicians performing surgical treatment of time-critical diseases like strokes and heart attacks. During a classical intervention computed tomography (CT) scans are taken with a specific frequency. They help the doctor localize the catheter. In the experimental set-up the CT scans are processed by a tracking algorithm that outputs the position of the guidwire tip. It has currently been tested on a vessel phantom made of acrylic glass. The coordinates are then given to the control algorithm which outputs commands. These commands will be carried out by the robotic manipulator [1].

A group of machine learning algorithms that has proven to be quite successful when it comes to teaching machines how to act in an intelligent manner is called reinforcement learning. Within this framework we want an agent to learn a behavior in a certain environment without providing it with explicit instructions. This means that learning by trial and error is encouraged. In order to let the agent know what it should learn it is necessary to provide rewards. A reward can be understood as either positive or negative feedback. In the beginning of the training phase the agent usually does not know anything about the environment. Neither does it know anything about which rules to follow. This is why the actions are chosen in a random manner. The rewards the agent obtains are used to optimize the manner in which it interacts with the environment. Repeating this process many times allows the algorithm to gradually improve, which in turn leads to the agent interacting with the environment based on experience rather than on randomness. The general principle of the training process is illustrated in Fig. 1. The agent executes an action which changes the environment. As a result it obtains a reward as well as a new state upon which it then acts. A classical example set-up is the Atari game Pong, in which the agent learns to control the paddle by observing image frames and receiving points as feedback.

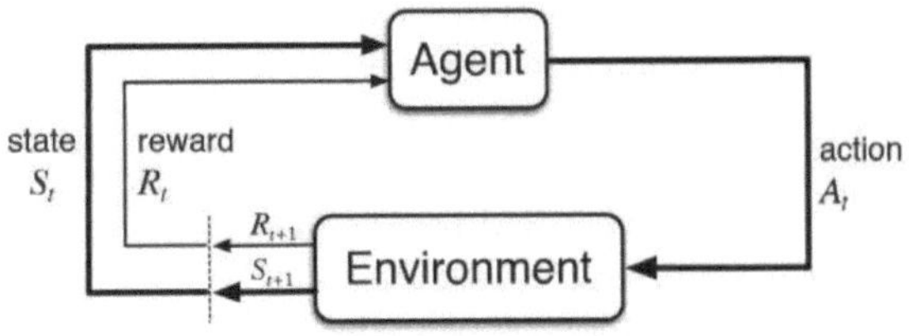

Figure 1: Training loop for an agent trained with reinforcement learning

The field of reinforcement learning has been growing rapidly within the last years which in consequence lead to many different approaches. One example is the combination of reinforcement learning and deep learning creating

the field of deep reinforcement learning, which is especially useful when interacting with complex environments.
The control algorithm that is used in STACIE belongs to the class of deep reinforcement learning algorithms and is called Deep Deterministic Policy Gradient (DDPG) together with Hindsight Experience Replay (HER) [1].
The aim of the paper is to identify a suitable deep reinforcement learning algorithm for STACIE based on constraints that are due to the properties of the project. The most important constraint imposed on the algorithm is based on the properties of the guide wire as well as the complexity of a human vessel tree. Another constraint is the fact that the newly trained agent should profit from experiences other agents have already made, e.g. during an intervention or during simulations. If the agent can profit from prior experiences it will learn a more robust behavior pattern. Furthermore the algorithm can then be easily parallelized which is another advantage as the simulation that is used to train needs a lot of computation time.

2 Material and Methods

2.1 Methods

Literature research was performed in order to find deep reinforcement learning algorithms that fulfill the criteria imposed by the project run by Fraunhofer IPA. The necessity to incorporate experiences other agents have made corresponds to the need of an off-policy algorithm. Off-policy algorithms sample data from a replay buffer in order to train the agent. There is therefore no need to obtain the data using the current policy, which could only be done by the agent itself. Instead when using an off-policy algorithm other experiences can be integrated in the training process. Another advantage of off-policy algorithms follows directly from this property. As more than one agent can collect experiences simultaneously those algorithms are easy to parallelize which improves the computation time of the training process [2]. The last constraint that is imposed by STACIE translates to a partially observable Markov decision process (POMDP). For many problems that are solved using reinforcement learning the Markov property holds. However for the described problem of catheter navigation the agent cannot tell in which direction the guide wire tip is rotated by taking into account the last observation only. Therefore in order to choose the next action the agent needs to consider past observations and past actions which contradicts the Markov property. Nevertheless note that the transition from one state to the next depends just on the last state. That is why the problem can be modeled as a POMDP. Hence the algorithm should ideally be compatible with recurrent neural networks to save past observations and past actions.
The chosen algorithms were then experimentally compared to the currently used approach using a toy problem. The original problem needs a long time for training and is therefore not suitable for the selection process. In order to compare the chosen algorithms we take a look at the average success rate depending on the number of episodes.

2.2 Experiment setup

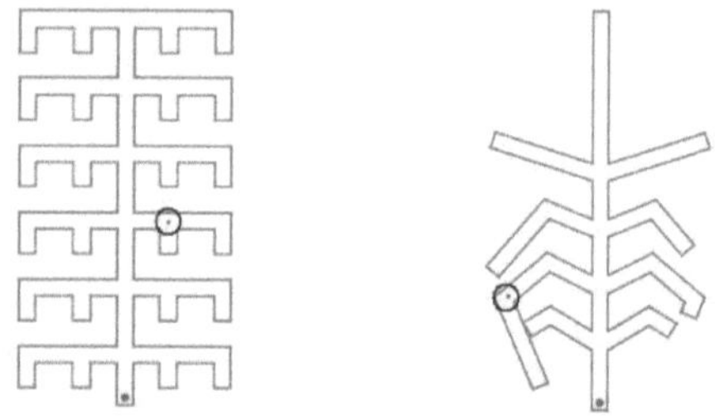

Figure 2: The two different tilt maze environments showing the ball at the starting point as well as the target. Manhattan maze (left), Trifurcation maze (right)

The aim of the experiments is to compare the algorithms to the current one used in the project in order to evaluate whether one of them could possibly yield better results. The Deep Deterministic Policy Gradient method is sensitive to hyperparameter tuning [5], which made it necessary to train an additional algorithm to obtain a benchmark. The Dueling deep Q network (DDQN) was used.
The algorithms that will be compared can be found in the next section. The toy problem consists of a two dimensional tilt maze. Each deep reinforcement learning algorithm was trained on both mazes that can be seen in Fig. 2. The agent needs to learn to tilt the maze plane in order to navigate the ball such that it reaches an arbitrary target goal within the maze. Two different environments were chosen in order to verify that an agent cannot only learn successful behavior in a specific case. The Trifurcation environment is similar to a very simple human vessel tree. This set-up will be useful when generalizing our findings to the catheter-based intervention problem STACIE.
The number of agents that work in parallel as well as the reward system are based on STACIE. However as the tilt maze problem is less complex the number of agents is reduced to 10. The reward system is dense meaning that the agent is given a negative feedback of -0.2 for each interaction step, a positive or negative feedback depending on the change of the distance from the target and a positive feedback of 100 once the target is reached [1]. The practical use of the recurrent neural network will be neglected for this toy problem as implementations are not included in one single framework and results might therefore not be comparable.

2.3 Material

The experiments were carried out on Lenovo ThinkPad equipped with Quadro K620M (GPU) and on a remote computer equipped with GeForceRTX 2070 (GPU) running Ubuntu 18.04 using the deep reinforcement learning framework Coach [6]. The employed algorithms are implemented in a single framework in order to ease future comparisons of the alternatives.

3 Results and Discussion

3.1 Results

Out of the various off-policy algorithms two of them have been identified to be compatible with recurrent neural networks. Both of these methods are actor-critical and have been recently developed. The first one is a successor of DDPG called Twin Delayed Deep Deterministic Policy Gradient (TD3) [4], [7]. The second one is called Soft Actor-Critic (SAC) [5], [3].
Fig. 3 and Fig. 4 show that for both maze environments

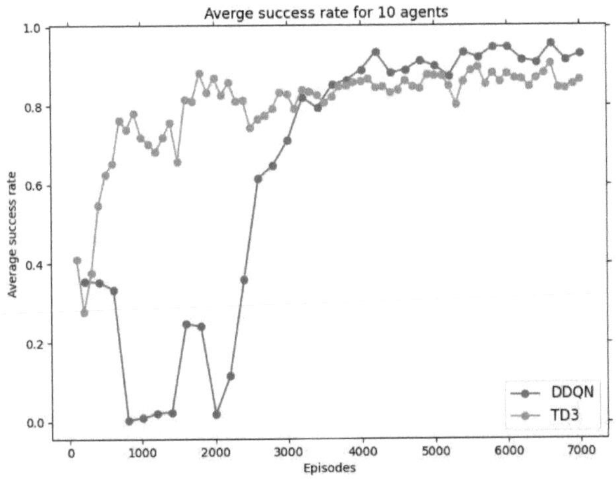

Figure 3: Results for DDQN and TD3 training on the Trifurcation maze environment. Both algorithms used 10 simultaneously working agents.

TD3 is capable of navigating the ball to a randomly chosen target point by tilting the maze plane. In both cases the chosen algorithm could not exceed the average success rate of the benchmark, but performance was promising nonetheless. The success rate is measured every 100 episodes. In contrast to DDQN the Twin Delayed Deep Deterministic Policy Gradient needed less than 1000 episodes to obtain an average success rate of more than 70% when training on the Trifurcation maze environment as can be seen in Fig. 3. In Fig. 4 we can see that TD3 gradually improves. The average success rate does not drop below 50% after episode 500.
Comparing both figures we observe that for TD3 it seems to be easier to learn a successful behavior within the Trifurcation maze environment. The average success rate of DDQN however decreases in both scenarios and then recovers again.
The Soft Actor-Critic method could not be trained with more than one agent as for now. Therefore the average success rate that can be seen in Fig. 5 fluctuates strongly. The amount of peaks might also be due to a learning rate that was chosen too high. Experimenting with tuned hyperparameters could possibly lead to even better results. The learning curves for the different maze environments is similar for SAC as can be seen in 5. Note that training with one agent only drastically decreases computation time. Thus

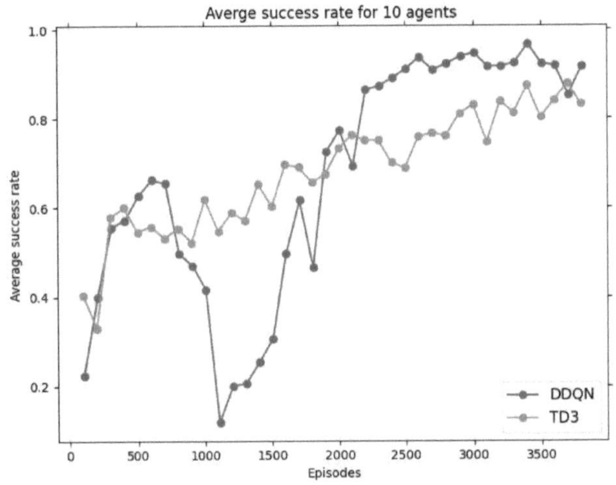

Figure 4: Results for DDQN and TD3 training on the Manhattan maze environment. Both algorithms used 10 simultaneously working agents.

in comparison to TD3 and the benchmark algorithm SAC needed a lot less time to obtain good results, which is a big advantage when it comes to the catheter-based navigation. As mentioned earlier for STACIE the simulation during training need a lot of computation time. That is why it makes a big difference if an algorithm has the advantage of learning successful behavior quickly.

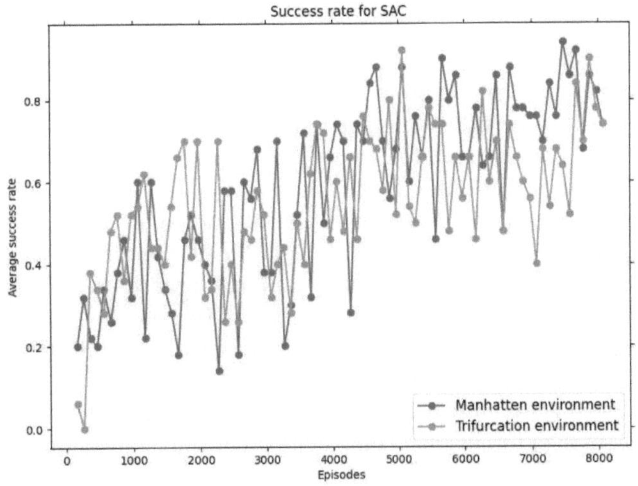

Figure 5: Results for SAC training on the Trifurcation and Manhattan maze environment. The algorithm was training one single agent.

3.2 Discussion

In contrast to DDPG together with HER which is the currently used approach the chosen algorithms TD3 and SAC do not seem to be as sensitive to hyperparameter tuning. Both algorithms yield good results in comparison to the benchmark method DDQN which nearly reached 100% in both maze environments. Even though we can observe good

results it is important to note that SAC and TD3 both have only been tested on the toy problem as for now. The tilt maze environment is a lot less complex than the environment used to simulate catheter-based navigation. Nonetheless because of the good results for the toy problem we are optimistic that both methods will yield good results for the set-up in STACIE as well. As a next step it is also important to investigate why SAC could only be run with one single agent. Its steep learning curve suggests that it might easily outperform the current algorithm DDPG together with HER when it comes to computation time.
As explained in Section 2 the use of recurrent neural networks has been neglected for the toy problem. As a next step we will make use of this property both algorithms have. Another idea that could be tested for the more complex set-up in STACIE is the use of pre-trained models. It takes a lot more time to train an agent to learn to navigate a catheter to a desired target point than to teach the agent how to tilt a simple maze plane. That is why the use of pre-trained models could especially be useful when it comes to complex environments. As the Soft Actor-Critic and the Twin Delayed Deep Deterministic Policy Gradient method are off-policy algorithms one can use a pre-trained model and additionally use all the data that was already sampled for the current replay buffer. In that way it can be made sure that the behavior that was learned during other simulations will not be forgotten.

4 Conclusion

In order to find a more suitable algorithm for a catheter-based intervention project called STACIE we analyzed different properties. Starting with a literature research we found two deep reinforcement learning algorithms working off-policy that fulfill all the criteria set up beforehand. The two promising algorithms are called Soft Actor-Critic and Twin Delayed Deep Deterministic Policy Gradient. TD3 is a successor of the algorithm currently used for STACIE, Deep Deterministic Policy Gradient. That is why it was easier to tune its hyperparameters. Because of the additions that were made to TD3 in comparison to DDPG it is less sensitive to the wrong choice of settings. Both algorithms were then trained and compared on our implementation of a simple tilt maze environment. TD3 could be compared to the benchmark and even though the average success rate was not quite as high as the one obtained by DDQN the results are promising. The algorithm seems to learn the right behavior quicker than the benchmark method. The hyperparameters of SAC were harder to tune as the algorithm is not a successor of the currently used DDPG. Furthermore the Soft Actor-Critic method could only be trained with one single agent as for now. That is why the success rate fluctuates a lot. Nonetheless the algorithm will be investigated further as positive behavior is learned very quickly in comparison to the benchmark and TD3.
The next steps will involve using the chosen methods for the catheter-based navigation project STACIE as well as further hyperparameter tuning especially for SAC. Both algorithms were chosen for their compatibility with recurrent neural networks, among other things. This property is very important as the problem of catheter-based intervention is a partially observable Markov decision process and thus needs information from previous states and previous actions. The recurrent neural network will operate as an efficient memory. To fully exploit the off-policy property of both algorithms we intend to build a database to collect all experiences any agent has ever made. Relevant experiences will then be placed in the replay buffer. Therefore new agents cannot only be trained in parallel but can also profit from experiences other agents have already made. The need to explore the environment increases and computation time decreases.

Acknowledgement

The work has been carried out at Fraunhofer Institute for Manufacturing Engineering and Automation IPA, Mannheim and supervised the Institute of Medical Informatics, Universität zu Lübeck.

Author's Statement

The authors state no conflict of interest. All co-authors have seen and agree with the contents of the paper. We certify that the submission is original work and is not under review at any other publication.

5 References

[1] T. Behr et. al. *Deep reinforcement learning for the navigation of neurovascular catheters.* Current Directions in Biomedical Engineering, Volume 5: Issue 1, De Gruyter, 2019.

[2] W. Jung, G. Park and Y. Sung *Population-guided parallel policy search for reinforcement learning.* ICLR Conference Paper, 2020.

[3] D. Han, K. Doya and J. Tani *Variational recurrent models for solving partially observable control tasks.* ICLR Conference Paper, 2020.

[4] S. Fujimoto, H. van Hoof and D. Meger *Adressing Function Approximation Error in Actor-Critic Methods.* ICML, 2018.

[5] T. Haarnoja et. al. *Soft Actor-Critic Algorithms and Applications.* arXiv, 2019.

[6] Caspi et. al. *Reinforcement Learning Coach.* https://github.com/IntelLabs/coach, 2017.

[7] R. Fris (2019) *The landing of a quadcopter on inclined surfaces using reinforcement learning* [Master Thesis, Delft University of Technology]. Institutional Repository at the Delft University of Technology. https://repository.tudelft.nl/.

Evolutionary computation towards adaptive gaits of legged robots

Eduard Buss[1] and Heiko Hamann[2]
[1] Robotics and Autonomous Systems, Universität zu Lübeck, eduard.buss@student.uni-luebeck.de
[2] Institute of Computer Engineering, Universität zu Lübeck, hamann@iti.uni-luebeck.de

Abstract

Technological advances could enable mobile robots to be integrated into our everyday lives. Thus, they could help us in various tasks. Legged robots have generally a higher adaptivity and maneuverability on uneven ground compared to wheeled robots. Our overall goal is to develop a wide variety of gaits for a six-legged robot. We use evolutionary computation methods, more specifically the Multi-dimensional Archive of Phenotypic Elites (MAP-Elites) algorithm, to train artificial neural networks (ANNs). We start with a classification problem as benchmark. Subsequently, ANNs are trained to control the movement of one simulated leg of the robot. MAP-Elites finds multiple high performing solutions, which occupy a defined space of interest as best as possible. Both experiments show an increasing fitness indicating that the approach is effective and thus provides the basis for gait development.

1 Introduction

Looking at human environments, such as their homes, they are filled with obstacles that are difficult for wheeled robots. Stairs, small steps, narrow places are easier to overcome by legged robots [1]. Walking on legs causes less damage to the ground and vegetation than traveling on wheels or chains. Through progress in artificial legged locomotion, robots may be able to support humans in a variety of tasks. Usually, each leg joint is actuated by one motor, which causes legged robots to have more actuated degrees of freedom (DOF) than wheeled robots [2]. Due to the high DOF and the complex mechanical structure, it is difficult to develop an accurate dynamic model. Strategies of evolutionary computation only need feedback from the environment to evaluate its performance, making it a model-free approach [1]. These machine learning algorithms are inspired by natural evolution [3]. For instance, one can define all weights of an ANN as a genome. This genome is one individual of a population. With strategies like mutation, crossover and selection, we are able to manipulate these genomes to find an individual that might be able to solve the task. Gait generation is a multi-constrained and multi-objective optimization problem [1]. The objectives can include tradeoffs between speed, stability, energy consumption, etc. For example, only a certain speed can be maintained while ensuring stability. One new approach is the MAP-Elites algorithm. Traditional search algorithms return one solution with the best performance [4]. In contrast, MAP-Elites provides an archive of solutions that, in the best case, cover a defined space of interest. Our overall goal is to develop gaits on a physical hexapod robot (PhantomX Metal Hexapod Mark III). So far, only intermediate goals can be achieved, which lead to promising results. Classification problems are common machine learning approaches. Therefore, we use a non-linear separable classification problem to study the algorithm. Afterwards, we simulate one leg of the hexapod to achieve a working toolchain and to train ANNs, with the objective to explore its entire motion space.

2 Material and Methods

The PhantomX Metal Hexapod Mark III build by Trossen Robotics is a six-legged robot (Fig. 1). It is made of aluminum and has a weight of approximately 2 kg. Each leg has 3-DOF, which totals to 18-DOF. All joints are actuated by DYNAMIXEL AX-12A servos. An existing model is used for the experiments involving simulations (available at https://github.com/HumaRobotics/phantomx_gazebo). All code is written in Python and available online, as well as further visualizations (available at https://github.com/ebuss81/Internship).

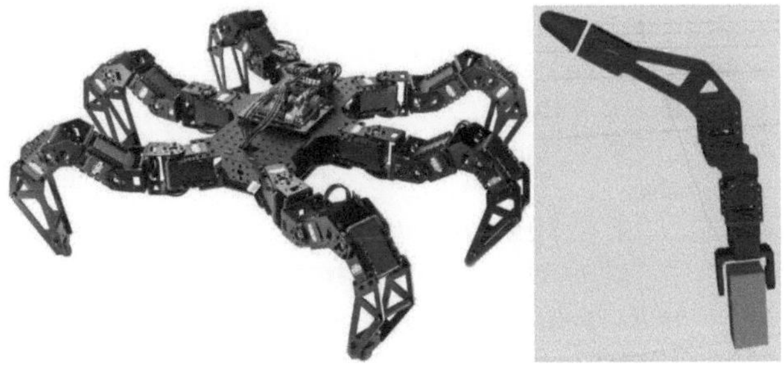

Figure 1: Left: PhantomX Metal Hexapod Mark III. Right: Simulated leg of the hexapod robot (black) attached to a fixed base (red).

ANNs and NetworkX ANNs are computational models abstracted from the biological nervous system [3]. These are able to convert sensory inputs into motor commands via a network of artificial neurons, which are arranged in layers. We are using feed forward ANNs in which signals are not transmitted between neurons within a layer or back to previous layers. To design and implement ANNs, we use the framework NetworkX. It is used to study complex networks. We choose this tool because each neuron and each connection can be given arbitrary properties. For example, each neuron is assigned an activation function and bias, each connection a weight and an activity. This activity will later be used to manipulate the architecture.

MAP-Elites Through local competition, the algorithm is able to find high performing solutions while maintaining a priority on diversity [4]-[5]. The first step is to define a performance measure $p(\mathbf{x})$ or fitness, which evaluates the solution $\mathbf{x}$. In our first experiment, it is the percentage of correct classified data. The search space is defined by all possible values of $\mathbf{x}$, for instance, all weighted connections of an ANN. The N-dimensional feature space ($\mathcal{B}$) is user-defined, domain-dependent, crucial for diversity and described by a feature descriptor $\mathbf{b}(\mathbf{x})$. Behavioral characteristics can be considered here, such as the number of legs used within a gait. After the features have been defined, the spanned space needs to be discretized (e.g., in a 2-D case: a grid). This allows to occupy the resulting grid cells with the best individuals depending on their feature values. Initially, we create an empty N-dimensional feature space $\mathcal{B}$ and performance space $\mathcal{P}$. Then, k random individuals are generated and their feature descriptors and fitness values are directly determined. If the cells $\mathcal{P}(\mathbf{b}')$ and $\mathcal{B}(\mathbf{b}')$ of the resulting features are not yet occupied with an individual, a randomly generated one is stored. If the cell is already occupied, the better individual is saved. After initialization, one of the individuals is taken randomly and changed, for example, by mutation or crossover. Features and fitness are calculated again and compared with the corresponding cell. This process is repeated until a termination criterion is reached, for example, a maximum number of iterations I.

Algorithm 1 MAP-Elites [4]

$\mathcal{P} \leftarrow \mathbf{0}, \mathcal{B} \leftarrow \mathbf{0}$
for $i = 1 \rightarrow I \ldots$ **do**
  if $i < k$ **then**
    $\mathbf{x}' \leftarrow random\ solution$
  else
    $\mathbf{x} \leftarrow random\ selection$
    $\mathbf{x}' \leftarrow random\ variation\ of\ \mathbf{x}$
  $\mathbf{b}' \leftarrow feature\ descriptor\ of\ \mathbf{x}'$
  $p' \leftarrow performance\ of\ \mathbf{x}'$
  if $\mathcal{P}(\mathbf{b}') = 0\ or\ \mathcal{P}(\mathbf{b}') < p'$ **then**
    $\mathcal{P}(\mathbf{b}') \leftarrow p'$
    $\mathcal{B}(\mathbf{b}') \leftarrow \mathbf{x}'$

Robot Operating Systsem (ROS) and Gazebo To minimize the risk of damaging the real robot and to test the algorithm we first simulate with the open-source software Gazebo (v.9) and ROS (ROS-Melodic). Gazebo is a simulation tool, which allows to test robotic systems in predefined environments. Due to shared memory, we are able to exchange, for instance, sensor values like joint angles or to send commands like goal positions of joints. Furthermore, it provides physics engines like Open Dynamics Engine (ODE), as used in our second experiment. ROS is the architecture, which allows communication between Python executables, Gazebo and ROS-packages [6].

Experiment 1: Classification The problem is defined by points, separated into 2 classes, in a 2-D space (Fig. 2). The biggest possible ANN includes an input layer without activation function or bias and two neurons, which receive the x- and y-coordinates as input. We integrate one hidden layer with a maximum of four neurons and sigmoidal activation functions. Since a distinction is only made between two classes, the output layer is defined by one neuron with a binary activation function. The feature space is defined by the connection cost and modularity of the ANN [7]. These features can be used to find ANNs with less connections and high modularity. An ANN with these properties could be more adaptive, since a rewiring of modules seems easier then a fully connected neural net. The feature space is discretized with a resolution of 50×50. The effects of mutation are based on the work of Clune, Mouret and Lipson (2013), which includes changes in the weights of the connections, the bias and the activity of connections [7]. Weights and bias are defined by a given range $[-10, 10]$ in steps of 0.1. Both are mutated independently with a probability of $2/n$ and 0.3, respectively, where n represents the number of active connections. When a modification is made, the current value is decremented or incremented with equal probability. The next mutation operator is used to add or remove a connection. With a probability of 0.3, one of the inactive connections is activated or one of the active connections is deactivated. The corresponding connection is chosen randomly.

Experiment 2: Simulation of one leg We simulate the motion of one leg of the hexapod model in our second experiment. For this purpose, we attach the coxa joint of the leg to a fixed base (Fig. 1). The fitness is calculated by comparing the traveled angular positions with all possible angles. If a new combination of all three angles is approached, 0.01 is added to the fitness (max. 128.68), otherwise it remains constant. The current joint angles [rad] serve as input, which lead to three input neurons without bias or activation function. A hidden layer with a maximum of four neurons is added again. The output layer contains three neurons that generate the target angles of the next iteration. Each neuron of the hidden and output layer receive a bias neuron as well as the hyperbolic tangent as activation function. The outputs [-1,+1] are multiplied by the respective maximum angle to achieve a direct mapping. The feature space is that of the first experiment, but the resolution is reduced to 10×10, due to increased computational complexity. The maximum values of the bias and the weights are fixed at -15 and +15. A Gaussian mutation with a mean of zero and a standard deviation of three is chosen for weights and biases [3].

3 Results and Discussion

As before mentioned, we start with a non-linear separable classification problem to study MAP-Elites. The algorithm in combination with Gazebo and ROS is then demonstrated on the basis of one hexapod leg. The goal is to evolve ANNs, enabling the leg to move in its entire motion space.

Experiment 1: Classification We generate 100 random individuals that may differ in the above aspects. They are evaluated and stored in cells, given the respective fitness and features. 46 individuals with an average fitness of 0.59 (max. 1) are saved, with the best having a fitness of 0.72. Afterwards 20,000 iterations are performed to manipulate these individuals and to occupy the grid as best as possible. We find 231 individuals each stored in one cell (Fig. 3). The average fitness increased to 0.89, with the 50 best individuals having a fitness of 0.99 (Fig. 2).

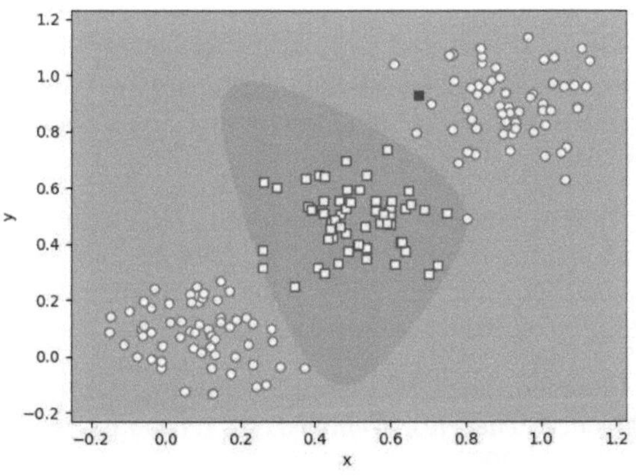

Figure 2: Classification of one best ANN. The classes are symbolized by red circles and blue squares. The class boundaries found by the ANN are marked by the corresponding colors. Incorrectly classified points are filled with color.

Experiment 2: Simulation of one leg We generate 500 random individuals, starting with a simulation time of 3 s. The resulting fitness is non-deterministic as it varies due to synchronization differences per evaluation with constant ANN. Therefore, three simulations per evaluation are performed and the average of the resulting fitnesses is stored. After initialization, 9 individuals with an average fitness of 0.25 are saved, with the best having a fitness of 0.70. We manipulate the random initialized individuals for approximately 48 h and 4700 iterations (Fig. 4). Once a better individual is found, it is stored as before and additionally its simulation time is increased by 1 s (max. 60 s). Since the simulation time depends on the fitness, the total time required is significantly reduced. The number of occupied cells remains constant, while the average fitness increased to 7.59. The best individual achieves a fitness of 12.94 with a simulation time of 60 s (Fig. 5).

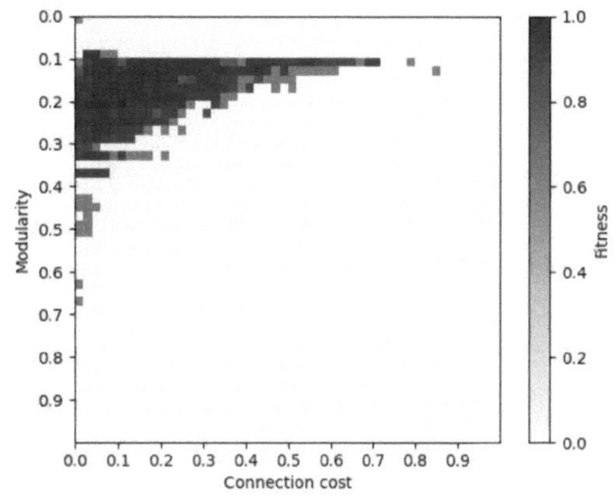

Figure 3: Classification benchmark: Generated grid after 20,000 iterations. The grid is spanned by the features of normalized modularity and normalized connection cost of ANNs with a resolution of 50×50 and its fitness as third dimension. No solutions are found within the white area.

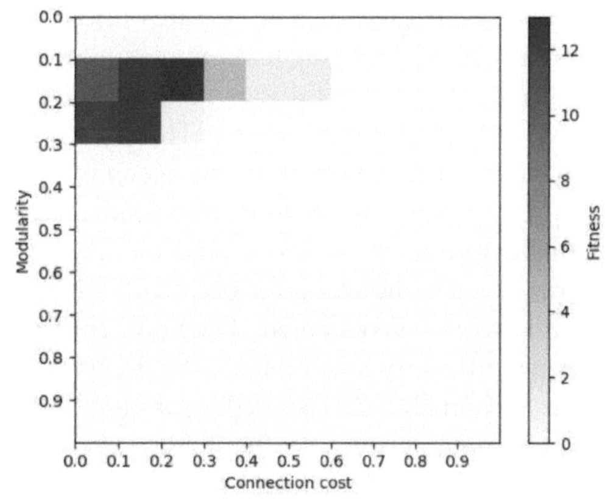

Figure 4: Simulation of one leg: Generated grid after 4,700 iterations. The grid is spanned by the features of normalized modularity and normalized connection cost of ANNs with a resolution of 10×10 and its fitness as third dimension. No solutions are found within the white area.

Discussion In our first experiment, only 1 of 175 data points is misclassified. Although a fitness of 1 could probably be achieved with additional neurons and layers, it would also lead to overfitting. Through MAP-Elites, a good classification has thus been achieved and, in addition, 50 high performing solutions have been found. The average fitness increased by 150 %, as well as the best fitness by 137 %

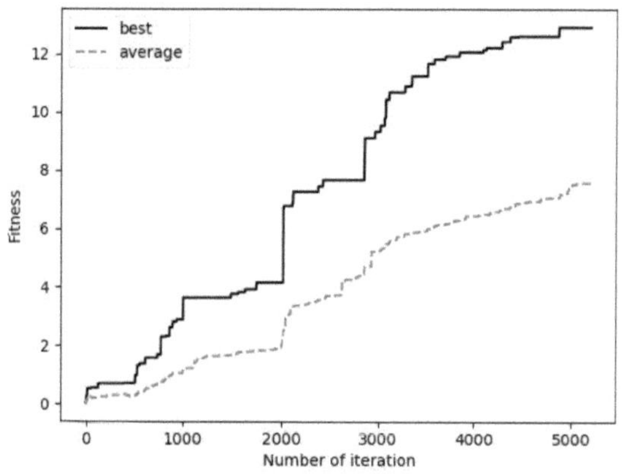

Figure 5: Simulation of one leg: Average and best fitness over the number of iterations. The first 500 steps includes the random initialization.

compared to the initialization. Nevertheless, only 10.82 % of the total feature space has been occupied. The maximum connection cost is only reached in the unlikely case of a fully connected ANN with maximum weights. The modularity depends on the size and the number of connections of the ANN. We found an individual with a modularity of 0, which only has one connected neuron pair. The found ANN with the highest modularity of 0.68 has three separated neuron pairs. Both are unlikely special cases, since none of them pass the input to the output. As a result, they achieve a low fitness, which excludes convergence to such ANNs. Another aspect is that both features influence each other. As already mentioned, the maximum connection cost can only be achieved with a fully connected ANN, which concurrently leads to low modularity. This eliminates the existence of individuals at both maxima. Keep in mind that the goal is not to occupy the entire feature space, the goal is to occupy the feature space as best as possible. A similar result can be observed in the second experiment, where only 9 % of the features space is occupied. The number of individuals found is significantly lower than in the first experiment, which can be attributed to the reduced resolution of the grid. This is also the main reason why the feature space was not further occupied after initialization. In addition, only 9.94 % of all possible angles were covered, which is due to the time limit. Nevertheless, the best and the average fitness increase with the number of iterations in both experiments. Both results prove that we are able to find a variety of good solutions with MAP-Elites together with Gazebo and ROS.

4 Conclusion

The overall goal is to develop gaits for a physical robot. In order to come closer to this goal, interim goals were set. First, the MAP-Elites algorithm is successfully tested and implemented on a non-linear classification problem. We found a diverse, high-performing solution set based on self-defined features. This suggests that with MAP-Elites and appropriate features, a variety of different gaits could be found. In order to exclude possible damage to the robot and to find efficient ANNs, we first evaluate the found solutions of MAP-Elites in simulation. We simulated only one leg of the robot to minimize the overall problem and to successfully connect the toolchain, consisting of Gazebo, ROS and MAP-Elites. The increasing best and average fitness shows that we can constantly improve the solutions. There are several possibilities to improve these results, for example, further mutation methods can be tested, the hyper parameters can be optimized or the architecture of the network can be changed. Nevertheless, these results serve as a good basis for the next steps, for instance, crossing the reality gap by doing experiments with the real leg or to simulate with the whole robot.

Acknowledgment

The work has been carried out and supervised at the Institute for Computer Engineering, Universität zu Lübeck.

Author's Statement

Conflict of interest: Authors state no conflict of interest.

5 References

[1] D. Gong, J. Yan, and G. Zuo, "A Review of Gait Optimization Based on Evolutionary Computation," *Applied Computational Intelligence and Soft Computing*, vol. 2010, p. 413179, 2010.

[2] P. Biswal and P. K. Mohanty, "Development of quadruped walking robots: A review," *Ain Shams Engineering Journal*, 2020. [Online]. Available: https://doi.org/10.1016/j.asej.2020.11.005

[3] D. Floreano and C. Mattiussi, *Bio-Inspired Artificial Intelligence: Theories, Methods, and Technologies*. The MIT Press, 2008.

[4] J.-B. Mouret and J. Clune, "Illuminating search spaces by mapping elites," *arXiv preprint arXiv:1504.04909*, 2015.

[5] J. K. Pugh, L. B. Soros, and K. O. Stanley, "Quality diversity: A new frontier for evolutionary computation," *Frontiers Robotics AI*, vol. 3, p. 40, 2016.

[6] K. Takaya, T. Asai, V. Kroumov, and F. Smarandache, "Simulation environment for mobile robots testing using ROS and Gazebo," *2016 20th International Conference on System Theory, Control and Computing (ICSTCC)*, pp. 96–101, 2016.

[7] J. Clune, J. B. Mouret, and H. Lipson, "The evolutionary origins of modularity," *Proceedings of the Royal Society B: Biological Sciences*, vol. 280, no. 1755, p. 20122863.

Implementing and altering the quadruped 12 dof robot by the Open Dynamic Robot Initiative

Martin Buchschuster [1], Ralf Bruder [2], Elmar Rückert [2]
[1] Robotics and Autonomous Systems, Universität zu Lübeck, martin.buchschuster@student.uni-luebeck.de
[2] Institute for Robotics and Cognitive Systems, Universität zu Lübeck {bruder, rueckert}@rob.uni-luebeck.de

Abstract

The Solo-12 Robot is an open-source quadrupedal robotic platform developed by the *open dynamic robot initiative*. It allows for cheap and easy testing of robotic algorithms and motion learning. It can be manufactured using 3D printing technology as well as off the shelve components. Such a robot was built for the *institute of robotics and cognitive systems* at the *University of Lübeck*. Some changes and improvements were made during the process. These are documented in this paper and in our GitHub repository [1]. In particular, a new magnetic Rotatory encoder and M3 belts and pulleys for the motor pulley and center pulley of the actuator module have been put in place. These aim to make the project cheaper and easier to build. Besides, some detailed comments and suggestions on the process are added in case the reader intends to recreate the Solo-12 Robot or any of the changes proposed here.

1 Introduction

Legged robots are an important new technology of our time. By being able to navigate terrain that is not accessible by tired or tracked vehicles enables new means of transportation. In particular, four-legged or *quadrupedal* robots are promised to navigate better in rough terrain than existing vehicles. Robotic research, such as by C. Dario Bellicoso et al. [2], therefore aims at finding algorithms to drive quadrupedal robots. The testing however, of such algorithms, often turns out to be imprecise. This requires researcher to work with real systems.

Related Work Numerous research labs have come up with their propiate platforms such as the StarlETH Robot [3] , the Oncilla Robot [4], or the Solo-12 Robot [5] by the *open dynamic robot initiative*. It has developed a low cost open-source robotic platform for a twelve degrees of freedom (12-dof) quadrupedal robot called *Solo-12*. The instruction manual is published on GitHub [6].

Contribution As a means of testing dynamic motion learning algorithms, the Institute of Robotics and Cognitive Systems of the University of Lübeck has issued the fabrication of one Solo-12 robot unit. Prior to the start of the project and along with the manufacturing process, some changes have been made to the original design of the robot which will be documented, described and evaluated here. For further reference and details please also see the GitHub page of the changes made [1]. These changes aimed mainly at trying to reduce the overall cost of the robot while utilizing more available material, reducing the complexity and simplify the manufacturing process.

Overview An overview of the computer aided design (CAD) model of the Solo-12 robot can be seen in Figure 1. It consists of four legs. Each leg has, from bottom to top, an *Lower Leg*, *Upper Leg*, *Hip AA* and *Hip FE* module. Each module consists of the same *acturator module*. An actuator module consists of one *brushless DC motor* that drives a 9:1 reduced two stage pulley system. Each motor's rotation is also monitored using an encoder.

2 Material and methods

Initially the manual as described by [6] was followed as is, in order to manufacture the Solo-12 robot. If the reader is not familiar with the project it is recommended to first have a look at the GitHub instructions before continuing reading. This is because the changes made rely on already existing implementations. Firstly the optical rotary encoder, used to measure the rotation of the motors and as feedback for the drivers, were exchanged for magnetic encoder integrated circuits (ICs). This also altered the motor shaft length, as well as the CAD drawings of the cover shell of the Upper Leg, Hip AA and Hip FE parts. Secondly, the pulleys and belts used in the original manual were exchanged for parts of equivalent size and strength, but different tooth profile. Consequently, the manufacturing instructions of the motor-pulley, the center pulley as well as the 3D printed center pulley and output shaft pulley CAD files were altered.

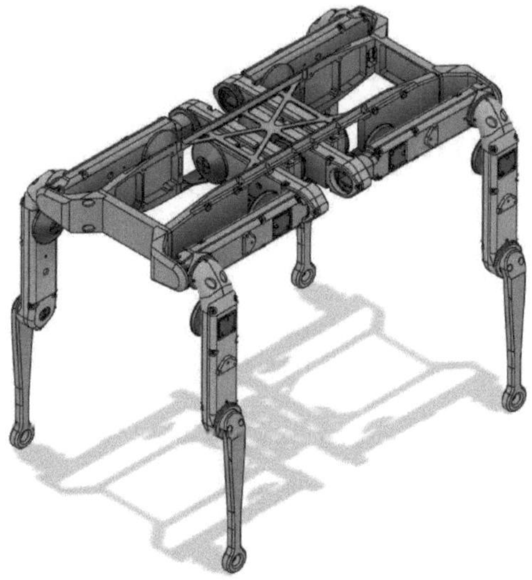

Figure 1: A CAD model of the assembled robot. The four legs, each consisting of three actuator modules can be seen. The front to back spans approximately 44 cm.

Table 1: An overview of the changes to each change in the actuator module showing the parts features before and after.

Element	Before	After
Motor Encoder	Broadcom AEDT-9810-Z00	AS5047 IC
Motor shaft	4 x 33.4 mm	4 x 30.1 mm
Motor pulley (10t)	3 mm pitch	HTD 3M
Center pulley (10t)	3 mm pitch	HTD 3M
Output Pulley (30t)	3 mm pitch	HTD 3M
First Stage belt	AT3 GEN III	HTD 3M
Second Stage belt	AT3 GEN III	HTD 3M

2.1 Magnetic encoder

The new encoder consisted of the *AS5047 IC* that was placed stationary above a diametrically magnetized magnet (see Figure 3 right). The magnet was fixed onto the end of the rotor shaft. The AS5047 was then able to translate the rotation of the magnets magnetic field into the quadrature-encoded (ABI) protocol for the μDriver.
In order to accommodate the magnet, as well as the circuit board at the end of the motor shaft without violating the width restriction of the parts, the bearing housing (e) was moved towards the motor by 3mm. This can be seen by (c) in Figure 2. This resulted in a shortened motor shaft (f) with the magnet places at its end (b). Its rotation can then be picked up by the *AS5047 IC* (a). As the position of the motor was not changed, but only the length of the shaft, the motor pulley (d) remained in its original position.

2.2 Pulleys and belts

We also modified the pulley and belt tooth profile. The original design featured special AT3 GEN 3 belts with custom made pulleys. The belts were exchanged for ones of equal size and number of teeth. The tooth profile was exchanged for a M3 tooth profile. This was done so that the metal pulleys for the motor shaft and the center shaft could be bought off the shelf and then only turned to size (see Figure 5). This was easier to manufacture than to cut custom pulley teeth. The M3 pulley is available as a standard part for 10 teeth in 9 mm and 15 mm. These were used for the motor pulley and center pulley respectively.
The files for the 3D printed center and output pulleys were also altered so that it matched the tooth profile of the new belts and pulleys. In addition to the machining instructions of the motor pulley and the center pulley, new machining instruction for the motor shaft were generated.

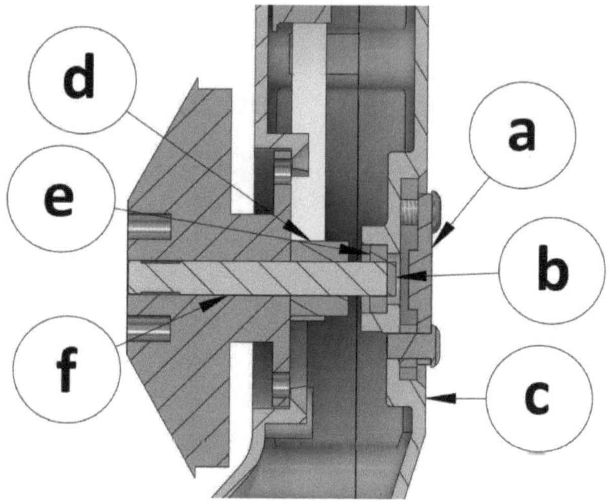

Figure 2: A cross section of the altered "Upper Leg" module. What can be seen is: (a) encoder PCB, (b) diametrically magnetized magnet, (c) outer shell case, (d) motor pulley, (e) motor shaft bearing, (f) motor shaft

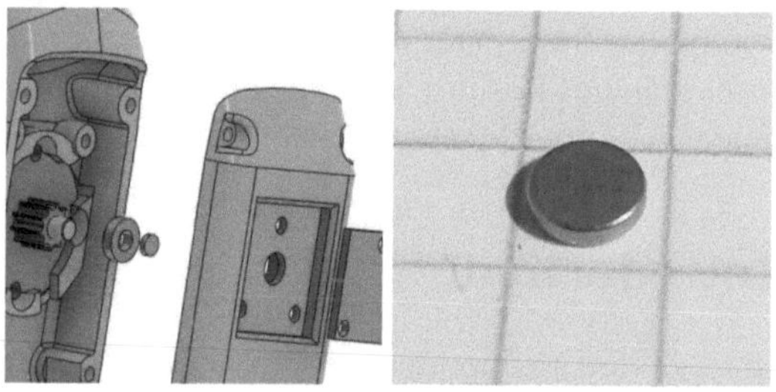

Figure 3: Exploded view of the motor and encoder assembly (left). Size of the small 4 mm magnet for reference (right).

2.3 Additional improvements

In addition, alternative suppliers for various parts could be identified. Some parts, such as the optical encoder wheel or the Hip AA bearings had to be ordered directly. By utilizing a 27 x 20 x 4 mm bearing instead of a 25 x 20 x 4 mm from an online supplier, all parts could be sourced in online stores. The required bearing shoulder was adjusted accordingly. A list of the updated suppliers can be found under

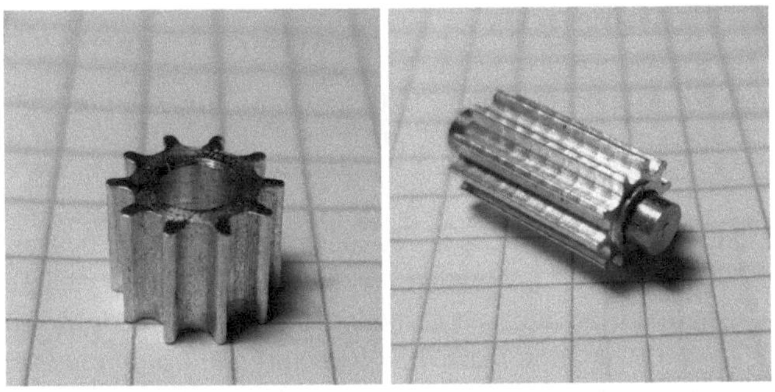

Figure 4: Close view of the new motor pulley (left) and the center pulley (right).

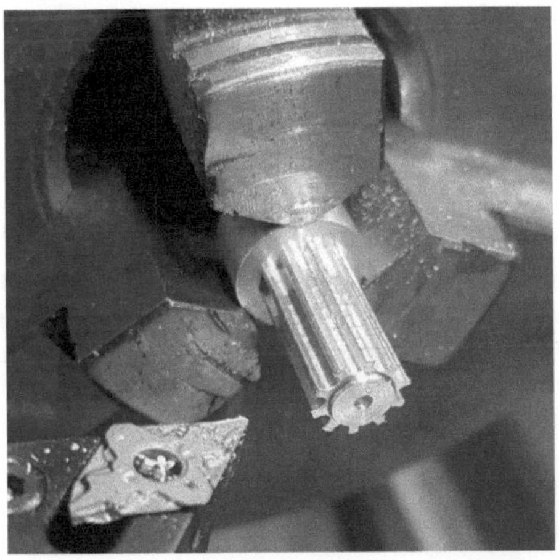

Figure 5: Photograph of the pulley being machined inside a manual lathe. The aluminum made it easy to machine.

[1]. The sensor cables for the foot contact switches were attached to the bed of the outer shell casing. This was done because no specific instructions, on how the wires should be fed through the Upper Leg, could be found. The attempted solution can be seen in Figure 6.

Table 2: An overview of the additional changes made to the robot apart from the ones mentioned in Table 1

Element	description
Hip AA bearing	Changed size to fit available bearings
Foot sensor cables	Fed below center pulley
Suppliers	Located online suppliers for various parts

3 Results and Discussion

The mentioned changes were implemented and evaluated. The observed results are presented in this section.

3.1 Encoder improvements

As of the publishing date of this paper, we did not find any effect of the changes that could be seen as a dis im-

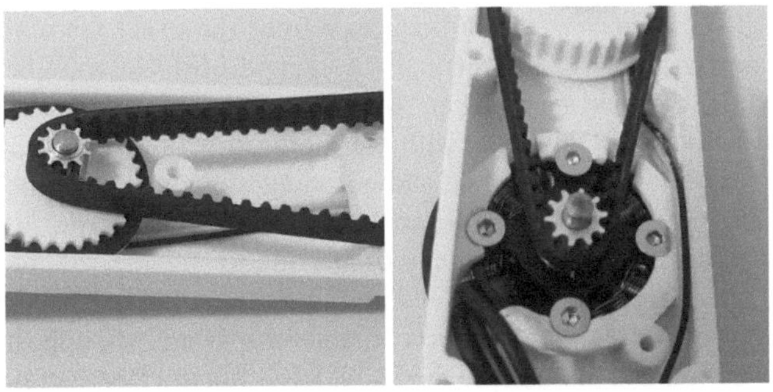

Figure 6: The black, white, gray wire of the foot contact switch can be seen running below the center pulley (left) and out on the side of the motor shaft (right).

provement to the previous solution. In addition we found that the encoder IC, as well as their printed circuit board (PCB), came out 149,52€ less as compared to the original encoders. Also, the *AS5047 IC* is capable of storing position data in non-volatile registers. This allows the encoders to store data throughout power cycles and therefore requires less calibration. Another advantage is the communication via serial peripheral interface (SPI), next to the rotary incremental encoder signal (ABI), which allows the encoder data to be used in a digital communication protocol. This, however, would require that the main controller (currently the master board) can process additional SPI inputs.

3.2 M3 belts and pulleys

The new belts and pulleys have not shown any signs of bad elastic behavior or accelerated aging of the actuator module. The power transmission of the new tooth profile had zero play and did not require any tensioners. That is to be said that a thorough side to side comparison of the old and new drive train has yet to be carried out. Also a prolonged test to show accelerated aging effects has also not been carried out. As for the pulleys, the simplified manufacturing only proved useful because a manual lathe was available. If mechanic parts have to be custom ordered, the more available M3 tooth profile has no effect on the cost or availability. If however the off the shelf components can be processed by yourself the cost can be cut drastically. Here an assumption of the cost reduction is difficult, because custom manufacturing may vary a lot based on the contractor. However some makers have made online arrangements to order the center and motor pulley in larger quantities [7]. This is to share the reduced cost per piece of batch productions among them. This may lead to the assumption that the processing of off the shelf M3 pulleys may be a legitimate cheap alternative.

3.3 μDriver and Master board

Establishing the communication of the master board and the μDriver has proven to be very challenging. Mainly compatibility issues between all participating software frameworks, such as the compilers and the python 2.7 and

3.8 standard, made it difficult to retrace the exact instructions as given in the manual. A second obstacle was the nature of the system design. In order to allow the computer system to communicate with the motor drivers, the master board relays all incoming and outgoing messages from the Ethernet/Wifi to the SPI port and vice versa. In order to assure fast round trip times of 0.2 ms to 1.2 ms [5] the higher layers and frames of the TCP/IP protocol are being ignored. This requires the computer hardware to support injection and monitoring mode, which is not always readily available.
From our perspective a solution based on the universal serial bus (USB) could achieve similar speeds while still providing an easier user experience. The μDriver expects a data cycle every 0.7 ms or about 1.5 kHz [8]. The 34 bytes of the motor communication frame and its answer of the same size for all 6 motors then requires approximately:

$$2 \cdot 32 \cdot 6 \cdot 1500 = 612 \frac{kB}{s} \quad (1)$$

This rate is covered the USB standard as stated in [9]. Such an attempt however has not been completed by us until now.

4 Conclusion

Being able to issue and manage all orders online has proven to be very useful in the light of the current global pandemic. With the original design being very new, it still shows some flaws. However, the changes made to the robot help to improve the overall performance and raise the value of the Solo-12 robot as a community project. Using the benefits of open-source this project can improve from the input of other makers. Especially a more diverse way of communicating with the μDrivers apart from the master board would enable other platforms like the NVIDEA® Jetson Nano™ to access a very powerful actuator.

4.1 Future work

The work on the Solo-12 robot is not yet finished. Our future work will include the fitting of appropriate foot contact sensors, as well as a more easily accessible computer interface. Any future addition can be followed via GitHub [1].

Acknowledgement

The work has been carried out at the University of Lubeck supervised by the Institute of Robotics and Cognitive Systems. This project has received funding from the Deutsche Forschungsgemeinschaft (DFG, German Research Foundation) - No 430054590 (TRAIN).

Author's Statement

Author states no conflict of interest.

5 References

[1] M. Buchschuster, "Github repo of the undergone changes," https://github.com/PRGeeesus/Solo12-Robot, January 2020.

[2] C. Dario Bellicoso, F. Jenelten, P. Fankhauser, C. Gehring, J. Hwangbo, and M. Hutter, "Dynamic locomotion and whole-body control for quadrupedal robots," in *2017 IEEE/RSJ International Conference on Intelligent Robots and Systems (IROS)*, 2017, pp. 3359–3365.

[3] M. Hutter, C. Gehring, M. Bloesch, M. A. Hoepflinger, C. D. Remy, and R. Siegwart, "Starleth: A compliant quadrupedal robot for fast, efficient, and versatile locomotion," 2012. [Online]. Available: http://infoscience.epfl.ch/record/181042

[4] A. Spröwitz, A. Tuleu, M. Ajaoolleian, M. Vespignani, R. Moeckel, P. Eckert, M. D'Haene, J. Degrave, A. Nordmann, B. Schrauwen, J. J. Steil, and A. J. Ijspeert, "Oncilla robot: a versatile open-source quadruped research robot with compliant pantograph legs," *CoRR*, vol. abs/1803.06259, 2018. [Online]. Available: http://arxiv.org/abs/1803.06259

[5] F. Grimminger, A. Meduri, M. Khadiv, J. Viereck, M. Wüthrich, M. Naveau, V. Berenz, S. Heim, F. Widmaier, T. Flayols, J. Fiene, A. Badri-Spröwitz, and L. Righetti, "An open torque-controlled modular robot architecture for legged locomotion research," *IEEE Robotics and Automation Letters*, vol. 5, no. 2, pp. 3650–3657, 2020.

[6] thomasfla, "Github repo of the open robot initiative," https://github.com/open-dynamic-robot-initiative, November 2020.

[7] O. group, "Group order on machined parts to reduce costs," July 2020. [Online]. Available: https://odri.discourse.group/t/group-order-on-machined-parts-to-reduce-costs/29

[8] J. Viereck, "Github repo of the open robot initiative," https://github.com/open-dynamic-robot-initiative/master-board/blob/master/documentation/BLMC_%C2%B5Driver_SPI_interface.md, 2020.

[9] "What are the usb data transfer rates and specifications?" Mar 2020. [Online]. Available: https://www.sony.com/electronics/support/articles/00024571

Improvement of Machine Learning Algorithms for Object Detection

Sven Benecke [1], Meik Frischke [2], Jasper Diesel [2], and Mattias Heinrich [3]
[1] Medical Engineering Science, Universität zu Lübeck, sven.benecke@student.uni-luebeck.de
[2] Corporate Technology and Innovation, Drägerwerk AG Co. KGaA, {meik.frischke, jasper.diesel}@draeger.com
[3] Institute for Medical Informatics, Universität zu Lübeck, heinrich@imi.uni-luebeck.de

Abstract

Object recognition and the detection of changes in an image have become increasingly important in recent years. Among the many approaches, neural networks have gained particular attention. The subject of this paper is the development of machine learning algorithms in the PyTorch environment, with a data pre procession using a Computer Vision Library. The finished networks are then ported using the ONNX - Open Neural Network Exchange format. It addresses the problem of processing data with a conventional computer vision toolbox while using the strengths of a different framework to solve a task in the best possible way. Furthermore, the impact of data pre-processing on the performance of the neural networks is investigated and compared. It has been observed that different levels of pre-processing have significant effects on the accuracy, especially on the speed at which the networks converge. Even with basic network architectures, the given data set could be nearly saturated.

1 Introduction

In recent years, neural networks have become a significant tool for many applications, including applications in the medical field. There, it is often a question of recognizing a certain object in medical images, for example, cancer, in a mammogram [1]. The basic problem is, as shown in this work, a binary classification based on image data. In the course of this project, a machine learning algorithm was designed and ported, which performs a binary classification. It recognizes whether a reddish discoloration, caused by a chemical reaction, is present in the form of a red bar or not. The images, taken by a smartphone camera, are cropped and down-sampled before being processed by the algorithm. The algorithm itself is divided into two main parts: the preprocessing of the image sections and the neural network itself, which takes the processed images as input. A similar algorithm already exists, which is based exclusively on conventional computer vision features. It was written in the computer language C++ and runs as a mobile application on smartphones. Thus, the pre-processing should be implemented in this environment as well. The problem is, that C++ is less established for developing machine learning algorithms. To get around this issue, the machine learning component is created in the PyTorch framework, which is specialized for developing and training neural network architectures. The goal is to port the trained neural network via the Open Neural Network Exchange (ONNX) interface [5] into the C++ environment to be embedded into the existing smartphone application. Before this, an internal benchmark with the previous and the new algorithm should be performed to compare both of them in terms of speed, accuracy, and robustness. Special requirements include the data pre-processing, performed with the library Open Computer Vision (OpenCV) [6] in Python as well as in C++. Moreover, the network architecture should be fast enough to run on older mobile phones as well.

2 Material and Methods

2.1 Related Work

Object recognition has been one of the main areas of computer vision for some time. Conventional algorithms have been outperformed in speed and accuracy in recent years, especially by deep neural network structures such as VGG Net [8] or GoogLeNet [7]. However, with increasing network depth and complexity comes computational expense, which makes such networks impractical to run on mobile devices. MobileNet [4] and PeleeNet [3] are architectures that are only slightly less accurate than state of the art networks while being 32 times smaller and up to 27 times less compute-intensive [4]. While MobileNet mainly focuses on depth-wise separable convolution, PeleeNet is a mixture of many different ideas, all to reduce model parameters to run fast on computationally weak devices.
The OpenCV library, whose features are used in the current algorithm, is also designed for computational speed and efficiency. This is why C++ was chosen for coding: to speed up computation as much as possible. On average, the current algorithm only requires approx. 0.1 seconds to process

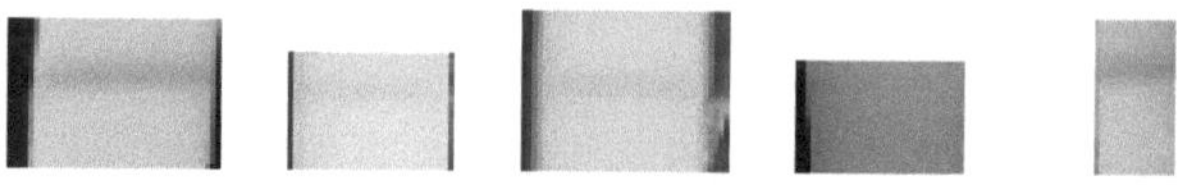

(a) (b) (c) (d) (e)

Figure 1: Examples of input images with different sizes, contrast, white balance, sharpness, and color cast. All of them are labeled as "true" but also the visibility of the red bar varies from image to image.

an image, but only achieves about 90 % accuracy.

2.2 Image Data

The images on which binary classification is performed are in Portable Network Graphics (PNG) format and contain RGB channels. They have an average size of about 35x40 pixels, but the size of each image may vary as shown in Fig. 1. Originally, they were taken with various smartphone cameras but cropped and down-sampled before being fed to the algorithm for greater computational efficiency. The data set includes 10,152 annotated images in total, 7,248 of them are annotated as "true", which means there is a red bar inside the white space.

Depending on the smartphone's camera with which the picture was taken, contrast, white balance, sharpness, and color cast vary from picture to picture. Furthermore, the red bar, if present, varies in strength depending on how strong the chemical reaction has taken place or if there was enough light while taking the photo. It's quite difficult to see the red bar with the naked eye in some images like in Fig. 1d).

2.3 Image Pre-Processing

As shown in Fig. 1, many of the images have a thick border that is much darker than the red line in the center. Therefore, it was investigated whether it is advantageous to increase the contrast in the center by pre-processing the images to better emphasize the red bar. To determine whether and how much pre-processing is needed, a few different stages of contrast enhancement were introduced. In order to hide the dark sides, the main idea is to crop out the inner, white quadrilateral of the image. This alone provides a significant increase in contrast and forms the basis for the following measures. The OpenCV library is used to handle the images and perform various calculations.

The contour of the white inner quadrilateral is found by the OpenCV function “findContours”, which performs a border following algorithm on binarized images to find the four vertices to be seen in Fig. 2 as starlike markers. These vertices are then shifted slightly towards the center to compensate for any inaccuracies to be seen in Fig. 2 as triangle markers. To finally obtain the inner region of interest (ROI), two fundamentally different approaches are chosen. The more precise method is to use the OpenCV function "warpPerspective", which applies a linear transform on the image to warp a section of it into the given size. This way, the shifted contour vertices can be used directly. In the second

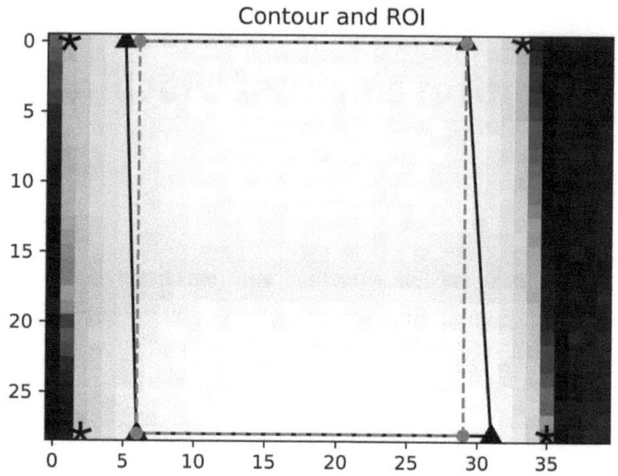

Figure 2: The obtained contour vertices are shown in starlike markers. The shifted contour, to make the region more accurate, is represented by the triangular markers with the solid line. And the region of interest (ROI) is shown in dashed lines with dot vertices. The inner rectangle can be obtained via cutting the edges or applying a linear transform.

option, only the parts of the image outside the quadrilateral are cut off. However, the sides must be orthogonal. Therefore, the smallest rectangle is extracted from the determined contour quadrilateral to be seen in Fig. 2 as dot markers and dashed lines.

After transforming or cropping the image, further methods to enhance contrast can be carried out. One such method is equalizing the image's color value histograms. This increases the contrast by spreading the color value range of the image to the entire available range to make differences more easily visible. Another option includes applying a contrast-limited adaptive histogram equalization (CLAHE), followed by bilateral filtering, which suppresses noise but preserves the edges, and finally equalizing the resulting histogram. The different results can be observed in Fig. 3 c) and d).

Several different filtering, thresholding, and histogram methods, such as Gaussian blur, differences of a Gaussian (DoG), adaptive thresholds on its own, Canny edge detection or speed up robust features (SURF) [2] was tried, but found not to be as effective as the methods named above.

2.4 Network Architectures

As already mentioned in section 2.1, there are many different approaches to neural network architectures for object recognition on mobile devices. However, since these are aimed at object recognition in the broader sense and not at simple binary classification - red bar present or not [1,0] - as in the present case, only basic architectures were examined to keep the complexity as low as possible. For comparison, three different concepts were tested. First, a multilayer perceptron (MLP). Second, a convolutional neu-

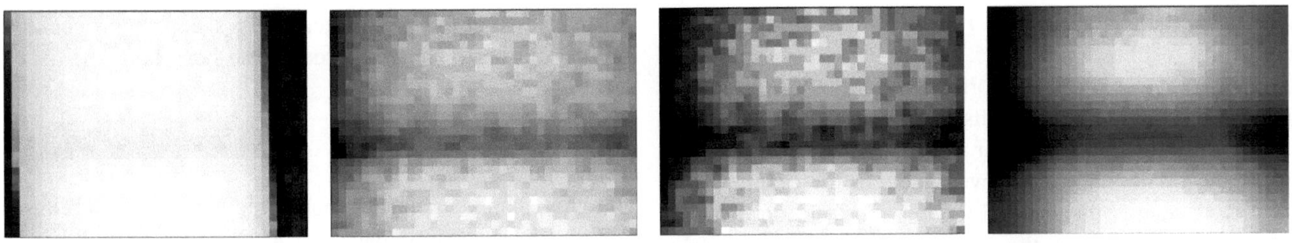

(a) Original Image (b) Inner quadrilateral (c) Histogram equalisation (d) CLAHE + Bil. filtering

Figure 3: The three main stages of processing the images. First, the inner quadrilateral is cut out (b). Subsequently, either contrast spreading using the histogram equalization method (c) or a combination of bilateral filtering and contrast limited adaptive histogram equalization (CLAHE) (d) can be performed.

ral network (CNN) with a global adaptive maximum pooling layer inside such that any kind of input size could be processed without any changes to the network parameters. And third, a standard CNN in two different depths. Every CNN ends with a linear classification layer followed by a softmax layer. All networks only contain square kernels, convolution-, linear-, pooling-, a batch norm layer with the momentum of 0.1, and a sigmoid layer in the end. After every convolution layer, a rectified linear unit (ReLU) as non-linearity is performed. The structure of the individual networks is explained in Fig. 4.

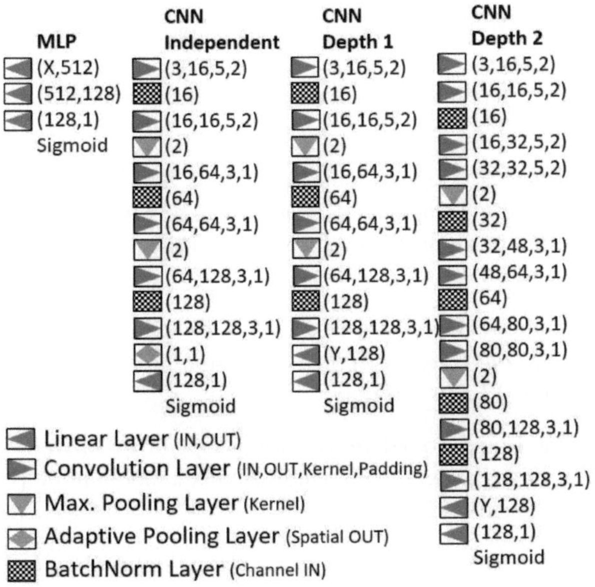

Figure 4: All different architectures from top to bottom. After every convolution layer, a ReLU is performed. "X" stands for the input size at the beginning and "Y" for the input size inside the network, which results from the original input.

2.4.1 Training

The training was carried out exclusively in PyTorch with a fixed split of training- and validation-data with a rate of 90/10. All nets were trained for 80 epochs with a batch size of 15. Since PyTorch cannot handle different input sizes of images with a batch size larger than one, all images were resized to 30x37x3 pixels. Two different input types were tested: only the processed image and the original and processed image stacked next to each other, resulting in an input size of 30x74x3. The goal is to gain information through the processed image version without discarding information from the original one. Eventually, it was not possible to use the version where both images are stacked behind each other, because OpenCV does not support images with more than four channels. The chosen optimizer was Stochastic Gradient Descent (SGD) with a momentum of 0.5 and the chosen metric was Binary Cross-Entropy (BCE) Loss. The learning rate started at 0.02 and was reduced to 0.01 at epoch 20, to 0.005 at epoch 35, and 0.001 at epoch 60.

3 Results and Discussion

Table 1: Network accuracy in % depending on the network architecture, the input, and the pre-processing mode. "Inp. 1" is only the processed image and "Inp. 2" is the original and processed image stacked side by side. With "a", cropping was done by the ROI and in "b" via warping. "0" means no processing, at "1" only cropping was done, "2" also has histogram equalization and with "3" CLAHE and bilateral filtering was done after cropping.

Mode	0	1a	1b	2a	2b	3a	3b
MLP							
Inp. 1	78,0	79,0	78,0	92,0	91,2	94,3	94,4
Inp. 2	80,0	89,0	89,0	91,6	92,2	92,0	91,7
CNN Ind							
Inp. 1	91,1	93,3	93,2	91,9	93,2	92,7	92,6
Inp. 2	92,7	94,5	95,0	93,9	93,6	93,5	93,0
CNN D1							
Inp. 1	93,2	95,3	95,0	93,1	93,5	94,7	93,0
Inp. 2	91,9	92,7	92,5	94,9	94,7	94,1	94,5
CNN D2							
Inp. 1	94,1	93,9	94,2	92,8	92,8	93,8	93,8
Inp. 2	94,0	94,1	94,4	94,4	94,1	93,9	94,1

It was shown that it is possible to port the proposed networks, via the ONNX format, into a C++ environment with the OpenCV library and run it there. Table 1 summarises the performances of all network types with all different input and pre-processing variants. It can be seen that all networks could achieve a similar maximum of about 94-95% accuracy, albeit this was achieved under different input conditions. It seems that the MLP finds the task too difficult without pre-processing the images, whereas the networks with increasing depth tend to prefer the images with little or no pre-processing to achieve good accuracy. The different crop types had little to no influence on the performance of the networks. Often, even the simpler method of cutting the sides was more successful regarding performance and computational efficiency. However, the 95% limit could not be exceeded by any of the networks, which could be due to the fixed split of the data, but also to the annotation of the images themselves. Looking at the images that were incorrectly classified according to the network shows that there is a certain amount of label noise. It was observed that the stability of the results is increasing when using a higher level of pre-processing. Other than that, the networks tend the converge much faster in training when ran with the processed images. All networks except the MLP already converged after about 40 epochs when processed images from mode "2" as in Fig. 3c) or higher as in Fig. 3d) were used. A disadvantage of all networks is the additional computational workload due to pre-processing and the complexity of the networks themselves, except the MLP. Due to limited time and the goal of demonstrating general feasibility, no hyper-parameter tuning was performed and no task-specific network architectures were developed. Instead, the extent to which a transfer learning approach with the MNIST data set would bring improvements was investigated. However, it turned out not to be effective or possible, as the two tasks are most likely too different.

4 Conclusion

One could show that without any further tuning the networks could achieve up to 95% accuracy. This is about 4-5% better than the previous algorithm. First tests show an increase in computational time, by a factor of ten in the C++ environment but could not be tested on a smartphone yet. Also, the benchmarking is to be done still. It was shown that it is possible to port pre-trained architectures from PyTorch to OpenCV using the ONNX format. The only restriction is that the channel size of the inputs must not be larger than four. The next steps could be to work on the performance by training with even more and especially noise-free data, performing random and label equalized data splits, optimizing the network's architecture, and use anisotropic filter kernel sizes. Finding an appropriate transfer learning data set to pre-train the network, fine-tune the hyperparameters, and use a different pre-processing if needed. One could also optimize the current pre-processing functions to run faster on mobile devices as well. Besides, one could investigate first to which degree pre-processing increases the performance to reduce computational workload. In conclusion, one can say that the general feasibility has been proven and the foundation for further research has been laid out.

Acknowledgement

The work has been carried out at the Coorporate Technology and Innovation department at Drägerwerk AG & Co. KGaA and was supervised by the Institute for Medical Informatics, Universität zu Lübeck. Special thanks to my supervisor, Meik Frischke, for providing guidance and feedback throughout this project.

Author's Statement

Conflict of interest: Authors state no conflict of interest. All authors contributed to the final manuscript.

5 References

[1] Azam Hamidinekoo, Zobia Suhail, Erika Denton, and Reyer Zwiggelaar, *Comparing the Performance of Various Deep Networks for Binary Classification of Breast Tumours*. Conference: Fourteenth International Workshop on Breast Imaging, July 2018.

[2] Herbert Bay, Tinne Tuytelaars, and Luc Van Gool, *SURF: Speeded Up Robust Features*. Computer Vision and Image Understanding 110(3):346–359, January 2008.

[3] Robert J. Wang, Xiang Li, Charles X. Ling, *Pelee: A Real-Time Object Detection System on Mobile Devices*. Conference on Neural Information Processing Systems, April 2018.

[4] Andrew G. Howard et al., *MobileNets: Efficient Convolutional Neural Networks for Mobile Vision Applications*. 17 Apr 2017.

[5] The Linux Foundation, *ONNX - Open Neural Network Exchange*. Available: https://onnx.ai/about.html [last accessed on 2021-01-17].

[6] OpenCV team, *OpenCV - Open(source) Computer Vision*. Available: https://opencv.org/about/ [last accessed on 2021-01-17].

[7] Christian Szegedy et al., *Going deeper with convolutions*. Computer Vision and Pattern Recognition, September 2014.

[8] K. Simonyan and A. Zisserman. Very deep convolutional networks for large-scale image recognition. International Conference on Learning Representations, 2015.

Segmentation of Cutaneous Lymphoma Lesions Using Convolutional Neural Networks

Jan Schladetzky [1], and Manuel Studer [2], and Heinz Handels [3]
[1] Medical Informatics, Universität zu Lübeck, jan.schladetzky@student.uni-luebeck.de
[2] imito AG, Zurich, ms@imito.ch
[3] Institute of Medical Informatics, Universität zu Lübeck, handels@imi.uni-luebeck.de

Abstract

The determination of the percentage of affected body surface area in cutaneous lymphoma patients is challenging and prone to intra- and inter-observer variability. The state-of-the-art method uses calculation by hand where parts of the patient's hand are used as reference areas to determine the size of all lesions. We trained a convolutional neural network (CNN) on 51 high-resolution skin images of patients with cutaneous lymphomas. Using a CNN decreases the intra- and inter-observer variability when obtaining the total body surface area affected (% BSA). Our model is able to segment the affected areas with a Dice score of 0.7656 and can therefore be used to reduce the variability. We also show how these results could be used to assist in calculating the "modified severity-weighted assessment tool" (mSWAT).

1 Introduction

Cutaneous lymphomas are cancers of lymphocytes that primarily involve the skin with an estimated incidence in Germany of 1 / 100.000 per year [1]. They commonly cause an itchy rash which can look like other common skin conditions like eczema or other chronic dermatitis. The manifestation of symptoms paired together with usually a slow growth often result in delayed diagnoses of up to several years. To assess the severity of these lymphomas and to track the success of treatments, medical practitioners often use metrics such as the percentage of skin area affected.

As a support for clinicians the St John's Institute of Dermatology in London created the mobile application Cutaneous Lymphoma Resource Tools which allows to calculate metrics such as the modified severity-weighted assessment tool score by making information material available on mobile platforms. Albeit helpful, the affected skin areas still need to be measured/estimated by hand introducing intra- and inter-observer variability into the process.

There has been research to automatically detect and segment skin lesions to support physicians in this task using conventional methods [2], machine learning such as support vector machines [3] or deep learning [4]. However, the focus in this research has been on segmentation of melanoma lesions because it is the type of skin cancer with the highest incidence and due to data availability. Recently the first work has been published dedicated to segmenting lesions of cutaneous lymphomas [5].

In this work we aim to expand the research of cutaneous lymphoma lesion segmentation by training a network on a newly created dataset consisting of high resolution images taken with a digital reflex camera and evaluating several different loss functions.

2 Material and Methods

2.1 Modified Severity-Weighted Assessment Tool

The modified severity-weighted assessment tool (mSWAT) is used to measure the cutaneous involvement in patients and assess the impact of treatments. The tool takes into account the percentage of total body surface area (% BSA) affected by lesion type (patch, plaque, tumor) where each type is weighted accordingly. As a reference for physicians the hand of the examined patient is used and defined as representing 1% of the total body surface area.

The patch type is defined as "any size lesion without induration or significant elevation above the surrounding skin", whereas plaques are defined as "any size lesion that is indurated or elevated" [[6]]. It defines tumors as "any solid lesion with at least one centimeter in diameter with evidence of deep infiltration in the skin and/or vertical growth". The weighting factors for each type and the average BSA of each body region can be seen in Table 1.

Albeit being recommended by the European Organization for Research and Treatment of Cancer (EORTC) [6] the method is not perfect because of its dependency on the examiner's performance. The manifestation of the disease can often pose a challenge due to many small lesions across the body resulting in a high intra- and inter-observer variability of the method.

Body Region	% BSA	Patch	Plaque	Tumor
Head	7			
Neck	2			
Anterior trunk	13			
Arms	8			
Forearms	6			
Hands	5			
Posterior trunk	13			
Buttocks	5			
Thighs	19			
Legs	14			
Feet	7			
Groin	1			
Weighting factor		1	2	4

Table 1: Modified Severity Weighted Assessment Tool to assess skin involvement in cutaneous lymphoma patients. The score equals the summation of all subtotal lesion BSA × factor.

2.2 Dataset

We used 51 RGB images with a size of 2000 by 3008 pixels from 3 patients with cutaneous lymphomas as the training dataset. Experts of the Department of Dermatology, Campus Kiel, University Hospital of Schleswig-Holstein manually segmented the images to obtain binary masks used as the ground truth.

After standardizing the images to have zero mean and a variance of 1 they were split up into smaller images the size size of 256 by 256 pixels and padded to a size of 284 by 284 pixels to fit the model.

Any images with fewer than five percent of lesion area were removed resulting in a dataset of 931 images. The dataset was then split with an ratio of 80:20 into a training and a validation set.

We investigated data augmentation as a mean to increase the available amount of training data by randomly flipping the images along both axes, cropping up to 20% at each side and changing the brightness by a maximum delta of 0.2.

2.3 Model architecture

As the model architecture we chose the U-Net as described in [7] due to its ability to accurately segment images with small training datasets.

It consists of two paths, a contracting and an expansive path, which together form the u-shape. In the contracting path the number of filters is doubled after each downsampling step to increase the feature information but decrease the spatial information. The expansive path then combines the feature information with the spatial information through concatenation use of up-convolutions.

Compared to the original architecture proposed by the paper we removed one up- and one downsampling step resulting in the highest number of filters being 512 (see Fig.1) and the model having 8557570 trainable parameters to reduce the complexity and size of the model. We implemented the model using the machine learning framework TensorFlow.

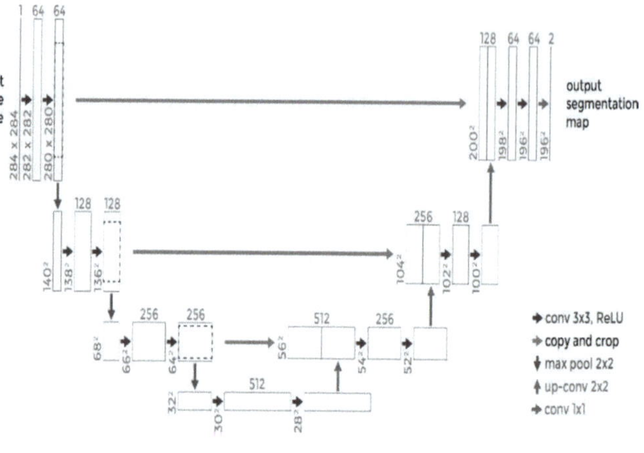

Figure 1: Model architecture with three up- and downsampling steps and 512 filters maximum.

2.4 Loss functions

We tested four different loss functions to examine their influence on the results:

Binary cross-entropy as defined as

$$L_{BCE}(y, \hat{y}) = -(ylog(\hat{y}) + (1 - y)log(1 - \hat{y})) \quad (1)$$

with $\hat{y}$ as the predicted value and y the ground truth.

The second loss function used was the Dice loss, an adaption of the Dice coefficient

$$DSC(y, \hat{y}) = \frac{2y\hat{y}}{y + \hat{y}}. \quad (2)$$

As the Dice coefficient is not defined for edge cases such as $y = \hat{y} = 0$ in the case of the Dice loss a constant ε is added to both numerator and denominator

$$DL(y, \hat{y}) = 1 - \frac{2y\hat{y} + \varepsilon}{y + \hat{y} + \varepsilon} \quad (3)$$

to eliminate the division by zero. In our work we set $\varepsilon = 1e - 6$.

We also tested the Log-Cosh Dice loss as proposed by [8]. Although widely used the Dice loss with its non-convex nature might fail in obtaining optimal results. Therefore the Log-Cosh Dice loss aims to solve this problem by encapsulating the loss in the logarithmic and the hyperbolic cosine functions as defined in (4).

$$L_{lc-dce} = log(cosh(DiceLoss)) \quad (4)$$

Lastly we tested the focal loss [9]. Especially with highly-imbalanced datasets it can improve the results because it down-weights the contribution of simple examples, therefore forcing the model to focus on the more difficult ones. The loss can be understood as a variation of cross-entropy. Starting with the formula for cross-entropy

$$CE = \begin{cases} -log(p) & \text{if } y = 1, \\ -log(1 - p) & \text{otherwise} \end{cases} \quad (5)$$

it defines the estimated probability of a class as

$$p_t = \begin{cases} p & \text{if } y = 1, \\ 1 - p & \text{otherwise} \end{cases} \quad (6)$$

for convenience purposes. Thus (5) can be written as

$$CE(p, y) = CE(p_t) = -log(p_t). \quad (7)$$

To down-weight simple examples and thus focus on the more difficult ones, two parameters α and γ are introduced so that the focal loss becomes

$$FL(p_t) = -\alpha_t(1 - p_t)^{\gamma} log(p_t). \quad (8)$$

α balances the classes while γ down-weights simple examples. In our tests we set $\alpha = 0.25$ and $\gamma = 2$ as proposed in the original paper[9].

3 Results and Discussion

3.1 Pipeline

We propose the following approach for reducing the intra- and inter-observer variability of the mSWAT as shown in Fig. 2.
In step 1 of the process, the physician photographs the patient. A full-body scanner or photogrammetry is used to obtain a complete scan of the patient. Alternatively, images taken from all sides can also be used. The downside of this approach is a reduced accuracy of the score when lesions are included in more than one picture. After obtaining the scan or images of the patient, the trained convolutional neural network is used to segment the affected skin areas. The expert can then make corrections of the segmentation results while also labeling each area with the corresponding lesion type patch, plaque or tumor. Every pixel that is not completely black is treated as body surface area. As a result, the mSWAT is then automatically calculated as the sum of all areas weighted by their respective labels. The higher the model's accuracy, the fewer corrections need to be done by the physician resulting in a lower variability of the resulting score.

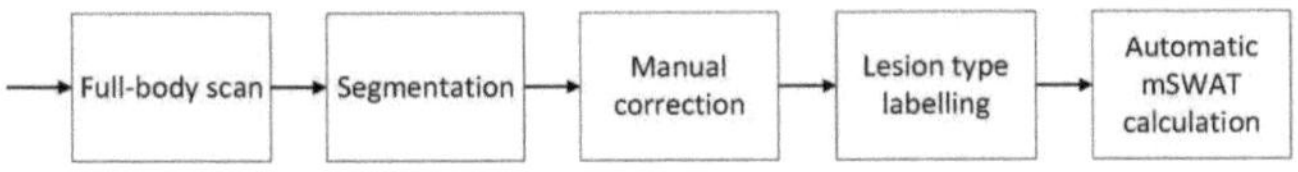

Figure 2: Our proposed pipeline for a semi-automatic mSWAT calculation.

3.2 Model results

The results were obtained with a 5-fold cross validation on the training images level after 2000 training steps and a batch size of 8. We used the Adam optimizer with default parameters and a learning rate of 0.001. Furthermore, training was performed on a single NVIDIA RTX 2070 GPU with the mixed precision implementation of the machine learning framework TensorFlow so that only certain parts of the model were kept as 32-bit floating point variables while the remaining parts used 16-bit floating point variables. This was done to reduce the memory footprint of the model and to allow larger batch sizes. Training used 5GB of VRAM and took 6 minutes to complete.

	Dice Coefficient	
	no augmentation	augmentation
Binary Cross-Entropy	0.7165	0.7607
Dice Loss	0.7167	0.7609
Log-Cosh Dice Loss	**0.7213**	**0.7656**
Focal Loss	0.6983	0.7130

Table 2: Comparison of loss functions and the effect of data augmentation for cutaneous lymphoma segmentation.

Table 2 shows that the Log-Cosh Dice loss performed best in the case without data augmentation with a Dice score of 0.7213 and a score of 0.7656 for training with augmentation. Our findings are in line with our expectations as the binary cross-entropy loss works best for datasets with an equal distribution among the classes. On the other hand, focal loss is best used for highly-imbalanced datasets explaining the low results in our tests. Since we filtered the smallest lesions out during our preprocessing and most of the remaining lesions representing an area of 30-70% of their respective images, our class distribution was only mildly imbalanced.
Additionally, the results show that data augmentation can

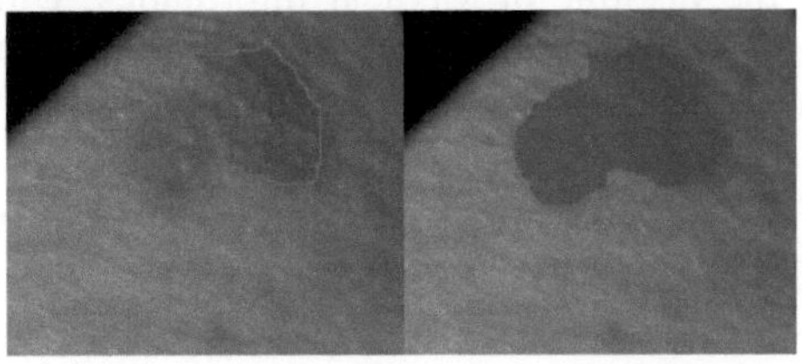

Figure 3: Segmentation results. Shown are the input image (left) with the ground truth mask (red) and the prediction overlayed onto the image (right).

improve results due to more training data being available, helping the model to better generalize. As seen in Fig. 3 segmentations in the best cases were nearly identical with their respective ground truth mask. Our model encountered problems in cases with crusted and advanced lesions where it was not able to predict sufficiently accurate masks in these cases (see Fig. 4). We expected these kind of errors as only a small proportion of our training images included these type of lesions. The need to manually review and correct the segmentation masks by physicians remains.

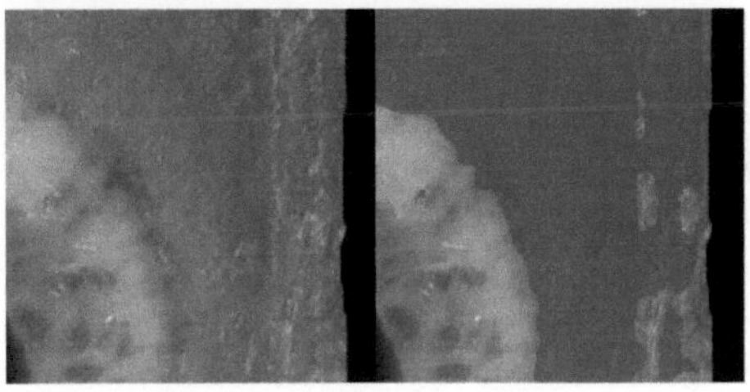

Figure 4: Segmentation of an lesion in an advanced stage.

4 Conclusion

The proposed pipeline can lower the variability and help objectify the assessment of the skin involved by cutaneous lymphomas. Our model is able to segment the lesions with a sufficiently high accuracy.
Since our dataset consisted of data from only 3 patients there is a need to increase the number of patients and to diversify the dataset in the future by including different skin types and color to increase the model's accuracy and to improve the evaluation.
As no extensive finetuning of the model's hyperparameters was done during training using this method should further increase the model's performance. In the future we will also look into multi-class segmentation to be able to also predict the lesion types. As our ground truth masks only included binary labels, we plan on expanding the dataset with multi-class labels to research the possibility of fully automatic segmenting of the lesion areas and calculation of the mSWAT score.

Acknowledgement

The work has been carried out at the imito AG and supervised by the Institute of Medical Informatics, Universität zu Lübeck. Furthermore, we would like to thank Dr. med. Ulrike Wehkamp for the medical supervision of the project.

Author's Statement

Conflict of interest: Authors state no conflict of interest.

5 References

[1] C. Assaf, S. Gellrich, M. Steinhoff, D. Nashan, F. Weiße *et al.*, "Cutaneous lymphomas in germany: an analysis of the central cutaneous lymphoma registry of the german society of dermatology (DDG)," *JDDG*, vol. 5, no. 8, pp. 662–668, aug 2007.

[2] A. Wong, J. Scharcanski, and P. Fieguth, "Automatic skin lesion segmentation via iterative stochastic region merging," *IEEE Transactions on Information Technology in Biomedicine*, vol. 15, no. 6, pp. 929–936, nov 2011.

[3] Y. He and F. Xie, "Automatic skin lesion segmentation based on texture analysis and supervised learning," in *Computer Vision – ACCV 2012*, K. M. Lee, Y. Matsushita, J. M. Rehg, and Z. Hu, Eds. Berlin, Heidelberg: Springer Berlin Heidelberg, 2013, pp. 330–341.

[4] Y. Yuan, M. Chao, and Y.-C. Lo, "Automatic skin lesion segmentation using deep fully convolutional networks with jaccard distance," *IEEE Transactions on Medical Imaging*, vol. 36, no. 9, pp. 1876–1886, sep 2017.

[5] Z. Liu, H. Pan, C. Gong, Z. Fan, Y. Wen *et al.*, "Multiclass skin lesion segmentation for cutaneous t-cell lymphomas on high-resolution clinical images," in *Medical Image Computing and Computer Assisted Intervention – MICCAI 2020*, A. L. Martel, P. Abolmaesumi, D. Stoyanov, D. Mateus, M. A. Zuluaga, S. K. Zhou, D. Racoceanu, and L. Joskowicz, Eds. Cham: Springer International Publishing, 2020, pp. 351–361.

[6] E. A. Olsen, S. Whittaker, Y. H. Kim, M. Duvic, H. M. Prince *et al.*, "Clinical end points and response criteria in mycosis fungoides and sézary syndrome: A consensus statement of the international society for cutaneous lymphomas, the united states cutaneous lymphoma consortium, and the cutaneous lymphoma task force of the european organisation for research and treatment of cancer," *Journal of Clinical Oncology*, vol. 29, no. 18, pp. 2598–2607, jun 2011.

[7] O. Ronneberger, P. Fischer, and T. Brox, "U-net: Convolutional networks for biomedical image segmentation," 2015.

[8] S. Jadon, "A survey of loss functions for semantic segmentation," *2020 IEEE Conference on Computational Intelligence in Bioinformatics and Computational Biology (CIBCB)*, Oct 2020. [Online]. Available: http://dx.doi.org/10.1109/CIBCB48159.2020.9277638

[9] T.-Y. Lin, P. Goyal, R. Girshick, K. He, and P. Dollár, "Focal loss for dense object detection," 2018.

Deep Learning of Cancer in Prostate MRI: Reducing the Impact of Incomplete Annotations

Ruben Schulze [1], Ievgen Korol [2]
[1] Medical Engineering Science, Universität zu Lübeck, ruben.schulze@student.uni-luebeck.de
[2] Fuse-AI, Hamburg, ievgen.korol@fuse-ai.de

Abstract

Magnetic resonance imaging plays a crucial role in the diagnosis of prostate cancer. Prostate cancer detection is a difficult task even for experienced radiologists. Support by a artificial neural network could improve diagnostic accuracy and speed. To successfully apply supervised learning, complete annotations are required. However, the annotations of radiologists are systematically incomplete. The proposed method improves prostate cancer detection based on such annotations. It changes the loss calculation by applying a mask to the model output during training. The method was 10-fold cross-validated and compared to conventional supervised learning. It is shown that using the mask improves detection accuracy, training stability and model generalization.

1 Introduction

Magnetic resonance imaging (MRI) plays a crucial role in diagnosis of prostate cancer. The Prostate Imaging Reporting and Data System (PI-RADS) allows standardization of prostate MRI interpretation. This is a difficult task due to heterogeneous signal changes from benign prostatic hyperplasia, inflammation and scarring after biopsy [1].

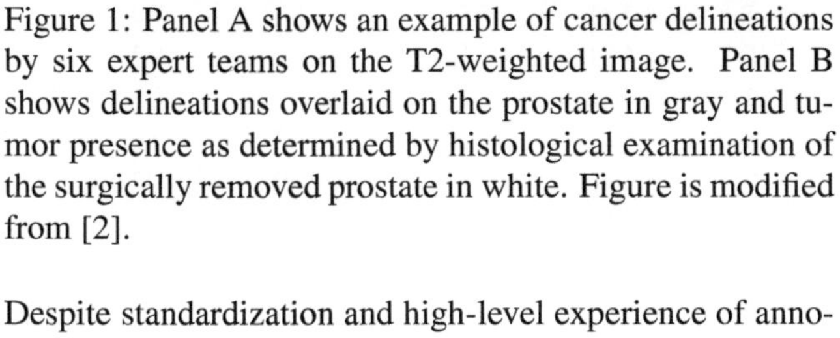

Figure 1: Panel A shows an example of cancer delineations by six expert teams on the T2-weighted image. Panel B shows delineations overlaid on the prostate in gray and tumor presence as determined by histological examination of the surgically removed prostate in white. Figure is modified from [2].

Despite standardization and high-level experience of annotators, inter-reader variability is an issue [2]. In study [2] all 6 radiologist teams missed 67 of 69 satellite malignant lesions, resulting in a systematically high false negative rate [2]. An example from this study is shown in Fig. 1. Despite that, the demand for prostate MRI interpretations is at an all time high [1].
Convolutional neural networks (CNN) approaches often exceed human level performance in natural image analysis. Therefore they could provide an opportunity to improve the diagnosis accuracy and duration by supporting the radiologist [1].
Training a clinically applicable CNN requires dependable annotations by subject matter experts. Since even expert annotations show a high false negative rate [2], it is expected that the model will be falsely penalized for correct cancer detection during training. To deal with this issue, a mask was developed that manipulates error calculation. It is hypothesized that by penalizing only the edges and region of the annotated lesion as well as the non-prostate regions, the model will learn more stably and make better predictions.

2 Material and Methods

2.1 Data

For this experiment bi-parametric MRI scans of 126 patients with one or more malignant prostate lesions were used. Prostate and lesions were annotated by one of 3 experienced radiologists. A T2-weighted image and the corresponding apparent diffusion coefficient image (ADC) were available to the radiologist for the delineation. The annotations were not validated by biopsy or histological examination. Therefore a high false negative rate is expected as in [2].
Since lesions are relatively small and often only occupy a single slice, the classes (background and lesion) are heavily imbalanced. Since imbalance has a detrimental effect on model classification accuracy, two methods were applied to decrease this imbalance [3]. The first is undersampling the background class. Even though undersampling does not improve accuracy, it reduces training time, provides better

understanding of model behavior and prevents favoring of the majority class [3]. Since the goal is not to obtain optimal model accuracy, but to show a relative increase in accuracy, the advantages of undersampling outweigh its disadvantages. To further decrease the effect of class imbalance a weighted loss function was used.

2.2 Model

The model used in the experiment is a CNN called U-Net. The U-Net is a type of artificial neural network often used in image recognition that is specifically designed for image segmentation. It consists of encoder and decoder, linked using skip connections. This allows the recovery of the original image resolution while providing voxel-based segmentations [1].

2.3 Mask Structure and Function

During each epoch the model prediction for a certain input is compared to the annotation of the radiologist. The difference between the two is determined using a loss function. This loss is then used to modify the model parameters to approach the correct output. This type of deep learning is known as supervised learning [4]. The proposed methods deciding difference from conventional supervised learning is masking the prediction before loss calculation. Based on the expert annotation, different regions in the mask were defined. Each region defines a modification of the prediction during training before loss calculation. A visualization of the mask structure is shown in Fig. 2. The original annotation is binary, deciding for each pixel if its background (0) or foreground (1, lesion). For the mask this classification is further differentiated. Every pixel lying outside of the prostate is considered background (0). Similarly the lesion itself is treated as foreground/lesion (1). The third region is the prostate located closely around the lesion. Since the radiologist separated the lesion from the rest of the prostate, this border is expected to contain no further lesions. Therefore it is treated as background (0). For every sample the border width was set to 6 mm. The prediction stays unchanged in these regions and the pixel values contribute to the loss as normal.

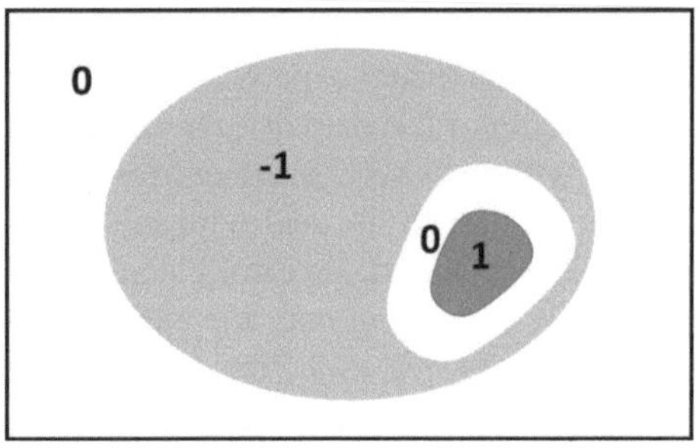

Figure 2: A Schematic of the Mask. The structure is based on the expert annotation. Outside the prostate, in orange, the background is set to 0. Lesion tissue, in blue, is marked as 1. The border region around the lesion is regarded as background. The rest of the prostate is marked -1.

For the rest of the prostate no prior knowledge can be used to safely assign a class (-1). Therefore each pixel of the prediction belonging to this region is set to 0. It does not contribute to the loss, letting the network find additional lesions ("false positive" in prediction/false negative in annotation) without being penalized. This reduces the amount of prostate-background pixels to the pixels inside the lesion border. Even though this is a strong reduction in information, it is hypothesized that only the close region around and in a lesion is needed to successfully identify it. By avoiding penalizing satellite lesions an improvement over training without masking can be expected.

2.4 Preprocessing

Each 3D case was split up into 2D slices. After cropping to the center, resizing and normalizing the images, a sample was generated by grouping the main T2-weighted slice with the neighboring slices and the corresponding ADC maps. This method allows context information from neighboring slices to be used for the detection. Additionally a binary prostate segmentation was concatenated, providing a probabilistic region the model learns to focus on. This simplifies the learning task [5].

2.5 Training Scheme

To ensure reliability, the method was ten-fold cross-validated [6].

Table 1: Amount of Patients and Slices per Fold. Each fold has a certain amount of cases used for training and validation. Each case data (3D) is split up and undersampled into a certain amount of 2D slices.

Folds	Patients Training	Patients Valid.	Slices Training	Slices Valid.
1	111	15	699	92
2	117	9	724	67
3	106	20	658	133
4	114	12	727	64
5	121	5	757	34
6	111	15	698	93
7	109	17	693	98
8	117	9	735	56
9	113	13	699	92
10	115	11	729	62
Mean	113.4	12.6	711.9	79.1

Before training, the dataset was divided into 10 folds. For each of the two methods studied, 10 trainings were conducted and evaluated. In each run, one of the folds was used for validation and all others for training. Each training was performed for 150 epochs. The amount of patients and slices per fold are shown in Table 1. The optimizer used was Adam (adaptive moment estimation) [7]. The learning stepsize was bound to 0.001.

2.6 Loss Function and Metrics

For evaluation three different metrics and the loss were tracked during training. The dice coefficient (dice) is the most used metric in validating medical volume segmentations. The dice is a measure of overlap between the ground truth and the model prediction. It provides a good baseline metric for segmentation quality. The metric returns values from 0 to 1, 1 representing a perfect match and 0 no overlap at all [8].
Since the dice is sensitive to class imbalance, another more robust metric was also used. The Matthews Correlation Coefficient (MCC) takes into account true and false positives and negatives and is generally regarded as a balanced measure which can be used even if the classes are imbalanced. It returns a value between -1 and +1. A coefficient of -1 represents total disagreement between prediction and observation, 0 means no better than random and +1 indicates a perfect prediction [9].
The loss function used to optimize the model is the Sensitivity-Specificity-Loss. It is based on the F_β-score, a generalized version of the dice, with a weight $\beta = 1.5$ to reduce the impact of class imbalance. It was smoothed for better differentiability with a log-cosh operation [10]. The loss is in range of $[0, 0.43]$.

3 Results and Discussion

3.1 Training Curves

The loss curve over all epochs is shown in Fig. 3. Two types of loss function curves can be identified. Either a sharp drop followed by a relative flat linear decrease or a sigmoidal decrease. For the first case, the model quickly learns to focus on the prostate. Using the mask accelerates this process, resulting in a steeper drop in loss, smaller changes along the epochs and a more optimal local minimum, compared to unmasked training.
For the second case, applying the mask tends to slow down the decay. The unmasked model plateaus earlier. However, the minimum that is reached after 150 epochs is comparable. Overall, smaller fluctuations can be seen in the curves with masking. The masked training is more stable and reaches the same loss values in training. This indicates better training stability and reliability.

3.2 Metric Evaluation

To compare metric values, Table 2 shows all folds with their corresponding maximum metric values over all epochs. On average the training dice and MCC with masking is 0.08 and 0.09 higher than without masking. The higher accuracy is also more consistent. In eight out of ten folds the maximum dice and MCC of masked training is higher. In three out of these eight the difference is more than twice then the average difference, exceeding 0.19. The masked training dice and MCC is the highest overall in fold 7 with 0.57 for both metrics.

Table 2: Maximum Dice and MCC per Fold. For each epoch the average dice and MCC were calculated. The per fold maximum of these values is compared in this table. The row-wise maximum is written in bold numbers. The over all folds maximum value is written in bold, cursive numbers.

	With Mask Training		Without Mask Training	
Fold	Dice	MCC	Dice	MCC
1	0.51	0.52	**0.53**	**0.53**
2	**0.47**	**0.49**	0.42	0.42
3	**0.53**	**0.54**	0.47	0.47
4	**0.52**	**0.53**	0.49	0.49
5	0.47	0.48	**0.53**	**0.53**
6	**0.54**	**0.55**	0.49	0.49
7	***0.57***	***0.57***	0.56	0.56
8	**0.48**	**0.49**	0.28	0.30
9	**0.52**	**0.52**	0.22	0.23
10	**0.53**	**0.53**	0.26	0.26
Mean	**0.51**	**0.52**	0.43	0.43

	With Mask Validation		Without Mask Validation	
Fold	Dice	MCC	Dice	MCC
1	**0.21**	**0.22**	0.08	0.08
2	**0.23**	**0.23**	0.19	0.18
3	**0.20**	**0.22**	0.20	0.18
4	0.11	0.14	**0.16**	**0.16**
5	0.00	0.00	0.00	0.00
6	**0.10**	**0.11**	0.02	0.03
7	**0.15**	**0.18**	0.13	0.14
8	0.18	0.18	**0.19**	**0.20**
9	0.24	0.25	***0.28***	***0.28***
10	**0.24**	**0.26**	0.14	0.14
Mean	**0.17**	**0.18**	0.14	0.14

High training coefficient values do not have to correlate directly with high validation values. This is especially prevalent for small training datasets. In this study, the independence is most pronounced for training without masking: In folds 1, 5 and 6 the predictions are close to random. In fold 9, the 0.28 reached in validation is higher than the corresponding value in training, indicating a statistical outlier. This is confirmed in the training curve, as seen in Fig. 3. In fold 5, none of the methods seems to have enabled the model to generalize.
The masked training performs better in validation. It performs on average 0.03 (dice) and 0.04 (MCC) better than the competitor. In 6 of 10 folds the metric values are higher. In all others, the gap is below 0.05.
These results show that masking has a positive effect on model performance: Model accuracy is more robust and less susceptible to statistical effects. Model accuracy increases on average for validation and training.

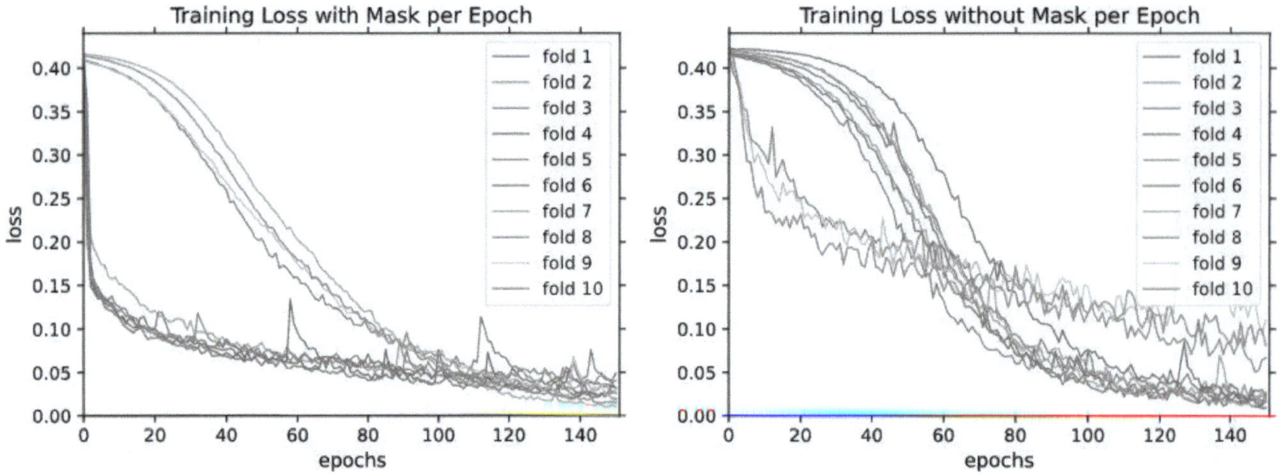

Figure 3: Each color belongs to a fold. The left panel shows the loss for training with mask. The right panel shows the loss for training without applying the mask.

4 Conclusion

It is shown that utilizing the mask improves detection accuracy, training stability and model generalization. Training becomes more stable and is less susceptible to statistical effects. A more optimal local minimum is reached more consistently. Model accuracy increases on average and is more consistent for validation and training. The proposed method improves supervised learning of prostate cancer in MRI. It mitigates the detrimental effect of systematically incomplete annotations.

The next step is to check the scalability of the mask. Another study is needed to verify, if the benefits are carried over to a larger dataset and setup. In other fields where images are only partially annotated, these images can now be used for learning by employing a similar mask. Since low quality annotations are usually cheaper and easier to obtain, this method offers a simple solution to make more data usable. The method can be applied independent of pipeline or architecture.

Acknowledgement

The work has been carried out at Fuse-AI, Hamburg and supervised by Prof. Mattias Heinrich, Institute of Medical Informatics, Universität zu Lübeck. The data used in this study was provided by Fuse-AI, Hamburg.

Author's Statement

Conflict of interest: Authors state no conflict of interest.

5 References

[1] P. Schelb et al., *Classification of Cancer at Prostate MRI: Deep Learning versus clinical PI-RAD Assessment*, Radiology, Heidelberg, pp.607–617, 2019.

[2] P. Steenbergen et al., *Prostate Tumor Delineation using multiparametric Magnetic Resonance Imaging: Interobserver Variability and Pathology Validation*, Elsevier, Radiotherapy and Oncology, 2015.

[3] A. Bria, C. Marrocco and F. Tortorella, *Addressing Class Imbalance in Deep Learning for small Lesion Detection on medical Images*, Elsevier, Biology and Medicine, 2020.

[4] R. Kishore and T. Kaur, *Backpropagation Algorithm: An Artificial Neural Network Approach for Pattern Recognition*, International Journal of Scientific & Engineering Research, Vol. 3, Issue 6, 2012.

[5] O. Oktay et al. *Attention U-Net: Learning where to look for the Pancreas*, arXiv:1804.03999v3, 1st Conference on Medical Imaging with Deep Learning, Amsterdam, The Netherlands, 2018.

[6] R. Kohavi, *A Study of Cross-Validation and Bootstrap for Accuracy Estimation and Model Selection*, Computer Science Department, Stanford University, 1995.

[7] D. P. Kingma and J. L. Ba, *ADAM: A Method for Stochastic Optimization*, arXiv:1412.6980v9, ICLR 2015, 2015.

[8] A. A. Taha and A. Hanbury, *Metrics for evaluating 3D medical Image Segmentation: Analysis, Selection, and Tool*, BMC Medical Imaging, 2015.

[9] S. Boughorbel, F. Jarray and M. El-Anbari, *Optimal Classifier for imbalanced Data using Matthews Correlation Coefficient Metric*, PloS ONE 12(6): e01777678, 2017.

[10] S. Jadon, *A Survey of Loss Functions for semantic Segmentation*, arXiv:2006.14822v4, IEEE Member, 2020.

Utilizing Embedded Deep Learning-based Object Detection for Visual Inspections of Medical Devices

Michael Lichtenhagen [1]
[1] Biomedical Engineering, Luebeck University of Applied Sciences, michael.lichtenhagen@stud.th-luebeck.de

Abstract

Inspired by 'Edge AI' this paper proposes the operationality of YOLO, a state-of-the-art real-time object detection model, embedded on a NVIDIA Jetson Nano SBC for visual inspection tasks in the medical industry. For the training, a custom data set was acquired from the actual process as well as pre-processed using Roboflow. The model training has been performed using the computational resources from Google Colab. The embedded implementation of the model has been validated against the manufacturer's statement. The experimental results have shown that deploying the model on reasonable although power-efficient edge devices does not compromise mean average precision (mAP) (91.3 %) and delivers an average performance of 13 fps. Thus, using the low-budget approach of utilizing embedded AI to detect, count and localize objects is applicable to many industrial applications.

1 Introduction

When humans look at images or videos, any object of interest can be recognized and located within a matter of moments. The goal of deep learning-based object detection is to mimic this intelligence utilizing computer vision and *artificial neural networks* (ANNs). The challenge of object detection is to locate the presence of objects with bounding boxes and assign class labels to these objects in an image. Over the past few years object detection has become popular for a variety of applications for example in medical imaging. Here the detection of cancer cells in images is often assisted by *artificial intelligence* (AI) in order to relieve radiologists in performing these challenging and time-sensitive tasks.

Since entering Industry 4.0 means starting the ongoing process of using smart technology, e.g. large scale *machine-to-machine* (M2M) communication and *internet of things* (IoT), object detection is widely considered in the automotive industry. The next decade is likely to see a rapid rise in the utilization of object detection in the healthcare industry. To mention some examples where it found application in healthcare:

- Surgical Robotics
- Workplace Automation
- Warehouse Management
- Flow Management
- Augmented Reality.

Use Case: In regulatory affairs, for example of the EU-regulated market, product compliance is often labelled with the CE mark. According to the market, and the individual customers there are different requirements on product marking. Therefore, in many visual inspections, checking that the product contains the appropriate labels, is a crucial process to prevent non-compliance and customer dissatisfaction, especially in the healthcare sector. Nowadays, the inspection process is carried out by hand in order to mitigate the risk of *defect on arrivals* (DEFOAs) due to missing or misplaced labels. Therefore, object detection can be utilized, checking the presence and position of certain labels on a medical device automatically. Based on this requirement, this paper describes the process of utilizing deep learning-based object detection embedded on an edge device and how well it performs based on a small-scale pilot. The challenge in accomplishing the requirements for implementing AI on the edge is to deliver high detection accuracy of the model while managing the limited resources of a device. Nevertheless, the innovations driven not least by the contributions of big companies like NVIDIA or Intel, involving performance increases of *central processing units* (CPUs) and *graphics processing units* (GPUs), has made it possible embedding AI on edge devices.

2 Material and Methods

Generally, edge AI is based on the concept that it can perform the inference process on an embedded system. Although, training process requires much more computational power. Therefore, it is not performed on the embedded system, rather on a dedicated cloud-based server. Then, the obtained weights are extracted and implemented in the model already deployed on the edge device.

There are plenty models that are used for object detec-

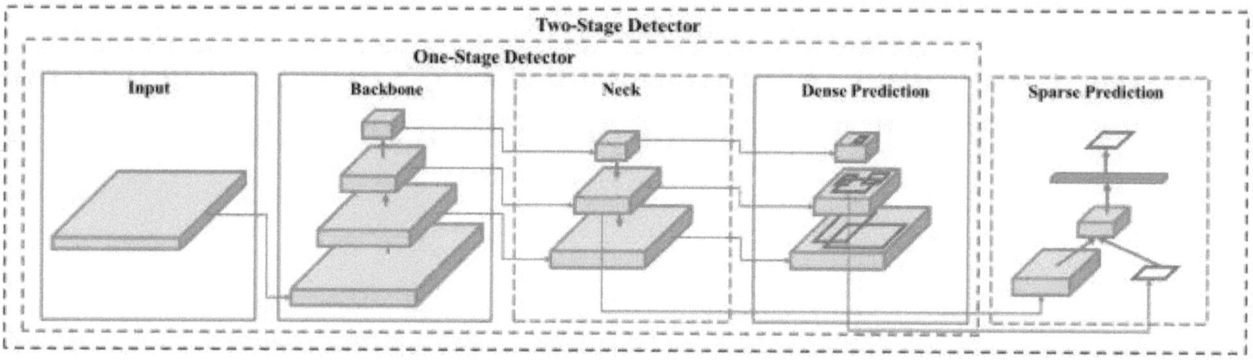

Figure 1: Architecture of the YOLOv4 framework and its composition of several parts [1].

tion. Each with trade-offs between speed, size, and accuracy. In this paper the most popular one has been picked: YOLO (You Only Look Once). In comparison to other models, YOLO has equal high detection average precision (AP) but runs significantly faster, which makes it state-of-the-art object detection. The first (of three versions) of YOLO was initially presented by Jospeh Redmon [2]. Thereafter, the further development of YOLO was maintained by Alexey Bochkovskiy, the Russian developer who built the YOLO Windows version, Chien-Yao Wang, and Hong-Yuan Mark Liao. Based on Redmond's algorithm they released YOLOv4 in 2020, which improves YOLOv3's AP and FPS by 10 % and 12 %, respectively [1].

For the embedded implementation of the model, an NVIDIA Jetson Nano 4GB SBC has been used. Tab. 1 shows a benchmark presented by the manufacturer between various selected models performing on the embedded hardware. From this, it can be seen that the Jetson Nano hardware is capable to run at least YOLOv3-tiny, which uses a lighter version of the YOLOv3 darknet model, with 25 FPS when using TensorRT optimized inference. On the other hand, community-based approaches often result in less fps (around 10).

Table 1: Performance of various models with Jetson Nano and TensorRT, using FP16 precision and batch size 1 [3].

Model	Framework	fps
YOLOv3-tiny	Darknet	25
SSD Mobilenet-V2	TensorFlow	27
SSD Resnet-18	TensorFlow	16

2.1 YOLOv4 Architecture Framework

YOLO is a new approach to object detection using the *Darknet* architecture. Darknet is a neural network written in C and CUDA and has been developed and trained on PascalVOC 2007 dataset by Redmon et al. [2]. Unlike other state-of-the-art approaches, YOLO frames object detection as a regression problem to spatially separated bounding boxes and associated class probabilities. The basic idea is that YOLO looks globally at the image only once. Therefore, it is capable of predicting all bounding boxes across all classes for an image simultaneously. As opposed to its bigger brother, YOLOv4-tiny uses a lighter counterpart of the Darknet-53 network. Therefore, it is dubbed "tiny" with the goal of having a faster computation with significant but not too much loss of accuracy. This makes the tiny version very suitable for AI applications at the edge with the use of embedded devices. YOLOv4 is a fully convolutional network, which means that is uses only convolutional layers in order to reduce the computational needs. As seen in Fig. 1, it consists of several components. It starts with the feature extractor or backbone dubbed CSPDarknet53 network. Its fundamental role is to extract features hierarchically, which starts from raw pixels coming from the input layer. The backbone ends in a final layer, where any pixel contains very compressed information of the image. The extracted representations are later used for the Dense Prediciton, where the prediction of labels for each pixel is performed. In contrast to YOLOv4, YOLOv4-tiny has a reduced number of convolutional layers in the *Cross Stage Partial (CSP)* backbone called CSPDarknet53-tiny [1].

The prediction process of YOLOv4-tiny method is the same with YOLOv4 method. Firstly, it also resizes the input image to make all input images have the same fixed size. Secondly, input images are divided into $S \times S$-grids, while every grid cell predicts multiple bounding boxes B by using predefined anchors. Therefore, $S \times S \times B$ bounding boxes are generated for a single input image. If the center of an object falls in a grid cell, the bounding boxes from this grid cell are very likely to predict the object [1].

To reduce the redundancy of bounding boxes in the prediction process, *Non-Maximum Suppression* (NMS) is applied. Therefore, the best bounding box with the maximal confidence score of having the object inside is identified and fixed. Then, it removes all other bounding boxes that have an *Intersection over Union* (IOU) greater than a certain threshold (typically 0.5). IOU measures the overlap between the ground truth box and other predicted bounding boxes. That means that it simply removes all duplicate bounding boxes that overlap the most with the chosen one [1].

Model performance evaluation was performed on a dataset

where 6 different classes were considered. Totally, 98 images were acquired with a 20 megapixels Canon IXUS 185 camera from randomly selected products from the same product family. The images were annotated by using *LabelImg*, an open-source tool [4]. Then, the dataset was uploaded to Roboflow, which is a browser-based data management tool that provides dataset organisation, preprocessing and augmentation techniques. Additionally it was used in order to extend the data set size to 230 by data augmentation (cropping images by 17 % and rotation of the images by $\pm 14°$). Moreover, the final dataset was split into train, valid and test sets with a ratio of 70 %, 20 %, 10 %, respectively. The training for the different models were performed on Google Colab, which provides a cloud-based version of Jupyter Notebook with free GPU-access. The batch size, epochs, learning rate, momentum and decay are 64, 120, 0.00261, 0.9 and 0.0005 for all methods, respectively.

2.2 Hardware Setup

NVIDIA's Jetson family is another uprising embedded hardware for AI applications, where a small form factor, low power consumption, and price is important. In June 2019, NVIDIA released the *Jetson Nano*, a 99$ *Single Board Computer* (SBC), which represents the lower segment of NVIDIA SBCs. However, it has the potential to outperform all other available SBCs, e. g. Raspberry Pi 3 with Intel Neural Compute Stick 2, and Google Edge TPU Coral Dev Board in terms of model compatibility and performance, see [3]. Key feature is the CPU-GPU heterogeneous architecture, where the quad-core 64-bit ARM CPU boots up the firmware. For hardware acceleration, the 128 CUDA-capable Maxwell architecture-based GPU is used, accomplishing complex machine learning algorithms with a peak performance of 472 GFLOPs [5]. The Nano has two versions which differ in RAM (2GB vs. 4GB) and count of available USB slots (2 vs 4 slots, respectively). In this work the 4GB LPDDR4 memory type with a 32 GB SD-card has been used. As it can be seen in Fig. 2, the board was built into a housing, which was designed specifically for the Nano. It also includes a mount for different types of cameras up to 180° roll angle. Likewise, an IMX219-120 Camera, with 8 Megapixels, 120° FOV was used. In order to provide wireless connection to the factory network, the AC8265 Wireless NIC module was added. It enables 2.4G / 5G WiFi and Bluetooth 4.2 connection on the device.

3 Results and Discussion

3.1 Quantitative Results: Model Performance

To understand the model performance, mAP is computed on the test dataset. Mean average precision is used to assess and score a model's accuracy in detecting objects. Therefore each predicted bounding box is compared with the ground truth and marked as true positive TP if the object is present. Moreover, IOU must be greater than a threshold.

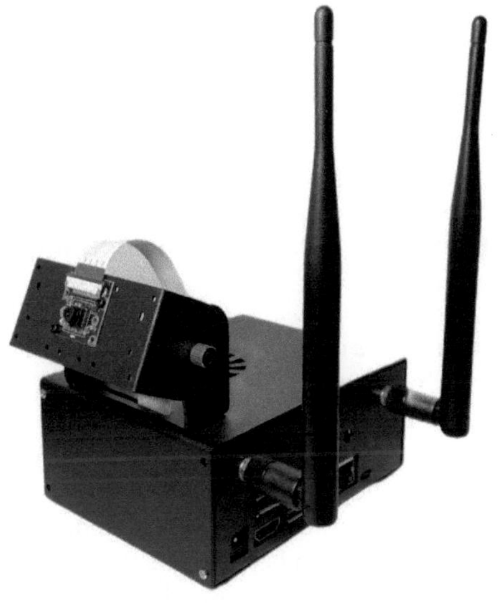

Figure 2: Edge Device Prototype with wide-angle camera and antennas for wireless connections.

If IOU is lower than the target or the object is not within the bounding box, the prediction is marked as false positive FP. Finally, non-detected objects are marked as missing predictions (false negative FN). The predicted bounding boxes are outputted only if they overcome a level of confidence. This is set up as a certain confidence threshold c, which was chosen as c=50 %. Therefore, it is possible to calculate the *precision* and the *recall* of the network:

$$Precision = \frac{TP}{TP+FP} \qquad Recall = \frac{TP}{TP+FN} \tag{1}$$

When associating precision and recall, the precision-recall trade-off can be plotted, which provides a comparable model-wide evaluation. Commonly, the graph is then smoothed in order to get a monotonically decreasing precision curve by using interpolation methods $p_{interp}(r) = max_{r'>r}\, p(r')$. Then the area under the curve (AUC) can be mathematically described, taking the interpolation into account, as:

$$AP = \sum (r_n - r_{n-1})\, p_{interp}(r) \tag{2}$$

For a multiple class detecting model, mAP contains information about the mean AP of all classes. With reference to the confidence threshold it is common to indicate this when giving results:

$$mAP_{.50} = \frac{\sum_{i=1}^{N_c} AP_i}{N_c} \tag{3}$$

Based on the validation set the model training achieved very good results, as seen in Tab. 2. In comparison to YOLOv4, the validation of YOLOv4-tiny resulted in a slightly lower mAP value. This is comprehensible, since it uses the thinner CSP backbone with less convolutional layers. Increasing the number of epochs, as well as fine-tuning the hyperparameters of the network could increment mAP for YOLOv4-tiny. However, for the current dataset this is a very reasonable starting point.

Table 2: Training Validation Results

Model	$mAP_{.50}[\%]$
YOLOv4	98.12
YOLOv4-tiny	91.3

3.2 Qualitative Results: Embedded Implementations

After the training, the model has been deployed on the hardware platform presented in section 2.2. Then, the hardware including the model was deployed in the visual inspection process. In order to test its overall performance in terms of model accuracy and frame rate, the model was run with input taken from the connected camera in real-time. An interesting comparison between the models is shown in Tab. 3. Even though, it is promised by NVIDIA that converting the Darknet-based model to TensorRT-based, using YOLOv3 could reach 25 fps [6]. Therefore, a higher performance can be expected after conversion. However, with the Darknet-based YOLOv4-tiny embedded in the NVIDIA Jetson Nano, an average frame rate up to 13 fps in 10 W mode has been achieved, which can still be an acceptable value for this small-scale pilot. This is in good agreement with the community's deployment results.

As expected, based on the test dataset (10 images) we could only achieve $mAP_{.50}$ scores of 96.67 % and 79.03 % for YOLOv4 and YOLOv4-tiny, respectively. To solve this, further data collection is required to improve training and robustness of the YOLOv4-tiny model, since only a small-scale dataset of 230 images was used.

According to [7], with the combination of Raspberry Pi SBC and the Intel's Neural Computing Sticks (NCS), the performance is lowered to five fps in the best case. Hence, the Intel Neural Sticks are reasonable edge devices as well, when a good price/performance ratio is needed. However, the final price of this setup is slightly higher compared to the Jetson Nano. Nowadays, if looking for a perfect balance between performance and cost in this range, the Jetson Nano seems to be a very good choice.

Table 3: Implementation Benchmark

Model	$mAP_{.50}[\%]$	$mAP_{.75}[\%]$	avgfps
YOLOv4	96.67	57.75	1.6
YOLOv4-tiny	79.03	52.51	13
TensorRT			
YOLOv4	*96.67*	*57.75*	*4.26*
YOLOv4-tiny	*79.03*	*52.51*	*25.5*

4 Conclusion

In conclusion, this paper has shown promising prospects utilizing a real-time object detection model on an edge AI-optimized device. For this, a model has been trained on a custom data set, acquired from a real use case, and tested under real circumstances. In order to highlight model performances on a custom dataset, experimental evaluations have been carried out. Good results have been demonstrated in terms of recall, precision and speed during detection of objects with different sizes. The tested system was capable to produce real-time high detection performance with minimal resources. However, to gain full potential of the Jetson Nano, it is necessary to optimize both Jetson hardware and training process. Better hardware performance could be achieved by Darknet to TensorRT conversion. Moreover, the methodology presented in this paper could be used with a bigger training dataset to improve model's performance.

In view of an extension of the presented work, these findings suggest that the methodology is not limited to label detection task, but could also be implemented for any applications where the detection of objects at the edge is needed.

Acknowledgement

The work has been carried out at Philips Medical Systems DMC GmbH, Hamburg Germany and supervised by Prof. Dr. A. Drews, Business Informatics, Universität of Applied Sciences Lübeck.

Author's Statement

Author state no conflict of interest.

References

[1] A. Bochkovskiy, C.-Y. Wang, and H.-Y. M. Liao, "Yolov4: Optimal speed and accuracy of object detection", 2020. arXiv: 2004.10934 [cs.CV].

[2] J. Redmon, S. K. Divvala, R. B. Girshick, and A. Farhadi, "You only look once: Unified, real-time object detection", *CoRR*, 2015. [Online]. Available: http://arxiv.org/abs/1506.02640.

[3] dustynv, "Jetson Nano: Deep Learning Inference Benchmarks", https : / / developer . nvidia . com / embedded / jetson - nano - dl - inference - benchmarks, Online Accessed: 12-Dec-2020.

[4] Tzutalin, "Labelimg – an open-source image annotation tool", https://github.com/tzutalin/labelImg, 2015.

[5] "Jetson Nano Dev Kit Specification Sheet", Januar 2020.

[6] J. Jung, "Tensorrt demos running on nvidia jetson or x86/64 pc platforms." https://github.com/jkjung-avt/tensorrt_demos, 2019.

[7] V. Mazzia, A. Khaliq, F. Salvetti, and M. Chiaberge, "Real-time apple detection system using embedded systems with hardware accelerators: An edge ai application", *IEEE Access*, 2020. DOI: 10.1109/ACCESS.2020.2964608.

Detection of Axonal Degeneration in Microscopic Image Time Series using a Deep Learning Approach

Niklas Auer [1] and Marietta Zille [2,3,4]
[1] Medical Engineering Science, Universität zu Lübeck, niklas.auer@student.uni-luebeck.de
[2] Institute of Experimental and Clinical Pharmacology and Toxicology, Universität zu Lübeck, m.zille@uni-luebeck.de
[3] Institute for Medical and Marine Biotechnology, Universität zu Lübeck
[4] Fraunhofer Research and Development Center for Marine and Cellular Biotechnology, Fraunhofer Research Institution for Individualized and Cell-Based Medical Engineering

Abstract

Axonal degeneration occurs in a number of neurological diseases. Previous experiments of our group have identified four different morphological patterns of axonal degeneration in the context of brain injury. To automatically detect and classify these in microscopic image time series of *in-vitro* experiments, a deep learning approach with a 3D convolutional neural network was tested in this study. We were able to detect degenerating axons, but the classification of the different patterns was challenging for the neural network. While the background was detected reliably (F1 score > 0.95), the differentiation of the morphological patterns (F1 score ≤ 0.73) sould be further improved. In the future, an enhanced version of this method may be used to automatically evaluate the extent of degeneration and time after which the four patterns occur in *in-vitro* experiments.

1 Introduction

Axonal degeneration is the disintegration of an axon, which occurs during nervous system development and aging, but also as an element of degenerative nervous system diseases. Many different morphological patterns of axonal degeneration have been described [1, 2, 3]. Our group previously identified four patterns: granular, retraction, swelling, and transport degeneration, which are being shown as segmented microscopy images in Fig. 1 [1]. Granular degeneration is characterized by the granular separation of (axonal) fragments. In retraction degeneration, the distal part of the axon retracts and ultimately degenerates granularly. Swelling degeneration is classified as the enlargement of axonal swellings and subsequent granular degeneration. Transport degeneration is degeneration in which axonal swellings of constant size, which do not enlarge, are transported along the axon resulting in granular degeneration.

It is important to understand these morphological changes of axonal degeneration to develop novel therapeutic approaches for neurodegenerative diseases [3, 4].

To support the evaluation of the degeneration patterns in experiments, a method was developed in this study to automatically detect and classify axonal degeneration in image time series with the ultimate goal to automatically obtain information about the time and extent of the different axonal degeneration patterns.

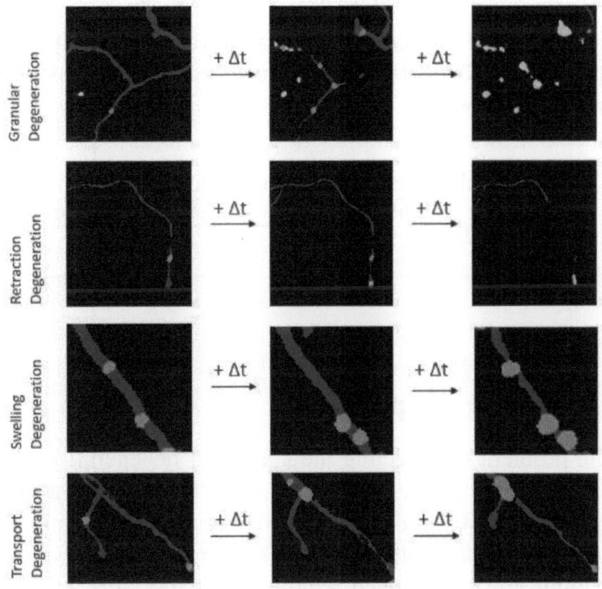

Figure 1: The four axonal degeneration pattern shown in already segmented microscopic images; axonal swellings in lighter grey, and axonal fragments in white.

For this reason, a deep learning approach can be used. To solve the problem of detecting and classifying degeneration, i.e., changes in image time series, it can be looked at problems from the fields of object detection and video classification. Since object detection is typically only done frame by frame in videos, a hybrid approach from both fields is important to efficiently use the temporal as well as spatial features because, for example, transport degeneration and swelling degeneration can not be distinguished by using only spatial features.

2 Material and Methods

2.1 Dataset and Preprocessing

To generate image time series, primary cortical neurons were prepared as previously described [1] and grown in a microfluidic device that allowed the observation of isolated axons in one compartment. After the administration of different doses of the cytotoxic hemolysis product hemin (oxidized heme), axonal degeneration was observed under the microscope. The image series were acquired by phase-contrast microscopy over a period of 24 hours at a 30-minute interval using an Olympus IX81 time-lapse microscope. This resulted in a series of images comprised of 47 images each (stack). The images were first segmented into background, axon, axonal fragment, and axonal swelling as previously described [1].
The dataset used for all experiments in this study consisted of 24 image stacks. In the image stacks, a total of 103 instances of degeneration were marked as regions of interest and classified by hand by experts. Each region belonged to up to three classes of degeneration at the same time, as different degeneration processes can occur one after the other or at the same time. Not all degeneration patterns are represented equally often in the dataset, making it highly class imbalanced (Table 1). These formed the training basis for the neural network.

Table 1: Number of samples for each degeneration pattern

	Granular	Retraction	Swelling	Transport
Number of samples	77	29	61	24

2.2 General Approach

The problem of detecting the classes of degeneration was solved in two steps. First, a 3D convolutional neural network (CNN) was trained to classify certain regions into the four degeneration patterns plus a background class. For this training, the 103 labeled regions of interest plus an additional 50 crops from the parts of the background of the 24 image stacks, which contained axons, were used. Because the network learns to distinguish foreground from background, in the second step, an approach similar to the Region Based Convolutional Neural Network (R-CNN) was used for the object detection [5]. This object detection network was the basis for much faster variants such as Faster R-CNN which introduced a Region Proposal Subnet (RPN) to the network architecture [6]. The addition of an RPN however has been demonstrated to be the main bottleneck in previous experiments with this dataset and has caused a significant drop in precision. Therefore, although the variant described in this study is notably slower, an RPN was not used.

2.3 Classification

For the classification of the four degeneration patterns, the SlowFast network architecture was utilized [7]. It is a 3D-CNN, which consists of (1) a slow pathway with low temporal resolution and a high number of channels and (2) a fast pathway with higher temporal resolution and fewer channels. Every second image of the stack was used as input for the fast pathway. Thus, this branch of the network got an input with a temporal resolution of one hour. For the slow path, every 16th image served as input, which means that the temporal resolution here was eight hours. The architecture of the model is shown in Table 2.

Table 2: Architecture of the SlowFast Model used for classification.

Stage	Slow Pathway	Fast Pathway	Repeats	Tensor Size (T x S^2)
input	-	-		Fast: 24 x 320^2 Slow : 3 x 320^2
conv1	1 x 7^2, 64 stride 1, 2^2	5 x 7^2, 8 stride 1, 2^2	1	Fast: 24 x 160^2 Slow : 3 x 160^2
pool1	1 x 3^2 max stride 1, 2^2	1 x 3^2 max stride 1, 2^2	1	Fast: 24 x 80^2 Slow : 3 x 80^2
res2	1 x 1^2, 64 1 x 3^2, 64 1 x 1^2, 256	3 x 1^2, 8 1 x 3^2, 8 1 x 1^2, 32	3	Fast: 24 x 80^2 Slow : 3 x 80^2
res3	1 x 1^2, 128 1 x 3^2, 128 1 x 1^2, 512	3 x 1^2, 16 1 x 3^2, 16 1 x 1^2, 64	4	Fast: 24 x 40^2 Slow : 3 x 40^2
res4	1 x 1^2, 256 1 x 3^2, 256 1 x 1^2, 1024	1x 1^2, 32 1 x 3^2, 32 1 x 1^2, 128	6	Fast: 24 x 20^2 Slow : 3 x 20^2
res5	1x 1^2, 512 1 x 3^2, 512 1 x 1^2, 2048	1x 1^2, 64 1 x 3^2, 64 1 x 1^2, 256	3	Fast: 24 x 10^2 Slow : 3 x 10^2
output	average pool, concatenate, fully connected layer			5 classes

The neural network was trained from scratch on one graphics processing unit (GPU) for 70 epochs with a batch size of four on a training subset. For the training, the Adam Optimizer was applied to a weighted binary cross-entropy loss function. The individual weights were chosen in a manner to compensate for the class imbalance of the dataset during training. In addition, a dropout of 0.5 before the classification layer was used during the training phase.
After training, the model was validated on a separate testset containing 50 of the 153 regions of interest with a class ratio comparable to the training set. For evaluation, precision, recall and F1 score were calculated for each class as follows [8]:

$$Precision = \frac{TP}{TP + FP} \tag{1}$$

$$Recall = \frac{TP}{TP + FN} \tag{2}$$

$$F1Score = \frac{2 * TP}{2 * TP + FP + FN} \tag{3}$$

TP denotes true positives, FP false positives and FN false negatives.

2.4 Detection

The detection of the regions of interest has been performed in most approaches of detection only in single images and not with the whole videos or image time series as an input. For the detection of regions of interest in the R-CNN architecture an algorithm named selective search, which works by over-segmenting the images, is used [5]. Since this approach is not well-suited for the already pre-segmented grayscale dataset, the selective search was replaced by another method in this study. Image differencing was used to generate images from the 3D data [9]. This simplified the problem of generating meaningful bounding boxes, which contain regions of interest and preserved relevant temporal information. The difference images (DI, Fig. 2) were generated according to the following equation:

$$\begin{aligned} DI &= |I(t=15) - I(t=0)| \\ &+|I(t=31) - I(t=15)| \\ &+|I(t=46) - I(t=31)|. \end{aligned} \tag{4}$$

I(t=0) denotes the image from the image time series at time zero. At the end, these images were normalized to the range [0, 1].

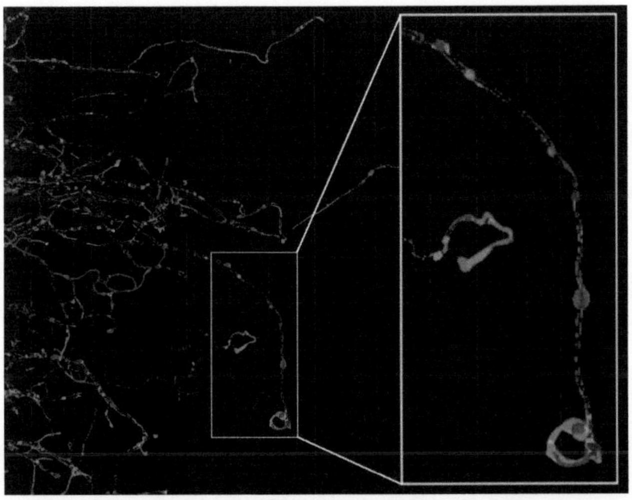

Figure 2: An example difference image from an image time series. Changes in the image in the first third are shown in red, changes in the second third in green and changes in the third third in blue. Intermediate colors result from changes in more than one third of the time.

To generate bounding boxes, which can then be classified by the SlowFast Network, so-called anchors, the centers of the bounding boxes, must first be distributed appropriately over the image. All pixel coordinates that fulfilled two conditions were used as anchors:

1. The pixel value is not zero.
2. The pixel is at least 7 pixels away from another anchor point in both image dimensions.

For each anchor point created in this way, eight bounding boxes were generated, each of them with a different combination out of two scales and four aspect ratios. These bounding boxes were then rescaled to a size of 320 x 320 pixels and classified by the SlowFast Network. All boxes containing one or more axonal degeneration patterns were saved. After all bounding boxes were classified, the best candidates were filtered out by non-maximum suppression and presented. For evaluation, all bounding boxes containing at least 80 % of the ground truth box were considered as correctly detected.

3 Results and Discussion

3.1 Classification

Classification on the test dataset achieved an overall F1 score of 0.72. The discrimination of background (axons which did not degenerate) and the axonal degeneration patterns achieved good results with an F1 score of 0.96 (Table 3). Thus, the SlowFast network learned to detect the degeneration of axons in general. This was the most important distinction for the later object detection in the whole image time series. Granular degeneration was almost always correctly detected, as the recall value of 0.94 shows. However, the precision value of 0.6 indicates that many samples that did not contain granular degeneration were nevertheless labeled as such. The low precision value was due to the fact that granular degeneration was the most frequent degeneration pattern in the dataset. This class imbalance causes the network to predict this class more often than it occured.

The classification of retraction and transport degeneration was more difficult for the algorithm with F1 scores of 0.57 and 0.44. Both classes have a precision value of 1 but recall values of 0.4 and 0.29. The neural network often classified samples showing swelling degeneration and transport degeneration as swelling degeneration only. This may mean that the SlowFast Network often did not detect the movement of axonal swellings along the axon that distinguishes the two patterns. Retraction degeneration was also not detected in samples with multiple labels and was hardly recognized by the neural network.

There are two conceivable approaches to improve this issue. First, to increase the temporal resolution in the two network branches even more, but this would require more computational effort and more memory. The second solution would be to increase the dataset most importantly with the underrepresented axonal degeneration patterns or with image sections with only one degeneration pattern for the network to learn the features of the currently underepresented classes better.

Table 3: Results of the classification experiment

	Precision	Recall	F1 score
Background	0.92	1	0.96
Granular Degeneration	0.6	0.94	0.73
Retraction Degeneration	1	0.4	0.57
Swelling Degeneration	0.7	0.7	0.7
Transport Degeneration	1	0.29	0.44

3.2 Detection

Fig. 3 depicts a section of an image from an image time series. In this example you can see that the boxes predicted by the network are larger than the ground truth boxes. This was a common detection error in the results.

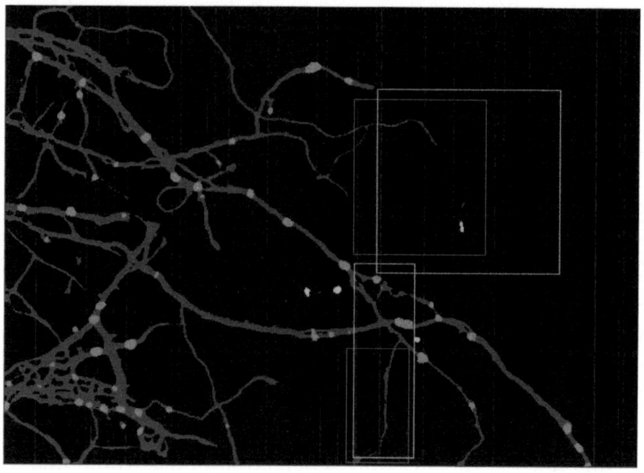

Figure 3: An example of the detection results in one image out of an image time series. The ground truth boxes are shown in blue and the network predictions are shown in yellow.

The recall value of the background boxes decreased from 1 to 0.78 compared to the simple classification because much more variation occurred in the background samples during the detection task than the variation which was presented to the network in the classification data set. This means that some locations in the image time series have been marked by the SlowFast network that did not show degenerating axons. The precision also decreased from 0.92 to 0.87, meaning that fewer degeneration instances were detected by the network. The classification results of the foreground boxes in the different morphological patterns of axonal degeneration were comparable to the results reported in the classification results. Overall, this detection approach showed first good results. In many cases, degenerating axons were distinguished from those that remained intact. The shape of the bounding boxes, on the other hand, was imprecise in some places and also contained parts of non-degenerating axons in addition to the degeneration sites.

4 Conclusion

The 3D-CNN described here was able to discriminate background from axonal degeneration. The classification of axonal degeneration, however, was more difficult. The more degeneration patterns were visible in an image section, the harder it was for the algorithm to correctly identify all of them. In the future, an improved SlowFast Network trained on a bigger dataset with the described method of detection may be used to improve the algorithm. This will help to better understand axonal degeneration in the context of health and disease.

Acknowledgement

The work has been carried out at the Institute for Neuro- and Bioinformatics, Universität zu Lübeck and the Fraunhofer Research and Development Center for Marine and Cellular Biotechnology of the Fraunhofer Research Institution for Individualized and Cell-Based Medical Engineering under the co-supervision of Amir Madany Mamlouk and Marietta Zille.
We would like to thank Alex Palumbo for providing the microscopic image time series dataset.

Author's Statement

Conflict of interest: Authors state no conflict of interest.

5 References

[1] A. Palumbo, P. Grüning, S. K. Landt, L. E. Heckmann, A. M. Mamlouk and M. Zille et al., *EntireAxon: Deep learning deciphers four distinct patterns of axonal degeneration.* bioRxiv, 2020.

[2] L. J. Neukomm and M. R. Freeman, *Diverse cellular and molecular modes of axon degeneration.* Trends in Cell Biology 24, 2014.

[3] N. Salvadores, M. Sanhueza, P. Manque and F. A. Court, *Axonal degeneration during aging and its functional role in neurodegenerative disorders.* Frontier in Neuroscience, 2017.

[4] S. Saxena and P. Caroni, *Mechanisms of axon degeneration: From development to disease.*. Progress in Neurobiology, 2007.

[5] R. B. Girshick, J. Donahue, T. Darrell and J. Malik, *Rich feature hierarchies for accurate object detection and semantic segmentation.* CoRR, 2013.

[6] S. Ren, K. He, R. Girshick and J. Sun, *Faster R-CNN: Towards real-time object detection with region proposal networks.* IEEE Transactions on Pattern Analysis and Machine Intelligence, 2015.

[7] C. Feichtenhofer, H. Fan, J. Malik and K. He, *SlowFast networks for video recognition.* IEEE/CVF International Conference on Computer Vision (ICCV), 2019.

[8] D. M. W. Powers, *Evaluation: from Precision, Recall and F-measure to ROC, Informedness, Markedness and Correlation.* Journal of Machine Learning Technologies, 2011.

[9] B. S. Karthik, *Change detection using image differencing: A study over area surrounding Kumta, India.* Second International Conference on Electrical, Computer and Communication Technologies (ICECCT), 2017.

Automatic Angle Determination of Feet in Images using Convolutional Neural Networks

Lennart Berkel [1], Dominik Mairhoefer [2], and Manuel Laufer [2]
[1] Medical Engineering Science, Universität zu Lübeck, Lennart.Berkel@student.uni-luebeck.de
[2] Institute for Neuro- and Bioinformatics, Universität zu Lübeck, {mairhoef,laufer}@inb.uni-luebeck.de

Abstract

The quality of x-ray images of ankle joints depends on the correct angular position of the foot. In practice the adjustment is based on personal experience and can result in varying image quality. The purpose of this research project was to automatically determine a foot angle in images with methods of machine learning. Therefore, a dataset was generated by recording several feet in different positions labeled with the foot angle. Afterwards a convolutional neural network was trained on three different image formats of the self-made dataset and evaluated in consideration of their informative value for angle determination. With the results of evaluation, we could show in this research project, that the angular position of feet can automatically be determined by neural networks which later potentially can be used in medical practice to optimize x-ray procedures.

1 Introduction

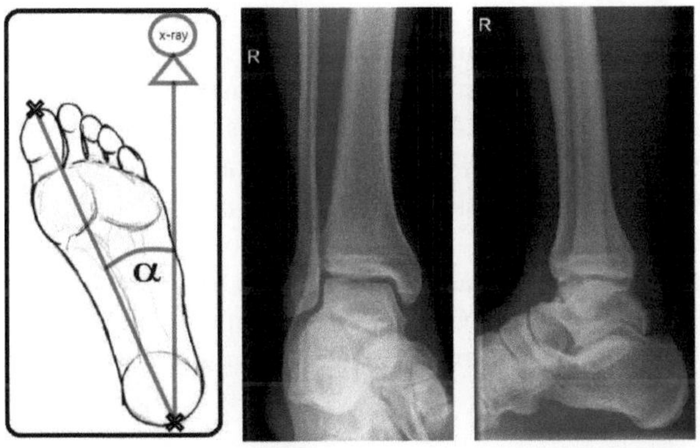

Figure 1: Acquisition scheme (left) and x-ray of an ankle in a.p. (middle) and in lateral direction (right) (modified figure from [1]).

The quality of an x-ray image of an ankle joint heavily depends on the correct angle of the foot. The angle adjustment must be precise to enable a diagnosis of possible small fractures. In practice this setting is done by a medical assistant and is based on learned rules regarding anatomical conditions, angles, and personal experience. Since this subjective parameters can result in varying image qualities and x-ray images are invasive, time consuming and costly, the purpose of this research project was to automatically determine a foots angle in images with machine learning methods to enable qualitative constant and reproducible imaging procedures. Especially the spatial representation given in Depth images by time of flight (ToF) cameras promised advantages for this computer vision task. In the first step a dataset had to be generated since there is no open source dataset of feet which are labeled with angles. Therefore, different feet were photographed in different angular positions. The second step considered machine learning methods to automatically determine the angular position of a foot. The PyTorch implementation [2, 3] of the ResNet-18 [4] was utilized for training and testing an the self-created dataset. Due to the data being acquired in the formats RGB, depth- and Infrared image, the networks performance was evaluated based on each image format. Machine learning methods are very powerful and can help in many different areas to increase quality and efficiency of processes and products. In this research project we could show that the angular position of feet can be automatically determined by neural networks which could later be used in medical practice to optimize x-ray procedures.

2 Material and Methods

2.1 Dataset

For the execution of the research a dataset was needed that contains pictures of feet in different angular positions labeled with the angle. And although the amount of open source datasets is constantly rising there was no available source with the required recordings and labels. For the acquisition of a new dataset the *Microsoft Azure Kinect* development kit [5] was used, whose sensor is often used for computer vision tasks. Therefore, the sensor includes a 1-MP depth sensor and a 12-MP RGB video camera outputting the captures in as RGB, depth and Infrared (IR) images. For a better comparison of the image formats with each other, the RGB images have been transformed to the viewpoint of the depth camera, unintentionally causing invalid points. As part of the actual data acquisition the feet of the persons were captured. Therefore, the leg was placed on an even horizontal surface allowing the leg to rotate freely, while the angular position was determined using a self-made device. This in complexity and accuracy limited instrument was made of a long rod that is attached to the big toe, projecting the angle of the foot onto an angle disk via a point of rotation. The cameras point of view was right from the front, set up with a distance of 50 cm. With a rotation of 20° lateral to 60° medial in steps of 1°, 81 angular positions were captured. Each angular position was recorded five times. The background was covered up. In total the acquired dataset comprises 1.620 captures of four different feet, thus partitioned into the sets foot no.1 (F1), foot no.2 (F2), foot no.3 (F3), and foot no.4 (F4), and accessible in the formats RGB, depth and IR image. Captures of the three formats in the angles 60° medial, 0° and 20° lateral are exemplified in the following Fig. 2.

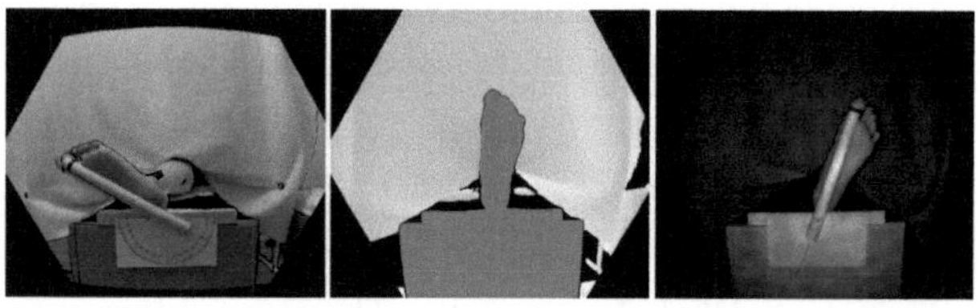

Figure 2: Representation of different image formats. Left: RGB; Middle: Depth image, langer distances relate to lighter colors; Right: IR image, using an infrared illumination. Invalid points appear in black.

2.2 Modeling

The goal of the presented project was to feed an image of a foot into a machine, which processes the input and outputs a number representing an angle. Due to the current superiority of CNNs in image processing the choice for the network architecture fell on the ResNet [4]. ResNet-18 is a CNN that consists of 18 consecutively 3 × 3 convolutional layers using strides of 2 for down sampling. This series is originally completed by a global average pooling layer and a 1000-way fully connected (FC) layer with a SoftMax function to solve a classification problem with 1000 classes. In this project we are handling the angle determination as a regression problem, due to the order of the classes and the resulting correlation between adjacent angles. Therefore the 18 convolutional layers are followed by a single output neuron without a SoftMax function, as one can see in Fig. 3.

The used loss function is the Mean Square Error (MSE), also known as the Quadratic Loss or the L2 Loss [7]. It is calculated as the sum of the squared distances between the predicted and the known value, thereby taking class order into account. Minimizing this loss function should lead the model to approximate the expected probability distribution.

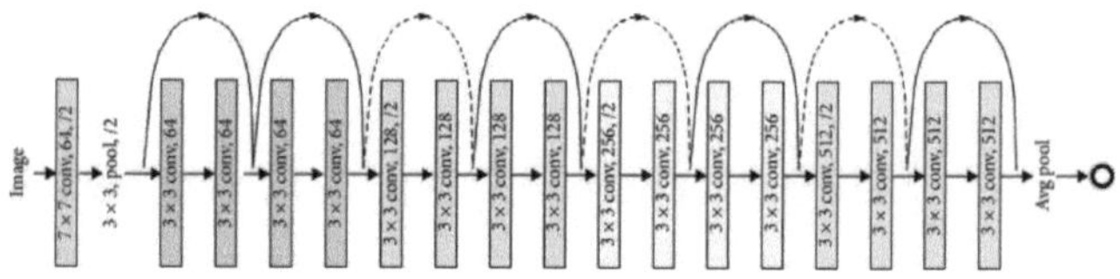

Figure 3: Modified ResNet-18 architecture for regression (modified figure from [6]).

2.3 Implementation

The utilized PyTorch implementation [2] follows the practice of the original paper [4]. Modifications were made in number of output classes, which was changed to one class related to the angle value itself. All image formats were feed as 3-channel input to the network, with the one-dimensional formats (Depth, IR) being concatenated three times. To overcome the sparsity of the given dataset augmentation was facilitated. Augmentation is used to increase the depth of information in a dataset by using slightly changed data as input and serves as a method of regulation [8]. Therefore the following geometric transformations encode invariances and prevent the model from learning irrelevant patterns. In training the image of size [576, 640] was randomly (I.) changed in brightness and contrast in the range of $(-0.2, 0.2)$, (II.) gaussian noise was added from a standard deviation of $(0.01 * 255, 0.06 * 255)$ with zero mean, (III.) blurred using a median filter with a random aperture linear size in the range of $(3, 7)$, (IV.) flipped horizontally and (V.) cropped to three quarters of its original height and width. All augmentations were applied with a probability of $50\,\%$. As well for training as for testing the image was rescaled to [202, 224] and its range of values normalized to $(-1, 1)$. Since no pretrained weights are used, the model is trained from scratch using the Stochastic Gradient Descent (SGD) initialized with a weight-decay of $1 \cdot 10^{-3}$, a momentum of 0.9 and a learning rate of $1 \cdot 10^{-3}$.

3 Results and Discussion

3.1 Experiments

The ResNet-18 was evaluated on all three image formats separately to compare their informative value with regard to the angle determination task. As training dataset, the partitions of the dataset associated with three of the four captured feet were used, resulting in a 75 / 25 split and a total of 1215 training and 405 testing images. In total each training of the regression model took $2 \cdot 10^5$ iterations while each iteration had a batch size of 8. For evaluation the MSE and the accuracy allowing $\pm 0.5, \pm 1, \pm 2, \pm 5, \pm 10$ degrees deviation were calculated as 4-fold cross validation. To support the evaluation each training run was illustrated in a scatter plot, showing the correlation between ground truth labeling and prediction.

Table 1: Accuracy on image formats

Data	Accuracy in %															
	±0.5°				±1.0°				±2.0°				±5.0°			
	RGB	Depth	IR	Mean	RGB	Depth	IR	Mean	RGB	Depth	IR	Mean	RGB	Depth	IR	Mean
F1	11.03	06.86	02.45	06.78	24.26	12.50	04.90	13.89	38.63	20.59	26.96	28.73	92.89	36.91	**100.0**	76.60
F2	10.29	12.99	29.51	17.60	16.91	21.32	77.70	38.64	33.58	35.93	**100.0**	56.50	63.63	96.57	**100.0**	86.73
F3	07.59	47.21	09.80	21.53	15.93	78.63	24.07	39.54	37.75	96.57	80.39	71.57	91.18	**100.0**	**100.0**	97.06
F4	**55.00**	03.43	42.06	**33.50**	78.53	16.91	**87.45**	**60.96**	95.20	56.67	98.53	**83.47**	**100.0**	**100.0**	99.75	**99.92**
Mean	**21.00**	17.62	20.96	-	33.90	32.34	**48.53**	-	51.29	52.44	**76.47**	-	86.93	83.37	**99.94**	-

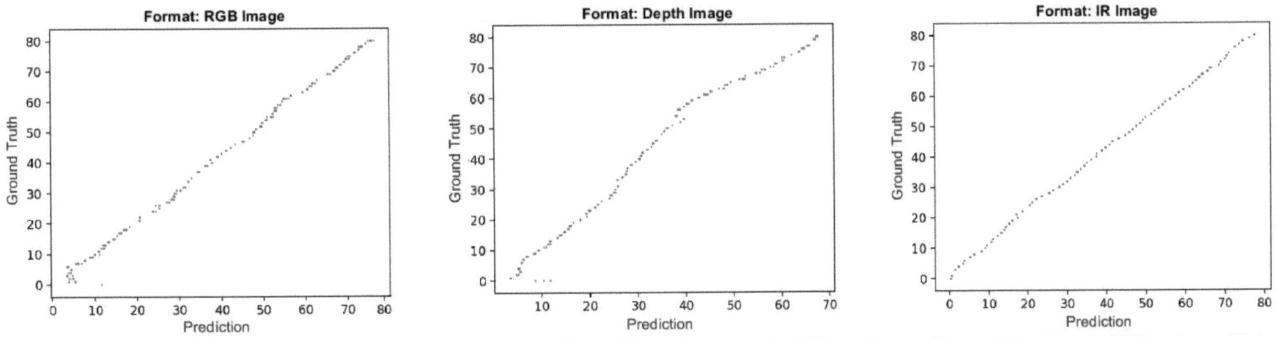

Figure 4: Evaluation of the F1 partition.

3.2 Results

Tables 1 presents the results of the model evaluations. Accuracies that were achieved with confidence intervals of ±0.5, ±1.0, ±2.0 and ±5.0 degrees are shown. For this, a differentiation was made between the results on the four partitions of the dataset (F1, F2, F3, F4), each being used in the cross validation as test basis. As the first table shows for accuracies with ±0.5° margins, the worst result of 2.45 % was made on the IR images of the F1 partition, while the highest score of 55.0 % was tested on the RGB format of the F4 partition. This result on the IR images is offset by a very good accuracy of 42.06 % on the F4 partition, leaving the mean accuracies on the RGB and IR images being the same with around 21 %. This means that mean results on RGB and IR images exceed the accuracy on the depth images by around 3 percentage points. Regarding the accuracy with a margin of ±1.0°, both the worst and the best accuracy value can be determined on the IR image format, with 4.90 % and 87.45 %, respectively. Looking at the average over all data sets, the mean accuracy of 48.53 % on the IR images stands out from the other image data, which come up with values of 33.90 % and 32.34 %. Even if the margin is increased to ±2°, the accuracies on IR data remain the highest. The ResNet-18 achieves 100 % accuracy on the IR images of the F2 partition, whereas the worst value of 20.59 % is achieved on the depth data of F1 partition. Here, too, the results on the IR image data surpass those of the other two data types. For confidence intervals of ±5.0°, the models achieve 100 % accuracy on almost all IR data, and top values of 90 - 100 % on the both other image formats. Overall, the ResNet-18 achieves higher levels of accuracy on the IR images. It should be mentioned that comparatively very high accuracies are achieved on the depth images of the F3 partition, while particularly low accuracies are measured on the ones of the F4 partition. Thus, the difference between the partitions of the dataset must be noted. The observed accuracy is always the highest on the F4 partition and lowest on the F1 partition. These results can be supported by the scatter plots shown in Fig. 4. These scatter plots are similar to the representation of a confusion matrix as they plot the predicted angles on the x-axis against the ground truth value on the y-axis. They visualize the performance of the model in terms of class prediction. A perfect prediction generates a diagonal, while prediction errors are represented by deviations from this diagonal. The distribution of the classes from 0 to 81 correspond to the distribution of the angles from 20° lateral to 60° medial. The performance of the ResNet-18 model is shown on the image types RGB, depth and IR, tested on the same dataset partition. The results on the IR images strongly approximate the diagonal with only minor deviations. Looking at the class distribution of the model tested on the RGB images, greater distances to the diagonal are observable, and especially the border areas from class 0 to 10 are distributed off the diagonal. The class prediction based on the depth images shows the greatest deviation from the perfect prediction. In addition, here only classes from 0 to 70 are predicted, which means that the model has not returned the highest 10 angles for any input. Overall, one can derive from the plots that the ResNet-18 has successfully learned angles from the pictures. It achieves highest accuracy on the IR images, followed by the RGB images and finally the depth images. The network shows weaknesses in predicting the limit classes.

3.3 Discussion

An explanation for the better performance of the model on the IR images could be that the IR images are less complex compared to the other two image types. The IR images are captures as gray-scaled image and are characterized by the fact that, due to the infrared illumination, the foot strongly dominates the background in terms of brightness, thus the model might focus more onto the foot instead of the barely visible background. The RGB image type contains more complexity as they depict the background and provide three color channels. In additions, during the transformation of viewpoints, invalid points arise that can disrupt the processing. In contrast, the depth images do not describe the detected brightness but the distance to the reflective layer, which creates a spatial representation. We had hoped that this spatial representation would facilitate the determination of the angle. However, the results cannot confirm this assumption. The reason for this could be invalid points that arise at interfaces that do not reflect the infrared light back onto the camera. It is also possible that this type of spatial data is not suitable for an architecture such as the ResNet. Architectures such as the PointNet are designed for the input of spatial data, such as point clouds. Furthermore, the fluctuations in the results on the individual feet or the different dataset partitions must be discussed. Since horizontal flipping of every second image as part of the augmentation ensures that images of right and left feet are trained in equal parts, an imbalance of left and right feet can be excluded. In particular, the accuracies with confidence intervals of ± 0.5 and ± 1.0 show strong deviations from one another on the individual partitions. This suggests that measurement errors were made when acquiring the dataset and creating the labels. In summary, it can be stated that the underlying dataset is subject to limitations in terms of the amount of data and the accuracy of the labels. Recordings of only two people are not sufficient as a basis for training and test datasets, since the left and right feet of a person may not differ significantly. These limitations affect the model in the form of fluctuating results. In addition, the influence of the rod of the measuring device on the result was not taken into account. Nonetheless, the ResNet-18 has learned, with a certain confidence interval, to derive angles from the feet images. A larger dataset with more different feet and recordings promises improvement. In addition, different architectures should be tested as network backbone, especially with regard to the depth images.

4 Conclusion

The research goal of this paper was to quantify the automatic angle determination of feet in images. For this purpose, a new image dataset was recorded, which served as the basis for training and evaluation. The widely used CNN architecture ResNet-18 was considered and evaluated on the self-created dataset. Furthermore, attention was paid to the informative value of three different image formats. The performance on RGB, depth and IR images were discussed with regard to limitations in the dataset and network modeling. Nevertheless, the results show that the automatic angle determination is possible with a limited accuracy, but the advantages of a spatial view could not be confirmed. As this research project is part of a continuing internship the following efforts on this research project will aim to improve the underlying dataset in terms of number of images and labeling accuracy and consider different network models.

Acknowledgement

The work has been carried out and supervised by the Institute for Neuro- and Bioinformatics, Universität zu Lübeck.

Author's Statement

Conflict of interest: Authors state no conflict of interest.

5 References

[1] M. Grunewald and C. Schramm and M. Uder, *Sprunggelenk.* Available: http://idr.med.uni-erlangen.de/orthorad/rta/sprunggelenk-rta [last accessed on 2021-01-25].

[2] PyTorch, *Torchvision.Models.* Available: https://pytorch.org/vision/0.8/models.html [last accessed on 08.02.2021].

[3] A. Paszke et al., *PyTorch: An Imperative Style, High-Performance Deep Learning Library.* In: Advances in Neural Information Processing Systems 32, Curran Associates, Inc., 2019.

[4] K. He and X. Zhang and S. Ren and J. Sun, *Deep Residual Learning for Image Recognition*, CoRR, 2015.

[5] Microsoft, *Azure Kinect DK.* Available: https://azure.microsoft.com/en-us/services/kinect-dk [last accessed on 2021-01-26].

[6] K. Almezhghwi and S. Serte, *Improved Classification of White Blood Cells with the Generative Adversarial Network and Deep Convolutional Neural Network.* Computational Intelligence and Neuroscience, 2020.

[7] I. Goodfellow and Y. Bengio and A. Courville, *Deep Learning.* Available: http://www.deeplearningbook.org [last accessed on 2021-01-24].

[8] C. Shorten and T. M. Khoshgoftaar, *A survey on Image Data Augmentation for Deep Learning.* Journal of Big Data, 2019.

13

eHealth

Market Analysis and User Evaluation of Input Devices for a Communication System in the Intensive Care Unit

Marina Ziewe [1], Börge Kordts [2] and Andreas Schrader [2]
[1] Medical Informatics, Universität zu Lübeck, marina.ziewe@student.uni-luebeck.de
[2] Institute of Telematics, Universität zu Lübeck, {kordts, schrader}@itm.uni-luebeck.de

Abstract

Improving communication can reduce the significant physical and psychological stress of weaning from mechanical ventilation, which is exacerbated by the limited ability to voice basic needs due to the breathing tube. One approach is the use of technical aids, such as the communication system used in project ACTIVATE, which is based on a novel interaction device tailored to the ICU context named BIRDY. Nevertheless, patients may benefit from alternative input devices due to the individual medical condition, personal preferences or previous experience. To this end, a market analysis based on various criteria (inter alia hygiene, battery life, availability, and costs) yielded three promising candidates (Kai, Leap Motion, and Litho). The devices were integrated into the ACTIVATE system and tested in a pilot study (n=6). The results point out Litho as the most promising candidate and further, stress the current limitations of the BIRDY prototype in development.

1 Introduction

Mechanically ventilated patients in intensive care units (ICU) struggle to impart their needs and feelings to nurses and family members. Verbal communication often cannot take place because of the ventilation, and nonverbal communication is also hampered by the patient's mental state and the medical equipment. As a result, these vulnerable patients are unable to adequately inform caregivers and family members about basic needs, such as perceived pain. Further possible consequences are Delir [1], anxiety, loss of identity, and feelings of unfamiliarity [2], [3].

The goal of the ACTIVATE project (`https://projekt-activate.de/`) is to support these vulnerable patients to overcome this issue. A new input device was developed for this purpose. BIRDY (Ball-shaped Interactive Rehabilitation Device) is a device tailored to the special requirements of ICU context. Because of its simplicity, it can be used by weaning patients dealing with limited cognitive and physiological abilities.

Despite the simple design and utility of BIRDY, other input devices potentially present a better choice for some patients or in certain situations. There may be other devices that are more familiar to the patient, so it makes sense to use one of these devices to achieve a low inhibition threshold for communication.

Especially in later stages of weaning, patients have higher awareness and can use increasingly complex input devices.

2 Methods

In order to find suitable input devices, a market analysis was first carried out. Subsequently, the promising candidates were implemented in the ACTIVATE context, followed by the evaluation of the input devices in a study.

2.1 Market Analysis

The devices researched in the market analysis were compared on the basis of various criteria, which aim at ensuring a smooth use of the devices in the ACTIVATE context (*range*, *market availability*, *hygiene*, *programm interfaces*, *battery life time*, *costs*, *haptics*, *complexity* and *security*).
Range: The range of wireless devices must be large enough to bridge the distance between the patient and the receiver or the ACTIVATE application.
Market availability: Devices that are not (no longer) available on the market could be excluded. An exception is BIRDY, which is only available at the institute.
Hygiene: In the hospital environment, and especially in the ICU environment, the hygienic requirements are particularly high in order to prevent infections. The input device should be easy to clean thoroughly and be waterproof so that it can also be disinfected.
Program interfaces: The device must have usable interfaces to allow it to communicate with the Reflection Framework, the underlying software platform of ACTIVATE.
Battery life time: For effective use, the device should work for at least one hospital staff shift without recharging.
Price: A price of less than 100€ is desirable.

Haptics: The device should feel as natural as possible for the patient and be easy to grasp. Haptic feedback for recognized inputs improves understanding and comprehensibility for the patient.
Complexity: The complexity of the input device should not be too high. A simple, low-stimulus design with no more than one button supports understanding of the device and reduces inhibitions in its use.
Security: Since the device is to be used in a medical context, technical security on the one hand and security in handling patient data on the other must be guaranteed.

2.2 Implementation

Since the system architecture of the ACTIVATE system is built on the Reflection Framework [4], the implementation of the input devices was also realized with it. This enables dynamic binding of the input devices with the ACTIVATE patient application. To enable communication between the Reflection Framework and the devices, a description of the devices was created using the *Smart Object Description Language (SODL)* [5]. The Leap Motion (`https://www.ultraleap.com/product/leap-motion-controller/`) implementation was realized using the Leap Motion Java SDK and the Device Template of the Reflection Framework. For the implementation of the Kai Controller (`https://kai.vicara.co/home`), the Python interface of the Kai Controller and the Python API of the Reflection Framework were used. Also the Kai Control Center is required. The interface to the Litho Controller (`https://www.litho.cc/`) was implemented using Unity Personal and the Reflection interface was implemented using the C# API.

2.3 Pilot Study

In the preliminary study, the selected input devices were compared with each other and with BIRDY. This involved investigating how the user experience of the respective devices was perceived. Subsequently, the devices were compared in a ranking according to various criteria and ultimately overall. For this purpose, experts in the field of computer science were asked to participate in the study, as this was expected to provide an affinity of new technologies and constructive feedback from the participants.
Six participants took part in the study. All were men and the average age was 31.5 years. Two participants had experience with the ACTIVATE patient application and BIRDY, one had experience with the Leap Motion, while the Kai Controller and Litho Controller were new to all participants.

2.3.1 Procedure for the Participants

For hygienic reasons, participants had to wear gloves when operating with the devices. Participants completed the same three tasks with each device to operate the ACTIVATE patient application. For the tasks, the patients lay in a hospital bed with the head section raised by about 30° to simulate the position of a patient in ICU. The first task was to communicate that they were fine by navigating through the application to that point. The second task was to communicate that the participant had level 2 (out of a maximum of 10) pain in their left leg. The integrated pain interface was used for this. In the third task, participants used the integrated text box and wrote the number sequence 1, 3, and 7, gaining experience using the text box. After each series of tasks, the participants evaluated the input device used with a questionnaire about their user experience with this device. Once all tasks were completed, participants filled out a ranking to compare all input devices. At the end, there was a questionnaire asking for demographic data such as age and previous experience with the devices and the ACTIVATE patient application.

2.3.2 Items of the Questionnaires

The questionnaire for the evaluation of each device after the participant finished the tasks had six items:

1. The operation of the input device has worked well (good functionality).
2. The operation of the input device was exhausting.
3. The operation of the input device was customized to the menu.
4. Completing the tasks was laborious.
5. The operation of the input device was easy to learn.
6. The operation of the input device was unfamiliar.

Each item could be rated with a value from one to five. 1 means *do not agree at all*, while 5 means *agree completely*. The ranking questionnaire has five questions. The last question is open-ended so that comments from the participants can be taken into account.

1. Which input device was the most comfortable to use?
2. Which input device had the best performance?
3. Which input device was easiest to use?
4. Thinking to all points. Which device was your favorite?
5. How do you justify your decision?

3 Results and Discussion

First, the results of the market analysis are presented and discussed. Then, the results of the preliminary study are considered and criticized.

3.1 Results and Discussion of the Analysis of Alternative Input Devices

The research and comparison of input devices showed that none of the devices available on the market met the stringent hygiene requirements needed for use in the ICU context.
Table 1 shows an excerpt of the results of the market analysis.
Because of the difficulties with the hygienic requirements for input devices, the requirements had to be relaxed to find potential alternatives to BIRDY. Thus, the Kai Controller and Litho Controller were selected even though they are not

Device Name	Range	Market availability	Hygiene	Program interfaces	Battery lifetime	Costs	Haptics	Complexity	Security
BIRDY	+	o	+	-	+	o	+	+	o
Gest	+	-	-	-	?	?	-	+	o
Kai Controller	+	+	o	o	+	o	+	+	o
Leap Motion	o	+	+	+	+	o	-	+	+
Litho Controller	+	+	o	o	o	o	+	+	o
Tap	+	+	o	o	+	o	+	+	o
Wave Ring	+	+	-	o	+	o	-	+	o

+: Criterion met well o: Criterion met -: Criterion not met ?: No information about this point

The criteria are explained in the section *Market Analysis*

Table 1: Results of the input device analysis at a glance

waterproof. The use of Gest and Wave was discarded due to the requirements not being met. Tap could not be looked at more closely due to time constraints. The Leap Motion initially seems to be a promising candidate.

3.2 Results and Discussion of Pilot Study

The results of the User Experience Questionnaire are presented first, followed by those of the ranking. This is followed by a reflection on the evaluation method and then on the operation of the devices.

3.2.1 Results of the User Experience Questionnaire

Some of the items in the user experience questionnaire were worded negatively. As a result, these items were changed to positive statements to facilitate the interpretation of the graph. Fig. 1 shows the results of the average score of the devices for each item. The Litho Controller achieved the best results. For the item *customized to menu*, all devices performed similarly. The Litho Controller has the best results in the items *easy to learn* and *not unfamiliar* due to the familiar handling of the touchpad, which is also used to operate the Litho Controller. The Leap Motion achieved the lowest rating in the study. The reason for this could be the learning curve of the device. In the short time to complete the tasks, the participants could not practice enough with the device to be able to use it optimally.

BIRDY performed slightly better. The participants mainly criticized the poor gesture recognition. Thus, it was noted in the free text comments that BIRDY often tended to unintentional inputs and that the operation was unfamiliar. As positive features, it can be concluded from the user experience questionnaire that the operation of BIRDY is not strenuous and is well adapted to the menu navigation.

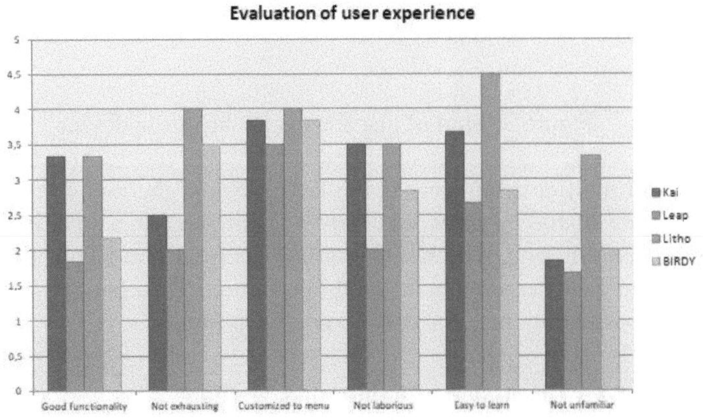

Figure 1: The average score of each item of the user experience questionnaire for each device in comparison

Overall, the Litho Controller has the best places, followed by the Kai Controller. Leap Motion and BIRDY were both mostly placed last.

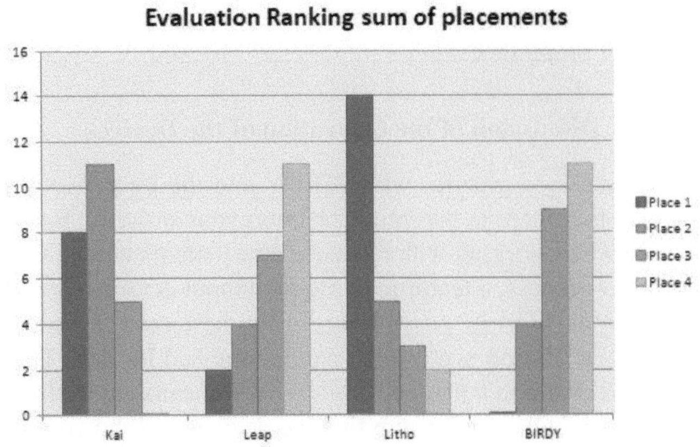

Figure 2: Sum of placements for all devices and questions

3.2.2 Results of the Ranking

Fig. 2 shows the sum of the rankings of all questions of the ranking questionnaire. The Litho Controller was most frequently ranked first. The Kai Controller was most often voted second. Leap Motion and BIRDY were chosen similarly often in 4th place. BIRDY was never placed first, and the Kai Controller was never placed fourth.

Fig. 3 shows the rankings of the devices in the last question of the questionnaire. A clear tendency can be seen here. The Litho Controller was voted first, the Kai Controller second, the Leap Motion third and BIRDY fourth.

Expressed with a reciprocal ranking (sum of placements with weight $1, \frac{1}{2}, \frac{1}{3}, \frac{1}{4}$ per place, beginning by Place 1), the

Litho Controller achieves a score of 18, the Kai Controller 15.17, the Leap Motion 9.08 and BIRDY 7.75.

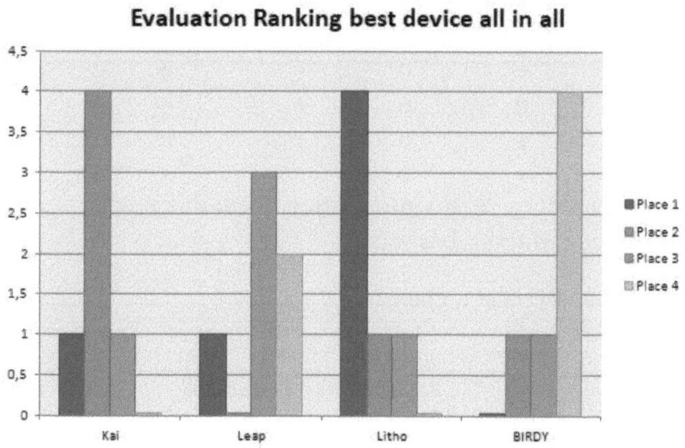

Figure 3: Sum of placements for favourite device

In the free comments in the last question, the recognition rate of the gestures was mostly mentioned as a justification criterion. The Kai Controller and the Litho Controller were both credited with good recognition. This, in turn, was mostly criticized for BIRDY and Leap Motion.

3.2.3 Discussion of Evaluation Method

The methodology of the preliminary study has room for improvement.
Especially, the number of participants was very small. In a further study, the subject group should be approximated to the target group, i.e. potential patients for ventilation in the intensive care unit. In this way, it can be checked whether the devices that performed well in the technology-savvy participants also perform similarly well in the target group. The proportion of women should ideally be 50% in order to be able to identify and balance out possible gender-specific preferences.

3.2.4 Discussion of the Operation of the Devices

The necessary practice with BIRDY and the Leap Motion shows that there is potential for improvement here. Especially when working with intensive care patients who have a short awareness, a learning phase with input devices should be kept as short as possible or, in the best case, avoided. The Leap Motion needs to be fixed to the bed for use. This is not realistic in a hospital context, as it means extra effort for the caregivers to ensure that the device is in the correct position all the time.
Wearing the gloves while completing the tasks, which was necessary for hygienic reasons, was perceived as annoying, especially in the case of the Litho Controller.

4 Conclusion

The research conducted for input devices showed that there are currently no realistic input devices for use in an intensive context on the market. In this respect, the development of BIRDY is a sensible consequence to change this. The biggest criticism of the prototype under development was the low recognition rate of gestures. This problem was already known prior to the study and is planned to be addressed.
The Litho Controller performed by far the best in the preliminary study and seems to be suitable in principle as an alternative input device. However, the problem of hygiene criteria must be addressed for realistic use in a clinical environment. Since the Litho Controller cannot be immersed in disinfectant, but is at least relatively easy to clean apart from the USB port for charging, the hardware would have to be adapted accordingly. Alternatively, the use of a single device per patient is conceivable. The Litho was probably preferred because of its touchpad operation. This indicates the potential of touch technology in general for the use in the intensive care context.
Overall, the three devices available on the market were better received than the BIRDY prototype, with the Litho Controller in particular being a suitable candidate.

Acknowledgement

The work has been carried out and supervised by the Institute of Telematic, Universität zu Lübeck.

Author’s Statement

Conflict of interest: Authors state no conflict of interest.

5 References

[1] Arbeitsgemeinschaft der Wissenschaftlichen Medizinischen Fachgesellschaften, S3-Leitlinie: Analgesie, Sedierung und Delirmanagement in der Intensivmedizin, 08/2015 - DAS Leitlinie, August 2015

[2] Alham Abuatiq. 2015. Patients’ and health care providers’ perception of stressors in the intensive care units. Dimensions of Critical Care Nursing, 34(4): 205-214, 2015.

[3] Louise Rose, Katie N Dainty, Joanne Jordan, and Bronagh Blackwood. Weaning from mechanical ventilation: a scoping review of qualitative studies. American Journal of Critical Care, 23(5):e54–e70, 2014.

[4] Daniel Burmeister. Selbstreflexive Geräteverbünde in smarten Umgebungen. Dissertation. Universität zu Lübeck. 2018.

[5] Andreas Schrader, Daniel Burmeister, Florian Burmann. The Smart Object Description Language: Modeling Interaction Capabilities for Self-Reflection. In: 2017 IEEE International Conference on Pervasive Computing and Communications Workshops (PerCom Workshops), 503–508, 2017.

Enabling Semantic Interoperability for Endoscopic Devices

Kathrin Pia Riech [1], Björn Andersen [2], Martin Kasparick [3], and Josef Ingenerf [4]
[1] Medical Informatics, Universität zu Lübeck, kathrin.riech@student.uni-luebeck.de
[2] Drägerwerk AG & Co. KGaA, Lübeck, bjoern.andersen@draeger.com
[3] Institute of Applied Microelectronics and Computer Engineering, University of Rostock, martin.kasparick@uni-rostock.de
[4] Institute of Medical Informatics, Universität zu Lübeck, josef.ingenerf@uni-luebeck.de

Abstract

In a modern operating room, there is a lack of networking of medical devices from different manufacturers. Communication standards enable a great variety of innovative medical devices and components to be combined. The scope of this work is to extend the IEEE 11073 standard series by detailed networking requirements for endoscopic camera systems and light sources. Device Specializations and Modular Specifications are developed to guide and support manufacturers in modeling their current and future devices' network representation. We defined term codes that shall extend the ISO/IEEE 11073-10101 Nomenclature to allow for devices to automatically interpret the exchanged information. Every element, measurement, setting, remote control function, and event of these highly complex devices is described. In this work, the structural interoperability of medical devices is improved through the unification of the devices' network representation. Semantic interoperability is achieved by adding endoscopy-specific term codes to the Nomenclature.

1 Introduction

Interoperability is a key factor in the networking of medical devices and is becoming increasingly important to meet the growing demands of a modern operating room (OR). The clinical need for greater safety, efficiency, and ergonomics is a constant driver for OR networking as the OR becomes more and more technologically advanced. One challenge so far has been the networking of devices from different manufacturers with each other. Only through standards is it possible to combine the large variety of innovative medical devices and components.
The research project „OR.NET - Secure and dynamic networking in operating room and hospital“ funded by the German Federal Ministry of Education and Research (BMBF) laid essential foundations in the form of a service-oriented communication protocol for the dynamic cross-vendor networking of medical devices. The project's results are now part of the *IEEE 11073 Service-oriented Device Connectivity (SDC)* series of standards [1]. So far, however, various manufacturers still model the network representation of very similar devices differently [2].
This is where the project "PoCSpec - Modular Specialisations for Point-of-Care Medical Devices", which started in January 2019 and is supported by the German Federal Ministry for Economic Affairs and Energy (BMWi), comes in: The project develops new standards to supplement the IEEE 11073 family of standards. These standards for certain device categories precisely define the networking requirements, i.e. the scope, structure, and meaning of the data and services offered in the network as well as the behavior of the device at runtime [3]. This enables devices from different manufacturers to be monitored and controlled uniformly over the network. The network requirements will be modeled exemplarily for two particularly complex device categories: Endoscopy and high-frequency surgery. This work focuses on the endoscopic camera and the endoscopic light source.
To achieve comprehensive interoperability, it is also necessary to extend the *IEEE 11073-10101 Nomenclature* with terms for modeling surgical devices. This requires new generic as well as specific term codes. The type of each element of the device description tree, down to each measurement and setting, should be described by a term code [4].
The goal is to achieve a higher level of interoperability and to enable the exchangeability of point-of-care medical devices (PoCD) from different manufacturers during operation by developing the Device Specializations (DevSpecs) and Modular Specifications (ModSpecs) and by extending the ISO/IEEE 11073-10101 Nomenclature.

2 Material and Methods

2.1 IEEE 11073 SDC

Communication between medical devices, healthcare devices, and external systems can be enabled by communication standards from the *ISO/IEEE 11073 Health informatics – Point-of-care medical device communication* series. Information about the patient, vital data, and operating data of the devices can be recorded automatically and in detail electronically [1].

The IEEE 11073 SDC standard series (see Fig. 1) specifies a communication protocol for medical devices used in high-acuity environments. Within the OR.NET project, the communication based on the Service-Oriented Architecture (SOA) paradigm was extended to a Services Oriented Medical Device Architecture (SOMDA).
Aiming for the interoperability of PoCDs, IEEE 11073 SDC covers cross-vendor device-to-device communication.

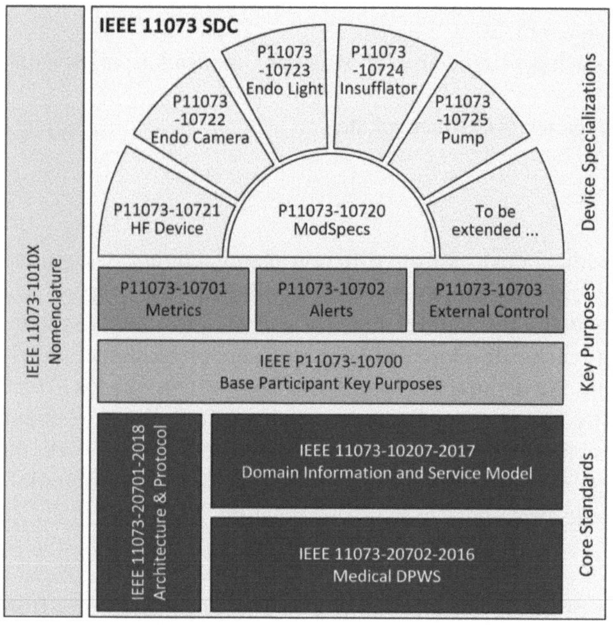

Figure 1: IEEE 11073 SDC standards family [5]

As shown in Fig. 1, the Core Standards of the IEEE 11073 SDC standard family include the *ISO/IEEE 11073-20702 Medical devices communication profile for web services (MDPWS)*, in which the use of web services and the underlying communication architecture is specified. Furthermore, the standard series contains the *ISO/IEEE 11073-10207 Domain information and service model for service-oriented point-of-care medical device Communication*. This standard is divided into the device description and the current device state of the PoCD and defines the structure of the exchanged data. The hierarchically organized relationship of elements is described as a so-called *containment tree*. As a root element, the medical device is represented by a *Medical Device System (MDS)* object, which can contain several *Virtual Medical Devices (VMD)* that represent the abstraction of a medical subsystem, e.g. modules. Below a VMD, *Channels* that are logical groupings of *Metrics* can be instantiated. Metrics represent the measurements and settings of the device. To enable machine interpretability, nomenclature terms are used for annotation at each level of the containment tree. The ISO/IEEE 11073-10101 Nomenclature is part of the ISO/IEEE 11073 standard series. This Nomenclature contains unique codes for specifying the semantics of measurement data, parameters, objects, and attributes and is relevant for all standards of the IEEE 11073 SDC standard family. Thirdly, IEEE 11073 SDC contains the standard *ISO/IEEE 11073-20701 Service oriented medical device exchange architecture and protocol binding*. Among other content, it provides a binding of the domain information and service model to the web service implementations, thereby specifying the SOMDA [1].
Further requirements for SDC participants in particular, in their roles as providers and consumers of metric data, alerts, and external control, will be defined in the Participant Key Purposes (PKP) standards [5]. The DevSpecs and the reusable ModSpecs developed in the PoCSpec project are based on the Core Standards and the PKPs. ModSpecs represent frequently occurring components of different devices and are intended to simplify and standardize these device descriptions.

2.2 Interoperability of Medical Devices

In the context of medical devices, interoperability is characterized by the exchange of information between independent, heterogeneous systems. This can be achieved by consistent standards that define the syntactic rules and semantic interpretations of information [6]. A distinction is made between four different types of interoperability. The foundational interoperability deals with the ability to exchange data. This is ensured by the transport technology standard ISO/IEEE 11073-20702 MDPWS. Structural interoperability describes the structure and format of the data to be exchanged. It is achieved by modeling each device and component on the network according to the Domain Information and Service Model and using the protocol bound to MDPWS. The ability of two or more systems to exchange, interpret, and use data describes the highest level: semantic interoperability. This level of interoperability is partly achieved by using value sets in the data model but mainly through a nomenclature. The use of Coded Values, which are well defined by a controlled vocabulary, allows for machine interpretability of the exchanged data. Safe and dynamic information exchange and remote control between devices in different clinical environments can only be enabled by using a nomenclature [1], [4]. The fourth level of interoperability, organizational interoperability, includes governance, policy, social, legal, and organizational considerations.

2.3 Modeling Device Specializations

DevSpecs define the structure of the capability descriptions of devices, the semantics of their functionality, the requirements for communication partners, and the patterns of interaction with other components to cover the common features and operating modes of current and future devices [3]. The basic idea behind this is to guide and support manufacturers in modeling their actual devices and to promote the inclusion of advanced functions in the network representation of the devices. For the *IEEE P11073-10720 Modular Specifications* standard, functionally similar subsystems being present in very different types of medical devices are collected and documented. This standard shall serve as a library of functional submodels.

By industry consensus, these new standards provide modular means to describe the capabilities and interaction modes of devices using the ISO/IEEE 11073-10207 Domain information and service model for PoCD [3]. In case a certain functionality is not covered by the standards, customer-specific extensions can be defined.

2.4 Extending the Nomenclature

To achieve the ability to automatically interpret the exchanged information of endoscopic devices, coding systems are needed. Usually, Coded Values are applied to annotate a data element with a machine-interpretable description. Coded Values typically consist of three identifiers: a term code with a well-defined meaning (code ID), the coding system in which the code is defined to specify the controlled vocabulary (coding system ID), and the version of this coding system to deal with several versions (coding system version) [4]. Term codes defined within this project shall extend the IEEE P11073-10101c Nomenclature. In previous extensions, terms from the surgical domain were not considered [4].

Each measurement, setting, and element of the containment tree must be described by a Coded Value. Due to the high complexity of an endoscopic camera and endoscopic light source, a lot of new specific term codes are necessary. Besides, remote control functions, commands, events, and device context states of networked devices, which were not considered before, have to be described. In previous nomenclature extensions, the device parameters were modeled individually for each device type. As suggested by Andersen et al. [4], properties that are common to many devices are defined more generally. Generic terms include, for example, operating parameters such as operating hours and operating cycles or settings such as brightness and contrast of device displays.

The results are systematically reviewed and developed by international endoscopy device manufacturers and connectivity experts.

3 Results and Discussion

3.1 Endoscopic Camera

The endoscopic camera model (Fig. 2) covers the entire image chain including the *endoscope*, *image acquisition*, *image processing*, *video output*, and *image documentation*. These logical components are modelled as Virtual Medical Devices (VMD). The VMD *endoscope* contains a channel *optical system*. The *optical system* projects light from the situs to the imager. Its physical properties influence the result of the *image acquisition*. The VMD *image acquisition* contains various channels. The channel *exposure* represents the logical grouping of metrics that determine the amount of light being processed by the image sensor. The channel *observation* represents the logical grouping of parameters that relate to the observation of the image. The third channel *illumination* represents the logical grouping of metrics that determine the illumination being calculated by the image sensor. The VMD *image processing* represents the processing of signals recorded as part of the *image acquisition* and contains one or more channel(s) *(processed) image*. Each of these channels represents the logical grouping of parameters that define the properties of the *(processed) image*.

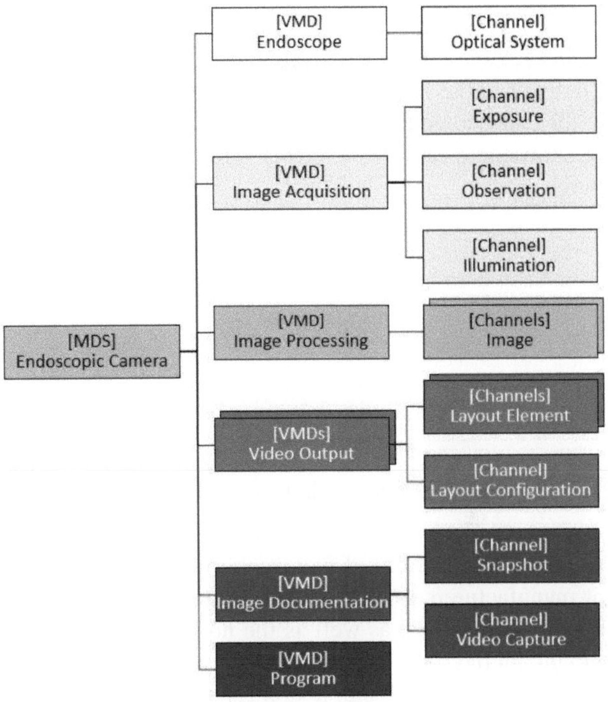

Figure 2: Endoscopic Camera Model

Additionally, the *endoscopic camera* model contains elements that are defined within the scope of ModSpecs. A *video output* ModSpec describes the individual display elements together with a layout configuration. Another ModSpec is the VMD *image documentation*, which allows capturing snapshots or video recordings. Finally, it contains a VMD *program* that allows presets for device settings that can be used in the context of a specific procedure or for a specific operator. The actual images and video streams are outside the scope of this standard as they are already covered by other standards such as DICOM. The nomenclature extensions for the endoscopic camera mainly includes six areas: Containment tree entries, Metrics, ProductionSpecifications, Valuesets, Alarms, and Operations. In these areas, more than 100 additional term codes have been defined and reviewed.

3.2 Endoscopic Light Source

An endoscopic light source enables the illumination of a surgeon's visual field. A light source can be a stand-alone device connected to the endoscope via a light fiber, or it can be integrated. To control the light source (automatically) via the camera interface, it can be connected to the Camera Control Unit.

For each (physical) lamp of the device, the MDS provides a VMD *lamp* (Fig. 3). Their channels *optical radiation* contain metrics representing the actual radiation, including light intensity and remote control. It also contains information about the physical characteristics of the optical radiation, e.g. spectrum, color rendering index, color temperature, and pulse length. Another VMD *composite*, to which a composite optical radiation channel is subordinated, bundles parameters that affect all lamps at the same time, if several are available, such as light intensity or spectrum. Also, the endoscopic light source contains the VMD *program* that is defined in the ModSpecs. The nomenclature extensions for the endoscopic light source include the same areas as for the endoscopic camera. 65 terms were defined for the light source.

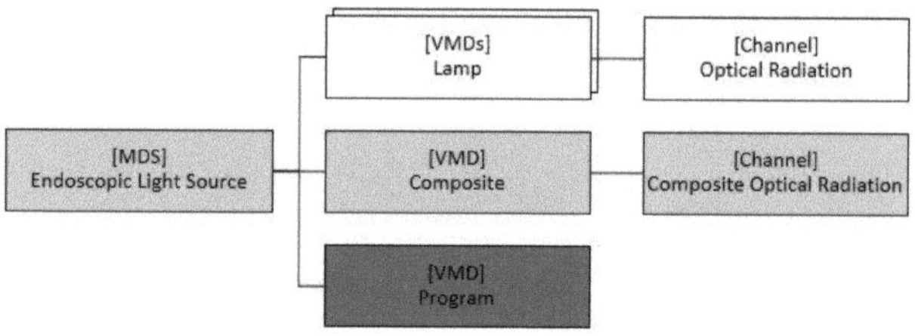

Figure 3: Endoscopic Light Source Model

We analyzed a variety of endoscopic devices from different manufacturers to achieve the results. The difficulty in creating the models, as well as the nomenclature codes, is to maintain the right level of specificity while remaining as general as possible. Manufacturers should be able to implement their current and future devices using the given models and find the properties of their devices in the containment tree without having to add new extensions. Likewise, existing term codes should describe these parameters specifically enough so that a manufacturer will not use a new one that other systems may be unable to interpret. We want to harmonize many devices from different manufacturers while respecting their intellectual property. To achieve this, reviews from as many international endoscopy device manufacturers and connectivity experts as possible are needed.

4 Conclusion

This work holistically addresses manufacturer-independent interoperability for endoscopic cameras and endoscopic light sources. Creating specific models for endoscopic camera systems and light sources extends the communication protocol standards family IEEE 11073 SDC. These models cover the features and operating modes of current devices and enable future functions by including extension points. The unification of the network representation of these devices promotes foundational and structural interoperability. The semantic interoperability of software systems is based on the use of coding systems. It is achieved in this work by adding endoscopy-specific terms to the ISO/IEEE 11073-10101 Nomenclature. The next step is the prototypical implementation of the devices whose manufacturers are involved in the PoCSpec project to further evaluate the models. The complete model designs and nomenclature codes can be viewed and discussed online in project's development management system [7].

Acknowledgement

The work has been carried out within the scope of the PoCSpec project and supervised at the Institute of Medical Informatics, University of Lübeck. The project is funded by the German Federal Ministry for Economic Affairs and Energy (grant number: 03TNH017).

Author's Statement

Conflict of interest: Authors state no conflict of interest.

5 References

[1] M. Kasparick, M. Schmitz, B. Andersen, M. Rockstroh, S. Franke, S. Schlichting, F. Golatowski, and D. Timmermann, "OR.NET: a service-oriented architecture for safe and dynamic medical device interoperability." *Biomedizinische Technik. Biomedical engineering*, vol. 63, pp. 11–30, Feb. 2018.

[2] B. Andersen, S. Baumhof, and J. Ingenerf, "Service-Oriented Device Connectivity: Device Specialisations for Interoperability." *Studies in health technology and informatics*, vol. 264, pp. 509–511, Aug. 2019.

[3] B. Andersen, M. Kasparick, K. Riech, S. Klöckner, A. Keller, L. Mündermann, J. Maier-Holzberg, D. Timmermann, and J. Ingenerf, "Service-Oriented Medical Device Connectivity: Particular Standards for Endoscopic Surgery*," in *IEEE EMBC*, Jul. 2020, pp. 5649–5652.

[4] B. Andersen, M. Kasparick, F. Golatowski, and J. Ingenerf, "Extending the IEEE 11073-1010X nomenclature for the modelling of surgical devices," in *IEEE BHI*, Feb. 2016, pp. 244–247.

[5] M. Kasparick, B. Butzin, F. Golatowski, J. Pabst, H.-J. Cappius, P. Westerhoff, B. Andersen, and D. Timmermann, "From IEEE 11073 SDC Device Specializations to Assistive Systems: Rule-based Data Analysis for Minimal Invasive Surgery," in *IEEE SmartNets*, Dec. 2019.

[6] Healthcare Information and Management Systems Society (HIMSS), "HIMSS Dictionary of Healthcare Information Technology Terms,Acronyms and Organizations, Fifth Edition," Productivity Press, 2019.

[7] B. Andersen, M. Kasparick, K. Riech, and M. Eichelberg, "Modular Specialisations for Point-of-Care Medical Devices," https://sourceforge.net/projects/pocspec/, 2021, last accessed 26.01.2021.

Visualization and Exploration of Integrated Patient Data

Sebastian Germer [1], Mohamed Lambarki [2], Hannes Ulrich [3], Josef Ingenerf [3,4] and Martin Lablans [2]

[1] Medical Informatics, Universität zu Lübeck, sebastian.germer@student.uni-luebeck.de

[2] Federated Information Systems, German Cancer Research Center (DKFZ), {m.lambarki, m.lablans}@dkfz-heidelberg.de

[3] IT Center for Clinical Research, Universität zu Lübeck, h.ulrich@uni-luebeck.de

[4] Institute of Medical Informatics, Universität zu Lübeck, josef.ingenerf@uni-luebeck.de

Abstract

Due to the increasing digitalization in the medical domain, more and more medical data becomes available for a secondary use in studies. On multiple clinical research sites in Germany so-called *bridgeheads* are deployed, which can be filled with integrated data to enable further data sharing. Statistical tools such as dashboards are often used for data exploration and especially for visualization to get a first impression of the integrated data and also to explore the data set to find medically interesting subgroups. In this paper we discuss two common used frameworks and evaluate them regarding to this use case with consideration of end user requirements. We propose a tool for data visualization and exploration which can be integrated in the existing bridgehead environment.

1 Introduction

Collaborative research takes place in a wide variety of disciplines. Federated information systems serve to link the participants of a network with each other and to provide a standardized infrastructure. The underlying common processes such as authentication, pseudonymization and data integration are the basis of cross-institutional data management. *Bridgeheads* are a central component in the federated information systems [1]. They are used to connect the sites to the respective network and to enable the data to be stored in a standardized format without uploading patient-related data to external sites. Bridgeheads provide a harmonized view of the source data using a local data management and a networking component, which is responsible for the controlled release of data derived from the local data management [1].

An example for a research network is the German Consortium for Translational Cancer Research (DKTK) with its Clinical Communication Platform (CCP). The aim is to bundle expertise and critical masses (e.g. of subjects and samples for studies) via the partner institutions to advance research into the mechanisms of cancer progression and the development of tools for cancer treatment and detection [2].

To get an overview of the data contained on one site, which is often aggregated from multiple primary systems, an automated visualization of the data is helpful [3]. Furthermore, in the context of secondary studies, it is important to search exploratively for interesting subgroups within the available data and to discover statistically relevant properties. In a next step, scientific hypotheses can be generated with the help of the filtered group.

2 Material and Methods

2.1 Data Visualization and Exploration

Data visualization is a matter of preparing raw, abstract data in such a way that they can be used as interactive images for further purposes such as exploration and analysis [4]. There are many types of visualization, depending on the type of data and the use case.

Data analysis describes a collection of statistical methods that can be used to extract information from collected data and to document it in tabular or graphical form [5].

Data exploration is a subfield of data analysis. It describes the process of interactively extracting knowledge from data without knowing exactly what one is looking for in advance. The goal is to formulate hypotheses so that new data can be collected or existing data is analyzed in more detail [3]. This is in contrast to traditional data processing, where it is usually assumed that users know exactly the underlying data model and can make queries to it concretely.

The use of dashboards is particularly suitable for data exploration. A dashboard is a collection of visualizations arranged in an application that presents the information important for a task [6]. In the past dashboards were used for the administration of servers. Over the years the range of applications has expanded. Meanwhile, dashboards are also used in numerous exploration scenarios (e.g. [7], [8]), which is why we decided to use dashboards in our scenario. There are various technologies and frameworks for creating dashboards. These can roughly be divided into two categories: In the first category are preconfigured frameworks that come with premade interfaces and display types, but are difficult to customize depending on the use case. An example of this is the Kibana framework from the company Elastic [9]. In the other category are frameworks that only provide the underlying backbone, so everything else has to be programmed. The Shiny framework based on R is a good example of this category [10].

2.2 Requirements Survey

In order to decide on a visualization and exploration framework, we collected different requirements for the framework. These are on the one hand of technical nature, such as the possibilities of data input. On the other hand we asked in expert interviews for concrete wishes for the tool from four stakeholders in collaborative research. These represent different user groups: A senior physician in the field of personalized oncology, a scientific coordinator of the CCP of the DKTK, a professor in the field of cohort research, and a professor of federated information systems. These user requirements can be classified in the categories *interactivity and usability*, *search functionality*, *visualizations* and *data output*.

3 Results and Discussion

First, the results of our framework evaluation are presented. Afterwards, a dashboard implementation based on the most suitable candidate is presented and discussed.

3.1 Framework Evaluation

The frameworks Kibana and Shiny were evaluated based on the collected requirements:

Technical Requirements

Data processing in R and therefore also in Shiny is mainly based on dataframes, which are table-like data structures. In order to transform data into such a dataframe, a whole series of functions exist for various data sources. XML files can be read in and structured in order to transform them into a dataframe. R can also retrieve data from an SQL database. This works both materialized and virtualized: Materialized, all data in the requested table is first loaded as a data frame into the R environment and so also into the local working memory, then filtered and aggregated on this basis in R itself. Virtualized, the filters and aggregations are first translated by R into SQL statements and then a collected query is issued to the database, so that the R environment always receives only the respective result of the query. This has the advantage that the complete data set is not queried from the database at any time. When connected to a data warehouse with about 12000 patients, we achieved a query time of 17 seconds with the virtual approach. A query of a server with Fast Healthcare Interoperable Resources (FHIR) can be done with the help of additional packages. R runs on all common operating systems, a use of Docker for deployment is also possible. Most packages for R are open source and available for free.

To use Kibana, the data must be materialized on an Elasticsearch server. For this materialization the user also needs to run the Logstash program with a configuration file that defines the input, possible transformation steps and the port of the Elasticsearch server. An import of JSON should be possible, but we did not succeed in loading a FHIR resource for testing purposes in a reasonable time. Kibana also runs on all common platforms and can also be set up as a Docker image. Only the core is open source, and many features require an additional subscription.

Interactivity and Usability

Interactive graphics can be programmed in R using the Plotly package [11]. In conjunction with the Shiny framework, these can also be used to interact with the rest of the program, for example to create filters. However, this is not trivial and involves more programming effort, since the associated methods only work with specific parameters, some of which are not documented. In addition, no errors are issued if the parameters are incorrect.

In Kibana, the graphics are also interactive and implemented as a filter option by default.

Search Functionality

Various filters can be programmed into the Shiny interface. With the help of packages the possibilities can be extended and improved, e.g. dropdown menus with a search function are possible. This is very helpful, for example, when searching for a specific diagnosis. However, the functionality of the filters must also be programmed in the background by the developer. Query languages are not directly supported in the interface itself; this could at most be realized via free text fields. An integration of the entity catalog, an external criteria catalog for oncology entities, is possible.

In Kibana, filtering is mainly done via a search bar, which filters according to the Elastic Query Language, and by clicking in the graphics themselves. There are also (experimental) dropdown menus for filtering. We did not find a way to additionally enter external criteria catalogs here.

Visualizations

With Shiny, many of the visualization packages that are available for R allow also the rendering of their visualizations on a web page. It is also possible to add and adjust visualizations at runtime, e.g. via buttons, but the logic behind this (especially in interaction with interactivity and filtering) has to be programmed. There is also a multitude of packages to create advanced visualizations like a patient timeline.

Also in Kibana there are numerous pre-programmed visualization types, where the user only has to specify which data element should be plotted in which way. This is done interactively via the user interface. Adding new visualizations at runtime is also possible. However, in contrast to Shiny, the dashboards are also changed on the server side. So if another user accesses the dashboard, these changes are visible to him. More complicated visualizations such as a patient timeline cannot be created in Kibana. Custom visualizations can be implemented theoretically, but are officially classified as experimental and only sparsely documented.

Data Output

Shiny applications can also be integrated as iFrame into other websites, if they are operated with a Shiny server, for example. It is also possible to save graphics in PNG or SVG format by the user. A data export e.g. as CSV file as well as a forwarding to an external API can also be programmed. Kibana dashboards can also be embedded as iFrame in other web pages, but they cannot be customized much. Reports as PDF or PNG can be generated with a paid subscription. A CSV export is possible, but no direct API export.

Evaluation Result

R in combination with Shiny, on one hand, has a much higher implementation effort, the interaction of inputs (filters) and outputs (graphics) as well as the interactivity among the outputs have to be programmed. For this, one can fall back on a very large number of extensions, both in terms of visualizations and input formats. Data retrieval can also be completely virtualized here without having to duplicate the data. In addition, virtually all packages and functions of R are available open source. Thus, one has more flexibility in design and is also more future-proof overall to deal with future requirements.

One the other hand, many functions are directly available in Kibana. No programming work is required here, only the type of input must be configured. However, this also leads to a disadvantage: the framework is quite rigid overall. Individual, more complex visualizations cannot be inserted easily, also the input must have a special format to be imported into the Elasticsearch store. Another serious drawback is that this Elasticsearch store is additionally required, thus necessitating duplication of data. This is difficult to keep synchronous with the primary data warehouse. Furthermore, multiple storing of patient data is not exactly in line with applicable data protection rules.

For these reasons, we constructed our dashboard using R and Shiny.

3.2 Implementation

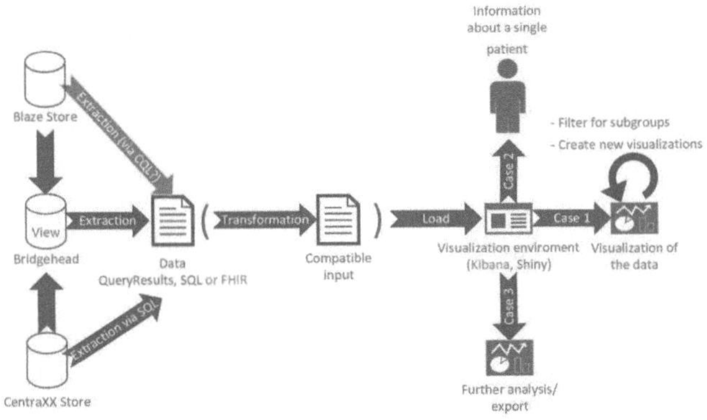

Figure 1: The implemented pipeline. The grayed out elements we either discarded or did not implement during this study.

The visualization pipeline we implemented is shown in Fig. 1. The DKTK project currently uses the CentraXX data warehouse [12], a relational database, as local data management in the bridgehead. In other projects, the use of FHIR is increasing. The Blaze Store is an example of a FHIR-based data warehouse used by the German Biobank Alliance. As test instance we connected our program to a CentraXX data warehouse using SQL. During the implementation, it was difficult to fulfill all user wishes and requirements at the same time, as they were also partly contradictory to each other. For example, on the one hand, the dashboard had to be as flexible as possible with respect to the imported data model and data source, and on the other hand, filters were desired that were already very specific to a particular data model (e.g., the entity catalog). Also, the difference between an external and an internal access was relevant. For these reasons, we designed two dashboards representing these different categories and then implemented them.

The first dashboard is adapted to the DKTK data model. The target group for this is especially people who should or want to get only an approximate insight into the data. First of all, there are different filter options to choose from in the sidebar. Here the user can which data element from the DKTK data model he wants to visualize. Afterwards, numerous filters are available: For example, filtering by gender, age, tumor diagnosis and tumor morphology is possible. Filters with multiple selection were used, which contain not only the classification code of the field but also its definition. Both can be searched for using a search box. We also integrated the entity catalog to simplify the search for cancer entities. In addition, a filter for tumor stages according to the criteria specified by the Union for International Cancer Control (UICC) can be set. While setting the filters, the user can see the result of the query on the right side: There are info blocks that display how many patients, diagnoses and treatment events have taken place in the filtered group. In addition, the frequency distribution of the selected element in the filtered group is displayed both as a bar chart and as a pie chart. Below this, there is also a sunburst chart, which displays the distribution hierarchically by gender, diagnosis and UICC stage. A possible setting within this dashboard can be seen in Fig. 2.

We designed the second dashboard relatively independent of the used data model, with freely adjustable filters and visualizations. This is intended for researchers who want to perform data exploration with the bridgehead data, for example to find interesting study populations for further analysis. Using a configuration file, the user can set how to access or import the data. After the data is loaded, adding new elements to the dashboard is possible. For this purpose, one can select a data element and an associated visualization type. Afterwards, the respective plot and a filter field are created. In this field the user can filter the respective characteristics as multiple selection. In the case of time histograms, one can also select the time periods over which the frequencies are to be formed. After the creation of several such elements, interactive filtering is available: One can select relevant characteristics in one plot, whereupon the other plots show only the frequencies that correspond to this selection. Once the user has done this with several plots and thus formed a group of interest for further analysis, he can either download the associated patient data as a JSON file or post it to an external API.

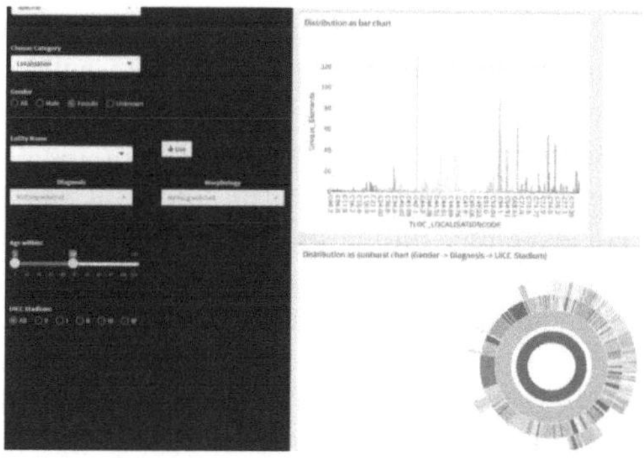

Figure 2: A detail of the DKTK dashboard.

3.3 Discussion

After a short analysis, we agreed to focus on connecting via SQL to a CentraXX store instead of using the FHIR resources of the Blaze store. The main reason behind this was that by the end of the study, only a few projects already had real data in FHIR, which would have made practical testing of our dashboard very difficult. However, we made sure during programming that the dashboards could be adapted to new data sources as easy as possible, so that a later extension to FHIR resources would require less effort. The decision to use R with Shiny instead of Kibana did involve significantly more effort in some cases. Nevertheless, as a more universal framework with a very large user and developer community, Shiny is considerably more flexible. Both input and visualizations can be easy exchanged for new components in the future and can be adapted to the respective needs. This also makes it more future-proof. Another advantage is the possibility of virtual data retrieval compared to an additional materialized memory. This allows the program to be used much more easy, also from a data protection point of view.

4 Conclusion

In this study, we have developed a program for exploring data in the bridgehead environment. For this, we talked to various end users and received feedback regarding desirable and required features. We compared existing frameworks in relation to these features and additional technical requirements and decided to build our tool based on R and Shiny. A virtual data query using SQL is possible. In the future the tool can be extended to deal with FHIR.

Acknowledgement

The work has been carried out at the German Cancer Research Center, Heidelberg and supervised by the Institute of Medical Informatics, Universität zu Lübeck.

Author's Statement

Conflict of interest: Authors state no conflict of interest.

5 References

[1] M. Lablans, E. E. Schmidt, and F. Ückert, "An architecture for translational cancer research as exemplified by the german cancer consortium," *JCO clinical cancer informatics*, vol. 2, pp. 1–8, 2018.

[2] S. Joos, D. M. Nettelbeck, A. Reil-Held, K. Engelmann, A. Moosmann, A. Eggert, W. Hiddemann, M. Krause, C. Peters, M. Schuler, K. Schulze-Osthoff, H. Serve, W. Wick, J. Puchta, and M. Baumann, "German cancer consortium (dktk) – a national consortium for translational cancer research," *Molecular Oncology*, vol. 13, no. 3, pp. 535–542, 2019.

[3] H. Bartsch, W. K. Thompson, T. L. Jernigan, and A. M. Dale, "A web-portal for interactive data exploration, visualization, and hypothesis testing," *Frontiers in neuroinformatics*, vol. 8, p. 25, 2014.

[4] M. Chen, H. Hauser, P. Rheingans, and G. Scheuermann, *Foundations of Data Visualization.* Cham: Springer International Publishing, 2020.

[5] U. Kamps, "Datenanalyse," 2013. [Online]. Available: https://wirtschaftslexikon.gabler.de/definition/datenanalyse-30331/version-164492 [last accessed on 14.12.2020]

[6] S. Few, *Information Dashboard Design: The Effective Visual Communication of Data*, 1st ed. Beijing: O'Reilly Media, Inc., 2006.

[7] J. Rogers, N. Spina, A. Neese, R. Hess, D. Brodke, and A. Lex, "Composer—visual cohort analysis of patient outcomes," *Applied Clinical Informatics*, vol. 10, no. 2, pp. 278–285, 2019.

[8] S. Paley, K. Parker, A. Spaulding, J.-F. Tomb, P. O'Maille, and P. D. Karp, "The omics dashboard for interactive exploration of gene-expression data," *Nucleic acids research*, vol. 45, no. 21, pp. 12 113–12 124, 2017.

[9] Elasticsearch B.V., "Kibana," 2021. [Online]. Available: https://www.elastic.co/guide/en/kibana/current/index.html [last accessed on 05.01.2021]

[10] W. Chang, J. Cheng, J. Allaire, Y. Xie, and J. McPherson, "Shiny: Web application framework for r," 2021. [Online]. Available: https://CRAN.R-project.org/package=shiny [last accessed on 17.01.2021]

[11] C. Sievert, *Interactive web-based data visualization with R, plotly, and shiny*, ser. Chapman & Hall/CRC the R series. Boca Raton, FL: CRC Press, Taylor & Francis Group, 2020.

[12] Kairos GmbH, "CentraXX," 2021. [Online]. Available: https://www.kairos.de/produkte/centraxx/ [last accessed on 18.01.2021]

Infinite Science
Publishing